HANDBOOK OF TUBERCULOSIS

Dr. Kedir Yahya Yasin

ALLIED HEALTH PRESS

Handbook of Tuberculosis

Author: **Dr. Kedir Yahya Yasin**

Allied Health Press
4164 Lakeshore Road
Burlington ON L7L 1A4
Canada
www.alliedhealthpress.com
Email: orders@arclereducation.com

ISBN: 978-1-77956-792-5

ABOUT THE AUTHOR

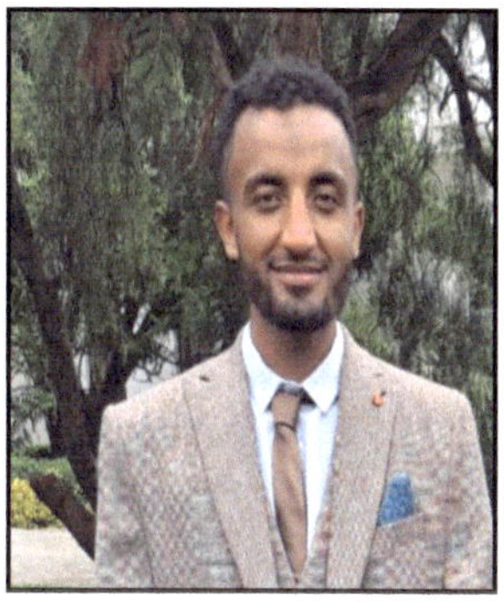

Dr. Kedir Yahya is a young medical doctor who is currently working in Asella teaching and referral hospital. He embarked on a journey to explore various fields within the medical landscape. With a versatile skill set and a commitment to lifelong learning, he has made significant contributions to healthcare across diverse specialities. Whether it's clinical practice, research, or teaching, he continues to strive for excellence in improving patient care and advancing medical knowledge.

Brief Table of Contents

Detailed Table of Contents

CHAPTER 10

Tuberculosis in Special Populations 311

CHAPTER 11

TB in Pregnancy and Other Special Situations 341

CHAPTER 12

Latent Tuberculosis Infection (LTBI) 371

CHAPTER 15

LIST OF FIGURES

PREFACE

Tuberculosis (TB) is a very old infectious disease that remains among the leading causes of illness and mortality in the present day. It is caused by the bacterium *Mycobacterium tuberculosis* (MTB) and mostly targets the lungs but can spread to bones, the central nervous system (CNS), lymph tissues, and other organs. Despite all the advances in the medical sector, problems such as poor access to healthcare, poverty, hunger, and the evolution of drug-resistant organisms have eroded the progress made toward the eradication of the disease. Knowledge of tuberculosis encompasses knowledge of its biology, host response, detection of infection, and successful treatment and prevention. By presenting these issues in plain, step-by-step terms, this book brings the reader face-to-face with the basic principles of contemporary tuberculosis research and clinical practice.

Handbook of Tuberculosis integrates the expertise of microbiologists, clinicians, epidemiologists, and public health specialists to provide a comprehensive reference for all phases of the disease. This text is evenly weighted between basic science and clinical practice. Clinical recommendations, derived from the most current World Health Organization (WHO) guidelines and recent peer-reviewed publications, guide decision-making in low-resource and high-technology environments. As a primary textbook for academic courses or desk reference for healthcare professionals, *Handbook of Tuberculosis* provides the tools to diagnose and treat this worldwide health problem.

The first five chapters lay the biological and clinical foundation for interpreting tuberculosis. Chapter 1 discusses *Mycobacterium tuberculosis's* microbiology: cell wall structure, growth needs, genetic variation, and culture in the laboratory. An explanation of acid-fast staining, colony morphology, and nucleic acid amplification tests (NAATs) with clarity permits readers to understand the limitations and strengths of various diagnostic methods. Chapter 2 covers how the bacterium causes infection, bypasses immune defenses, and forms the typical granulomas of active disease. Major host responses; macrophage activation, cytokine signaling, and cell-mediated immunity are discussed along with mechanisms used by the pathogen to survive in phagosomes. Chapter 3 deals with diagnostic approaches, from the historic tuberculin skin test (TST) to interferon-gamma release assays (IGRAs) and newer-generation molecular tests identifying drug-resistance mutations. It also examines the role of radiography, computed tomography (CT), and ultrasound in detecting pulmonary and extrapulmonary involvement. Chapter 4 treats the clinical presentations of pulmonary tuberculosis (PTB): pattern of cough, hemoptysis, weight loss, fever, and night sweats, and chest X-ray and computed tomography presentations. Chapter 5 discusses extrapulmonary and disseminated presentations, describing lymph node (LNs), pleural, meningeal, osseous, and genitourinary presentations, and emphasizing that symptoms depend on site and immune status.

Chapters 6 through 10 introduce therapeutic techniques and unique clinical challenges. Chapter 6 contains step-by-step treatment of drug-susceptible tuberculosis (DS-TB) using initial antibiotics, dosing frequency, hepatotoxicity monitoring, and ways to encourage compliance. Practical guidance on side effects and patient counseling by directly observed therapy (DOT) contributes to practical application. Chapter 7 then deals with drug-resistant tuberculosis (DR-TB), including the genetics of resistance, diagnostic algorithms for multi-drug resistant and extensively drug-resistant (XDR) forms, and new treatment regimens that include new agents as well as repurposed drugs. Chapter 8 examines HIV co-infection, in which both pathogens alter the other's course. Integrative models of care, timing of antiretroviral therapy (ART), and management of immune reconstitution inflammatory syndrome (IRIS) are treated with reference to high-prevalence and resource-limited settings. Pediatric tuberculosis is a focus of Chapter 9, discussing differences in disease presentation among infants and children who are older, age-related diagnostic strategies, dosing adjustment, and challenges with preventive therapy delivery. Chapter 10 covers tuberculosis in special populations, such as the elderly, individuals with diabetes or chronic kidney disease, and those on immunosuppressive therapy, detailing how co-existing conditions impact disease course and treatment strategies.

The final five chapters address preventive measures, public health measures, and directions for future research. Chapter 11 deals with tuberculosis in pregnancy and other special clinical conditions, that is, organ transplant or silicosis, and offers recommendations on balancing mother and child safety versus treatment success. Chapter 12 describes the definition and control of latent tuberculosis infection (LTBI), risk stratification, screening guidelines for healthcare workers and high-risk groups, and current preventive regimens. Chapter 13 outlines national and global tuberculosis program organization, such as surveillance methods, contact tracing, outbreak response, and financing structures. It elaborates on the Stop TB Strategy and End TB Strategy, contrasting aims, metrics, and issues encountered by different areas. Chapter 14 reports on vaccination and non-drug prevention: the *Bacillus Calmette-Guérin* (BCG) vaccine, research into new vaccine candidates, and community interventions such as housing upgrade and dietary supplementation. Finally, Chapter 15 monitors advances in treatment and diagnosis: point-of-care molecular diagnostics, digital technologies for drug-taking adherence, host-directed therapies (HDTs) to alter immune responses, and the pipeline for drugs that could shorten therapy or circumvent resistance.

The book is for general readership. Medical, dental, and nursing students will find it rewarding to have plain language descriptions that form a basis of information. Internal medicine, pediatric, infectious disease, and public health trainees will be grateful for up-to-date clinical guidelines and presentation of programmatic challenges. Clinicians in practice, pulmonologists, obstetricians, pediatricians, and primary care provider, can utilize this as a convenient reference for diagnosis and management. Public health workers, epidemiologists, and program managers will appreciate the policy, surveillance, and community intervention chapters. Laboratory scientists and microbiologists will appreciate in-depth reviews of diagnostic methods and microbial genetics. Finally, immunology, pharmacology, and vaccine research personnel will gain from understanding pathogenesis and new technology.

Chapter 1

MICROBIOLOGY OF MYCOBACTERIUM TUBERCULOSIS

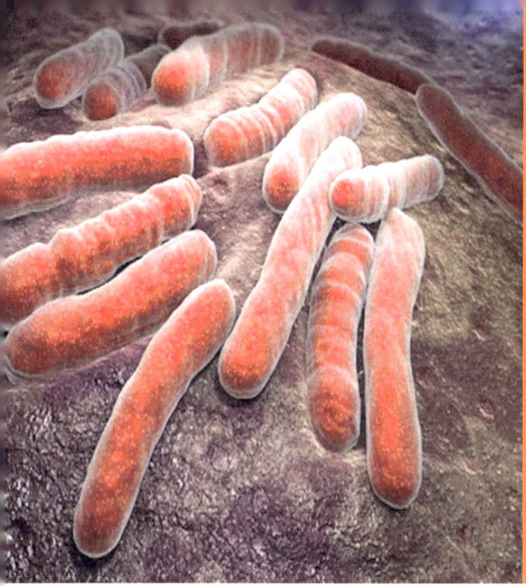

Contents

Introduction

The research of infectious diseases has for centuries been at the heart of studying human health, with those caused by bacterial pathogens that have complex survival mechanisms and life cycles being of paramount importance. *Mycobacterium tuberculosis* (MTB) is one of those pathogens that best represent an example of a pathogen that causes tuberculosis (TB), a disease with significant global health implications. Its peculiar biological attributes, such as its sluggish growth and capacity for survival in adverse conditions within host cells, are factors responsible for its pathogenicity and pose complexities in treatment. Microbiological research continues to deconstruct the molecular and structural elements of MTB, yielding knowledge of crucial importance in formulating new therapeutic methodologies and diagnostic measures for the effective management of tuberculosis. At the heart of the virulence and survival of MTB is its unique cell wall structure, which is key to its drug resistance and pathogenicity. The complex cell wall contains a mycolyl-arabinogalactan-peptidoglycan structure that is central to structural integrity as well as impermeability to numerous antibiotics. Research on the biosynthesis pathways of these cell wall polymers has shown several enzymatic targets for antitubercular drugs, including the arabinofuranosyltransferases responsible for assembly of arabinogalactan. The elucidation of these molecular processes has enabled the discovery of new drug targets, as with the arabinofuranosyltransferases C enzyme whose inhibition would inhibit essential branching in cell wall synthesis and thus potentially improve treatment efficacy (Birch et al., 2008). These advances highlight the importance of microbiological studies in controlling tuberculosis. In addition to the cellular and molecular features of MTB, advances in molecular biology and diagnostic science have revolutionized our detection and analysis capability for mycobacterial infections. Methods like polymerase chain reaction (PCR) and DNA fingerprinting have played a crucial role in separating pathogenic mycobacteria from closely related types, facilitating early diagnosis and allowing for epidemiological surveillance. Sensitive and accurate detection is essential, as a result of the latent and frequently asymptomatic character of infections, which makes disease control and eradication attempts more challenging. Though specific to *Mycobacterium paratuberculosis*, concomitant advances in PCR technologies, such as enhanced sample pre-treatment and incorporating internal controls, demonstrate the wider potential of molecular testing in mycobacterial research (Englund et al., 2002). These technological innovations continue to mold the overall picture and control of tuberculosis globally.

Overview of Mycobacterium Tuberculosis (MTB)

To elucidate the pathogenic processes of MTB, one needs to look at its molecular constituents that play a role in virulence and intracellular persistence. One such interesting aspect is the presence of Forkhead-associated (FHA) domains, which are phosphopeptide-binding motifs essential for signal transduction. MTB has six proteins harboring these domains, but notably, the Rv1747 gene product is an ATP-binding cassette (ABC) transporter with two FHA modules. Rv1747 mutations cause reduced bacterial burden in murine models and compromised growth in macrophages and DCs but do not influence growth *in vitro.* This points towards a dedicated function of Rv1747 to mediate infection within host immune cells by phospho-dependent interaction, especially with the serine-threonine protein kinase PknF. These interactions highlight an important signaling pathway critical to the virulence and adaptation of the bacterium in host environments (Curry et al., 2005). These molecular processes are pivotal to the ability of the pathogens to maintain persistence and to cause disease. The macrophage serves as the major cellular niche that is targeted by MTB, where the bacterium uses mechanisms to survive and multiply in the presence of host immune defenses. The conventional macrophage systems lack high genetic tractability, so host-pathogen interactions at the molecular level cannot be studied. Progress in conditional immortalization of myeloid progenitors, in the form of ER-Hoxb8 cell differentiation from Cas9-expressing transgenic mice, has offered a strong model for analyzing these interactions. Conditionally immortalized macrophages are stable and retain the functional properties of bone marrow-derived macrophages, which allow for precise genetic manipulation and stable and reproducible infection studies. Implication of this model to MTB has identified key host genes and pathways controlling bacterial intracellular persistence and immune system modulation, thus shedding more light on MTB pathogenesis in the host immune microenvironment (Roberts et al., 2019). The complex interaction between MTB and cellular host processes underscores its advanced mechanisms for persistence. Outside of signal transduction and cellular invasion, the bacterium's ability to manipulate host immune responses is vital in the establishment of latent infections. By living inside macrophages, MTB escapes extracellular immune processes, manipulating phagosome development and antigen presentation to evade clearance. This intracellular lifestyle relies on specialized proteins like Rv1747 and kinases like PknF, which coordinate adaptive responses by phosphorylation-dependent signaling cascades. These molecular features enable survival under a permissive host, enabling MTB to remain viable for years and re-activate when immunosuppressed. Understanding these microbiological characteristics is crucial for creating targeted therapeutics and effective vaccines against tuberculosis's long-standing global health crisis (Roberts et al., 2019; Curry et al., 2005) (Figure 1.1).

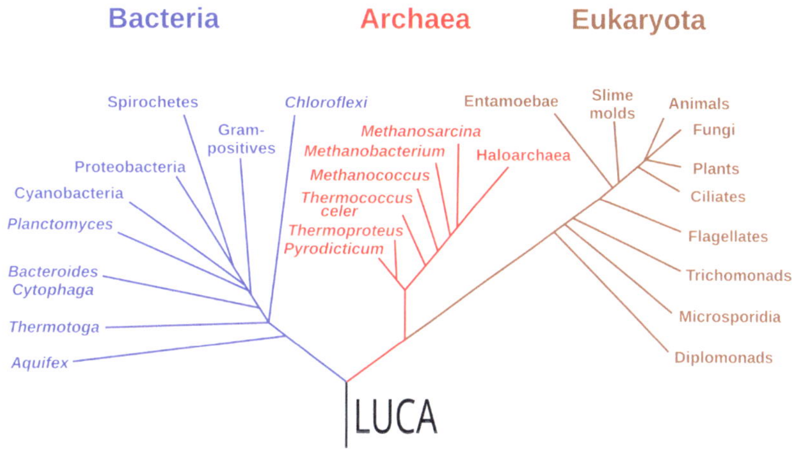

Figure 1.1. Bacteria use molecular machines to move proteins, including toxins, across cell membranes. *M. tuberculosis*, which kills more than 1 million people a year, uses the ESX-4 type VII secretion system to transport its potent exotoxin.

Source: By Chiswick Chap - Own work, CC BY-SA 4.0, https://commons.wikimedia.org/w/index.php?curid=118210187

Importance of Studying Tuberculosis

The microbiology of tuberculosis (TB) is of great importance, particularly in the context of its persistence as a significant public health issue. Despite medical progress, TB continues to be a major cause of death, most notably in immunocompromised individuals in whom opportunistic infections are compounded by disease severity. Knowledge of MTB microbiology allows scientists and medical professionals to decipher the complex pathogenicity of MTB, resistance mechanisms, and host immune interactions. The complex interaction of TB with co-infections, including fungal infections in patients with compromised immunity, highlights the importance of thorough studies. For example, new data illustrate instances of simultaneous infections from pathogens such as *Trichoderma pseudokoningii* combined with *Mycobacterium bovis*, where new aspects of TB pathology both in human and veterinary medicine come to light (Khalifa & Torky, 2012). These perspectives underscore the imperative to advance our microbiological understanding to enhance diagnostic, therapeutic, and preventive measures against complex infectious landscapes. Historically, TB microbiology is rooted in the wider history of germ theory and microbiological science. The development of bacteriology was dominated by trailblazing scientists like Robert Koch, who confirmed the cause-and-effect relationship between MTB and tuberculosis. In addition to evolutionary models that prevail in contemporary microbiology, germ theory gave the applied foundation for disease identification and control of infectious diseases. Koch's method relied on careful classification and description of pathogens within a creationist paradigm that mirrored the varied currents of thought informing early disease research (Gillen et al., 2010). Understanding this historical perspective enhances modern studies by reminding present-day researchers of the value of empirical observation and isolate-based approaches that continue to be at the core of MTB research. Knowledge of such core contributions enables ongoing studies to draw upon a solid scientific foundation, fostering advances against one of humankind's oldest infectious foes. Additionally, the significance of tuberculosis research extends beyond fundamental science and impacts global public health policy and intervention programs. TB persistence, aggravated by drug resistance and co-morbidities like HIV/AIDS, makes control tougher globally. Molecular and microbiological research gives evidence on pathogen diversity, drug resistance mechanisms, and vaccine design, all essential in the efficient management of the disease. Such studies also guide surveillance systems that evolve according to changing epidemiologic trends for timely response and containment. In addition, knowledge of the microbial ecology of MTB and its relationship with other pathogens and environmental reservoirs informs overall strategies in human and animal health fields. The integrated strategy stresses that the control of TB needs to be achieved through persistent scientific research as well as integrated public health measures to minimize the disease burden and avert future epidemics (Gillen et al., 2010; Khalifa & Torky, 2012).

1.1. Taxonomy and Classification

Classification of bacterial species into taxonomic groups forms the basis for their biology and clinical significance. *Mycobacterium tuberculosis* (MTB), a species of the genus *Mycobacterium*, belongs to the family Mycobacteriaceae, with distinctive cell wall structures containing high concentrations of mycolic acids. The genus comprises pathogenic and non-pathogenic species varying greatly in rates of growth and ecological niches. Classification is also dependent on molecular methods addressing conserved genetic markers like 16S rRNA genes that distinguish slow-growing pathogenic strains like MTB from environmental mycobacteria. Molecular tests have shown complexities within the genus, for instance, closely related species with shared phenotypic characteristics, thus making it necessary for sophisticated genomic studies for clarification on species delineation. Therefore, taxonomy is more than a hierarchical tag but an ever-changing mirror of genetic, physiological, and environmental characteristics that are important for diagnosis and therapeutic approaches.

The separation of pathogenic mycobacteria from environmental analogs is of significant difficulty due to genomic similarities and coincidental biochemical characteristics. For example, *Mycobacterium avium* subsp. *paratuberculosis*, the causative agent of Johne's disease in cattle, is genetically homologous to other mycobacteria, making detection and classification challenging. Current molecular investigations have highlighted the necessity for gene targets other than conventional sequences such as IS900, since very closely related organisms can contain homologous elements that provide false positives in PCR-based diagnostics. Methods like PCR-based fingerprinting with enterobacterial intergenic consensus sequences have been established to enhance discrimination between mycobacterial species with improved sensitivity and specificity in diagnostic processes. This is a reflection of the dynamic nature of taxonomy that employs molecular biology tools not just for classifying, but also for identifying clinically important strains of utmost importance for the control of disease and epidemiology (Englund et al., 2002). In addition to pathogenic species, the taxonomy of environmental mycobacteria enhances knowledge of the diversity of the genus and the ecological functions of the bacteria. Recent developments have utilized next-generation sequencing (NGS) and targeted molecular analyses to evaluate fast- and slow-growing mycobacterial diversity across different soil environments. These studies uncovered a wide range of mycobacterial species, a number of which slow-growing taxa are linked to pathogenicity, in essence revealing hidden populations that standard culturing techniques miss. Quantitative analysis supported high gene target densities in environmental samples, highlighting the ubiquity of mycobacteria in natural reservoirs. The molecular view contrasts with conventional schemes for classification by uncovering complex communities with clinically relevant species and non-pathogenic relatives, highlighting the significance of environmental context for taxonomy and implications for the transmission dynamics and efficacy of vaccines (Pontiroli et al., 2013).

1.1.1. Classification Within the Mycobacteriaceae Family

In the wider context of bacterial taxonomy, precise classification is crucial to deciphering pathogenic mechanisms and diagnostic tool development. The Mycobacteriaceae family, to which MTB belongs, is marked by complex genetic and phenotypic variability. Such variability resists simplistic taxonomic classification and requires an integrative approach employing molecular biology tools. Different species in this family, such as the pathogenic MTB and related environmental mycobacteria, share specific genomic signatures that are useful for differentiation. For example, molecular methods like PCR amplification using specific DNA sequences have made it easier to detect and characterize related species, such as *Mycobacterium avium* subsp. paratuberculosis, the causative agent of long-term infections in animals, which is generally difficult to diagnose because it is closely related genetically to other members (Englund et al., 2002). These advances emphasize the need for the refinement of classification schemes through molecular markers to enhance clinical and epidemiological outcomes. Phylogenetic analysis of gene sequences has emerged as a key tool for understanding the evolutionary relationships in the Mycobacteriaceae family. Current research emphasizes the division of mycobacteria into clearly distinguished clades, each differentiated through typical domain structures and regulatory mechanisms at the molecular level. Notably, the cysteine biosynthetic pathway, with the enzyme serine acetyltransferase (CysE), exhibits structural variability in mycobacterial species. The phylogenetic grouping of this enzyme mirrors the general taxonomic structure, dividing mycobacteria into well-separated groups aligned with their evolutionary history and functional specialization. These findings, based on comparative genomics and molecular phylogeny, enable more accurate classification and the determination of possible drug targets by uncovering complex relationships between structure, function, and taxonomy (Gupta et al., 2022). The complex taxonomy of Mycobacteriaceae also calls for reassessing diagnostic approaches and taxonomic criteria. The application of insertion sequences such as IS900 for identifying members such as *M. paratuberculosis* has been hindered by the finding of closely related organisms with similar sequences and minor differences. This finding calls for the establishment of alternative PCR systems that recognize different genetic markers to minimize misidentification and increase diagnostic accuracy. Moreover, molecular fingerprinting methods employing specific primer sets allow differentiation between closely related species, aiding in more detailed classification. This resolution based on molecules is not just important for epidemiology but also for the customization of treatments and comprehending pathogen evolution within the family. Combined, these tools and methods keep refashioning our concept of Mycobacteriaceae taxonomy as well as its relevance in clinical contexts (Englund et al., 2002) (Figure 1.2).

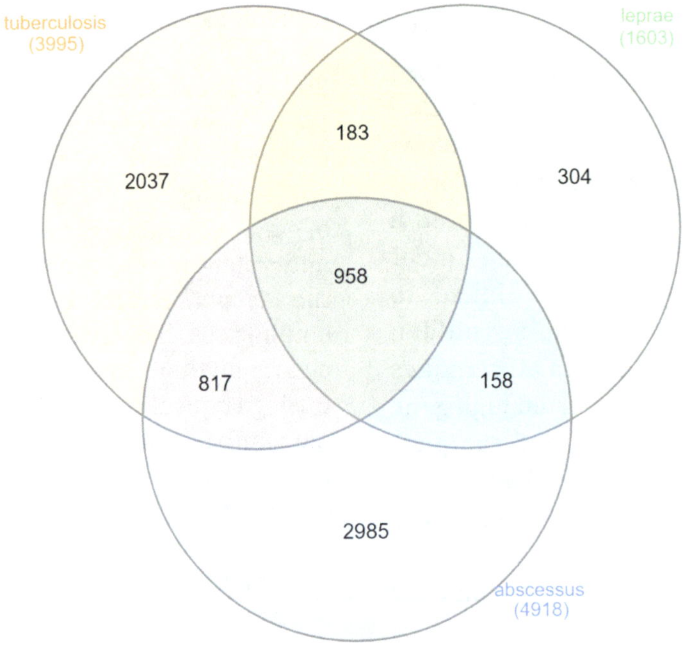

Figure 1.2. Mycobacteriaceae family.

Source: By Tkon13 - Own work, CC BY-SA 4.0, https://commons.wikimedia.org/w/index.php?curid=131649769

1.1.2. Characteristics of Mycobacterium tuberculosis (MTB)

The singular cell architecture of *Mycobacterium tuberculosis* (*M. tuberculosis*/*Mtb*) is the basis of its characteristic microbiology and virulence. The waxy, hydrophobic nature of its cell wall, which is rich in mycolic acids, plays a part in its desiccation and many standard drugs' resistance. The cell wall makes the staining process difficult, necessitating acid-fast methods for detection because of the organisms' ability to retain dyes despite acid alcohol decolorization. The retarded growth rate of *Mtb*, which takes weeks for colony formation to be evident, mirrors its complex metabolic adaptations and presents a challenge for clinical diagnosis. The aerobic metabolism of the bacterium and affinity for the oxygen-rich environment within the lung alveoli enable its infectious niche in human hosts. These traits together facilitate the pathogen's persistence in inhospitable conditions, leading to its capability to produce latent infections as well as avoid immunity, thereby providing efficient transmission and continuous infection cycles. Besides cell wall structure, *Mtb* is also highly phenotypically plastic, facilitating survival within host macrophages. Intracellular, the bacterium can resist oxidative bursts and acidic pH, in part by its capability to manipulate phagosomal maturation and prevent lysosomal fusion. The secretion of complex virulence factors, such as the ESX-1 secretion system, enables *Mtb* to modulate host immunity, facilitating granuloma development and chronic infection. Its slow growth is consistent with the long clinical course of tuberculosis, indicating a balance between replication and immune evasion strategies. Interestingly, the genome of the bacterium codes for multiple stress response proteins and lipid metabolism enzymes to allow adaptation to the hypoxic environment experienced during the process of granuloma formation. These molecular and physiological characteristics highlight the complex host-pathogen interactions of the pathogen and the challenge in designing therapeutics and vaccines against tuberculosis. The ecological and molecular diversity in the *Mycobacterium* genus reinforces the uniqueness of *Mtb* compared to environmental and opportunist strains. Molecular diagnostic progress has enhanced species discrimination, utilizing specific genomic markers other than the standard IS900 target to prevent misidentification, as cited in similar mycobacterial studies (Englund et al., 2002). While *Mtb* is slow growing akin to other pathogenic mycobacteria, environmental mycobacteria have wider growth phenotypes and genetic diversity as uncovered by recent molecular tests on 16S rRNA genes (Pontiroli et al., 2013). These studies show that slow-growing mycobacteria have unique genomic signatures enabling unambiguous identification, which is important for clinical and environmental research. Knowledge of these unique growth rates, genomic markers, and ecological distributions improves our understanding of *Mtb* traits and guides public health measures in tackling its transmission and pathogenicity (Figure 1.3).

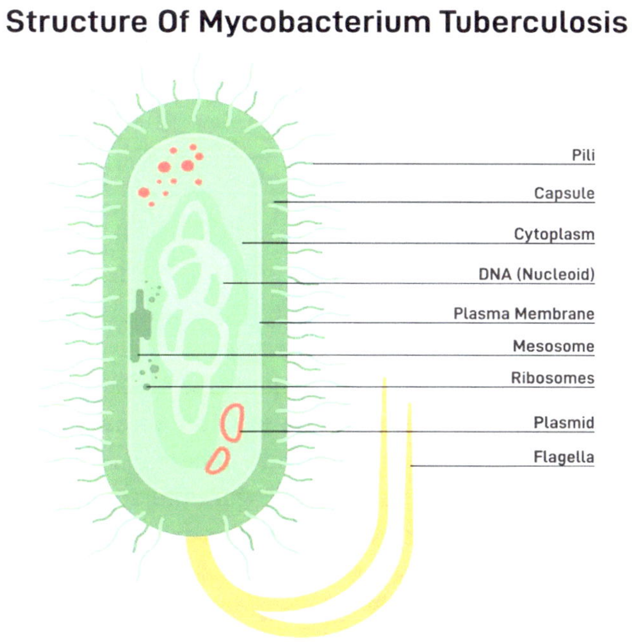

Figure 1.3. Structure of *Mycobacterium tuberculosis (*MTB*)*.

Source: Dreamstime. (n.d.). *Mycobacterium tuberculosis bacteria causative agent microorganism cell structure laboratory research concept.* https://thumbs.dreamstime.com/b/mycobacterium-tuberculosis-bacteria-causative-agent-microorganism-cell-structure-laboratory-research-concept-flat-vector-263240618.jpg.

1.1.3. Comparison with Other Mycobacterium Species

The *Mycobacterium* genus includes a wide variety of species, several of which have similar morphological and physiological characteristics but vary greatly in potential to cause disease and ecological niche. MTB is a human pathogen primarily causing pulmonary tuberculosis and extrapulmonary tuberculosis (EPTB) but has other species like *Mycobacterium leprae* and *Mycobacterium avium* complex (MAC) with separate clinical presentations and interaction with the host (Figure 1.4).

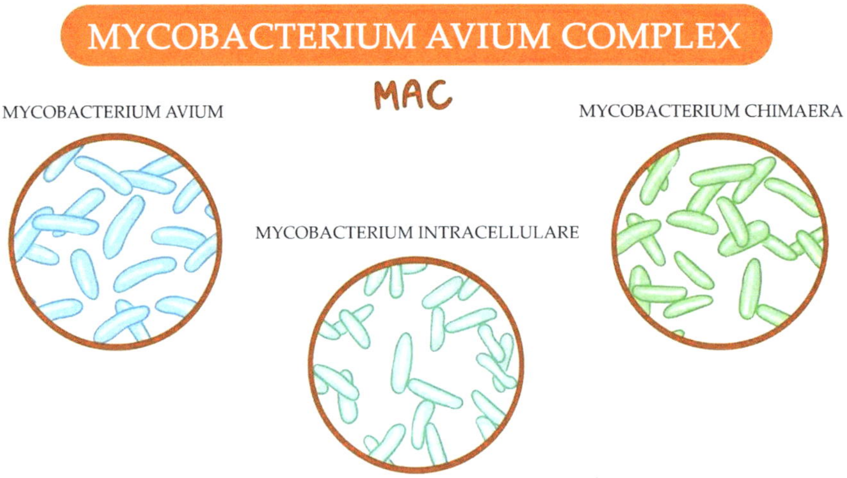

Figure 1.4. *Mycobacterium avium* complex (MAC).

Source: Cloudfront. (n.d.). *Mycobacterium avium complex (MAC): Mycobacterium avium, Mycobacterium intracellulare, Mycobacterium chimaera.* https://d16qt3wv6xm098.cloudfront.net/m55myolZQZeefc9R5czbN1x7TPKFPDPp/_.jpg.

In contrast to *Mtb*, which is slowly growing with specific culture requirements, certain environmental mycobacteria are more fastidious and opportunistic pathogens. These distinctions make diagnosis and treatment more challenging, emphasizing *Mtb*'s singular characteristic of being able to remain latent in host macrophages. The comparative study also uncovers variations in cell wall lipid content, impacting virulence and immune evasion across species. These differences are important for creating targeted therapeutic agents and enhancing molecular diagnostic instruments specifically for *Mtb*. As a consequence of advances in genome sequencing, comparative genomics has emerged as an essential instrument for distinguishing between *Mycobacterium* species at the molecular level. Whole-genome sequencing (WGS) technologies have uncovered extensive genetic differences within the genus, including single nucleotide polymorphisms and gene deletions that confer species-specific characteristics. Advanced bioinformatics software, including those that predict antimicrobial susceptibility from genomic information, is increasingly used to describe *Mtb* and its kin. Although the software has been found to be reliable in predicting resistance patterns in a number of bacterial species, it is still underutilized in the case of mycobacteria owing to complex mechanisms of resistance and genomic variability specific to the genus (Bortolaia et al., 2020). Continuous optimization of databases and interpretation algorithms will increase the comparability of *Mtb* with other mycobacteria, enabling better diagnosis and treatment on the basis of genomic profiles instead of phenotypic assays alone. Attempts to taxonomically place *Mycobacterium* species have been transformed by genome-based phylogenetic analysis that incorporates large data sets and advanced computational tools. Applications such as the type (strain) genome server (TYGS) facilitate high-throughput, accurate classification through the comparison of *Mtb* genomes with homologous species, with distinct species and subspecies boundaries (Jan et al., 2019). Such genome-scale methods resolve taxonomic uncertainty, which conventional phenotypic strategies commonly are unable to clarify because of homologous features between mycobacteria. These methods also shed light on evolutionary relationships and illustrate subtle genomic differences that are critical to epidemiology and pathogen biology. Knowledge of the taxonomic and genetic differences between *Mycobacterium* species is critical for clinical microbiologists and scientists who wish to engineer new diagnostics, vaccines, or therapies that capitalize on species-specific weaknesses and pathogenic processes.

1.2. Morphology and Structure

The special features of MTB are mainly due to its unusual cellular structure, which is responsible for its survival and virulence. In contrast to normal bacteria, *Mtb* has a complicated cell envelope, a waxy, hydrophobic layer that is laden with mycolic acids, long-chain fatty acids that impart a hydrophobic character and resistance to chemical damage. This lipid-rich barrier not only retards the entry of many antibiotics but also plays a key role in how the bacterium can resist host immune systems. In addition, the morphological uniformity of these bacilli, which are thin, aerobic rods measuring around 2–4 micrometers in length, aids in their survival in adverse environments like inside macrophages. This singular structural intricacy makes the diagnosis and treatment of tuberculosis more difficult, highlighting the necessity of understanding its cell morphology more deeply in microbiological studies. The structural structure at the molecular level of *Mtb*'s cell wall is the focal point for its functional adaptations. While the peptidoglycan layer may be thinner compared to some other bacteria, it plays a key scaffold role, attaching the arabinogalactan polysaccharide and giving rigidity as required. This is overlying the mycolyl-arabinogalactan-peptidoglycan complex, which also imparts pathogenic acid-fastness—a critical diagnostic character targeted by Ziehl-Neelsen staining protocols. Incorporated within this complex matrix are numerous glycolipids and lipoglycans, which not only stabilize the complex but also regulate immune interaction. These distinct molecular components have been the target of drug development, since disruption in their synthesis leads to disturbance in cell wall integrity and bacterial viability, showing how *Mtb* morphology is closely entwined with its structural biochemistry. Progress in pharmacological studies has favored the targeting of *Mtb*'s morphological components to counter drug resistance problems. For example, ATP synthase enzyme complex located in the cell membrane is crucial in the bacterium's energy metabolism. Compounds such as bedaquiline block the c-ring of the proton-translocating F0 sector of ATP synthase, preventing ATP synthesis critical in cell functions. But mutations in the atpE gene, which codes for the c subunit of this enzyme, have conferred resistance, prompting research into new drug candidates that are capable of adapting to structural changes in the protein complex. Revolutionary methods using molecular dynamics simulations and virtual screening have revealed molecules like L136, which exhibit highly effective binding affinity across wild-type and mutant ATPc proteins, indicating improved efficacy and reduced toxicity profiles (Roy et al., 2024). Moreover, computational models incorporating quantitative structure-activity relationships help in predicting compound activity against *Mtb*, accelerating drug discovery processes through correlating molecular shape with function (Ekosputri et al., 2024). These findings highlight the essential need to comprehend bacterial shape and structural changes in devising effective treatments.

1.2.1. Cell Wall Composition and Its Significance

The cell wall architecture is a characteristic of pathogenicity, essentially defining its mode of interaction with the host immune system. In contrast to normal bacterial cell walls, MTB consists of an complex arrangement of glycolipids, specifically mycolyl arabinogalactan, a polymer made of arabinofuranoside and galactofuranosides esterified by long-chain mycolic acids. This complex scaffold not only imparts unparalleled resistance against chemical attacks but also regulates the permeability of antibiotics and plays a role in the notorious drug resistance of the pathogen. The specific arrangement of arabinofuranoside motifs, such as varying α and β linkages and the presence of cyclopropanated fatty acids, regulates the self-assembly and physical properties of the cell wall. These molecular nuances have a pivotal impact on the morphology of cell wall constructs and the bacterium's capacity to survive in hostile host environments, highlighting their biological significance (Hotha et al., 2025) (Figure 1.5).

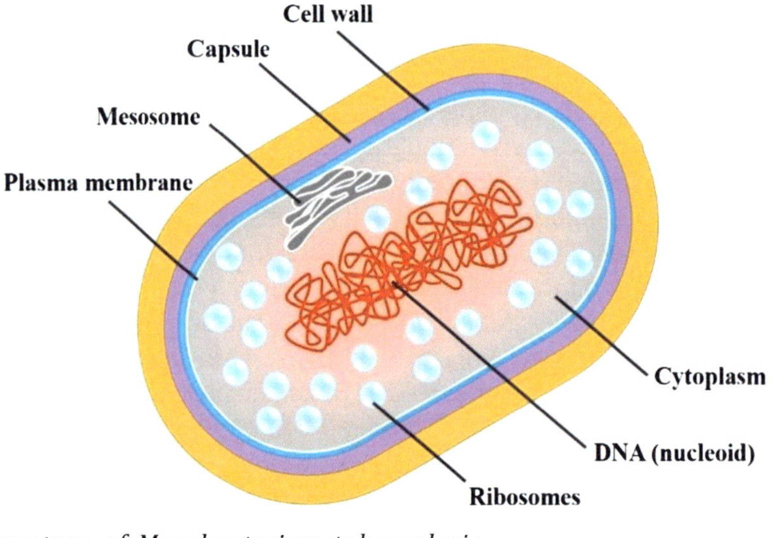

Figure 1.5. Cell structure of *Mycobacterium tuberculosis.*

Source: Wang Y, Shi Q, Chen Q, Zhou X, Yuan H, Jia X, Liu S, Li Q and Ge L (2022) Emerging advances in identifying signal transmission molecules involved in the interaction between Mycobacterium tuberculosis and the host. Front. Cell. Infect. Microbiol. 12:956311. doi: 10.3389/fcimb.2022.956311

The importance of the MTB cell wall reaches beyond its role of structural integrity to its dynamic function in immune evasion and intracellular persistence. The hydrophobic outer lipid layer restricts hydrophilic molecule access and shields the *Bacillus* from host-derived reactive oxygen and nitrogen radicals. In addition, the cell wall components actively participate in host-pathogen interactions through modulation of immune signal transduction. For example, glycolipids that are released from the cell wall can regulate macrophage activation, repressing effective immune clearance and promoting chronic infection. These lipids of the cell wall are involved in the biogenesis of extracellular vesicles (EVs) and MTB makes use of them to secrete bioactive molecules that can change host immune responses. Such vesicle communication is a reflection of the strength and flexibility of the cell wall composition that is pivotal in the survival mode of the pathogens inside the host (Alipoor & Elieh-Ali-Komi, 2024). Insight into the distinctive composition and functional relevance of the MTB cell wall provides invaluable information on new therapeutic targets.

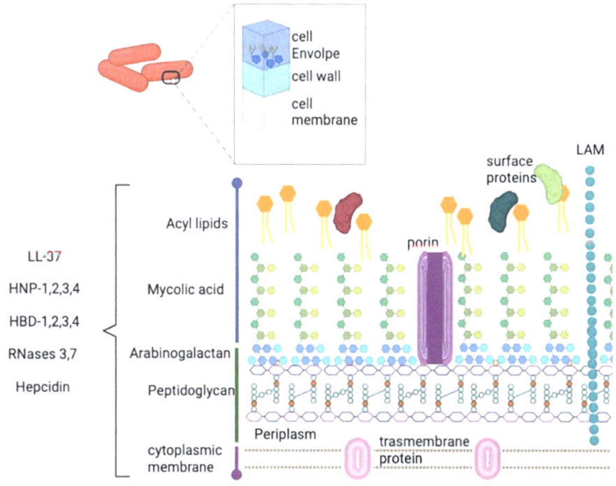

Figure 1.6. *M. tuberculosis* cell wall. The *Mtb* cell wall is composed of several complex layers, including the cell envelope, cell wall, and cell membrane.

Source: Jacobo-Delgado YM, Rodríguez-Carlos A, Serrano CJ and Rivas-Santiago B (2023) Mycobacterium tuberculosis cell-wall and antimicrobial peptides: a mission impossible? Front. Immunol. 14:1194923. doi: 10.3389/fimmu.2023.1194923.

The complex matrix of mycolic acids, arabinogalactan, and linked glycolipids offers difficult but potentially valuable targets for drug development. Interfering with the biosynthesis or organization of these elements compromises cell wall integrity and increases the susceptibility of the pathogen to antibiotics. Moreover, therapeutic interventions that hinder EV formation and release, regulated by cell wall molecules, may boost host immune effectiveness and restrict pathogen spread. Hence, the cell wall not just represents a physical envelope but also a center of pathogenicity and a vital interface for host-pathogen interactions, whose comprehensive definition is essential in the pursuit of tuberculosis treatment (Alipoor & Elieh-Ali-Komi, 2024; Hotha et al., 2025) (Figure 1.6).

1.2.2. Microscopic Appearance and Staining Techniques

Identification of MTB by microscopy is particularly challenging because of its characteristic cellular structure and staining features. Most bacteria differ from *Mtb* in that they have a lipid-rich waxy cell wall composed of mycolic acids, which makes them resistant to standard staining procedures.

This feature requires special staining procedures, for example, the Ziehl-Neelsen acid-fast stain, which takes advantage of the bacterium's acid-fastness. When stained, *Mtb* does not lose the red dye carbol fuchsin even after acid-alcohol treatment, unlike most other bacteria that lose the dye and become blue after taking up a counterstain. Differential staining is very important for microscopic diagnosis, particularly in sputum smears where bacterium concentration can be variable. Nonetheless, even with the extreme specificity of acid-fast staining towards *Mtb*, sensitivity is still low, thus the requirement for additional methods to enhance detection rates (Widhyasih et al., 2019). Improved culturing techniques supplement microscopic staining in the diagnosis of tuberculosis through improved timely detection of *Mtb*. Conventional culture on Löwenstein-Jensen (LJ) solid media enables easy visualization of typical rough, buff-colored colonies following growth but is slow, taking several weeks. Later developments have involved liquid-based micro-broth culture systems that allow microscopic observation of bacterial growth in microplate wells. These liquid cultures present earlier visual confirmation of microbial growth with the quick detection of acid-fast bacilli (AFB), lowering turnaround times significantly over solid media. These methods enable quicker confirmation of microscopy findings and enhance the overall sensitivity of diagnosis in clinical specimens. This transformation to liquid culture and microscopy improves diagnostic processes by providing faster and more precise detection of *Mtb*, which is critical for initiating early treatment (Kidenya et al., 2013). Even with the benefits of microscopic inspection and culture-based methods, some limitations impact the precision and quickness of tuberculosis diagnosis. The microscopic identification of AFB requires good-quality sputum samples and skilled technicians since there is a risk of false negatives when bacterial loads are low. False positives can also result from the presence of nontuberculous mycobacteria (NTM) or staining artifacts, making interpretation difficult. New immunochromatographic assays identifying specific antigens like ESAT-6 and CFP-10 have become tools to complement microscopy for these challenges, but their clinical use needs to be further ascertained. Combining better staining protocols with newer culture techniques and detection of antigens can potentially overcome these diagnostic limitations, minimizing delays in identifying *Mtb* and enhancing patient outcomes in tuberculosis-endemic settings (Kidenya et al., 2013; Widhyasih et al., 2019) (Figure 1.7).

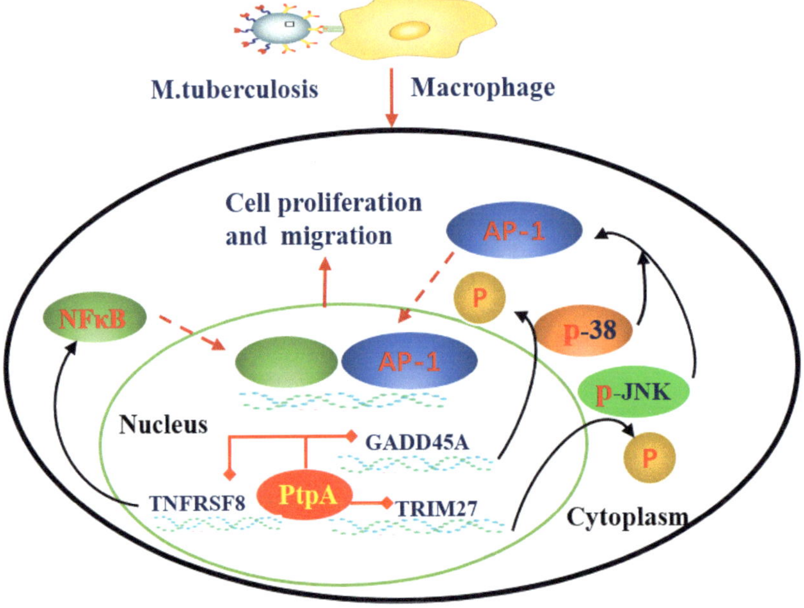

Figure 1.7. The mechanism by which MTB-PtpA enters the host cell nucleus to inhibit natural immune function. MTB-PtpA is secreted into the host cell to bind ubiquitin molecules and is activated, and the activated PtpA can inhibit the transcription of *TNFRSF8* in the host nucleus, thus inhibiting the NF-κB signaling pathway.

Source: Wang Y, Shi Q, Chen Q, Zhou X, Yuan H, Jia X, Liu S, Li Q and Ge L (2022) Emerging advances in identifying signal transmission molecules involved in the interaction between Mycobacterium tuberculosis and the host. Front. Cell. Infect. Microbiol. 12:956311. doi: 10.3389/fcimb.2022.956311

1.2.3. Growth Characteristics and Culture Requirements

The complex biology of MTB makes it difficult to culture and investigate, especially as a result of its sluggish growth rate and stringent nutritional needs. As opposed to the vast majority of bacterial pathogens, MTB has a long generation time, which is generally 15 to 20 hours to divide, and thus a long incubation period when cultured. This gradual replication is also partly due to its multi-layered cell wall structure that is rich in mycolic acids, which also affects its oxygen requirements and makes it an obligate aerobe. Growth of this pathogen usually requires specialized media like *Lowenstein–Jensen* or *Middlebrook 7H10* agar that are supplemented with growth factors to supply the necessary nutrients like fatty acids, vitamins, and trace elements. These rigorous requirements are essential to facilitate MTB's metabolism and replication, highlighting the organism's stringent *in vitro* nature and the delicate balance necessary for its cultivation. Production of viable cultures of MTB in the lab places not only nutritional requirements but also particular environmental conditions. The temperature has a significant impact on bacterial development, and MTB grows best at 37°C, very similar to the human body environment in which it occurs naturally. Also, the pathogen's need for an elevated oxygen tension mirrors its affinity for the well-oxygenated parts of the lungs of its host. The bacterium's ability to survive under hostile environments, like oxidative stress in macrophages, correlates with the advanced DNA repair systems it possesses that are differentially activated during various stages of infection (Roberts et al., 2019). These molecular mechanisms help MTB survive oxidative insults during infection and thereby impact its culture viability by reducing environmental stress. In addition, recent developments in macrophage-like cell models have made it easier to genetically study MTB as they offer a controlled environment to monitor bacterial growth and adaptation (Roberts et al., 2019). MTB's pathogenicity is linked closely to its slow and insidious growth modes both *in vivo* and *in vitro*, which requires careful culture methods. The longer incubation periods necessary for the development of visible colonies are difficult for standard diagnostic protocols and experimental schedules, calling for patience and exacting laboratory organization. Furthermore, the stringent containment requirements that must be observed in the culture of this high-risk organism complicate culture. Bacterial growth on liquid media, for example, *Middlebrook 7H9* broth, may involve additives such as glycerol and OADC (oleic acid, albumin, dextrose, and catalase) to further maximize bacterial growth. Knowledge of such growth features not only assists in optimizing culture techniques but also improves understanding of MTB's behavior at latent infection stages, where replication of bacteria is low but continuous (Gorna et al., 2010). Such knowledge is critical in designing better therapeutic interventions that target the survival mechanisms of the bacterium.

1.3. Pathogenesis

The course of MTB infection in the host represents a multifaceted interaction between the survival mechanisms of the pathogen and the immune defense of the host. After inhalation, MTB is exposed to the hostile pulmonary alveoli environment, where it needs to resist killing by resident macrophages. Through the inhibition of phagosome-lysosome fusion in macrophages, the bacterium can survive intracellularly and develop a niche for replication. This early survival initiates an avalanche of immune responses that may result in granuloma formation, a defining characteristic of tuberculosis pathology. Granulomas are a double-edged sword—though they contain the infection, they also create a microenvironment conducive to bacterial latency and reactivation. These phases of infection subject MTB to oxidative stress and

DNA damage, requiring efficient repair systems that are closely associated with its pathogenicity and host persistence (Gorna et al., 2010). Part of the pathogenic success of MTB lies in its high-grade molecular machinery for repairing DNA damage that occurs during infection. Unlike many bacteria, MTB lacks certain conventional DNA mismatch repair systems but compensates with efficient nucleotide excision repair, base excision repair, and homologous recombination pathways.

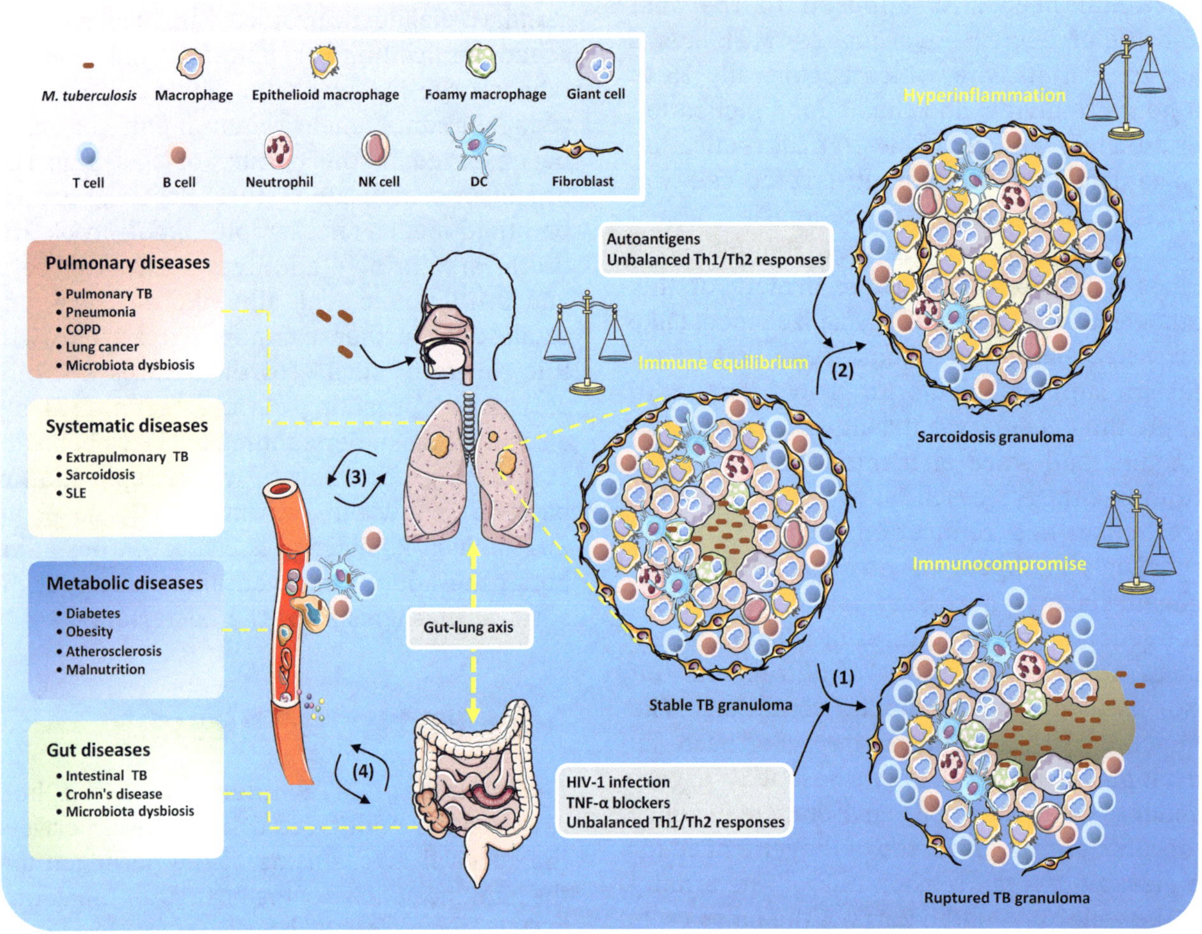

Figure 1.8. Disease progression of *Mycobacterium tuberculosis*.

Source: Chai Q, Zhang Y and Liu CH (2018) Mycobacterium tuberculosis: An Adaptable Pathogen Associated With Multiple Human Diseases. Front. Cell. Infect. Microbiol. 8:158. doi: 10.3389/fcimb.2018.00158

These pathways play a vital role in safeguarding genomic integrity against the oxidative and nitrosative stress inflicted by the host's immune machinery. Impressively, MTB up-regulates various DNA repair genes conditionally based on the stage of infection as a testament to an adaptation strategy toward the changing intracellular condition. The capacity for DNA lesion repair not only aids bacterial survival but can also affect drug resistance development and latency, highlighting the crucial role of DNA repair in MTB pathogenesis (Gorna et al., 2010). Although MTB and its closely related species have pathogenic characteristics in common, differences in molecular diagnostics reflect the challenge involved in comprehensively understanding their pathogenesis. For example, the difficulty in distinguishing *Mtb* from other mycobacteria such as *M. paratuberculosis*, which infects ruminants and causes Johne's disease, emphasizes the need for accurate molecular tools for diagnosis and epidemiological investigations. Improvements in DNA amplification and PCR-based fingerprinting methods have improved the detection and characterization of disease-causing mycobacteria, providing a basis for understanding their infection patterns. Such molecular information aids in understanding the nature of how varied mycobacterial species interact with their hosts, potentially affecting their pathogenicity and guiding enhanced therapeutic measures (Figure 1.8).

1.3.1. Mechanisms of Infection and Transmission

The ability of *Mycobacterium tuberculosis* complex (MTBC) microorganisms to infect is directly associated with their distinctive cell wall structure, which provides them with resistance to adverse environmental conditions and host immune responses. The composite lipid-laden cell envelope, especially the presence of mycolic acids, provides acid-fastness and robust protection against dehydration and chemical aggression. These characteristics allow the pathogen to survive in respiratory secretions that are coughed or sneezed out and so enable airborne transmission. Upon inhalation, the bacilli avoid initial immune clearance by alveolar macrophages using several virulence mechanisms, such as inhibition of phagosomal maturation. The interaction of mycobacterial virulence factors with host immune mechanisms then determines the course and establishment of infection. Typical granuloma development is indicative of a host's effort to encapsulate the pathogen, yet also signifies a bacterial survival and latency niche (Sawyer et al., 2023). Environmental perseverance of these species also facilitates intermittent spreading through indirect contact, for instance, contaminated fomites or ingestion, widening avenues for transmission. MTBC, especially *Mycobacterium bovis*, transmission dynamics reveal the multifaceted nature of infection pathways beyond direct host-to-host transmission. Epidemiological data emphasize respiratory droplets as the main means of transmission; nevertheless, studies show that environmental reservoirs such as water and soil may support viable bacteria for prolonged periods. Environmental persistence is a cause for concern regarding indirect means of transmission, for example, via contaminated water sources or pastures, particularly in livestock and wildlife settings. Furthermore, contacts with environmental amoebae such as *Dictyostelium discoideum* unveil further mechanistic dimensions through which *M. bovis* will survive predation and take advantage of other microenvironments beyond mammalian hosts (Rachel et al., 2019).

These amoebae-related mechanisms, such as evading destruction and phagocytic escape, recapitulate strategies adopted within mammalian macrophages, highlighting the pathogen's evolutionary strategies that augment both infection establishment and spread in various ecological niches. At the molecular level, virulence factors like the ESX-1 secretion system and lipid transporters are key factors in facilitating *Mtb* infection and transmission. The ESX-1 locus contains a type VII secretion machinery essential for bacterial escape from host cell membranes and host immune modulation. ESX-1-disrupting mutations correlate with compromised intracellular survival and impaired dissemination, highlighting its central role in pathogenesis (Rachel et al., 2019). Also, lipid-associated proteins, such as those implicated in sulfolipid biosynthesis and the PE/PPE protein families, are involved in immune evasion and persistence in host tissues. These proteins facilitate mycobacteria to modulate host cell signaling and establish a supportive environment for replication and transmission. Understanding these molecular mechanisms is critical to appreciate how *Mtb* sustains its infectious cycle and to building effective targeted interventions to cut off chains of transmission (Rachel et al., 2019; Sawyer et al., 2023).

1.3.2. Host Immune Response to Mycobacterium tuberculosis (MTB)

The complex interplay between MTB and the host immune system lies at the heart of tuberculosis pathogenesis. On inhalation, MTB is engulfed by alveolar macrophages as the primary defense mechanism. The bacterium has, however, developed advanced mechanisms of immune evasion, involving hijacking of antimicrobial processes of macrophages. New understanding points toward the contribution of microRNAs (miRNAs) in this regard, as they regulate host immune responses post-transcriptionally. Certain miRNAs like miR-155 and miR-29a modulate macrophage activation and cytokine release, thus determining the inflammatory environment pivotal for limiting or perpetuation of infection. In addition, exosomal miRNAs released by infected macrophages have the potential to modify surrounding cell functions, potentially biasing local immune responses toward bacterial persistence. These small regulatory RNAs are a promising area of research not only in the study of TB immunopathology but also in the design of new diagnostic and therapeutic instruments (Mukhtar et al., 2024). Protein acetylation also appears to be another key mechanism regulating the host immune response to MTB.

Both the pathogen and host cells undergo massive post-translational modifications that affect disease progression. Bacterial protein acetylation controls virulence, drug resistance, and metabolism to promote MTB survival under stressful intracellular conditions. On the other hand, MTB causes acetylation modifications in host proteins, which have effects on modulating immune signaling pathways. This two-way acetylation is essential in determining the state of macrophage activation and the effectiveness of host defense mechanisms. Elucidating the way MTB exploits host protein acetylation to inhibit protective immune responses may uncover new avenues for therapeutic intervention, especially in the area of improving antimycobacterial immune effectiveness (Huang et al., 2023). The immune response of the host to MTB infection is characterized by a fine balance between control and disease progression, mediated through both innate and adaptive immunity. Macrophages, dendritic cells (DCs), and T lymphocytes collaborate to develop granulomas, organized immune environments that contain the bacteria but can also act as reservoir sites for latent infection. Imbalanced immune reactions, mediated by aberrant expression of certain miRNAs or modifications in protein acetylation, can disturb this equilibrium and result in active tuberculosis along with tissue destruction. Exploring how MTB leverages host molecular regulators to subvert immune surveillance will be fundamental to the evolution of therapeutic approaches. These molecular findings form the basis of next-generation vaccines and host-directed therapies (HDTs) to restore protective immune responses while avoiding pathological inflammation (Huang et al., 2023; Mukhtar et al., 2024) (Figure 1.9).

Disease	Correlation to TB	Relevant findings	References
PULMONARY DISEASE			
Pneumonia	TB infection as a potential etiology	TB infection increases susceptibility to secondary bacterial pneumonia in young children	Oliwa et al., 2015a
COPD *	Increases the risk of active TB; TB infection as a potential etiology;	TB infection leads to remodeling of the lung architecture, such as extensive fibrosis, cavitation, traction bronchiectasis, bronchostenosis, or parenchymal lung destruction; the development of bronchiectasis in patients with COPD causes active TB	Dheda et al., 2005; Chakrabarti et al., 2007; Jordan et al., 2010
Lung cancer	TB infection as a potential etiology	TB infection establishes chronic and persistent inflammation; induces production of NO and ROS to bring about DNA damage; develops pulmonary fibrosis	Ardies, 2003; Sharma et al., 2004; Shin et al., 2008
AUTOIMMUNE DISEASE			
Sarcoidosis	TB infection as a potential etiology	*M. tuberculosis* HSP16 and HSP70 participate in the etiopathogenesis of sarcoidosis; activation of TLRs signaling caused by *M. tuberculosis* infection involves in the pathogenesis of pulmonary sarcoidosis	Dubaniewicz et al., 2006; Gabrilovich et al., 2013
SLE *	Increases the risk of active TB; TB infection as a potential etiology;	Cross-reactivity between mycobacterial and host self-antigens; antigenic resemblance between mycobacterial glycolipids and host DNA; immune abnormalities and immunosuppressive therapy lead to active TB development	Amital-Teplizki et al., 1989; Yun et al., 2002
METABOLIC DISEASE			
DM *	Increases the risk of active TB; promotes TB progression	Promotes mycobacterial proliferation; enhances $CD4^+$ Th1/Th17 responses and reduces frequencies of Treg cells in active TB patients; reduces Th1/Th17 responses in latent TB patients	Martens et al., 2007; Kumar et al., 2013, 2014
Obesity	Decreases the risk of active TB	The adipose tissue may have immunomodulatory functions against TB infection; the mechanisms are still largely unknown	Wieland et al., 2005; Ordway et al., 2008; Abella et al., 2017
Atherosclerosis	TB infection as a potential etiology	*M. tuberculosis* HSP65 accelerates the progression of atherosclerosis; both of two diseases accumulates foamy macrophages in the lesion	Peyron et al., 2008; Zhang et al., 2012; Chinetti-Gbaguidi et al., 2015; Wick et al., 2017
Hypovitaminosis D	TB infection as a potential etiology	Vitamin D is essential for production of antimicrobial peptide and promotion of autophagy and phagosomal maturation; the mechanisms of *M. tuberculosis*-induced hypovitaminosis D is still unclear	Liu et al., 2006; Campbell and Spector, 2012; Azam et al., 2016; Wang J. et al., 2017
CO-INFECTION			
HIV-1	Increases the risk of active TB; TB infection results in increased viral replication	Depletes *M. tuberculosis*-reactive T cells; inhibits phagocytosis and autophagy; induces cell death and tissue necrosis	Bell and Noursadeghi, 2017
Helicobacter pylori	Decreases the risk of active TB	Enhances host Th1-type responses with higher level of IFN-γ, IL-2, TNF-α, and CXCL-10	Perry et al., 2010
Helminth	Commonly occurs in TB patients; disturbs host immune responses to either of infectious pathogens	Reduces *M. tuberculosis*-antigen specific immune responses; lowers Th1/Th17 responses and elevates Th2 responses	Babu and Nutman, 2016

**COPD, chronic obstructive pulmonary disease; SLE, systemic lupus erythematosus; DM, diabetes mellitus.*

Figure 1.9. A schematic representation of the immune response of the host to infection with *Mycobacterium tuberculosis* (*Mtb*). *Mtb* is inhaled through aerosols and is transferred to the lung, where it is engulfed by alveolar macrophages and destroyed by multiple pathways, such as apoptosis and autophagy. When bacterial growth is halted but not killed in the initial phase of infection, the disease is in a latent state without clinical tuberculosis (TB) in 90–95% of patients.

Source: Chai Q, Zhang Y and Liu CH (2018) Mycobacterium tuberculosis: An Adaptable Pathogen Associated With Multiple Human Diseases. Front. Cell. Infect. Microbiol. 8:158. doi: 10.3389/fcimb.2018.00158

1.3.3. Factors Influencing Virulence and Disease Progression

The interaction between MTB and the host immune system plays an important role in determining the outcome of infection, affecting both virulence and disease progression. Initial infection tends to invoke innate immune responses; nevertheless, *Mtb* has a repertoire of virulence factors that facilitate the ability to evade or subvert these defenses, for example, the inhibition of phagosome-lysosome fusion in macrophages. This pathogen's survival within host cells causes the duration of the latent phase to be long, with metabolic activity in bacteria fluctuating widely, representing a dynamic balance rather than a resting stage. Environmental pressures, host genotype, and immune status determine critically whether the pathogen remains sequestered or progresses to active disease. This heterogeneity supports the range of clinical presentations seen, from latent infection to active disease, influenced by the interplay between bacterial persistence and host immune response (Aslam et al., 2018). This complex interplay between host and pathogen highlights the complexities of *Mtb* virulence that are more than just basic bacterial multiplication. The genetic heterogeneity between MTB strains is also responsible for varying virulence and regulating pathways of disease progression. Strain-dependent differences in cell wall constituents, secretion mechanisms, and stress response systems regulate the pathogen's ability to endure abusive host environments and cause diverse immunopathological effects. Additionally, the development and spread of multi-drug resistant strains are a major concern since resistance functions can influence bacterial fitness and virulence, making treatment harder and extending the duration of infection. The abuse of antibiotics speeds up the development of resistance, thus increasing virulence in certain situations by exerting selective pressures that benefit more tolerant variants. This interaction between antimicrobial resistance (AMR) and virulence not only makes clinical control more difficult but also underscores the importance of multidisciplinary intervention involving new therapeutic and preventive measures to limit disease progression (Aslam et al., 2018). Assessment of these genetic and pharmacological determinants is crucial for optimal tuberculosis control. Rising evidence of the tuberculosis disease spectrum refutes conventional latent and active infection dichotomies, highlighting intermediate clinical phases that modulate virulence behavior and risk for disease progression. Identifying incipient and subclinical tuberculosis provides a more dynamic framework that accommodates changing bacterial metabolic activity and immune reaction during infection. These states are key windows for intervention because bacterial replication starts to rise without apparent symptoms, potentially resulting in transmissible active disease if not controlled. Therefore, the pathogen's potential for remaining in a metabolically variable condition expresses adaptive virulence strategies that are consistent with evasion and survival in the host. Such a continuum highlights the significance of the early diagnostic and therapeutic interventions specific to these intermediate stages to avoid full disease development and community spread (Paul et al., 2018). This conceptual change in tuberculosis pathogenesis improves our knowledge about virulence factors modulating disease courses.

1.4. Epidemiology

The determinants and patterns of infectious diseases are important for understanding their effects on public health. For MTB, epidemiology not only directs diagnosis and treatment guidelines but also informs prevention. Tuberculosis continues to be a global health burden, disproportionately striking low-income areas with poor access to healthcare. Transmission is mainly by airborne droplets from active pulmonary TB patients, necessitating early detection and isolation. Additionally, epidemiological studies highlight the increased susceptibility among immunocompromised individuals, such as those suffering from chronic liver diseases, in which invasive infections are at higher risk due to compromised host immunity and imbalance of cytokines, thus making it easier for MTB infections to progress (Bunchorntavakul et al., 2012).

Surveillance statistics provide different incidence and prevalence rates of tuberculosis in diverse geographic and demographic environments. Of significance is the fact that in hospital settings, caution is needed since nosocomial transmission complicates the control of outbreaks. Co-pathogen studies carried out in the field of epidemiology confirm that MTB tends to occur concomitantly with other bacterial pathogens in immunocompromised individuals. For example, the incidence of TB in patients with systemic infection corresponds to difficulty in choosing proper empirical antibiotics, making the localized resistance pattern critical. Contrasting TB with other infections, such as septic arthritis, reveals differing pathogen distributions, highlighting microbiological diversity and drug susceptibility critical for individualized treatment regimens (Clerc et al., 2011).

Knowledge of the epidemiology of MTB also helps identify disease severity or transmission-relevant risk factors. Socioeconomic status, HIV co-infection, and existing comorbidities have a strong impact on epidemiological trends. As a result, control programs bring together epidemiologic surveillance and public health interventions to decrease TB occurrence. These measures consist of targeted screening, vaccination, and antimicrobial stewardship to avoid the development of drug resistance. The epidemiological model thus gives essential information regarding TB's burden, informing clinical decision-making and resource prioritization to reduce its effect in the world and among vulnerable populations (Bunchorntavakul et al., 2012; Clerc et al., 2011) (Figure 1.10).

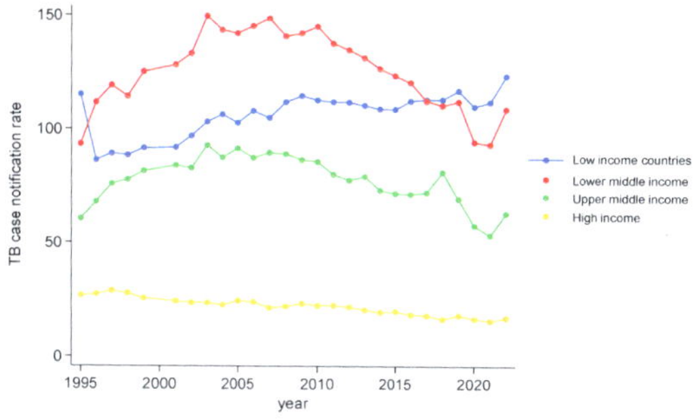

Figure 1.10. Estimated tuberculosis cases, 2007.

Source: Koura KG, Harries AD. The Trend of Tuberculosis Case Notification Rates from 1995 to 2022 by Country Income and World Health Organization Region. *Tropical Medicine and Infectious Disease*. 2024; 9(12):294. https://doi.org/10.3390/tropicalmed9120294

1.4.1. Global Prevalence and Incidence Rates

The epidemiology of MTB is determined by a multifaceted interplay among sociopolitical, economic, and healthcare determinants that differ significantly across regions. In the Republic of Moldova, longitudinal surveillance data show fluctuating trends that highlight the problems of tuberculosis control. Between 2015 and 2019, there was a decrease in both incidence and prevalence, which mirrors effective public health interventions. Yet the time period involving the COVID-19 pandemic witnessed an increase of 17% in global tuberculosis incidence, rising from 56.68 to 66.34 per 1,00,000 population, at the same time emphasizing the susceptibility of tuberculosis programs amidst global health emergencies. Nevertheless, the mortality rates showed a trend of decreasing in recent years, reflecting the enhancement of treatment outcomes. These epidemiological dynamics demonstrate the need for continued, responsive strategies specific to local environments in global tuberculosis control (Lesnic & Todoriko, 2025). Prevalence and incidence rates of tuberculosis are vastly different within the Eastern Mediterranean Regional Office (EMRO) and Middle East and North Africa (MENA) regions due to heterogeneous demographic and socioeconomic conditions.

United Arab Emirates surveillance records over 12 years show a relatively low incidence of tuberculosis, as compared to surrounding countries. Most tuberculosis in the UAE occurs among foreign nationals who are residents of high-burden countries like India, Pakistan, and the Philippines. The population structure highlights the need for accounting for migration and travel dynamics in the epidemiology of MTB. In addition, the appearance of drug-resistant tuberculosis (DR-TB) strains, such as rifampicin-resistant ones, albeit at low rates, necessitates sustained AMR surveillance and appropriate treatment regimens in this region (Thomsen et al., 2024). At the global level, MTB infection incidence reflects continued inequalities based on socioeconomic factors, healthcare setup, and population mobility, which add complexity to uniform control efforts. Significant gains have occurred in some low-burden nations, but high-burden areas remain plagued with challenges of multi-drug resistant tuberculosis (MDR-TB) and disruptions in regular care fueled by crises such as the COVID-19 pandemic. The interplay between declining prevalence in some places and rising incidence in others highlights the dynamic nature of tuberculosis epidemiology. This requires ongoing improvement in diagnostic capacity, surveillance networks, and public health responses for both latent and active tuberculosis infections. Insight into global incidence and prevalence patterns through such extensive regional analysis forms a basis for optimizing microbiological research and guiding overall tuberculosis control schemes globally (Thomsen et al., 2024; Lesnic & Todoriko, 2025) (Figure 1.11).

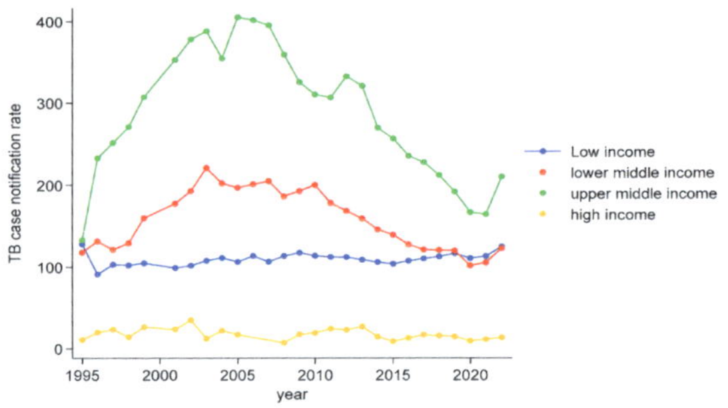

Figure 1.11. Tuberculosis (TB) epidemiology data per country: (a) TB prevalence per 1,00,000 population per year; (b) TB mortality per 1,00,000 population per year; (c) multi-drug resistant TB (MTB-TB) percentage; and (d) rifampicin-resistant TB (RR-TB).

Source: Koura KG, Harries AD. The Trend of Tuberculosis Case Notification Rates from 1995 to 2022 by Country Income and World Health Organization Region. *Tropical Medicine and Infectious Disease*. 2024; 9(12):294. https://doi.org/10.3390/tropicalmed9120294

1.4.2. Risk Factors Associated with Tuberculosis Infection

The complex interaction of social, environmental, and biological determinants has a crucial effect on the risk of MTB infection. Immunosuppression, caused by HIV/AIDS, malnutrition, or certain drugs like corticosteroids, is reported to reduce host defenses, making hosts more vulnerable to infection. Crowding, inadequate ventilation, and close housing promote airborne *Mtb* transmission, hence the role of socioeconomic determinants in disease dissemination. Furthermore, geographic areas that have poor access to healthcare tend to have increased tuberculosis incidence as a result of lower rates of diagnosis and treatment. The persistence and virulence of *Mtb* complicate these risks further, particularly in developing nations where endemic infection makes public health interventions difficult. It is imperative to recognize these complex risk factors in fighting tuberculosis worldwide and reinforce the microbiological information needed to control the pathogen (Dartois & Rubin, 2022). Antibiotic resistance amplifies the problem of tuberculosis infection, introducing an additional factor of risk at both individual and population levels. Development of multi-drug resistant (MDR) and extensively drug-resistant (XDR) tuberculosis strains arises through treatment courses that are incomplete or defective, raising the possibility of treatment failure and ongoing transmission. Since *Mtb* infects lung tissue, the ability of the bacterium to withstand inhospitable environments and resist immune killing attests to the resilience of the pathogen. New inhibitors of bacterial energy metabolism, including cytochrome bd oxidase inhibitors in conjunction with currently available drugs like Q203, are being explored to defeat drug tolerance and resistance, especially in those persistent, non-replicating subpopulations of bacteria (Lee et al., 2020). These developments highlight the importance of taking microbial biology and mechanisms of resistance into account as key risk factors when planning effective control of tuberculosis. Some physiological and demographic traits also increase tuberculosis risk, with age, comorbidities, and lifestyle being key factors. Infants, the aged, and those suffering from diabetes mellitus (DM) or chronic respiratory conditions commonly have compromised immune status facilitating easier infection establishment and disease progression. In addition, smoking and drug use are linked with lung injury and systemic immunosuppression, leading to increased susceptibility to *Mtb*. Low oxygen tension and nutritional deprivation under which the bacterium survives within granulomas make it difficult to eradication. Treatments that target these stable physiological states with new combinations of drugs against the bacterial oxidative phosphorylation pathway have the potential to significantly lower infection risk and enhance cure rates (Lee et al., 2020). Therefore, clinical and demographic risk factors need to be incorporated into the microbiological knowledge regarding *Mtb* to control effectively tuberculosis infection (Figure 1.12).

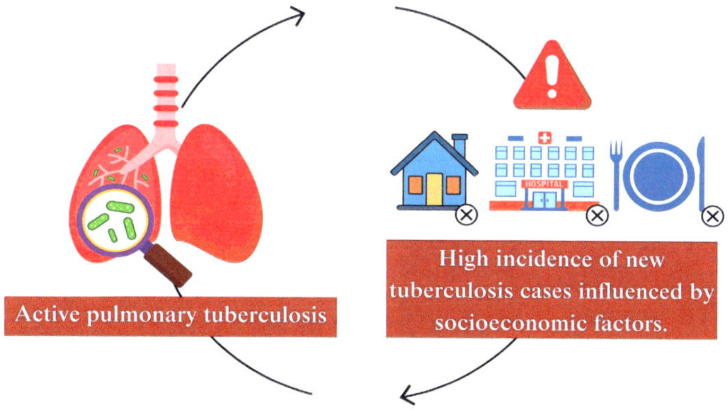

Figure 1.12. Risk factors for tuberculosis infection and disease.

Source: Mendes YC, Dourado ALL, de Oliveira PV, Rezende AdO, Sales ACdS, de Sousa GP, Pereira EdA, Sousa ELC, Lindoso MCCM, Júnior RdMR, et al. Nutritional Factors and Food and Nutrition Insecurity in Patients with Tuberculosis. *Nutrients*. 2025; 17(5):878. https://doi.org/10.3390/nu17050878

1.4.3. Impact of Socioeconomic Factors on Tuberculosis Spread

The complex interaction between infectious disease and economic conditions has had a long-standing impact on disease propagation and severity patterns. Tuberculosis (TB), which is caused by MTB, is highly influenced by conditions of poverty, crowding, and restricted access to medical care. Substandard living conditions, exemplified by poor ventilation and close living quarters among persons, provide optimal conditions for aerosol transmission of the *Bacillus*. In addition, malnutrition, commonly associated with lower socioeconomic status, compromises immune function, promoting susceptibility to infection and conversion to active disease. Such vulnerabilities are further heightened by limited access to healthcare, with delays in diagnosis and treatment, which facilitates community transmission. Microbiological properties of MTB, such as its slow rate of replication and latent infection potential, cross paths with these socioeconomic factors, further synergizing the public health burden of tuberculosis. Health system inequalities further heighten the epidemic of tuberculosis in poor communities. Inadequate provision usually means spasmodic diagnostic facilities and an insufficiency of useful drugs, which hinders early diagnosis and adherence to therapy. Discontinuity in treatment leads to the development of drug-resistant MTB strains, which are harder to treat and necessitate extended therapeutic cycles. Moreover, stigma and illiteracy about TB among vulnerable populations act as obstacles to obtaining healthcare, for facilitating hidden transmission. Such determinants of social environment emphasize the importance of dealing with TB in the context of an integrated approach consisting of enhanced socioeconomic status and effective healthcare provision. Such holistic strategies are vital to stem the microbiological persistence of MTB in high-risk groups and avert additional expansion of resistant strains in the general population (Gwenan et al., 2021). Past and present global public health efforts have proven that the development and deployment of vaccines can reduce tuberculosis incidence, yet socioeconomic obstacles continue to hamper universal coverage. The *Bacillus Calmette-Guérin* (BCG) vaccine is the sole widely applied intervention, and its variable efficacy is partially attributed to environmental and host determinants influenced by socioeconomic status. Limited access to vaccines in low-resource environments sustains inequities in TB control, underscoring the need for equitable healthcare policies. The evolution of vaccine science, guided by progress in microbiology, holds the promise of improved immunization tools. Yet, without looking at root socioeconomic disparities, such technological advance threatens to advantage only a fraction of populations. Successes in the past fighting infectious diseases using vaccines highlight the necessity of reconciling microbial biology with social determinants to stem tuberculosis worldwide (Hussein et al., 2015).

1.5. Diagnosis

Technological advancements in molecular biology have significantly revolutionized the diagnostics of MTB, overcoming centuries-old limitations based on its sluggish growth rate and complicated cell envelope. Conventional culture techniques, limited by the pathogen's doubling time of about 24 hours, tended to procrastinate timely clinical action. Nevertheless, the introduction of rapid culture systems such as BACTEC has speeded up detection, enabling quicker therapeutic choices. In addition, molecular diagnostic methods such as polymerase chain reaction (PCR) and DNA hybridization assays have increased sensitivity and specificity for detecting *Mtb* directly from clinical specimens. These molecular diagnostic methods not only enable early diagnosis but have made it possible to determine drug resistance by identifying certain mutations causing antibiotic resistance. For instance, the use of PCR-based assays with sequencing or real-time PCR has transformed resistance profiling and given a vital advantage in dealing with MDR-TB strains (Boruń-Popławska et al., 2005). The use of these molecular diagnostics is a major step in the direction of controlling tuberculosis globally. Venturing into biochemical profiling further, this has also proved to be a very valuable addendum for tuberculosis detection. Of particular interest, the mycolic acid analysis, a critical element of the mycobacterial cell wall, offers a new diagnostic option. By employing electrospray ionization tandem mass spectrometry, scientists have detected distinctive profiles of mycolic acids that distinguish *Mtb* from NTM. It exploits aimed multiple reaction monitoring of prevailing lipid species with the potential to make precise species-level identification. The clinical research has shown the diagnostic capability of this technique through rapid analysis of sputum for active tuberculosis, which presented higher sensitivity and specificity compared to traditional methods. The potential to provide results in hours, with minimal preparation of the sample or brief culture, reflects the potential for incorporating lipidomic methods into clinical diagnostics to enhance speed and efficiency (Szewczyk et al., 2013). Such developments have much potential for augmenting case detection in endemic areas. The convergence of molecular and biochemical diagnostic approaches provides an overarching strategy for addressing tuberculosis diagnosis, especially among areas weighed down by drug-resistant forms of the disease. In addition to speeding identification, these newer methods enable epidemiologic insight via strain typing and mutation mapping. This is realized in targeted research on Polish clinical isolates, where new insertion sequences and resistance-linked mutations have been enumerated, and in support of streamlined public health actions. As with the creation of assays like the DIG-PCR ELISA, these developments reinforce the trend toward approaches that are sensitive, specific, and amenable to direct testing of clinical samples. Together, these diagnostic technologies equip clinicians and microbiologists to institute timely, accurate, and efficient treatment procedures that directly influence patient outcomes and limit disease spread (Boruń-Popławska et al., 2005). Thus, the ongoing development and utilization of both genetic and cell wall-directed diagnostic methods continue to be imperative in the combat of MTB.

1.5.1. Traditional Diagnostic Methods (e.g., Tuberculin Skin Test [TST])

TB diagnosis is challenging, particularly in children where it may be difficult to obtain microbiologic confirmation. Under these conditions, the long-established diagnostic techniques, such as the tuberculin skin test (TST), are still important because of their wide availability and lack of invasiveness. The TST quantifies immune reaction to purified protein derivative (PPD) administered intradermally, which is an indirect marker of infection by MTB. Despite not being able to distinguish latent infection from active disease, its high specificity enables clinicians to safely rule out TB when the result is negative. Yet, TST sensitivity is poor, especially in immunocompromised patients and young children, causing possible false negatives. Even with these drawbacks, TST is still a mainstay of TB diagnosis in resource-poor environments, used by clinicians together with symptomatology assessment, radiographic studies, and other tests to make a clinical decision (Soto et al., 2025). It goes beyond just diagnosis; insight into the epidemiology of MTB is owed to an understanding of traditional methods placed in the practice of medicine. The TST, especially in combination with clinical symptoms and chest radiography, can increase diagnostic accuracy by giving valuable immune response information to complement epidemiological studies. This is particularly important in regions where access to sophisticated molecular diagnostics is limited. Although more recent modalities like nucleic acid amplification methods and automated culturing systems provide sensitive and accurate detection, these are resource- and infrastructure-intensive and not necessarily available universally. Thus, the persistence of the use of TST reflects its pragmatic relevance in a variety of healthcare settings. Its specificity and negative predictive value render it an economical strategy, facilitating efficient screening and early treatment, all contributing to the overall public health strategy against TB (Mohamed et al., 2024). Advances in conventional diagnostic methods have sought to improve the rapidity and accuracy of MTB detection but with the TST remaining central. Despite improvements in culture-based and molecular methods yielding quicker growth detection and sensitivity profiles in a matter of days, TSTs function cannot be replaced because of its ease of use and practicability in field conditions. Especially in pediatric diagnosis, where the symptoms can be nonspecific and microbiological confirmation infrequent, TST has been found to be clinically useful in excluding disease when used with symptom assessment and radiologic evidence. Its validity may be affected by nutritional status and age, impacting immune responsiveness and interpretation of test results. Thus, incorporating TST with detailed clinical assessments continues to hold key value for proper diagnosis and management of TB infection, reaffirming its continued relevance in MTB microbiology (Soto et al., 2025) (Figure 1.13).

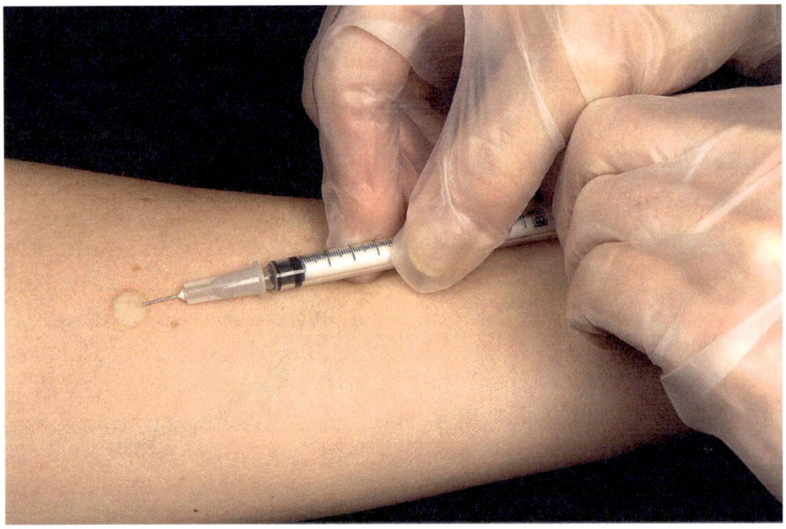

Figure 1.13. The Mantoux tuberculin skin test (TST).

Source: Wikimedia Commons. (n.d.). *Mantoux tuberculin skin test being administered.* https://upload.wikimedia.org/wikipedia/commons/thumb/f/fa/Mantoux_tuberculin_skin_test.jpg/1200px-Mantoux_tuberculin_skin_test.jpg.

1.5.2. Advanced Techniques (e.g., Molecular Diagnostics)

Advances in diagnostic techniques have greatly improved the detection and identification of MTB, transforming the microbiological paradigm. Conventional culture-based techniques, although accurate, are time-consuming and delay effective management of patients. Molecular diagnostics in this setting offer rapid, sensitive alternatives by specifically targeting genetic markers of *Mtb*. Methods like PCR and nucleic acid amplification tests (NAATs) allow the direct detection of bacterial DNA from clinical specimens without the need to go through long culture times. The methods have very important advantages, particularly in detecting latent infections and low load cases. Molecular techniques also make the characterization of drug resistance mutations possible, which directly guides treatment options. While tuberculosis remains an ongoing global public health issue, incorporating these sophisticated methods into their standard diagnostics is vital for early intervention and prevention of disease transmission. Molecular diagnostics of tuberculosis microbiology has a promising potential application in mycolic acid analysis, which are distinctive cell wall components of the mycobacterial cell. With electrospray ionization tandem mass spectrometry, scientists can quickly profile such long-chain fatty acids to differentiate *Mtb* from nontuberculous mycobacterial species. This method, which involves the combination of targeted multiple reaction monitoring with liquid chromatography, provides rigorous species-specific profiles after hours of sample preparation or following brief culture times. The sensitivity and specificity of this method are higher than most traditional methods, allowing for early and specific diagnosis. Such developments not only enhance laboratory confirmation but also show potential for utility in clinical practice by decreasing diagnostic turnaround times. The ability to consistently differentiate species on the basis of mycolic acid signatures adds strength to epidemiological surveillance and facilitates individualized patient management programs (Szewczyk et al., 2013). Nevertheless, despite such advances, there are overwhelming challenges to tuberculosis diagnostics in developing effective point-of-care tests that are rapid, cost-effective, and feasible in resource-constrained settings. Existing gold-standard tests require sophisticated laboratory facilities, delaying diagnosis and treatment onset. Inadequate precise, quick diagnostics constrain measures to control transmission, particularly in high-transmission communities. New advances involve new biomarker identification and molecular tests for detecting latent infections and drug-resistant strains. Yet the technical and operational complexity of these tests delays their universal adoption. Continuous political will, investment in healthcare infrastructure, and continuous research are crucial to bridge these molecular advances into practice. Integrated strategies in diagnostic accuracy, affordability, and accessibility alone can make global tuberculosis control a success (McNerney et al., 2012) (Figure 1.14).

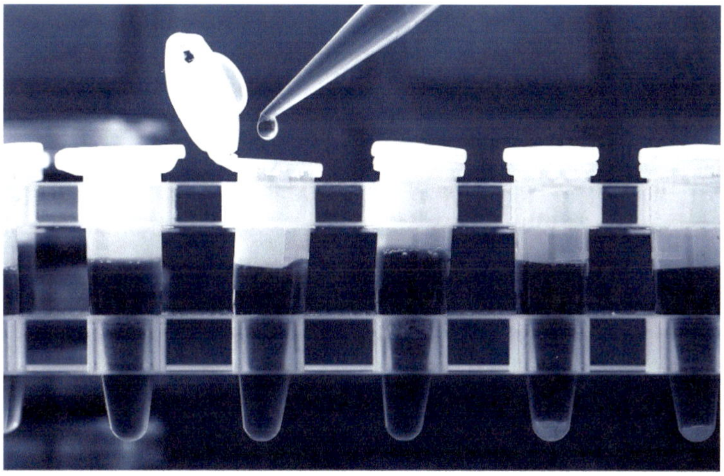

Figure 1.14. A simple blood-based PCR test can predict the progression of tuberculosis.

Source: Infectious Disease Advisor. (n.d.). *PCR test process involving pipetting into sample tubes in a laboratory setting.* https://www.infectiousdiseaseadvisor.com/wp-content/uploads/sites/16/2019/01/pcrtestg639553007_1432490.jpg.

1.5.3. Challenges in Accurate Diagnosis

Correct diagnosis of MTB is still a major challenge in tuberculosis control, particularly in areas with scarce healthcare resources. The microbiological complexity of *Mtb*, coupled with its slow rate of growth, most often results in delayed detection and diagnosis. The existence of coinfections, especially with human immunodeficiency virus (HIV), further complicates diagnosis. HIV-associated immunosuppression veils the characteristic clinical presentation of tuberculosis, leading to unusual manifestations that make it difficult to diagnose active disease. This interaction not only is detrimental to prompt diagnosis but also increases the risk of treatment failure by leading to the wrong therapeutic choices through diagnostic errors. It is imperative to comprehend these interacting pathogen-host processes for enhancing diagnostic methods and in turn designing efficient interventions for the affected individuals (Rangaraj et al., 2025). To differentiate MTB from NTM species is another important challenge in the correct diagnosis of tuberculosis. As the phenotypes are similar and their clinical symptoms overlap, standard diagnosis methods are usually unable to accurately differentiate the two mycobacterial infections. This differentiation is important because treatment strategies for MTBC and NTM infections are quite different. Molecular diagnostic devices, including PCR-based tests, also possess greater sensitivity and specificity but are still hampered by some limitations in specific clinical conditions. As an example, the performance difference between commercially provided PCR kits in detecting NTM versus MTBC underscores the need for ongoing testing and validation of the diagnostic platforms, especially under high-burden, low-resource settings (Castro-Rodr et al., 2024). The diagnostic challenges are also exacerbated by comorbidities and drug interactions that muddy the microbial picture. Illnesses like DM and immune reconstitution inflammatory syndrome (IRIS), which are often encountered in cases of MTB–HIV coinfection, may be modulating host immunity and disrupting the diagnostic markers. Also, combined toxicities due to simultaneous anti-TB and antiretroviral treatment may stimulate cytotoxic activities, which hinder clinical evidence. Therefore, an integrated approach, incorporating molecular diagnostics with exhaustive knowledge of immunological dynamics and pathogen interactions, is essential. Meeting these challenges calls for innovation in diagnostic approaches that can handle the complexity of comorbidities and coinfections to facilitate more accurate and timely identification of *Mtb* infections (Rangaraj et al., 2025).

1.6. Treatment and Management

Treating MTB infections requires a coordinated effort based on precise diagnosis, successful antimicrobial therapy, and monitoring of patients. Diagnostic technologies that are rapid and specific have profoundly impacted therapeutic approaches, with molecular tests like the CSF-Truenat allowing for rapid detection in severe forms of tuberculosis such as tubercular meningitis. The value of such assays is that they can minimize diagnostic delays and thus facilitate timely initiation of therapy, which has the potential to decrease morbidity and mortality. No test, however, is adequate; microbiological confirmation of the bacilli frequently proves difficult; hence, clinical acumen together with radiological and laboratory data continues to be the basis of informed decisions. The diagnostic sensitivity and specificity of Truenat, with its positive values, characterize its use in therapy guidance and cost-effectiveness, describing how improvements in microbiological methods reflect directly on therapy results in tuberculosis control (Nanda et al., 2024). Treatment protocols for MTB are complicated and should be individualized to the site, severity, and drug susceptibility patterns of the infection. Conventional antitubercular therapy (ATT) is generally a combination of drugs for prolonged periods to avoid resistance and induce sterilization. For tuberculosis of the spine, or tuberculous spondylitis, treatment includes antimicrobial therapy in accordance with pathogen identification and susceptibility testing, often supplemented with immobilization in an attempt to minimize spinal complications. With the potential for neurological deterioration and deformity, timely detection using magnetic resonance imaging (MRI) and accurate microbiological assessment, including biopsy where appropriate, maximizes therapeutic decision. Advanced cases with complicating factors such as abscess formation, instability, or neurological compromise are treated with surgery, demonstrating the subtle balance between medical management and surgery in the overall treatment of EPTB manifestations (Park, 2024). Treatment adherence and follow-up over the long term are essential challenges in tuberculosis control because of the ability of the pathogen to persist and cause relapse or resistance development. Regular close clinical monitoring facilitates early identification of failure of treatment and adverse drug reactions (ADRs), which can affect continuation of therapy and outcome in patients. Additionally, tuberculosis burden is increased in those who are immunocompromised and elderly, where management must be tailored to their comorbidities and drug interactions. On-going clinical research continues to explore new diagnostic methods, reduced therapy regimens, and HDTs to improve treatment efficacy and compliance. In total, the multifaceted method combining cutting-edge microbiological diagnostics, suitable pharmacological treatment, and close clinical observation reflects the complexity of treating MTB infections and the demand for ongoing innovation in this field (Nanda et al., 2024; Park, 2024) (Figure 1.15).

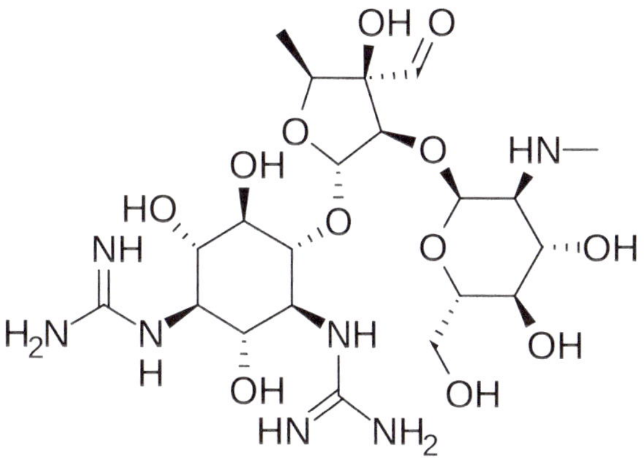

Figure 1.15. Treatment of tuberculosis.

Source: By User:Innerstream - Own work, Public Domain, https://commons.wikimedia.org/w/index.php?curid=155616907

1.6.1. Standard Treatment Regimens for Tuberculosis

Treating tuberculosis (TB) is largely based on standardized antibiotic regimens that have been optimized over several decades of clinical trials. The treatment regimens are formulated to achieve effectiveness while avoiding drug resistance and relapse of the disease. The initial treatment typically consists of a mixture of several drugs for two months, that is, isoniazid, rifampin, pyrazinamide (PZA), and ethambutol. This intense phase is designed to quickly decrease bacterial numbers and limit transmission, in both infective and resting populations of MTB. The subsequent four-month continuation phase uses isoniazid and rifampin to clear the lingering bacteria. This bifurcated regimen not only maximizes treatment success but also reduces the risk of MDR-TB strain development. These regimens highlight the multifaceted microbiological issues presented by *Mtb*, which requires prolonged and multidrug therapy to counteract the pathogen's distinctive cellular and metabolic protective mechanisms (Tzelios et al., 2022). Tailoring standard ATT is critical in the clinical arena owing to disease presentation variability and host immune response variability. Female genital tuberculosis, as a case in point, is a diagnostic challenge because it is indolent and in its paucibacillary state of infection, is only revealed following evaluation for infertility. Despite these challenges, the recommended therapy is concordant with the standard regimen, highlighting the importance of a two-month intensive phase and four-month continuation phase. Initiating treatment early is essential for avoiding irreversible organ damage and favorable clinical outcomes. In addition, treatment adherence is critical to avoid relapse or advancement of the disease, particularly in types of TB that involve extrapulmonary locations. This is reason enough to determine the microbiological dynamics of *Mtb* in various tissues to maximize therapy and counter the dramatic health and social consequences of the disease (Tzelios et al., 2022).

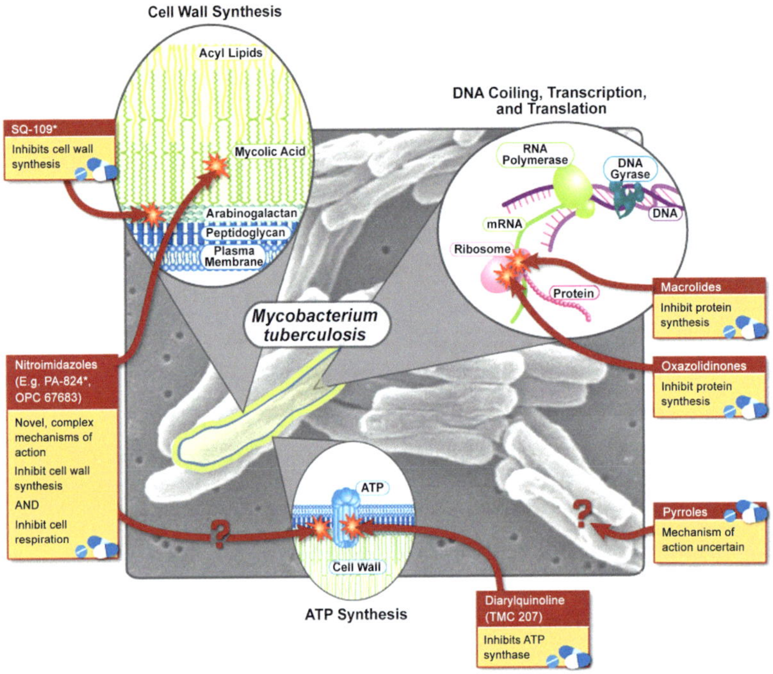

Figure 1.16. Several new types of TB drugs currently under development are shown here, along with their mechanisms of action.

Source: Wikipedia. (n.d.). *Mechanisms of action of tuberculosis drugs targeting Mycobacterium tuberculosis: Cell wall synthesis, protein synthesis, ATP synthesis, and DNA processes.* https://en.wikipedia.org/wiki/Management_of_tuberculosis#/media/File:Tuberculosis-drugs-and-actions.jpg.

Continued investigation of rifamycin antibiotics is an indication of attempts to improve the effectiveness of tuberculosis therapy and minimize regimen length. Although rifampin is still a mainstay of TB therapy, investigations into other rifamycins, like rifapentine, indicate dose-related enhancement of clinical and microbiologic outcomes without therapeutic ceiling achievement at increased dosage. While these results are extrapolated from highly related mycobacterial infections such as Buruli ulcer, similarly needing extended antimicrobial courses, they provide insights into possible improvement in TB treatment. Increased rifamycin effectiveness and optimal dosing schemes will enable shorter and less painful treatment regimens in the future, overcoming hurdles of adherence and cost of healthcare. Such pharmacological interventions are essential to the management of TB, especially in resource-constrained settings where long-duration treatment is a major challenge (Figure 1.16).

1.6.2. Issues of Drug Resistance and Its Implications

The development of drug resistance in MTB populations poses major challenges to tuberculosis control at the global level. Mutations related to resistance to first-line agents such as isoniazid have been recognized as key initial events during the evolution of multi-drug resistant strains. WGS-based studies have shown that isoniazid resistance tends to be followed by rifampin resistance, which points out its central role in the sequential process of developing more advanced forms of drug resistance. Despite molecular diagnostic progress, isoniazid monoresistance detection is still complex in nature owing to the variably mutated genes. This makes early correct detection and consequent effective treatments regimes impossible, leading to worse patient outcomes and additional resistance mechanisms. Additionally, whereas regular treatment of isoniazid-monoresistant tuberculosis can deliver comparable success to drug-susceptible tuberculosis under ideal circumstances, heterogeneity in resource-poor environments continues to increase treatment failure rates, highlighting ongoing clinical management gaps (O'Donnell, 2018). Concurrent with pressure caused by drug-resistant mutations, the limited nature of therapeutic interventions for addressing resistant strains builds on public health alarms. The emergence of XDR and completely drug-resistant MTB strains has threatened the effectiveness of traditional antitubercular regimens. While new drugs like bedaquiline, delamanid, and newer fluoroquinolones have increased the therapeutic armamentarium, their introduction into standard regimens is limited until clinical endorsement. Significantly, the threat of resistance to such newer drugs continues to offer a potential for perpetuation of the cycle of ineffective treatment and strain evolution. This situation underlines the imperative for prompt and conclusive diagnostic tools to customize treatment and stem resistance spread. Recent developments in molecular diagnostics—from liquid culture automation to NAATs such as the Xpert MTB/RIF assay—are promising for rapid drug susceptibility testing (DST), essential for starting effective regimens in cases of resistant tuberculosis (Chakravorty et al., 2012).

The consequences of drug resistance in MTB are not limited to individual patient outcomes but have far-reaching implications for public health strategies and resource allocation. The endurance of drug-resistant strains hinders efforts toward tuberculosis eradication because treatment failures enhance the chances of transmission of more virulent, drug-resistant organisms. Delayed diagnosis and inadequate DST in healthcare facilities that are limited in resources exacerbate disease control and sustain cycles of infection in resource-limited countries. Diagnostic innovations, such as new PCR-based assays and immunodiagnostic tests like interferon-gamma release assays (IGRAs), hold promise for improved sensitivity and specificity of tuberculosis diagnosis, especially in extrapulmonary and conditions with low bacillary load. However, successful drug resistance management depends on concerted efforts to integrate molecular diagnostics with maximized treatment strategies and efficient surveillance systems to avert resistance escalation and enhance global health outcomes (Chakravorty et al., 2012).

1.6.3. Public Health Strategies for Tuberculosis Control

Control of tuberculosis (TB) on the public health level requires multi-faceted approaches that go beyond mere clinical interventions. With the advanced microbiology of MTB, successful control strategies need to incorporate diagnostic innovations as well as specific therapeutics to stem transmission and enhance treatment outcomes. Early detection of cases, aided by molecular diagnostic technologies with the ability to discriminate among subspecies within the MTBC, is critical. This is particularly imperative in areas where zoonotic strains, e.g., *Mycobacterium orygis*, are responsible for bovine tuberculosis and potentially have risks of infecting humans, thus making epidemiological patterns complicated (Maqsood et al., 2024). Strong surveillance systems with molecular typing can allow for the correct identification of *Mtb* strains, allowing for specific public health responses. Furthermore, public health programs need to tackle the problem of latent and subclinical infection by using community screening and preventative treatment, so that latent reservoirs cannot continue to fuel the active disease cycle. Appearance and dissemination of multi-drug resistant (MDR) and XDR tuberculosis strains pose important challenges for TB control programs globally. Public health measures thus need to incorporate the creation and deployment of new drugs targeting vital bacterial processes, particularly those that augment bactericidal activity against both growing and resting forms of *Mtb*. Recent development in targeting the bioenergetic machinery of the pathogen is a prime example of this strategy, whereby dual inhibition of the cytochrome *bcc:aa3* and cytochrome bd terminal oxidases shows improved potency in eliminating antibiotic-tolerant mycobacteria (Lee et al., 2020). Incorporation of these novel drugs into drug regimens has the potential to dramatically decrease therapy duration as well as decrease resistance emergence. At the same time, public health infrastructure needs to prioritize adherence support, DST, and treatment monitoring so that gains from these advances are followed by measurable reductions in TB incidence and mortality. Most importantly, any effective public health approach to tuberculosis control needs to take a comprehensive framework that looks at socio-economic determinants as much as microbiological challenges. TB targets disproportionately vulnerable populations with poor access to health care and is worsened by conditions like malnutrition, crowding, and co-infection with HIV. The control programs thus require integrating medical interventions with community-based interventions aimed at better living conditions, education, and nutrition. In addition, zoonotic transmission routes discovered in places where livestock are reservoirs underscore the significance of One Health strategies that incorporate human, animal, and environmental health interventions (Maqsood et al., 2024). Multifaceted efforts to break transmission at varied ecological levels, backed by molecular epidemiology and emerging pharmacotherapy like that outlined in front-running drug candidates (Lee et al., 2020), portend a holistic and responsive model for TB burden minimization on a global scale.

Summary

The complex genetic heterogeneity of MTB has a vital function in its epidemiology and pathogenicity. Research with molecular methods like the multiple-locus variable number tandem repeat analysis (MLVA-VNTR) has demonstrated extensive heterogeneity among clinical isolates, particularly in heterogeneous populations. Such genetic heterogeneity highlights the complexities of controlling tuberculosis, since differences may impact transmission dynamics, virulence, and treatment response. The absence of clustering among tested isolates indicates a wide dispersion of unique strains instead of outbreaks restricted to particular areas, and this underscores the need for regional surveillance and specific public health interventions. The evidence underscores that molecular epidemiology is important in the management of tuberculosis to monitor sources and progression of infection, eventually informing targeted containment and prevention strategies (Farnad et al., 2021). Lab diagnostic advancements have also played a key role in enhancing the detection and control of tuberculosis. The combination of microscopic examination of cord formation and use of mycobacteria growth indicator tube (MGIT) cultures is very sensitive and specific for presumptive identification of the MTBC. This can permit quick distinction between tuberculous and NTM, thus allowing for prompt DST, which is essential for managing proper treatment regimens. Increased diagnostic precision helps to improve clinical outcomes and minimizes laboratory workload through simplified workflows and reduced turnaround times, thus directly influencing patient care and resource utilization (Pinhata et al., 2018). These innovations buttress the necessity of incorporating sophisticated microbiological techniques in routine tuberculosis programs. In conclusion, microbiological research on MTB clarifies both the strain-level genetic diversity of the organism and the need to accurately diagnose it. Capitalizing on the molecular genotyping methods coupled with enhanced culture-based technology allows us to better understand tuberculosis transmission dynamics and enable more rapid and accurate identification. This multi-pronged microbiological strategy is crucial for public health intervention refinement and patient management strategies. Future work must remain directed toward the development of regional genetic surveillance information and the application of rapid diagnostic procedures globally. Ultimately, the transition of microbiological science to clinical practice is imperative to enhance tuberculosis control and global health outcomes. The convergence of these views is the basis for future innovation in the fight against this chronic infectious disease (Pinhata et al., 2018; Farnad et al., 2021).

The MTB biology is highly complex and significantly determines its pathogenicity as well as the difficulties in treating tuberculosis. At the center of this complexity is the bacterium's capacity to remain in a nonreplicating, persistent phenotype inside host tissues, which renders it highly resistant to standard antibiotics. This persistence, or persister-like phenotype, enables the bacterium to survive various stresses such as immune reactions and pharmacological treatment. Recognizing these resistant subpopulations from clinical specimens like sputum points to the challenge of eliminating the infection and the need for novel therapeutic modalities aimed at both actively growing and latent bacilli (Garton et al., 2008). Elucidation of this process enhances understanding of the chronicity of tuberculosis and accounts for the lengthy treatment periods. Additional complexities arise from the spatial heterogeneity found within tuberculosis lesions, where MTB is present in varied microenvironments influenced by the host immune response. These granulomatous formations contain various types of immune cells, such as macrophages and foamy macrophages, that create niches conducive to the long-term survival of bacteria.

Studies that have applied sophisticated imaging methods have shown that the distribution and penetration of antibiotics within these lesions are extremely variable and dependent on conditions like macrophage density, the presence of necrotic tissue, and distance from lesion edges (Blanc et al., 2018). Such results highlight the critical role of microenvironmental context in drug delivery and action, underscoring the necessity for pharmacologic strategies aimed at the heterogeneous localization of the pathogen in infected lung tissue. In conclusion, the microbiology of MTB is multifaceted, with challenges arising from its mechanisms of persistence and heterogeneity of lesions. The bacterium's capacity to enter a drug-tolerant, latent state makes treatment regimens more complex, with longer antibiotic regimens and new drug designs aimed at these recalcitrant populations. At the same time, tuberculosis lesions' immune pathology is multifaceted and affects drug distribution, and a deeper understanding of lesion microenvironments is needed to maximize therapeutic interventions (Garton et al., 2008; Blanc et al., 2018). Collectively, these are important in moving forward the management of tuberculosis and highlight the necessity of ongoing research that combines microbial biology with pharmacology and immunopathology to better address current treatment shortfalls.

CLOSER LOOK

WHOLE-GENOME SEQUENCING (WGS)

WGS has become an effective tool against tuberculosis (TB), a bacterial infection caused by MTB. WGS enables the entire genomic analysis of the bacterium, which gives complete information regarding the genetic constitution of the pathogen. In contrast to conventional testing that can take weeks and provide limited information, WGS gives high-resolution data within days, allowing accurate drug resistance mutation identification, transmission patterns, and strain typing.

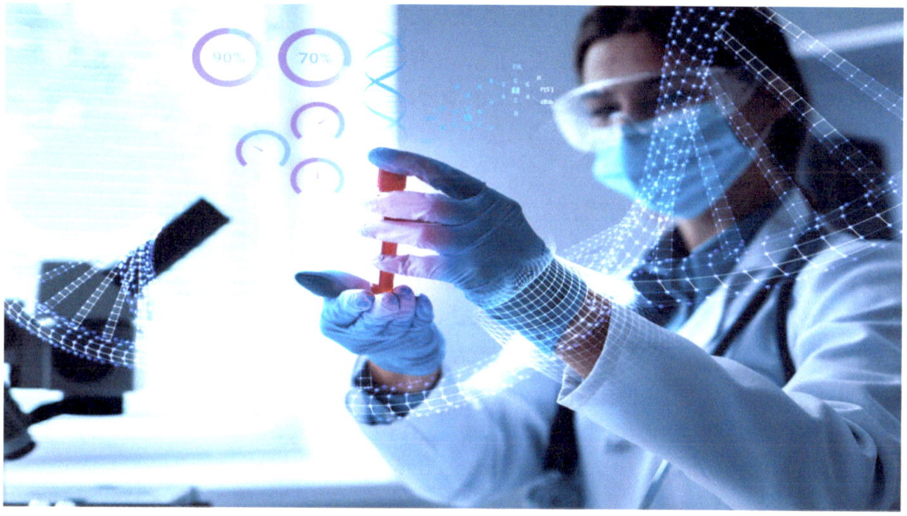

Source: BioSpectrum India. (n.d.). *Scientist analyzing test samples in a laboratory using advanced genomic data visualization.* https://www.biospectrumindia.com/uploads/articles/wgs-24408.jpeg.

One of the most important uses of WGS in TB treatment is identifying drug-resistant strains at a rapid rate. Through detecting resistance-associated mutations to first- and second-line anti-TB medications, WGS informs clinicians on how to choose effective treatments, which is vital in the management of MDR-TB and XDR-TB. The genomic method improves patient outcomes and assists in preventing the transmission of resistant strains.

In public health, WGS facilitates the comprehension of transmission chains and outbreak investigations. WGS is able to separate reactivation of latent infections from new transmissions, allowing epidemiologists to monitor and control TB outbreaks more effectively. WGS also underpins global surveillance by facilitating cross-border comparisons of TB strains, helping to inform the global effort against TB.

Though there are challenges to implementing WGS in low-resource environments, including cost, infrastructure, and technical expertise, continuous developments are making the technology more feasible. Handheld sequencers and streamlined bioinformatics pipelines are making it easier to include WGS in standard TB control programs.

References

1. Gorna, A. E., Bowater, R. P., & Dziadek, J. (2010). DNA repair systems and the pathogenesis of Mycobacterium tuberculosis: varying activities at different stages of infection. *Clinical science (London, England : 1979)*, *119*(5), 187–202. https://doi.org/10.1042/CS20100041 (accessed on 10 May 2025).

2. Birch, H. L., Alderwick, L. J., Bhatt, A., Rittmann, D., Krumbach, K., Singh, A., Bai, Y., Lowary, T. L., Eggeling, L., & Besra, G. S. (2008). Biosynthesis of mycobacterial arabinogalactan: identification of a novel alpha(1-->3) arabinofuranosyltransferase. *Molecular microbiology*, *69*(5), 1191–1206. https://doi.org/10.1111/j.1365-2958.2008.06354.x

3. Alipoor, S. D., & Elieh-Ali-Komi, D. (2024). Significance of extracellular vesicles in orchestration of immune responses in *Mycobacterium tuberculosis* infection. *Frontiers in cellular and infection microbiology*, *14*, 1398077. https://doi.org/10.3389/fcimb.2024.1398077(accessed on 10 May 2025).

4. Garton, N. J., Waddell, S. J., Sherratt, A. L., Lee, S. M., Smith, R. J., Senner, C., Hinds, J., Rajakumar, K., Adegbola, R. A., Besra, G. S., Butcher, P. D., & Barer, M. R. (2008). Cytological and transcript analyses reveal fat and lazy persister-like bacilli in tuberculous sputum. *PLoS medicine*, *5*(4), e75. https://doi.org/10.1371/journal.pmed.0050075

5. Arbab Nasr, M. H., Hasan, A. N., Alnour, T. M. S., & Ahmed, E. H. (2024). Evaluation of newly modified potassium nitrate containing media in detection and antibiogram of *Mycobacterium tuberculosis*. *SVOA Microbiology*. https://www.semanticscholar.org/paper/74ce515657be3e8968cc935b2b8453af8fe50ef4 (accessed on 10 May 2025).

6. Aslam, B., Wang, W., Arshad, M., Khurshid, M., Muzammil, S., Rasool, M. H., Nisar, M. A., et al. (2018). Antibiotic resistance: A rundown of a global crisis. *Infection and Drug Resistance, 11*, 1645–1658. https://doi.org/10.2147/idr.s173867.

7. Roberts, A. W., Popov, L. M., Mitchell, G., Ching, K. L., Licht, D. J., Golovkine, G., Barton, G. M., & Cox, J. S. (2019). Cas9[+] conditionally-immortalized macrophages as a tool for bacterial pathogenesis and beyond. *eLife*, *8*, e45957. https://doi.org/10.7554/eLife.45957

8. Blanc, L., Daudelin, I. B., Podell, B. K., Chen, P. Y., Zimmerman, M., Martinot, A. J., Savic, R. M., Prideaux, B., & Dartois, V. (2018). High-resolution mapping of fluoroquinolones in TB rabbit lesions reveals specific distribution in immune cell types. *eLife*, *7*, e41115. https://doi.org/10.7554/eLife.41115Bortolaia, V., Kaas, R. S., Ruppé, É., Roberts, M. C., Schwarz, Š., Cattoir, V., Philippon, A., et al. (2020). ResFinder 4.0 for predictions of phenotypes from genotypes. *Journal of Antimicrobial Chemotherapy, 75*, 3491–3500. https://doi.org/10.1093/jac/dkaa345.

9. Boruń-Popławska, M., Brzostek, A., Dziadek, J., & Sajduda, A. (2005). *Mycobacterium tuberculosis*– The 10 years of epidemiological and diagnostics studies. Folia Biologica et Oecologica 2: 17-34 (Acta Univ. Lodz., Folia Biol. Oecol.) https://core.ac.uk/download/71981248.pdf (accessed on 10 May 2025).

10. Butler, R. E., Smith, A. A., Mendum, T., Chandran, A., Wu, H., Lefrançois, L. H., Soldati, T., et al. (2019). The great escape: Dissecting the interactions between *Mycobacterium bovis* and the soil amoeba *Dictyostelium discoideum*. *Access Microbiology*. Volume 1. Issue 1;

https://doi.org/10.1099/acmi.ac2019.po0260. https://www.semanticscholar.org/paper/dcdbf63c1d7eed6cbb3a070de379ec35c5ad945c (accessed on 10 May 2025).

11. Curry, J. M., Whalan, R., Hunt, D. M., Gohil, K., Strom, M., Rickman, L., Colston, M. J., Smerdon, S. J., & Buxton, R. S. (2005). An ABC transporter containing a forkhead-associated domain interacts with a serine-threonine protein kinase and is required for growth of Mycobacterium tuberculosis in mice. *Infection and immunity*, *73*(8), 4471–4477. https://doi.org/10.1128/IAI.73.8.4471-4477.2005(accessed on 10 May 2025).
12. Castro-Rodríguez, B., Franco-Sotomayor, G., Rodriguez-Pazmiño, Á. S., Cardenas-Franco, G., Orlando, S., Hermoso de Mendoza, J., Parra-Vera, H., et al. (2024). Rapid and accurate identification and differentiation of *Mycobacterium tuberculosis* and non-tuberculous mycobacteria using PCR kits available in a high-burden setting. *Frontiers in Public Health, 12.* https://www.semanticscholar.org/paper/b3bca9d27c524490d251962f4a6a84138be3870c (accessed on 10 May 2025).
13. Kidenya BR, Kabangila R, Peck RN, Mshana SE, Webster LE, Koenig SP, et al. (2013) Early and Efficient Detection of *Mycobacterium tuberculosis* in Sputum by Microscopic Observation of Broth Cultures. PLoS ONE 8(2): e57527. https://doi.org/10.1371/journal.pone.0057527 (accessed on 10 May 2025).
14. Widhyasih, R. M., Hanifah, A. H., Chairlan, C., & Inderiati, D. (2019). Detection of Mycobacterium tuberculosis by Microscopic Technique of Sputum AFB and ICT (Cocktail Antigen) TB. *Medical Laboratory Technology Journal*, *5*(2), 124–130. https://doi.org/10.31964/mltj.v5i2.246 (accessed on 10 May 2025).
15. Chakravorty, Soumitesh, Boehme, Catharina, Lee, Jongseok, Tuberculosis Diagnostics in the New Millennium: Role in TB Identification and Control, *Tuberculosis Research and Treatment*, 2012, 768603, 2 pages, 2012. **https://doi.org/10.1155/2012/768603** (accessed on 10 May 2025).
16. Clerc, O., Prod'Hom, G., Greub, G., Zanetti, G., & Senn, L. (2011). Adult native septic arthritis: A review of 10 years of experience and lessons for empirical antibiotic therapy. *The Journal of Antimicrobial Chemotherapy, 66*(5), 1168–1173. https://www.semanticscholar.org/paper/973b3a35edfc0dae160a78f8decf88808c68e72a (accessed on 10 May 2025).
17. Drain, P. K., Bajema, K. L., Dowdy, D. W., Dheda, K., Naidoo, K., Schumacher, S. G., Ma, S., et al. (2018). Incipient and subclinical tuberculosis: A clinical review of early stages and progression of infection. *Clinical Microbiology Reviews, 31*. https://doi.org/10.1128/cmr.00021-18.
18. Ekosputri, A. J., Ardianti, A., Anggreainy, M. S., Artanto, B., Fitriawati, N., Valentina, F. A., & Santoso, V. K. (2024). *Random Forest Based QSAR Model Analysis for Predicting Drug Effectiveness Against Mycobacterium Tuberculosis Bacteria*. 1–5. https://doi.org/10.1109/iciss62896.2024.10750957(accessed on 10 May 2025).
19. Englund, S. (2002). Molecular biology techniques as a tool for detection and characterisation of *Mycobacterium avium* subsp. *paratuberculosis*. Acta Universitatis Agriculturae Sueciae. Veterinaria 2002, number: 123. Publisher: Swedish University of Agricultural Sciences. ISBN: 91-576-6366-1. https://core.ac.uk/download/11694594.pdf (accessed on 10 May 2025).
20. Farnad, M., Momtaz, H., Mosavari, N., Khosravi, Y., & Tadayon, K. (2021). Insight into population structure of *Mycobacterium tuberculosis* isolates in the multiethnic province of Alborz, Iran. *Iranian Journal of Microbiology, 13*, 58–64. https://www.semanticscholar.org/paper/18f6fab8665d382c0fa5c4ccbef90f2c759f97fe (accessed on 10 May 2025).

21. Gillen, Alan L.; Oliver, Douglas; and Sherwin, Frank, "Robert Koch, Creation, and the Specificity of Germs" (2010). *Faculty Publications and Presentations*. 140. https://digitalcommons.liberty.edu/bio_chem_fac_pubs/140 (accessed on 7 May 2025).
22. Gupta, S., & Gupta, V. (2022). Unveiling the structural features of CysE: A novel target for therapeutic interventions against persistent mycobacteria. Unveiling the structural features of CysE: a novel target for therapeutic interventions against persistent mycobacteria. (2022). *Journal of Applied and Natural Science, 14*(2), 531-542. https://doi.org/10.31018/jans.v14i2.3461 https://core.ac.uk/download/534912584.pdf (accessed on 10 May 2025).
23. Hajj Hussein, I., Chams, N., Chams, S., El Sayegh, S., Badran, R., Raad, M., Gerges-Geagea, A., et al. (2015). Vaccines through centuries: Major cornerstones of global health. *Frontiers in Public Health, 3*. https://doi.org/10.3389/fpubh.2015.00269.
24. McNerney, R., Maeurer, M., Abubakar, I., Marais, B., McHugh, T. D., Ford, N., Weyer, K., Lawn, S., Grobusch, M. P., Memish, Z., Squire, S. B., Pantaleo, G., Chakaya, J., Casenghi, M., Migliori, G. B., Mwaba, P., Zijenah, L., Hoelscher, M., Cox, H., Swaminathan, S., ... Zumla, A. (2012). Tuberculosis diagnostics and biomarkers: needs, challenges, recent advances, and opportunities. *The Journal of infectious diseases, 205 Suppl 2*, S147–S158. https://doi.org/10.1093/infdis/jir860 (accessed on 10 May 2025).
25. Hotha, S., Joshi, P., & Srinidhi, V. (2025). Synthesis of glycolipid library reminiscent of mycobacterial cell wall motif A and its significance by microscopy. *Angewandte Chemise*. https://www.semanticscholar.org/paper/620c3e990fa75bcb68689d0a377159865a8f83d0 (accessed on 10 May 2025).
26. Huang, Y., Zhu, C., Pan, L., & Zhang, Z. (2023). The role of *Mycobacterium tuberculosis* acetyltransferase and protein acetylation modifications in tuberculosis. *Frontiers in Cellular and Infection Microbiology, 13*. https://www.semanticscholar.org/paper/233f98d2bc6556b590d5c4faf9f4dbe4ea6822c6 (accessed on 10 May 2025).
27. Szewczyk, R., Kowalski, K., Janiszewska-Drobinska, B., & Druszczyńska, M. (2013). Rapid method for Mycobacterium tuberculosis identification using electrospray ionization tandem mass spectrometry analysis of mycolic acids. *Diagnostic microbiology and infectious disease, 76*(3), 298–305. https://doi.org/10.1016/j.diagmicrobio.2013.03.025 (accessed on 10 May 2025).
28. Khalifa, E., & Torky, H. (2012). *Trichoderma pseudokoningii* Rifai isolation from Egyptian immunocompromised cattle with *Mycobacterium bovis* infection. https://core.ac.uk/download/pdf/1569929.pdf (accessed on 10 May 2025).
29. Knight, G. M., Glover, R. E., McQuaid, C. F., Olaru, I. D., Gallandat, K., Leclerc, Q. J., Fuller, N. M., et al. (2021). Antimicrobial resistance and COVID-19: Intersections and implications. *eLife, 10*. https://doi.org/10.7554/elife.64139.
30. Lee, B. S., Hards, K., Engelhart, C. A., Hasenoehrl, E. J., Kalia, N. P., Mackenzie, J. S., Sviriaeva, E., et al. (2020). Dual inhibition of the terminal oxidases eradicates antibiotic-tolerant *Mycobacterium tuberculosis. EMBO Molecular Medicine, 13*. https://doi.org/10.15252/emmm.202013207.
31. Lesnic, E., & Todoriko, L. (2025). Dynamics of the epidemiological indicators of tuberculosis in the Republic of Moldova during different periods and during the COVID-19 epidemics. *Infusion & Chemotherapy*. https://www.semanticscholar.org/paper/44f3ed223f097e123f9fcafa0a4fbebb438aef16 (accessed on 10 May 2025).
32. Maqsood, R., Duffy, S. C., Rashid, H. B., Gill, S. S., Jabeen, C., Arshad, N., Umbreen, G., et al.

(2024). Molecular detection and characterization of the *Mycobacterium tuberculosis* complex subspecies responsible for bovine tuberculosis in Punjab, Pakistan. *Microbiology Spectrum, 12.* https://doi.org/10.1128/spectrum.02692-23.

33. Meier-Kolthoff, J. P., & Göker, M. (2019). TYGS is an automated high-throughput platform for state-of-the-art genome-based taxonomy. *Nature Communications, 10.* https://doi.org/10.1038/s41467-019-10210-3.

34. Mukhtar, F., Guarnieri, A., Brancazio, N., Falcone, M., Di Naro, M., Azeem, M., Zubair, M., Nicolosi, D., Di Marco, R., & Petronio Petronio, G. (2024). The role of *Mycobacterium tuberculosis* exosomal miRNAs in host pathogen cross-talk as diagnostic and therapeutic biomarkers. *Frontiers in microbiology, 15,* 1441781. https://doi.org/10.3389/fmicb.2024.1441781 (accessed on 10 May 2025).

35. Murray, C. J. L., Ikuta, K. S., Sharara, F., Swetschinski, L. R., Robles Aguilar, G., Gray, A. P., Han, C., et al. (2022). Global burden of bacterial antimicrobial resistance in 2019: A systematic analysis. *The Lancet, 399*, 629–655. https://doi.org/10.1016/s0140-6736(21)02724-0.

36. Nanda, S., Bansal, M. K., Singh, P., Shrivastav, A. K., Malav, M. K., & Prakash, C. (2024). Evaluation of the cerebrospinal fluid (CSF)-Truenat assay: A novel chip-based test in the diagnosis and management of tubercular meningitis at a tertiary care hospital. *Cures, 16.* https://www.semanticscholar.org/paper/3857c3272a09ffbf8c554456851f11106963749f (accessed on 10 May 2025).

37. O'Donnell, M. (2018). Isoniazid monoresistance: A precursor to multidrug-resistant tuberculosis? *Annals of the American Thoracic Society, 15*(3), 306–307. https://www.semanticscholar.org/paper/1b346651c5db66674f8d26a5d5ec58a214828baa (accessed on 10 May 2025).

38. Omansen, T. F., Almeida, D. V., Converse, P. J., Li, S. Y., Lee, J., Stienstra, Y., van der Werf, T. S., et al. (2018). High-dose rifamycins enable shorter oral treatment in a murine model of *Mycobacterium ulcerans* disease. *Antimicrobial Agents and Chemotherapy, 63.* https://doi.org/10.1128/aac.01478-18.

39. Park, K. (2024). Epidemiology and management of infectious spondylitis in Korea: A narrative review. *The Ewha Medical Journal.* 2024;47(3):e37. Published online: July 31, 2024

40. DOI:https://doi.org/10.12771/emj.2024.e37. (accessed on 10 May 2025).

41. Pinhata, J., Felippe, I. M., Gallo, J. F., Chimara, E., Ferrazoli, L., & de Oliveira, R. S. (2018). Growth characteristics of liquid cultures increase the reliability of presumptive identification of *Mycobacterium tuberculosis* complex. *Journal of Medical Microbiology, 67*(6), 828–833. https://www.semanticscholar.org/paper/06ef841a6e41e20c4a18afde668e184a1e9d7b15 (accessed on 10 May 2025).

42. Pontiroli, A., Khera, T. T., Oakley, B. B., Mason, S., Dowd, S. E., Travis, E. R., Erenso, G., Aseffa, A., Courtenay, O., & Wellington, E. M. (2013). Prospecting environmental mycobacteria: combined molecular approaches reveal unprecedented diversity. *PloS one, 8*(7), e68648. https://doi.org/10.1371/journal.pone.0068648 (accessed on 10 May 2025).

43. Rangaraj, S., Agarwal, A., & Banerjee, S. (2025). Bird's Eye View on *Mycobacterium tuberculosis*-HIV Coinfection: Understanding the Molecular Synergism, Challenges, and New Approaches to Therapeutics. *ACS infectious diseases, 11*(5), 1042–1063. https://doi.org/10.1021/acsinfecdis.4c00870 (accessed on 10 May 2025).

44. Roy, A., Banerjee, P., Paul, I., Ghosh, R., & Ray, S. (2024). Integrating structure-guided and fragment-based inhibitor design to combat bedaquiline resistant *Mycobacterium tuberculosis*: A molecular dynamics study. *Journal of Biomolecular Structure & Dynamics*, 1–39. https://www.semanticscholar.org/paper/4ba76468209adaa952e89d1015b2dffb6b66ec20 (accessed on 10 May 2025).

45. Sawyer, J., Rhodes, S., Jones, G. J., Hogarth, P., & Vordermeier, H. (2023). *Mycobacterium bovis* and its impact on human and animal tuberculosis. *Journal of Medical Microbiology, 72*(11). https://www.semanticscholar.org/paper/abd5692dcbebec0880c39fd135dfe1cd3ca7dcf1 (accessed on 10 May 2025).

46. Sosa Soto, G., Hossain, F., Rahman, T., Rahman, M., Kulkarni, S., Roy, T., Malik, A. A., et al. (2025). P-791. Contribution of tuberculin skin test for diagnosing tuberculosis disease in paediatric patients in Bangladesh. *Open Forum Infectious Diseases, 12*. https://www.semanticscholar.org/paper/9a1ec47b84dddde89b10ffb6f04268d1885268af (accessed on 10 May 2025).

47. Thomsen, J., Abdulrazzaq, N. M., Nyasulu, P., Al Hosani, F., Habous, M., Weber, S., Jabeen, F., et al. (2024). Epidemiology and antimicrobial resistance of *Mycobacterium* spp. in the United Arab Emirates: A retrospective analysis of 12 years of national antimicrobial resistance surveillance data. *Frontiers in Public Health, 12*. https://www.semanticscholar.org/paper/2be2ab6d8d1e5221b924a24b949a82014e07f4b4 (accessed on 10 May 2025).

48. Tzelios, C., Neuhausser, W., Ryley, D. A., Vo, N. H., Hurtado, R., & Nathavitharana, R. R. (2022). Female genital tuberculosis. *Open Forum Infectious Diseases, 9*. https://doi.org/10.1093/ofid/ofac543.

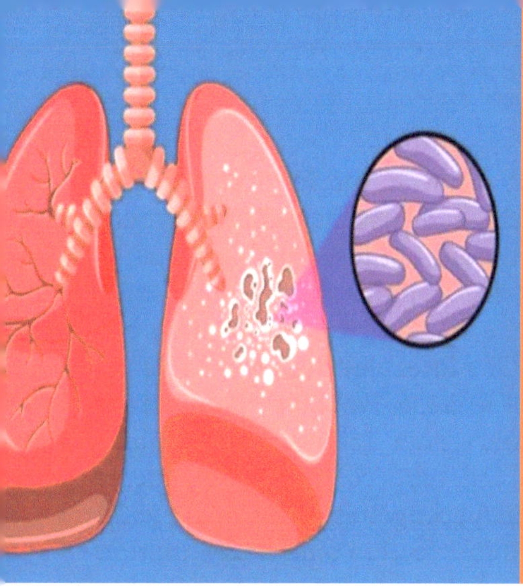

Chapter 2

PATHOGENESIS OF TUBERCULOSIS

Contents

Introduction

Tuberculosis (TB) is among the most powerful infectious diseases in the world, presenting a great challenge to public health despite the progress of medicine. TB predominantly targets the respiratory system but can spread to other organs with diverse clinical presentations. Its causative organism, *Mycobacterium tuberculosis* (MTB), infects the host's respiratory tract, setting in motion a multidimensional interaction between the pathogen and host immune system. It is vital to understand the pathogenesis of TB in unraveling how the infection advances from early exposure to active disease or latent infection. Scientific inquiry into the mechanisms of infection, immune evasion, and tissue damage offers insights necessary for the formulation of effective diagnostic, therapeutic, and preventive measures. Broaching these aspects in an introductory context lays down bases of knowledge essential for understanding the complexities involved in TB pathogenesis. The pathogenesis of TB includes a series of processes starting with the inhalation of airborne droplet nuclei harboring *Mtb*. Once in the alveoli, the bacteria are engulfed by resident macrophages, which under usual conditions would inactivate invading microbes. *Mtb* has specific adaptations to survive within these phagocytic cells, inhibit lysosomal fusion, and subvert host immune responses. This intracellular survival allows for the development of granulomas—structured aggregations of immune cells to contain infection but also as a niche in which the bacteria can cause latency and growth. The interplay between bacterial virulence determinants and host immunity decides the outcome of disease, whether containment or progression to active disease or dissemination to extrapulmonary sites (Stamp et al., 1952). Investigating these early processes is central to understanding the tuberculosis pathogenesis complexity and its related clinical aspects. Additionally, tuberculosis pathogenesis reaches beyond human health, since bovine tuberculosis also demonstrates analogous infection and dissemination mechanisms within animal populations and supports the zoonotic nature of the disease. Bovine tuberculosis research offers useful comparative insights, demonstrating how abattoir findings and pulmonary pathology reveal mechanisms of infection and immunity in animals. Primary infection usually involves the bronchial tree, and granulomatous lesions are seen in lung tissue, reflecting human pathological patterns. An assessment of these similarities helps in identifying transmission patterns and disease development between species and is important for planning integrated control mechanisms. Aspects gleaned from veterinary research enhance the general picture of tuberculosis pathogenesis and highlight the importance of a One Health response in fighting this chronic pathogen (Stamp et al., 1952).

Definition of Tuberculosis (TB)

Tuberculosis (TB) is a multifaceted infectious illness caused mostly by the bacterium MTB. It mainly targets the lungs but can infect other organs as well, making it a systemic disease in certain instances. The disease is still a major public health issue globally because it can remain in a latent form before developing into active disease. TB is spread by airborne droplets emitted when a person with the infection coughs or sneezes and propagates the bacteria in close-contact populations. The unique ability of the pathogens to suppress the immune response, along with its slow growth rate, are factors that contribute to the chronicity of the disease, making it different from most other bacterial infections. It is important to understand the rudimentary nature of TB to understand its pathogenesis, which entails complex interactions between the *Bacillus* and host defenses, ultimately determining disease outcomes. Fundamental to the definition of TB is its designation as a contagious bacterial disease by the presence of granulomatous inflammation. Granulomas develop as a host defense reaction to confine the mycobacteria in structures made up of immune cells, mainly macrophages and T lymphocytes. These granulomatous lesions are characteristics of TB and represent the active balance between pathogen survival and immune containment. The clinically heterogeneous but insidious development of TB is characterized by variable presentation from asymptomatic latent infection to active disease with tissue damage and systemic manifestations. In addition, host genetic determinants and environmental factors influence susceptibility and the course of disease. For instance, genetic variability in human drug-metabolizing enzymes such as NAT2 may impact therapy outcomes and risk for adverse events such as hepatotoxicity in the course of therapy, further indicating the complex interplay between pathogen, host, and treatment (Xiang et al., 2014). Strategies for vaccination have long been part of the control of TB, although they are subject to varying efficiency and need ongoing assessment within the larger pathogenic context of disease. The *Bacillus Calmette-Guérin* (BCG) vaccine, used to confer immunity against tuberculosis, actually prevents extensive forms in children from developing instead of providing adult humans with full immunity against pulmonary TB. The protective efficacy of this vaccine has been shown to vary depending on geographic region, age at vaccination, and strain variation. Though initially developed to combat TB, BCG has proven cross-protection for other mycobacterial infections such as leprosy, indicating immunological pathways with far-reaching implications beyond tuberculosis itself (Cunha et al., 2010). Grasping these subtleties is key to understanding the multipronged assault required to address TB pathogenesis and control, involving vaccination, drugs, and host-pathogen interactions.

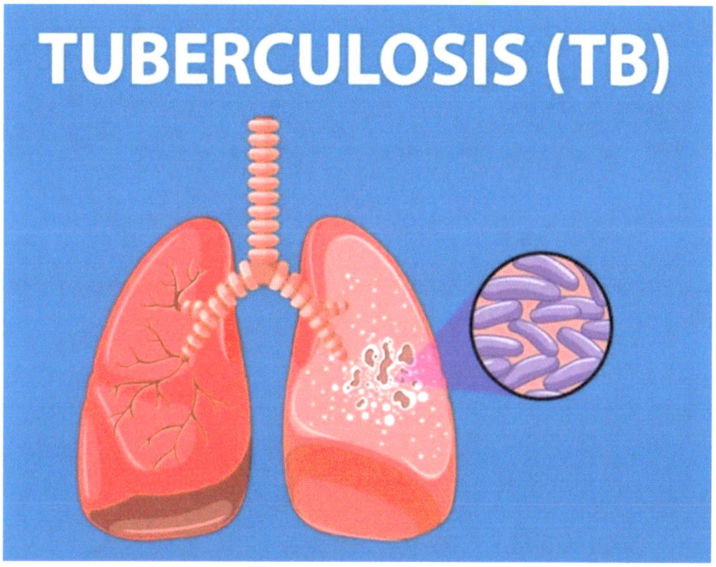

Source: Metropolis India. (n.d.). *Illustration of tuberculosis (TB) infection in lungs with magnified view of Mycobacterium tuberculosis.* https://www.metropolisindia.com/upgrade/blog/upload/24/01/Tuberculosis1705674281.webp.

Historical Context of TB

The history of tuberculosis (TB) as a worldwide health issue is profoundly entwined with human history, depicting a complicated interaction between host susceptibility and pathogen evolution. Ancient evidence proposes TB has affected humanity for thousands of years, and it is traced back to historic civilization using skeletal remains and historical documents. The onset of the Industrial Revolution provided the critical shift, where urbanization and dense living allowed MTB to disperse quickly. In this period, limited medical understanding and primitive public health interventions made TB a primary cause of death. The later identification of the tubercle *Bacillus* by Robert Koch in 1882 accelerated additional scientific investigations, facilitating improved knowledge regarding its pathogenesis and mode of transmission. Despite these advances, TB was tenaciously resistant, speeding up initiatives for effective drugs and preventive measures, which are ongoing to date as new drug resistance and co-infections emerge. The historical resistance to TB emphasizes the need for novel therapeutic techniques in contemporary medical research (Vijaya et al., 2023). Scientific research over the 20th century established the mechanistic basis of TB pathogenesis, demonstrating the persistence of the bacterium within host macrophages and the manipulation of immune responses. The complex interaction between immune modulation and TB infection was additionally complicated in the late 20th and early 21st centuries by the HIV pandemic. HIV coinfection resulted in dramatically faster progression of TB, posing a critical public health concern, particularly in those areas with high HIV prevalence. Studies have explained that TB modifies macrophage function, especially by modulating the type I interferon (IFN) pathway, which may enhance HIV pathogenesis by compromising antiviral immunity. Identifying these molecular interactions indicates the pathogen's potential to manipulate host immune responses for its benefit, making treatment in co-infected patients more challenging. This convergence between HIV infection and TB's pathogenesis is still an important therapeutic target and disease control area (DuPont et al., 2022).

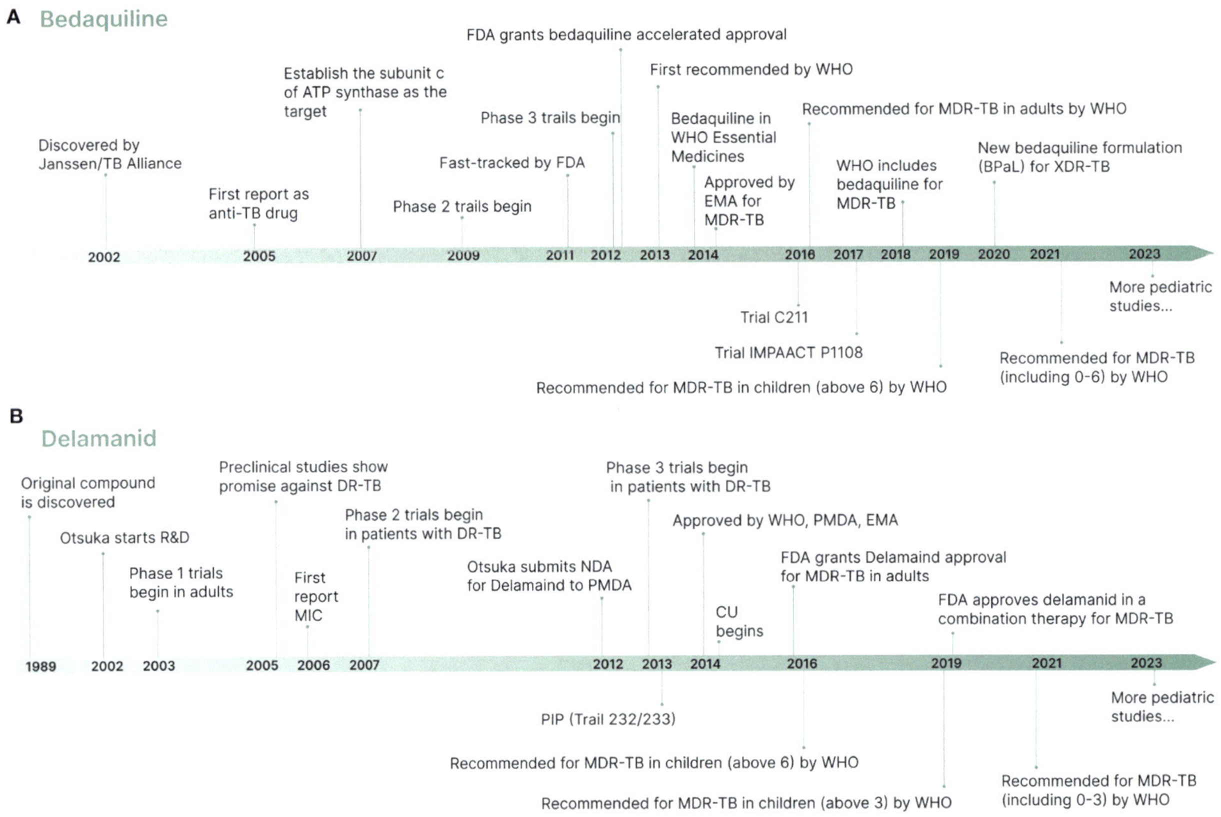

Figure 2.1. TB history timeline.

Source: Zhu H, Zhou X, Zhuang Z, Li L, Bi J and Mi K (2023) Advances of new drugs bedaquiline and delamanid in the treatment of multi-drug resistant tuberculosis in children. Front. Cell. Infect. Microbiol. 13:1183597. doi: 10.3389/fcimb.2023.1183597

Due to the persistent worldwide burden of tuberculosis, past treatment models have increasingly utilized adjunctive approaches, such as the investigation of natural products possessing immunomodulatory activity. Of these, plant-derived bioflavonoids have attracted increasing attention for their wide-ranging activities in augmenting host immunity and inhibiting mycobacterial virulence mechanisms. Traditional ethnobotanical medicine used diverse plant extracts to treat TB, a strategy being revisited today under contemporary scientific study. Studies find that bioflavonoids inhibit biofilm development, decrease mycobacterial virulence mechanisms, and affect host inflammatory mechanisms, possibly reducing tissue injury and increasing antimicrobial action. These features make bioflavonoids a highly potential adjunct to the traditional therapies, especially in curtailing drug resistance and treatment length issues. The convergence of historical and modern insights on natural medicines adds strength to the strength against TB, demonstrating the ways in which history inspires novel means to counter this relentless infection (Vijaya et al., 2023) (Figures 2.1 and 2.2).

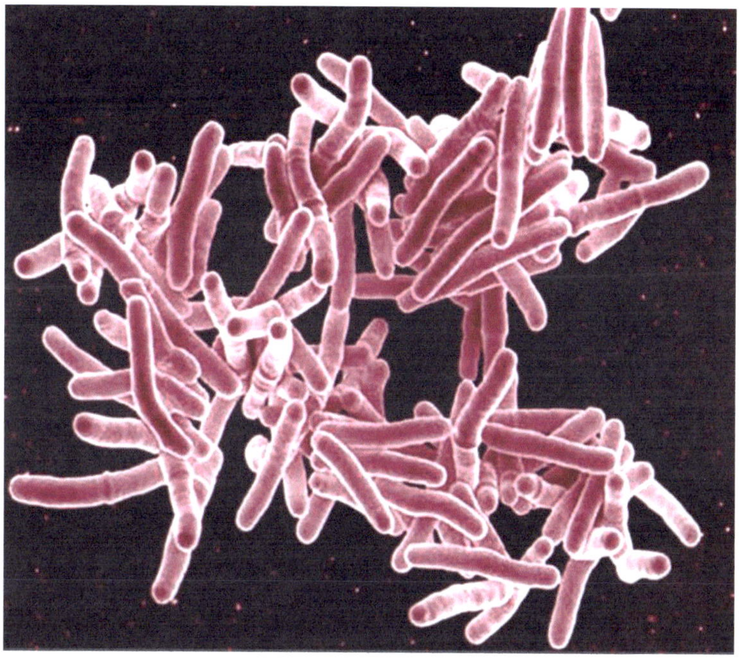

Figure 2.2. *Mycobacterium tuberculosis* is a pathogenic bacterial species in the family Mycobacteriaceae and the causative agent of most cases of tuberculosis.

Source: https://commons.wikimedia.org/wiki/File:Mycobacterium_tuberculosis_Bacteria,_the_Cause_of_TB_%285149398656%29.jpg

Importance of Studying TB Pathogenesis

Knowing the detailed mechanisms of infectious diseases continues to be the foundation for moving medical science and public health forward. Tuberculosis (TB), due to MTB, is a chronic worldwide health problem that requires careful investigation of its pathogenesis for the establishment of effective interventions. Exploring TB's cause unravels the complex host-pathogen interactions, specifically how the bacterium subverts immune defenses to cause infection. Knowledge developed using experimental models, including the macaque model, has been extremely useful in this endeavor. These models mimic human disease progression, making it possible for researchers to examine pathogenic processes and immune responses that are otherwise challenging to study directly in humans (Gardner & Luciw., 2008). A complete comprehension of these processes helps to recognize possible therapeutic targets and optimize vaccine approaches, highlighting the exigent necessity of analyzing TB pathogenesis to stop the disease burden worldwide. Furthermore, the molecular-level analysis of TB pathogenesis holds deep-seated significance for the design of accurate diagnostics and treatments. Pathogenic mycobacteria evolve to survive in host macrophages by manipulating gene expression that promotes intracellular persistence. Using advanced methods, for example, cDNA-total RNA subtractive hybridization, scientists have determined important bacterial genes that are upregulated during infection of macrophages, for example, those associated with the assembly of complex cell envelope structures critical to virulence (Wood et al., 2001).

Identification of these molecular strategies clarifies how *Mtb* can sustain chronic infection and evade host immunity. Therefore, understanding these molecular pathways is essential to identify new drug targets that can interfere with bacterial survival mechanisms, ultimately improving therapeutic efficacy and minimizing the global health burden of tuberculosis. Beyond basic science, the relevance of understanding TB pathogenesis extends into public health strategy development and personalized medicine. TB's complex nature, with different host and bacterial factors, requires an integrated approach to understanding disease evolution and patient-to-patient heterogeneity. Probing the immune evasion strategies and regulation of bacterial genes obtained from animal models and molecular research promotes next-generation vaccine and immunotherapy designs specific to different stages of infection. Such targeted interventions become obligatory to fight drug-resistant bacteria and heterogeneous clinical presentations of TB. In addition, this knowledge guides public health practice in policies to control the transmission and enhance patient outcomes, emphasizing the importance of studying TB pathogenesis to translate the findings of science into effective clinical and epidemiological solutions (Wood et al., 2001; Gardner & Luciw., 2008).

2.1. Causative Agent

Tuberculosis continues to be a serious worldwide health problem primarily due to the distinctive biological properties of its etiologic agent, *Mycobacterium tuberculosis* (MTB). As an intracellular pathogen, MTB has a high degree of genetic variation, making it hard to clarify its epidemiology and pathogenicity. High genomic sequencing of epidemic MTB strains demonstrates a highly conserved core genome but also many breaks in coding sequences, resulting in a smaller number of universally active genes. Such genetic diversity is a reflection of continuous evolutionary forces, both selective and background selection, acting on its capacity to adapt within various host environments. The genes that encode the cell wall and membrane show strong selective forces, indicating their pivotal importance in host-pathogen interactions and immune evasion. These adaptations highlight the advanced mechanisms MTB uses to survive in hosts and emphasize the intricacy of creating successful interventions against its molecular machinery (Zhou et al., 2024). Central to MTB's pathogenic success is its ability to hijack host cell pathways, guaranteeing its survival and replication in macrophages. Current research places a focus on the function of extracellular vesicles (EVs), nanoscale particles released both by the bacteria and host cells upon infection. These vesicles transport an assortment of bioactive molecules, some of which are MTB-derived, that can modulate host immune responses for bacterial persistence. By hijacking EV biogenesis pathways, MTB selectively packages virulence factors into these vesicles, thus molding the host environment to promote immune evasion and persistent infection. The temporal diversity of EVs varies depending on the host's physiological and nutritional context, evidencing a very adaptive strategy. Comprehension of this complex interaction unlocks new therapeutic avenues and gives insight into the intracellular life of the pathogen (Alipoor & Elieh-Ali-Komi,

2024). The genetic constitution of the causative agent and its use of EV-mediated communication have a fundamental impact on tuberculosis pathogenesis. MTB's capacity to finely modulate host immune defenses through genetic remodeling and EVs speaks to a well-developed co-evolution with humans. This multimodal strategy allows the bacterium to escape clearance, remain in latency, and, under appropriate circumstances, reactivate to produce active disease. Such sophistication makes vaccine development more challenging and requires greater investigation into the molecular mechanisms utilized by MTB. Ongoing investigation of how particular genetic variants modulate EV composition and function holds the promise to define key determinants of virulence and immune modulation. Eventually, a detailed understanding of MTB as the etiologic agent—incorporating both its genomic characteristics and interaction with host microenvironments—is essential in formulating novel strategies to counteract tuberculosis (Alipoor & Elieh-Ali-Komi, 2024; Zhou et al., 2024) (Figure 2.3).

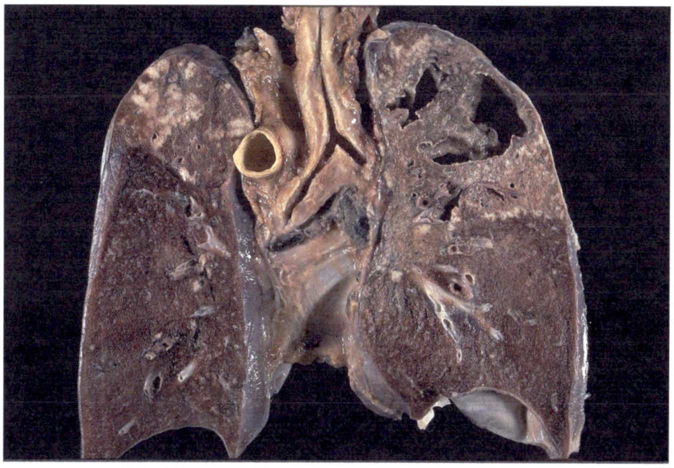

Figure 2.3. Your lungs are infected with tuberculosis bacteria when you have tuberculosis.

Source: By Yale Rosen - https://www.flickr.com/photos/pulmonary_pathology/6572343713/in/set-72157628551443837/, CC BY-SA 2.0, https://commons.wikimedia.org/w/index.php?curid=18560989

2.1.1. Mycobacterium tuberculosis (MTB) Characteristics

The capacity of *Mycobacterium tuberculosis* (M. tuberculosis/*Mtb*) to survive and create disease is precisely linked to its special structural and biochemical characteristics. Contrary to the majority of the bacterial pathogens, this bacterium has a complicated, lipid-containing cell wall that is constituted mainly by mycolic acids, which grants a unique acid-fast nature. This lipid envelope is an effective shield against host immune mechanisms and many antibiotics, thereby reinforcing the bacterium's tenacity in adversarial environments. In addition, *Mtb* is rather slow-growing relative to other bacteria, which makes immune recognition as well as therapeutic intervention more complex. The low rate of replication enables *Mtb* to avoid rapid clearance and promotes a long latent phase typical for tuberculosis pathogenesis. These architectural idiosyncrasies not only affect the clinical progression of the disease but also form the basis on which the bacterium hijacks host cell mechanisms to evade killing, a testament to its evolutionary selection as a human pathogen. Apart from the cell wall, *Mtb* has specialized metabolic mechanisms that facilitate its survival in the oxygen-variable and nutrient-poor conditions found in the host. The bacterium can grow on varied carbon substrates and adjust its metabolism following the granulomatous milieu developed during infection. Metabolic adaptability is vital in maintaining bacterial viability during the latent phase when oxygen availability is low, and nutrient supply is limited. In addition, *Mtb* takes advantage of the processes inhibiting host cell autophagy, a cell degradation process that would normally contribute to clearing intracellular pathogens. By disrupting autophagy, *Mtb* sustains a replicating niche within macrophages, evading innate immune defenses. These metabolic and immunomodulatory features elucidate how the pathogen persists and provide potential targets for therapeutic intervention directed at restoring host clearance pathways (Daniel et al., 2021). In addition to complicating disease control, *Mtb* has evolved such advanced mechanisms of immune evasion and modulation to increase its pathogenicity. *Mtb* can manipulate host immune signaling for its own survival by inducing granuloma formation, which sequesters bacteria but protects them from immune clearance. The secretion systems of the pathogen provide effector proteins that interfere with phagosomal maturation and antigen presentation so it can survive inside macrophages without triggering effective bactericidal reactions. Also, the bacterial adaptations are resistant to reactive nitrogen and oxygen species derived from activated immune cells. These interactions point to the pathogen-host virulence-defense equilibrium that characterizes tuberculosis development. With the persistent socio-economic burden of tuberculosis and increased emergence of drug-resistant populations, studies of *Mtb*'s peculiarity continue to be important to the development of better therapeutic and preventive strategies (David et al., 2020) (Figure 2.4).

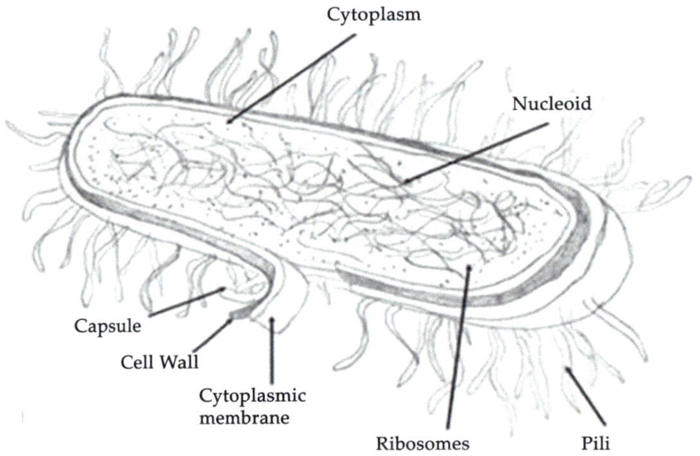

Figure 2.4. The structure of *M. tuberculosis.*

Source: Jabir, R. A., Rukmana, A., Saleh, I., & Kurniawati, T. (2018). The Existence of Mycobacterium tuberculosis in Microenvironment of Bone. InTech. doi: 10.5772/intechopen.69394

2.1.2. Transmission Methods of TB

The pathogenesis of tuberculosis (TB) essentially starts with its transmission, which is mainly due to airborne droplets emitted by persons with active pulmonary TB. When the patient coughs, sneezes, or speaks, they expel droplet nuclei with MTB into the air, where it becomes available for inhalation by susceptible hosts. These airborne infectious aerosols will remain suspended in confined or poorly ventilated areas over a long duration, making transmission easy. The infective dose to create infection can be incredibly low, allowing the pathogen to invade new hosts even with transient exposure. Moreover, specific zoonotic pathways exist, like transmission of bovine tuberculosis among farm animals and possibly to humans, highlighting the multifaceted epidemiology of TB. For example, in Swedish reindeer herds, the introduction of *Mycobacterium bovis* via imported animals precipitated an outbreak, illustrating the importance of cross-species transmission in specific situations (Wahlström et al., 2004) (Figure 2.5).

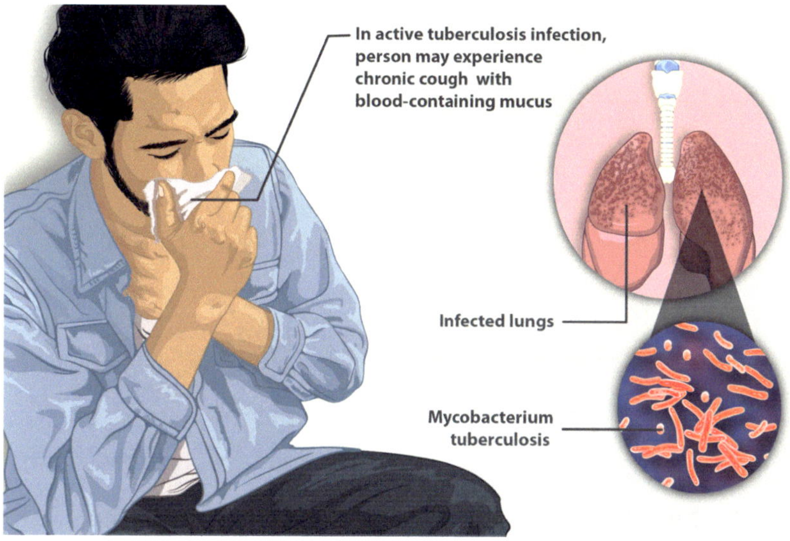

Figure 2.5. Mode of transmission of tuberculosis.

Source: By https://www.myupchar.com/ - https://www.myupchar.com/en/disease/tuberculosis-tb, CC BY-SA 4.0, https://commons.wikimedia.org/w/index.php?curid=82880185

These events underscore the varied pathways by which TB can spread among both human and animal populations. TB transmission dynamics also rely on environmental and host determinants of bacterial dissemination from the host and the probability of inhalation. Crowding, ventilation, and the immune status of exposed individuals modulate infectivity and susceptibility. In densely populated environments such as hospitals, prisons, and shelters, intimate and prolonged exposure increases the risk of transmission. Additionally, latent infection is a key phase where MTB is within host cells dormant, undiscovered by the immune system. The pathogen's resistance to host defenses via effective DNA repair processes at different stages of infection indirectly affects its transmission capacity by facilitating persistence and subsequent reactivation (Gorna et al., 2010). Knowledge of these processes explains how TB is able to sustain transmission chains in populations, which leads to its global persistence despite immune clearance in most cases. Apart from primary human-to-human transmission, TB is disseminated through indirect routes that hamper control initiatives. Animal reservoirs, particularly cattle and deer, serve to sustain *Mycobacterium bovis* in the environment and, by extension, infect humans upon close contact or ingestion of infected animal products. This zoonotic reservoir requires specialized control and surveillance measures beyond the conventional human public health response. Control in wildlife, for example, in large Swedish deer populations, depends on diagnostic testing and other methods such as meat inspection to detect and contain outbreaks (Wahlström et al., 2004). This measures the fact that effective TB control has not only to take into account all avenues of transmission, those between species included, to target pathogen reservoirs and interrupt transmission cycles. Therefore, the complexity of the spread of TB highlights the importance of integrative approaches that take into consideration environmental, animal, and human factors involved in tuberculosis pathogenesis (Figure 2.6).

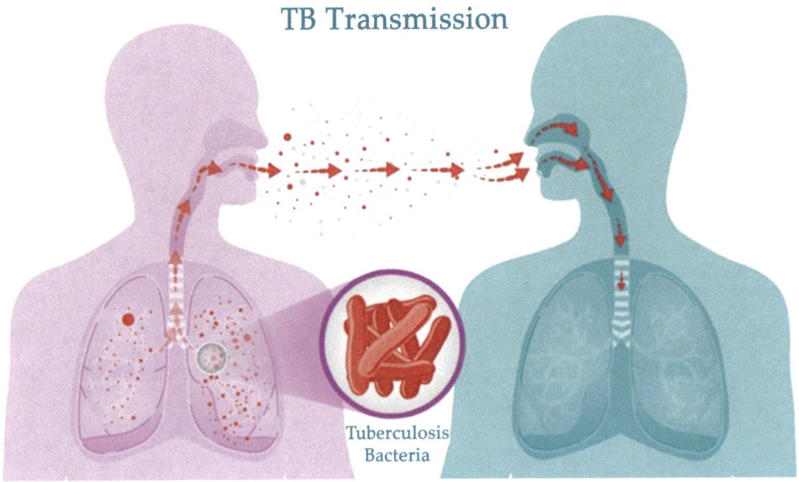

Figure 2.6. TB germs spread through the air from one person to another.

Source: Centers for Disease Control and Prevention (CDC). (n.d.). *TB transmission from infected to healthy individual via airborne droplets.* https://www.cdc.gov/tb/media/images/TB_transmission.PNG.

2.1.3. Virulence Factors of Mycobacterium tuberculosis (MTB)

The pathogenic capability of *Mycobacterium tuberculosis* (*Mtb*) is closely related to its extensive repertoire of virulence factors that allow survival in the host. They allow immune evasion and sustain persistence in hostile niches like the macrophage phagosome. Among the most important are cell wall components such as mycolic acids, which provide desiccation and chemical resistance. Additionally, *Mtb* produces proteins like ESAT-6 and CFP-10 that are capable of disrupting host cellular membranes, facilitating bacterial escape and spread. Virulence is also affected by genetic variability between *Mtb* strains since recent phylogenetic analyses have revealed several lineages with varying pathogenic characteristics and transmissibility, highlighting the intricacy of host-pathogen interactions (Napier et al., 2020). Recognition of these molecular arms helps explain how *Mtb* can cause chronic infections and is essential for designing effective diagnostic and therapeutic approaches. Virulence of *Mtb* is additionally optimized by its manipulation of host immune cells, specifically macrophages, which are the central niche for bacterial replication. On inhalation, *Mtb* infects alveolar macrophages and causes their conversion into lipid-filled foamy macrophages, providing an intracellular niche favorable for bacterial survival (Shim et al., 2020). These foamy macrophages define the granulomatous lesions that are the hallmark of tuberculosis pathology. Virulence factors actively subvert macrophage lipid metabolism and immune signaling pathways, repressing competent immune responses and maintaining a chronic inflammatory state. Such metabolic reprogramming not only protects *Mtb* from host defense but also causes tissue damage, which promotes disease progression. *Mtb*'s capacity to hijack the host's immune response is a prime example of its evolved survival strategies and remains a central focus area in tuberculosis pathogenesis research. In addition to direct interaction with host cells, *Mtb* virulence factors modulate disease outcomes through intervening in environmental adaptation and immune modulation within the granuloma. The pathogen's type VII ESX secretion system facilitates the export of effector proteins that influence host cell death and facilitate bacterial spread. Genetic studies emphasize new mutations and lineage-specific SNPs associated with these virulence characteristics and expose sophisticated mechanisms that regulate *Mtb*'s persistence in various host groups (Napier et al., 2020). These molecular changes make it difficult to control tuberculosis, as they are capable of modifying host immune recognition and response. Therefore, targeting these virulence determinants, in addition to traditional antimycobacterial treatments, is a promising approach for host-directed therapies looking to break *Mtb*'s pathogenic niche in foamy macrophages and granulomas (Shim et al., 2020). Such integrative knowledge is crucial for the development of tuberculosis control and eradication programs (Figure 2.7).

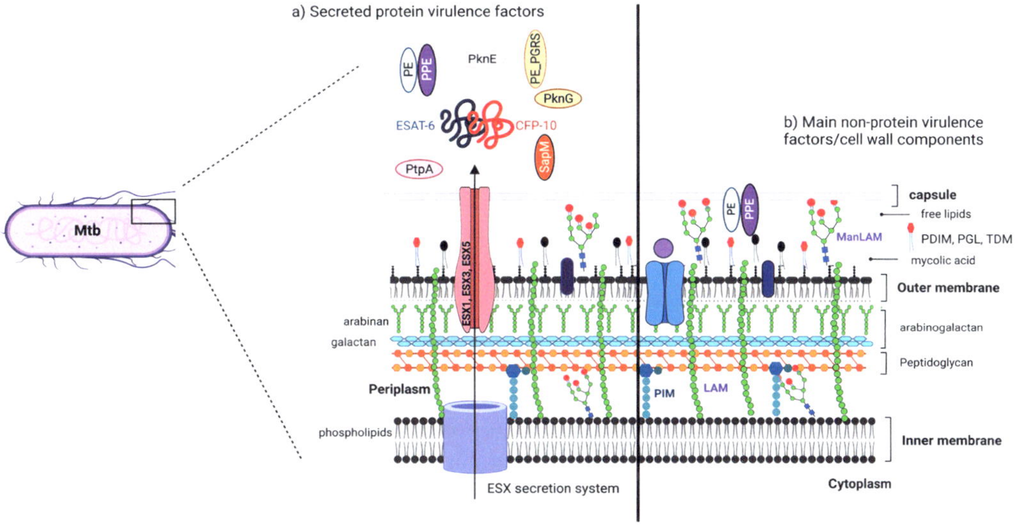

Figure 2.7. Virulence factors of *M. tuberculosis*.

Source: Ramon-Luing LA, Palacios Y, Ruiz A, Téllez-Navarrete NA, Chavez-Galan L. Virulence Factors of *Mycobacterium tuberculosis* as Modulators of Cell Death Mechanisms. *Pathogens*. 2023; 12(6):839. https://doi.org/10.3390/pathogens12060839

2.2. Host Immune Response

The sophistication of the host immune response to *Mycobacterium tuberculosis* (*M. tuberculosis*/ *Mtb*) is a reflection of an active interplay between host defense mechanisms and bacterial evasion mechanisms. Following inhalation, *Mtb* infects mainly alveolar macrophages, which represent the first line of defense by trying to phagocytose and confine the pathogen. *Mtb*, however, has developed mechanisms to survive inside macrophages through inhibition of phagosome-lysosome fusion and subsequent avoidance of destruction. This intracellular persistence provokes a more general immune response that entails the recruitment of diverse immune cells, such as dendritic cells (DCs), neutrophils, and T lymphocytes, to create granulomas. Granulomas are a containment mechanism to localize infection but also can create a niche to facilitate bacterial latency. The equilibrium between bacterial growth and containment by the immune system dictates disease advancement or regulation, highlighting the double-edged nature of the host immune response in tuberculosis pathogenesis.

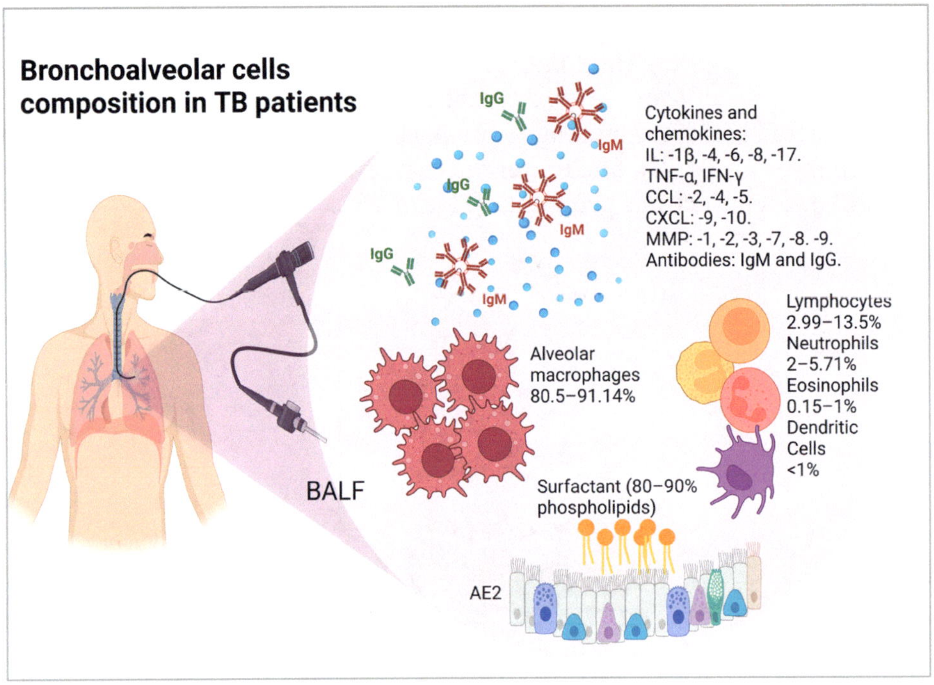

Figure 2.8. Regulation of the immune response during *M. tuberculosis* infection. Following infection with *Mtb*, specific regulatory pathways that normally serve to limit host-induced immune pathology may inadvertently promote pathogen persistence. Two such regulators include IL-10 and regulatory T cells.

Source: Herrera MT, Guzmán-Beltrán S, Bobadilla K, Santos-Mendoza T, Flores-Valdez MA, Gutiérrez-González LH, González Y. Human Pulmonary Tuberculosis: Understanding the Immune Response in the Bronchoalveolar System. *Biomolecules*. 2022; 12(8):1148. https://doi.org/10.3390/biom12081148

At the center of the initial immune signaling in tuberculosis is type I interferons (IFNs), a family of cytokines whose multifaceted effects on the outcome of infection are pertinent. Although type I IFNs are classically known for their antiviral activity, newer transcriptional data have shown their ability to regulate immunity in response to *Mtb* infection. The induction of type I IFNs can also inhibit pro-inflammatory responses which are required to control bacterial growth, thus enabling persistence and worse disease pathology. However, new evidence is also accumulating to indicate that in some immunological contexts, type I IFNs can be enhanced to induce host resistance by eliciting antimicrobial activity. This paradoxical function suggests that the timing, magnitude, and cellular environment of type I IFN signaling are crucial in determining whether host response promotes bacterial growth or limitation. Elucidating these mechanistic subtleties is crucial for the design of immunomodulatory therapies against tuberculosis (Moreira-Teixeira et al., 2018). Clinical translation despite progress in defining immune pathways engaged by tuberculosis has remained problematic, in part due to a lack of adequate integration of experimental and clinical information. Significantly, ethical revelations and financing transparency have emerged as essential factors in the publication of research results, upholding the validity and replicability of scientific work. Recent accounts underscore collaborations between pharmaceutical firms and researchers in tuberculosis immunology, emphasizing the need for impartial peer review and compliance with authorship guidelines when presenting immune response research. This level of rigor is critical in making therapeutic targets valid, including those that regulate type I IFN pathways or macrophage activity. As such, upholding rigorous research ethics and openness fills the gap between experimental understanding and clinical utility, which is imperative to progress in treating tuberculosis as well as developing vaccines (Dick et al., 2018) (Figure 2.8).

2.2.1. Innate Immune Response to TB

The first contact of MTB with the host takes place in the alveolar cavities of the lung, where innate immunity plays a key role in either controlling or exacerbating the infection. Upon entry through inhalation, *Mtb* is quickly identified by host cells like macrophages and DCs, which bear pattern recognition receptors (PRRs). These recognize conserved microbial molecules called pathogen-associated molecular patterns, allowing for an immediate host response. PRR activation initiates signaling cascades that result in pro-inflammatory cytokine, chemokine, and antimicrobial molecule production. Early bacterial growth is restricted by this quick detection and response, and the recruitment of other immune cells to the infection site is initiated. Nevertheless, the innate immune system also includes sensing damage-induced danger-associated molecular patterns, which may enhance inflammation or participate in tissue pathology, showing the complex balance among protective and harmful processes in early *Mtb* infection (Modlin, 2012). The part played by IFNs in tuberculosis pathogenesis is a good example of the double-edged nature of the innate immune response. Although type I IFNs are universally known for their antiviral action, their action during *Mtb* infection is paradoxical. Transcriptional profiling of patients and animal models has shown that high type I IFN signaling is associated with higher bacterial burden and poor outcomes in the disease, proposing an adverse role in tuberculosis. The cytokine family alters the expression of many genes that play roles in immune regulation, sometimes dampening beneficial inflammatory responses necessary for mycobacterial containment. However, new evidence also points to contexts in which type I IFNs could have positive effects, possibly through the modulation of immune cell activation or augmentation of antimicrobial pathways. Thus, the effect of type I IFN in *Mtb* infection relies on a multifaceted interaction between infection phase, host genetics, and environmental factors (Moreira-Teixeira et al., 2018). Assessment of the multilayered innate immune environment of tuberculosis is critical to the understanding of mechanisms affecting disease progression or control. Innate immune cells beyond PRRs and type I IFN, however, execute many effector activities, such as phagocytosis, autophagy, and production of reactive nitrogen and oxygen intermediates. These functions are meant to limit *Mtb* replication in host macrophages. Yet, the pathogen has developed advanced mechanisms to circumvent these defenses, including blocking phagosome maturation and hijacking antigen presentation to suppress effective innate responses. Further, overactivation or dysregulation of innate pathways can cause pulmonary tissue damage, thus underlining the need for an exquisitely controlled immune balance. Deciphering these intrinsic pathways has deep implications for the creation of new diagnostics, vaccines, and immunotherapies aimed at the early stages of tuberculosis infection (Modlin, 2012; Moreira-Teixeira et al., 2018) (Figure 2.9).

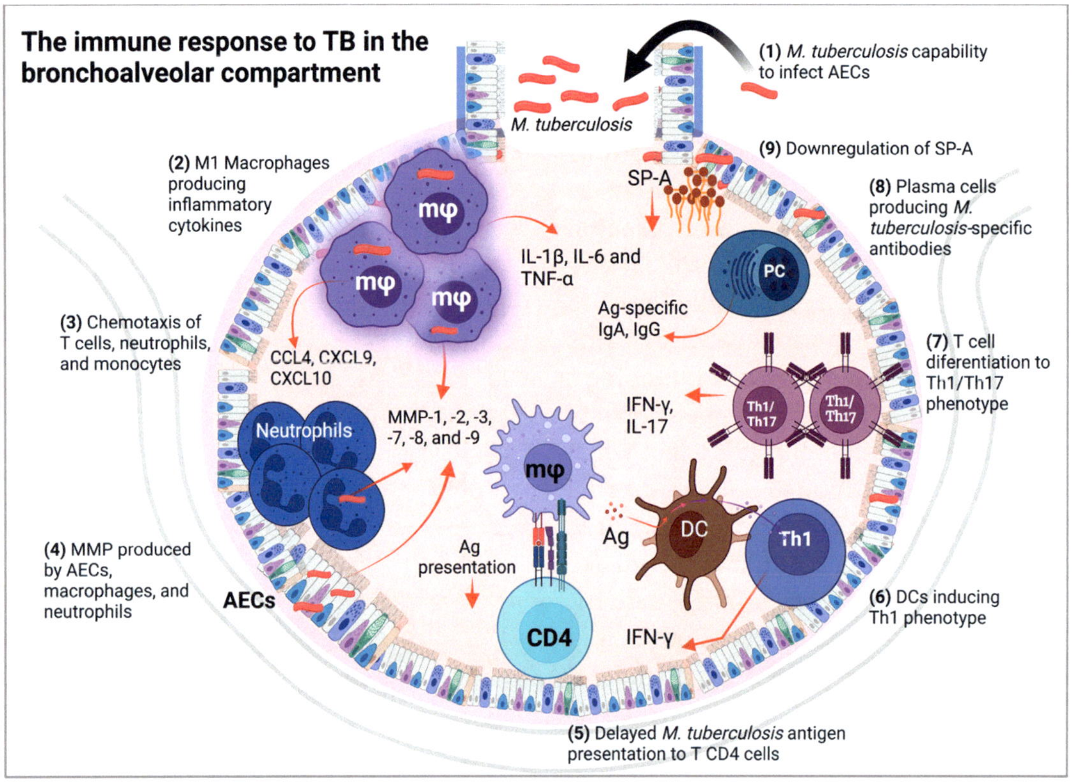

Figure 2.9. Infection of the alveolar macrophages is tuberculosis's first step.

Source: Herrera MT, Guzmán-Beltrán S, Bobadilla K, Santos-Mendoza T, Flores-Valdez MA, Gutiérrez-González LH, González Y. Human Pulmonary Tuberculosis: Understanding the Immune Response in the Bronchoalveolar System. *Biomolecules.* 2022; 12(8):1148. https://doi.org/10.3390/biom12081148

2.2.2. Adaptive Immune Response to TB

The immune response to MTB is a multifaceted interaction of cellular events which ultimately either result in infection resolution or progression. Initially, the innate immune response tries to hold back *Mtb*, but the bacterial replication needs to be controlled by the adaptive immune response to avoid disease advancement. The key to this process is the recruitment and activation of T lymphocytes in granulomatous lesions. These tissues act as sites of pathogen containment and antigen presentation. IRF-8 has come to play a critical role in the orchestration of these immune dynamics. IRF-8 deficiency interferes with organized granuloma formation and tertiary lymphoid structure formation in the lung, causing uncontrolled bacterial growth and acute tuberculosis pathology. IRF-8 loss abolishes homeostatic chemokine balance and reduces protective T-cell infiltration, whereas neutrophil prevalence dominates later infection phases, thus underlining IRF-8's pivotal role in sustaining an organized adaptive response to *Mtb* (Dorhoi et al., 2013). Genetic susceptibility contributes importantly to inter-individual differences in tubercular susceptibility, specifically through immune cell function genes. AspA1 variants that modulate cytoskeletal rearrangement have been associated with elevated TB susceptibility through disrupted DC migration. These APCs play a critical role in adaptive immune response initiation by carrying *Mtb* antigens from infected tissues to LNs, thereby stimulating T cells. Decreased ASAP1 expression impairs DC mobility and their ability to efficiently prime T cells, which could result in delayed or insufficient adaptive response. The defective migration later results in the failure of the immune system to establish granulomas and limit bacterial dissemination, thus highlighting the interface of host genetics and adaptive immunity in TB pathogenesis (Apt et al., 2015).

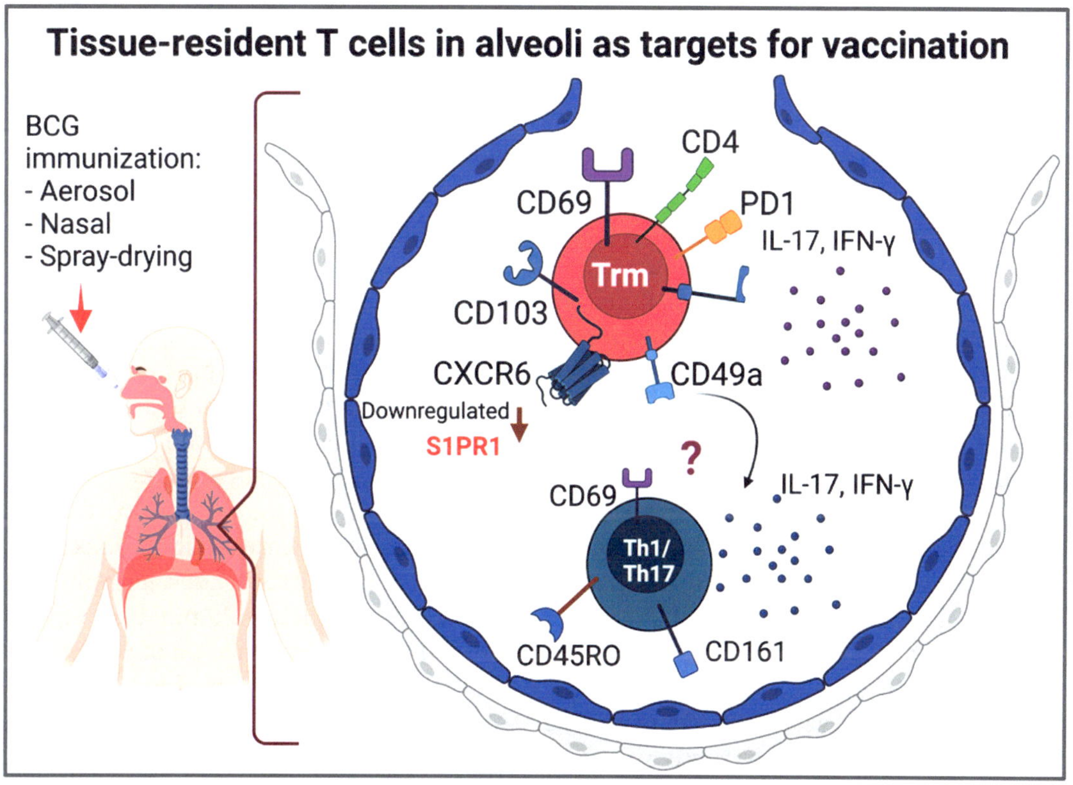

Figure 2.10. A complex composition of cells of the innate and adaptive immune system is found in bronchoalveolar lavage fluid (BALF) obtained from TB patients, 90% of which comprises alveolar macrophages.

Source: Herrera MT, Guzmán-Beltrán S, Bobadilla K, Santos-Mendoza T, Flores-Valdez MA, Gutiérrez-González LH, González Y. Human Pulmonary Tuberculosis: Understanding the Immune Response in the Bronchoalveolar System. *Biomolecules*. 2022; 12(8):1148. https://doi.org/10.3390/biom12081148

In the adaptive immune environment, CD4+ T cells and their interferon-gamma (IFN-γ) secretion are a foundation of host defense against *Mtb*. IFN-γ turns on macrophages to increase intracellular killing of mycobacteria as well as maintain granuloma integrity. Nevertheless, the immune response needs to be precisely regulated; overactive or deregulated T-cell responses can lead to tissue damage and disease progression. The development of lymphoid tissues in the infected lung compartmentalizes immune responses but needs chronic lymphocyte recruitment and appropriate chemokine signaling. Disruptions in these processes, which are determined by either IRF-8 deficiency or genetic determinants influencing APCs, hinder bacterial control and facilitate pathological inflammation. Thus, the adaptive immune response is a double-edged sword, critical for TB control but at the risk of driving immunopathology when homeostasis is disrupted (Apt et al., 2015; Dorhoi et al., 2013) (Figure 2.10).

2.2.3. Mechanisms of Immune Evasion by Mycobacterium tuberculosis (MTB)

The relationship between MTB and the host immune system is an ongoing war that plays a major role in the course of disease. *Mtb* uses advanced mechanisms to evade host defenses, which allows it to survive inside macrophages, cells usually responsible for clearing pathogens. One major mechanism is preventing phagosome-lysosome fusion, which inhibits the acidic and enzyme-mediated destruction usually fatal to pathogens. *Mtb* also regulates cytokine patterns to bias immune responses toward its survival. For instance, it can bring about the secretion of anti-inflammatory cytokines that inhibit effective immune activation. These mechanisms of evasion enable *Mtb* to establish a niche within macrophages, evading detection and killing. Additionally, smoking conditions worsen this immune suppression by abating macrophage phagocytic activity and raising proinflammatory cytokines in an unregulated manner, further hijacking the host's capacity to clear the *Bacillus* (Aryanpur et al., 2016). *Mtb* persistence inside host cells is also enabled by its capability to control antigen presentation and adaptive immune responses. Through the change in the expression of molecules that are essential for T-cell activation, *Mtb* slows down or suppresses the priming of effective cellular immunity, which is crucial for limiting the infection. This dysfunction leads to the development of latency, where bacteria are in a dormant but viable state, escaping immune clearance during prolonged periods. The latent reservoir poses an insurmountable challenge to worldwide eradication, since the bacteria may reactivate when the conditions are favorable, for example, immune suppression. The intricacy of such host-pathogen interactions places emphasis on an in-depth understanding of the mechanisms through which *Mtb* evades immune detection (Zumla et al., 2011). In addition, Its capacity to induce an uncontrolled inflammatory environment facilitates its evasion and pathological persistence. While it initiates the secretion of proinflammatory cytokines such as TNF-α and CXCL-8, which are critical for the granuloma, this response will be counterproductive when overblown to the point of causing tissue destruction and failure to contain. Protective inflammation and destructive immunity are finely tuned, and *Mtb* takes advantage of this to contribute to ineffective host defense. Disturbance of the usual functions of macrophages by factors like exposure to tobacco smoke exacerbates this imbalance, promoting immune evasion even further. Such multi-level approaches explain why tuberculosis continues to be one of the major infectious killers and underscores the necessity of therapeutic strategies restoring immune balance in addition to antimicrobial therapy (Aryanpur et al., 2016).

2.3. Pathophysiology of TB Infection

The complex interplay of MTB with the host immune system sets off a cascade of cellular events that underlies tuberculosis infection. After inhalation, MTB bacilli are engulfed by alveolar macrophages, which play the role of both the initial line of defense and the key niche for bacterial survival and replication. This pathogen-host encounter elicits macrophage activation and the production of inflammatory cytokines like TNF-α and CXCL-8, critical mediators in orchestrating immune responses. The functional potential of these macrophages is compromised in smoking patients, as indicated by impaired phagocytosis, thereby retarding bacterial clearance. Smoking worsens the inflammatory environment through increased levels of serum TNF-α and CXCL-8, tipping the balance between proinflammatory and anti-inflammatory mediators in favor of chronic infection and tissue damage (Aryanpur et al., 2016).

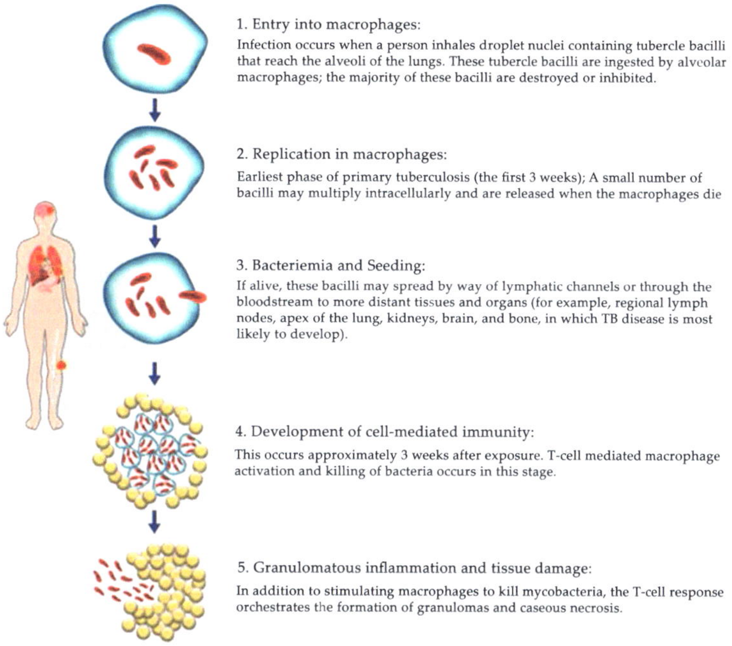

Figure 2.11. Pathogenesis of tuberculosis.

Source: National Tuberculosis Elimination Program (NTEP). (n.d.). *Pathogenesis of tuberculosis: From macrophage entry to granulomatous inflammation and tissue damage.* https://ntep.in/node/358/CP-pathogenesis-tb.

It emphasizes the susceptibility of specific patient groups and indicates the subtle regulation of immunity critical to TB pathophysiology. Cell biology is more important when lipid metabolism is recognized as an important immunomodulator of tuberculosis infection. Cholesterol-enriched microdomains, or lipid rafts, allow MTB entry and regulate macrophage activation, highlighting the pivotal role of lipids in pathogen-host interactions. Dysregulated cholesterol metabolism may interfere with membrane dynamics and immune signaling cascades, leading to immune dysfunction typical of TB and other infections. Cholesterol in the diet also influences cellular cholesterol homeostasis and inflammatory status, possibly modulating disease susceptibility and disease progression. The delicate interplay between immune response and lipid metabolism is particularly relevant in light of the recent changes in dietary guidelines, emphasizing the importance of elucidating how cholesterol and the associated metabolic processes affect tuberculosis pathogenesis and host immunity (Andersen et al., 2018). This interaction between metabolism and immunity creates openings for specific therapeutic interventions. In addition, tuberculosis pathophysiology is a constant state of balance between bacterial persistence and host defense mechanisms. While macrophages strive to quench MTB by phagocytosis and cytokine production, the bacteria use intracellular niches and immune evasion mechanisms to persist. The impaired phagocytic function caused by environmental exposures like cigarette smoking worsens this standoff, facilitating continued bacterial growth and formation of granulomas. Granulomas, once protective, can become zones of necrosis and tissue destruction if immune homeostasis is lost, highlighting the precarious immunopathological equilibrium central to TB development. The increased TNF-α and CXCL-8 secretion induced by MTB infection, especially with the added effect of smoking, highlight inflammatory injury while inadequately eliminating the pathogen (Aryanpur et al., 2016). These multifactorial dysfunctions characterize the complex pathophysiological terrain of tuberculosis infection, uncovering pivotal targets for intervention and control (Figure 2.11).

2.3.1. Initial Infection and Granuloma Formation

The initiation of MTB infection starts when inhaled bacilli arrive in the alveoli, where they are engulfed by resident macrophages. This first contact is pivotal, since *Mtb* has developed mechanisms to persist and grow within phagocytic cells and to escape early immune clearance. The ability of the bacterium to survive inside macrophages creates the background for a dynamic host-pathogen interaction that coordinates the following immune response. This includes the activation of the recruitment of more immune cells to the infected site, eventually determining the typical granulomatous structure housing the bacilli and mitigating tissue damage. It is important to clarify these early occurrences to describe the pathogenesis of tuberculosis (TB) and developing interventions. The central position of immune cell recruitment in the lungs, partly by interferon regulatory factors, is critical to the development of protective granulomas and lymphoid aggregates, central to containing *Mtb* infection (Dorhoi et al., 2013). The granuloma is the diagnostic hallmark of tuberculosis, acting as both a physical barrier to restrict mycobacterial growth and an active site of immune cell interaction. At the structural level, granulomas are composed of a central cluster of infected macrophages covered by layers of different immune cells such as lymphocytes, neutrophils, and DCs. These cells' recruitment and organization are orchestrated by chemokines and cytokines that react to bacterial antigenic stimuli. Abnormalities in these regulatory mechanisms may lead to inefficiency in the formation of granulomas, promoting bacterial dissemination and increased disease severity. In model systems, a lack of critical factors such as IRF-8 abrogates immune cell homing and granuloma stability, resulting in unchecked bacterial replication and acute development of disease, demonstrating the importance of balanced immune environment during this phase (Dorhoi et al., 2013). This serves to emphasize the granuloma not only as a point of bacterial containment but also of immune modulation. Although most infected persons with *Mtb* acquire a latent infection with stable granulomas and asymptomatic bacteria containment, the outcome of the infection is determined by the early immune response as to whether to remain controlled or lead to active disease. Phagocytosis by macrophages and the neogenesis of granulomas are key determinants of infection outcomes during early immune events. The capacity of the pathogen to modulate host cell reactions within granulomas enables persistence in a latent form, evading clearance but limiting tissue damage. Under most circumstances, immune compromise or dysregulation serves to tip this balance toward the breakdown of granulomas and active disease presentation. Progress in understanding tuberculosis immunopathogenesis, particularly host-pathogen interaction during the early stages of infection and the process of granuloma formation, holds the promise of guiding new drug and vaccine regimens necessary for the battle against TB internationally (Figure 2.12).

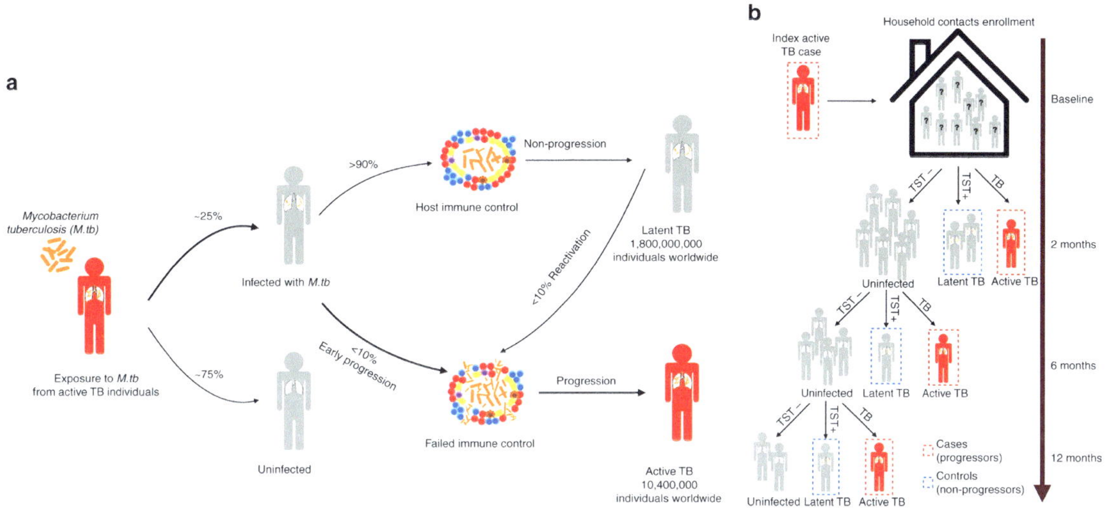

Figure 2.12. Overview of phases of *Mycobacterium tuberculosis* (MTB) infection and sample collection. (a) Pathophysiology of TB. Major steps following initial exposure to MTB are outlined, with the percentages of individuals progressing between steps taken from the WHO TB report. (b) Schema of cohort collection. In this study, we focus on a genetic comparison between recently exposed active pulmonary TB cases (progressors) and subjects with tuberculin skin test (TST) positive results who did not progress to active TB (non-progressors).

Source: Luo, Y., Suliman, S., Asgari, S. *et al.* Early progression to active tuberculosis is a highly heritable trait driven by 3q23 in Peruvians. *Nat Commun* **10**, 3765 (2019). https://doi.org/10.1038/s41467-019-11664-1

2.3.2. Progression to Active TB Disease

The shift from latent MTB infection to active tuberculosis disease is regulated by complex host-pathogen relationships that destroy the immunological harmony of latency. While latent infection, the host immune response successfully confines bacterial proliferation, mostly by organizing granulomas limited by adaptive immunity. Yet, disruptions in this immune balance can result in granuloma destruction and bacterial spread. Recent data from mouse models of human TB pathology suggest that active disease progression is associated with an increased IFN response and recruitment of neutrophils, with a simultaneous reduction in effector lymphocyte numbers including B cells, natural killer (NK) cells, and T cells. These immune changes seem to create a milieu that promotes bacterial growth and tissue destruction, thus promoting active disease development. Such cellular and transcriptional profiles, occurring both in susceptible mice and in human progressors before clinical diagnosis, illustrate the predictive and pathogenic functions of such immune changes in TB development (Moreira-Teixeira et al., 2020). Transcriptomic profiling has markedly enhanced knowledge of molecular processes leading to active tuberculosis, implicating distinct immunological signatures for risk and protection. Whole blood transcriptomics, specifically, has mapped IFN-γ-vitamin D-dependent signaling pathways that control antimicrobial defense in latent infection.

Recognizing IL-32 as a mediator in this axis highlights a characteristic immunologic protective mechanism that suppresses bacterial growth. Abrogation of these antimicrobial responses, on the other hand, can allow disease progression and cause harm. Large-scale transcriptomic datasets combined with comprehensive analyses continue to unravel the mechanisms of the complex gene networks and immune pathways involved in TB pathogenesis. Such systems biology strategies that integrate multiple disciplines are important for deciphering mechanistic determinants of progression from latent to active disease, providing potential early biomarkers of detection as well as targets for new therapeutic interventions (Deffur et al., 2015). Even with advances in delineating immune correlates, the development of active tuberculosis continues to be determined by varied host genetic, environmental, and microbial determinants that together regulate disease outcome. Differential immune signatures between resistant and susceptible subjects indicate differences in the host's ability to maintain protective responses, potentially modulated by demographic factors and comorbidities like HIV disease. Also, heterogeneity in the circulating immune cell compartment makes interpretation of transcriptomic biomarkers challenging, requiring precise inclusion of rich patient metadata to disentangle causal from correlational signals. Further development of refined integrated OMICS platforms and open data availability will increase reproducibility and the ability to identify strong correlates of protection and progression. Finally, a sophisticated assessment of such factors contributing to TB pathogenesis is crucial for the development of precision medicine interventions that prevent progression to active TB (Deffur et al., 2015; Moreira-Teixeira et al., 2020) (Figure 2.13).

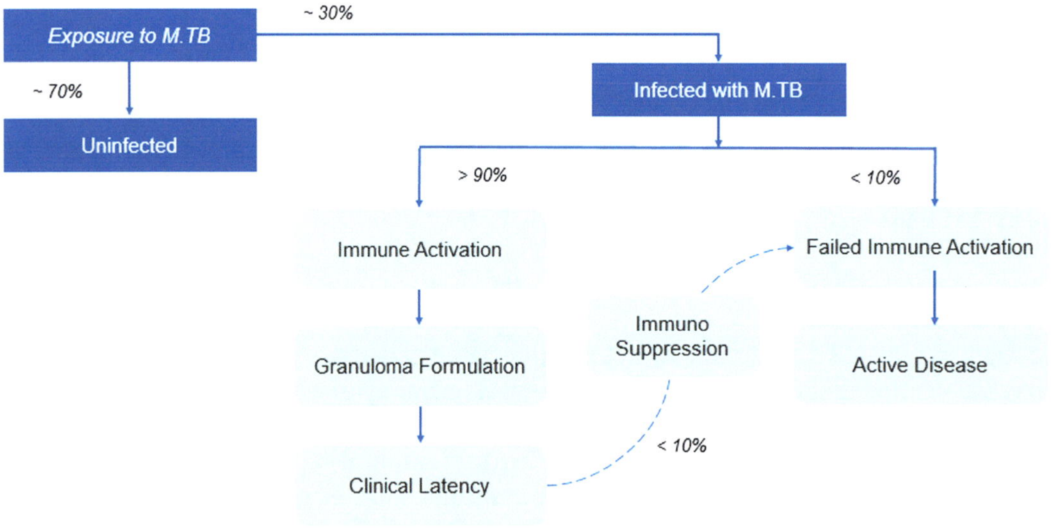

Figure 2.13. Flow chart for TB disease progression.

Source: National Tuberculosis Elimination Program (NTEP). (n.d.). *Progression of tuberculosis disease: From M. tuberculosis exposure to immune response, latency, and active disease.* https://ntep.in/te/node/509/CP-progression-tb-disease.

2.3.3. Impact of Latent Tuberculosis Infection (LTBI)

The worldwide burden of tuberculosis is inextricably associated with the immense reservoir of latent MTB infection, which exists in some one-third of the world's population. This latent form, where there are dormant bacilli without any evident clinical symptoms, is the most daunting obstacle in TB control and eradication programs. Persons with latent tuberculosis infection (LTBI) are a chronic reservoir source for future reactivation of disease, which may be induced in the presence of immune suppression or other risk exposures. Therefore, the latent form has emerged as a quiet but major driving force for continued transmission and new active TB case incidence worldwide. Notably, the latency of TB emphasizes the sophistication of host-pathogen relationships and an equilibrium state in which the bacilli are contained but not cleared by the immune system. In light of this dynamic, the certainty of latent infection requires a reevaluation on a critical basis of existing prevention and treatment measures for the successful management of this covert epidemic and the transition beyond mere control to ultimate eradication (Zumla et al., 2011). Immunologically, the LTBI establishes a singular niche in which MTB has a precarious existence in host macrophages, avoiding full immunity clearance without inhibiting uncontrolled replication. Recent studies illustrate the bivalent function of host immune responses, in this case, using IFNs, that are simultaneously able to increase bacterial growth and help in protective immunity, depending on the circumstances. The intricacy of such immune regulation superimposes levels of complexity in delving into the mechanisms of latent infection pathogenesis. Although IFNs are classically recognized for antiviral activities, their role in TB highlights the capacity of the pathogen to hijack host immunity for its benefit, facilitating persistence and occasionally disease exacerbation. Assessment of these subtle immunological interactions is important for the development of new therapeutic approaches that can tip this balance in a more desirable direction, preventing latent infection from progressing to active disease (Moreira-Teixeira et al., 2018). In a public health context, LTBI greatly inhibits the control of tuberculosis, creating a cycle of disease and infection that thwarts global efforts. Screening and chemoprophylaxis for latent TB have been effective to some extent but are limited by incomplete effectiveness and the potential for drug resistance. In addition, the biological heterogeneity of latent infection, which can range from total dormancy to low-level bacterial activity, makes identification and treatment schedules challenging. This heterogeneity suggests that one-size-fits-all strategies can be inadequate, requiring individualized management based on a better assessment of latent TB pathogenesis and its interaction with host factors. As emphasized by current controversy and unsolved issues in latent TB control, subtle policy driven by sound scientific research is essential to convert latent TB into a manageable disease from a worldwide reservoir of infection (Zumla et al., 2011).

2.4. Risk Factors for TB Development

The evolution of latent MTB infection to active tuberculosis illness is under the control of a multifactorial interaction of host and environmental factors. Although most infected patients harbor the bacteria in a latent state (about 90%), some 10% of them develop active TB, with an indication of the importance of certain risk factors that disrupt this equilibrium (Colombo et al., 2018). Immunocompromising diseases like HIV infection significantly enhance the risk of TB activation by downregulating the cellular immune response of the host, especially in macrophages and monocytes where *Mtb* exists and multiplies. Malnutrition, diabetes, and smoking also weaken immune defenses, creating an environment for bacterial growth. Socioeconomic conditions, such as overcrowding and poor ventilation, enable transmission and cycles of reinfection, which aggravate TB development on a population level. Knowledge of these risk determinants is essential to focused prevention strategies and enhancing curative outcomes in settings with heavy burdens of tuberculosis disease. The immune response's contribution to regulating tuberculosis infection identifies why specific predispositions of a clinical or genetic nature enhance disease susceptibility. Sophisticated transcriptomic studies confirm that immune regulators like IFN-γ and the vitamin D pathway are important in sustaining MTB containment (Deffur et al., 2015). Disturbance of these pathways by genetic polymorphisms or external insults such as vitamin D deficiency is detrimental to macrophage activation and antimicrobial activity, thus facilitating the conversion from latent to active TB. Transcriptomic data also indicate differential gene expression for inflammation and immune regulation genes that are associated with risk stratification in infected populations. These observations on immune correlates show that risk factors, far from being external, are closely embedded in the molecular processes that control host-pathogen interactions. This identification of individuals with weakened immune profiles could guide precision medicine strategies toward TB prevention. Environmental and demographic factors further synergistically add to the risk of developing tuberculosis, frequently synergizing with host immunological weaknesses. Epidemiological findings highlight that populations residing in crowded or resource-constrained environments have a greater TB incidence owing to chronic exposure and poor access to healthcare (Colombo et al., 2018). Another important aspect is age; infants and the elderly have diminished immune capacity, making them more susceptible to active disease. Concurrent concomitant diseases like diabetes mellitus (DM) provide a pro-inflammatory environment favoring *Mtb* growth, whereas drug abuse and low compliance with treatment enhance the risk of treatment failure and the development of resistant organisms. These multifactorial risks underscore the importance of an holistic public health approach that brings social determinants together with biological susceptibility in the fight against tuberculosis. Unless all these layered influences are tackled, attempts at controlling TB pathogenesis are incomplete (Figure 2.14).

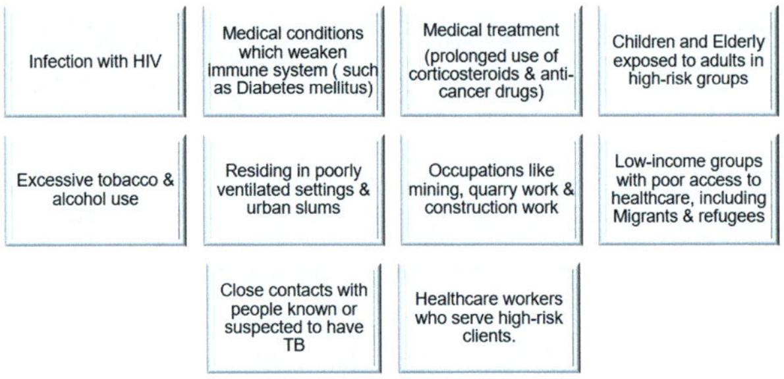

Figure 2.14. Risk factors for developing active TB.

Source: National Tuberculosis Elimination Program (NTEP). (n.d.). *Risk factors for tuberculosis disease: Medical, environmental, occupational, and social determinants.* https://ntep.in/node/326/CP-risk-factors-tb-disease.

2.4.1. Socioeconomic Factors

Socioeconomic status has a significant impact on the pathogenesis of tuberculosis by creating the environments in which MTB interacts with human hosts. Poor living conditions and poor ventilation, usually common in low socioeconomic communities, allow for airborne transmission of the *Bacillus*, with rates of exposure and risk of infection being higher. Malnutrition, usually found in low socioeconomic status, further weakens the immune defenses of the host, with the ability to keep latent infections under control compromised and susceptibility to active disease heightened. These variables intersect with general social determinants of limited healthcare access, delayed diagnosis, and treatment breaks, all aggravating the advancement and spreading of disease. Hence, the socioeconomic environment provides fertile soil for the bacterium's evolutionary adaptation and maintenance in susceptible populations, highlighting the need for holistic strategies that tackle both biological and social aspects of tuberculosis control (Lin & Koskella, 2014). In addition to physical risk factors, psychosocial stressors that are common among low socioeconomic populations have a strong modulatory impact on immune responses pertinent to the pathogenesis of tuberculosis. Mental unwellness, social loneliness, and chronic stress have been shown to weaken cellular immunity, which is pivotal in limiting MTB infection. There is evidence that negative psychosocial climates can reduce the effectiveness of vaccines, especially the BCG vaccine, and shift the biomarker profile of the host toward infection resistance. Positive psychosocial elements like social support have also been found to be associated with increased immune responsiveness. These observations underscore the importance of taking psychosocial dimensions on board as an integral part of host-pathogen interactions in tuberculosis, exposing an added mechanistic dimension through which socioeconomic conditions affect disease outcomes (Hayward et al., 2019). The complex interaction between socioeconomic determinants and pathogenesis of tuberculosis clarifies the multifaceted nature of challenges in disease prevention and control. Poverty-related environmental exposures not only enable primary infection and reinfection but also intersect psychosocial stress pathways that dampen immunity and activate disease. These interconnected influences require interventions beyond the purview of medical therapy, calls for social protection programs that alleviate economic distress, enhance living standards, and address mental health. Incorporating socioeconomic factors into tuberculosis research and public health policy can facilitate an understanding of the pathogen's persistence in poor populations as well as enhance outcomes through intervention on upstream social determinants. This integrated view is consistent with evolutionary perspectives on host-bacterial dynamics, highlighting that the bacterium's pathogenicity is shaped by immediate biological determinants as well as more extensive socioeconomic conditions (Lin & Koskella, 2014; Hayward et al., 2019;).

2.4.2. Co-Morbid Conditions (e.g., HIV)

The interaction of TB with co-morbid conditions contributes meaningfully to the natural history and outcome of TB disease. Of these, HIV infection is a leading risk factor that modifies the immune environment, promoting the reactivation of latent TB and hastening the course of disease. Immunosuppression caused by HIV lowers the ability of the host to hold MTB at bay, promoting a more virulent and disseminated presentation of TB. Therefore, TB continues to be the leading cause of death in HIV-infected individuals, making both diagnosis and treatment complicated. This double burden increases public health issues, especially in high-prevalence areas of both infections, highlighting the importance of combined management approaches. Additionally, the co-existence of other comorbidities, including DM, further aggravates disease severity by inhibiting immune function, resulting in delayed bacterial clearance and enhanced vulnerability to severe disease in TB patients. The introduction of highly active antiretroviral therapy (HAART) has revolutionized the clinical profile of HAART-HIV and TB co-infected patients. HAART improves immunity and decreases HIV viral burden, which subsequently contributes to better control of TB infection. Studies have documented that renal function significantly improves in HAART-treated HIV-positive patients, even when HIV-associated nephropathy is present, a prevalent co-morbid condition among these patients (Rahmanian et al., 2015). However, the initiation of HAART in TB-HIV co-infected patients is still key; early treatment will prevent immunosuppression but could enhance the risk of immune reconstitution inflammatory syndrome (IRIS), which exacerbates TB pathology. Therefore, knowledge of the immune interactions and complications resulting from the presence of comorbid conditions is crucial for maximizing therapeutic interventions and survival rates among this at-risk population. The intersection of TB and HIV infection enhances mortality and poses special challenges in disease pathogenesis management and outcome treatment worldwide. Deaths due to TB continue to be significant in developing nations, wherein HIV prevalence enhances vulnerability to poor tuberculosis and associated mortality (Olaleye & Beke, 2018). The impairment of HIV on cell-mediated immunity allows for unchecked mycobacterial dissemination that precipitates extrapulmonary tuberculosis (EPTB), which is more difficult to diagnose and treat. In addition, HIV co-morbid conditions like chronic kidney disease add complexity to disease management in terms of drug metabolism and tolerance. An intensive knowledge of the pathogenesis in the context of TB-HIV co-morbidity will help inform public health policy and formulate targeted interventions designed to tackle these concordant epidemics, ultimately curbing TB morbidity and mortality globally (Figure 2.15).

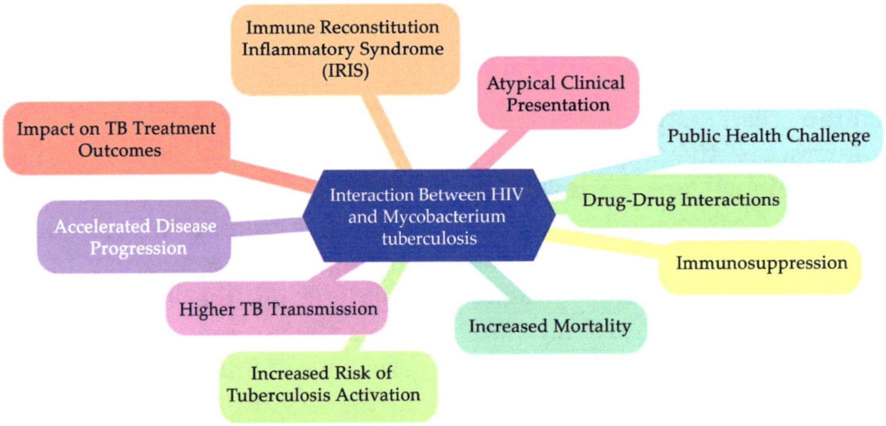

Figure 2.15. The interaction between HIV and *Mycobacterium tuberculosis.*

Source: Patel A, Pundkar A, Agarwal A, et al. (September 06, 2024) A Comprehensive Review of HIV-Associated Tuberculosis: Clinical Challenges and Advances in Management. Cureus 16(9): e68784. doi:10.7759/cureus.68784

2.4.3. Environmental Factors Influencing TB Spread

The complex interaction between the pathogen's biology and its environmental context significantly impacts tuberculosis's progression and transmission. MTB, the TB-causing organism, is exposed to several adverse environmental conditions after being expelled from the host via aerosols. The bacilli become subject to several conditions after being aerosolized, including humidity, temperature, and ultraviolet light, which decisively influence their viability for infecting new hosts. Within the human host, MTB is exposed to an ever-changing environment dependent upon immune reactions and tissue microenvironments producing a wide range of DNA-damaging entities. These stressors require strong bacterial DNA repair, which is utilized by MTB to maintain viability and resilience throughout stages of infection. The dynamic regulation of DNA repair genes during infection underscores the pathogen's capacity to adjust to these fluctuating environmental stresses, hence enabling persistence and successful transmission between host populations (Gorna et al., 2010). Such adaptive resilience attests to the multifaceted nature of environmental factors in TB pathogenesis.

Human behaviors and animal-human contact tend to lead to environmental conditions that enable tuberculosis transmission, especially at the wildlife-livestock interface. Where cattle and wildlife live together, like the Queen Elizabeth National Park in Uganda, illegal grazing and common grazing or watering points set the stage for interspecies encounters. While frequent aerosol transmission between wildlife, such as African buffalo, and cattle is unlikely because of the lack of close proximity, indirect avenues of transmission are still possible. Frequent aggregation of several cattle herds at shared facilities creates a network for possible disease transmission. These environmental conditions control the epidemiology of bovine tuberculosis, making control in multi-host systems more challenging. It is important to understand these dynamics because interventions focusing on the wildlife-livestock interface can have minimal effects on disease control when eradication is not possible, demonstrating the importance of environmental context in TB transmission (Meunier et al., 2017).

In addition to biotic determinants, structural and socioeconomic settings within human populations are equally important in influencing TB transmission patterns. The conditions of overcrowding, inadequate ventilation, and poor sanitation provide favorable environments for MTB airborne transmission. Urban slums and high-density populations place individuals at greater risk as close contact overcrowding with infected people favors spread. Furthermore, malnutrition and environmental pollutants are detractors of host immunity, which in turn boosts susceptibility to infection and disease development. These factors are what guide public health responses aimed at enhancing living conditions and lessening the risk of exposure. All these environmental determinants, which vary from microbial survival strategies through wildlife interactions and human socio-ecological environments, ultimately provide a holistic framework that is necessary to grasp the pathogenesis and control of tuberculosis.

2.5. Treatment and Management

Successful treatment and control of tuberculosis depend on the early detection and prompt initiation of correct antimicrobial therapy. The recommended first-line therapeutic regimen utilizes a combination of antitubercular drugs to counteract the organism's intracellular persistence and avoid drug resistance development. With extrapulmonary manifestations like tuberculous meningitis (TBM), therapeutic complexity is heightened because of the challenge of attaining sufficient drug penetration into the CNS. Adjunct corticosteroid therapy has proven to modulate the inflammatory process and lower mortality in TBM, emphasizing the importance of such management strategies being tailored according to disease presentation. New diagnostic technologies, such as next-generation sequencing (NGS), also assist in the early identification of drug-resistant strains, allowing for better, tailored treatment strategies. Even with these developments, there are significant challenges, especially in resource-poor contexts where delays in diagnosis lead to worse outcomes (Oo & Agarwal et al, 2025). Post-tuberculosis lung disease (PTLD) management highlights the long-term consequences of tuberculosis beyond microbiological cure. Residual pulmonary impairment from fibrosis, bronchiectasis, and cavitation tends to leave chronic respiratory symptoms necessitating continuing clinical management. Pulmonary rehabilitation is an important intervention for restoring functional capacity and enhancing the quality of life in patients with PTLD. Effective pharmacological therapy to control symptoms and prevent secondary infections must also be modified according to the extent of lung damage and comorbidities of the patient. Surgical therapy can be indicated in certain situations where localized disease importantly impairs respiratory mechanics. The issue is with full follow-up and care that goes beyond microbiological resolution, which places stress on the need for integrated health strategies in tuberculosis control schemes (Yadav et al., 2024). Host-directed therapies (HDTs) are a promising future in tuberculosis treatment and management by modulating the host immune system to augment clinical care. These adjunctive techniques are designed to maximize the effectiveness of antimicrobial therapies by modulating inflammation, minimizing tissue injury, and promoting pathogen removal. For TBM, experimental treatments such as nanoparticle drug delivery and intrathecal delivery attempt to maximize drug bioavailability in the CNS. Antioxidant and immune modulator application also have promise in reducing neural damage resulting from granulomatous inflammation. While welcoming the initial encouraging results, bringing these new treatments into standard clinical practice demands strong evidence from large clinical trials. In the meantime, tackling social determinants and compliance with multidrug regimens continue to be key to the effective treatment of tuberculosis and its complications (Oo & Agarwale, 2025).

2.5.1. First-Line Anti-TB Medications

Grasping the efficient control and cure of tuberculosis (TB) requires a wide-ranging analysis of antibiotics as the pillar for disease management. The first-line anti-TB drugs play a pivotal role in arresting the development of both latent and active TB, particularly pulmonary tuberculosis (PTB), which accounts for most infections. These medications, such as isoniazid, rifampicin, ethambutol, and pyrazinamide (PZA), focus on different aspects of the MTB disease pathogen's biology, inhibiting its ability to grow and survive within the macrophages of the host. The significance of these drugs not only lies in their bactericidal action but also in the fact that they shorten the infectious phase, hence restricting transmission among communities. The stringent treatment regimens required to avoid relapse and resistance emphasize the intricacy of TB pathogenesis and attest to the need for compliance with such protocols to achieve successful eradication of the disease (Al-Asady & Ali, 2023).

Lines	Grouping	Drugs	
First-line anti-TB drugs	Group 1 (oral)	Isoniazid (H/INH)	
		Rifampicin/rifampin (R/RIF)	
		Pyrazinamide (Z/PZA)	
		Ethambutol (E/EMB)	
		Rifapentine (P/RPT)	
		Rifabutin (RFB)	
Second-line anti-TB drugs	Group 2 (injectable)	Aminoglycosides	Streptomycin (S/STM)
			Kanamycin (KM)
			Amikacin (AMK)
		Polypeptides	Capreomycin (CM)
			Viomycin (VIM)
	Group 3 (oral and injectable; fluoroquinolones)	Ciprofloxacin (cfx)	
		Levofloxacin (lfx)	
		Moxifloxacin (mfx)	
		Ofloxacin (OFX)	
		Gatifloxacin (GFX)	
	Group 4 (oral)	Para-aminosalicylic acid (PAS)	
		Cycloserine (DCS)	
		Terizidone (TRD)	
		Ethionamide (ETO)	
		Prothionamide (PTO)	
		Thioacetazone (THZ)	
		Linezolid (LZD)	
Third-line anti-TB drugs	Group 5 (oral and injectable)	Clofazimine (CFZ)	
		Linezolid (LZD)	
		Amoxicillin plus clavulanate (AMX/CLV)	
		Imipenem plus cilastatin (IPM/CLN)	
		Clarithromycin (CLR)	

Figure 2.16. First-line anti-TB drugs.

Source: Al-Humadi HW, Al-Saigh RJ and Al-Humadi AW (2017) Addressing the Challenges of Tuberculosis: A Brief Historical Account. Front. Pharmacol. 8:689. doi: 10.3389/fphar.2017.00689

The mode of action by which first-line anti-TB drugs act is closely related to the distinctive cellular structure and metabolic activities of

MTB. Isoniazid, for instance, inhibits mycolic acid synthesis, a vital cell wall component of the bacterium that provides resistance to inimical host environments (Figure 2.16).

Rifampicin inhibits DNA-dependent RNA polymerase and consequently stops transcription and bacterial replication. PZA interferes with energy metabolism and membrane potential, with special activity against latent bacterial populations within acidic niches like within macrophages. Ethambutol inhibits the polymerization of arabinogalactan and thereby the integrity of the cell wall. These complementary but unique mechanisms emphasize the effectiveness of modulating the pathogen's biological vulnerabilities to counter TB infection and thereby demonstrate their applicability in both the therapeutic treatment of the disease and deciphering its pathogenesis (Al-Asady & Ali, 2023). The therapeutic use of first-line anti-TB drugs needs to take challenges from drug resistance and patient compliance into account.

Drug classification	Groups	Anti-TB drugs	Mechanism of action	Target TB	Efficacy	Mechanism of resistance	References
Cell envelope synthesis inhibitor	Peptidoglycan	Cycloserine	Inhibit 2 enzymes forming D-alanine residues	MDR, XDR	High	Mutations in *alrA*	Patel et al., 2012
		Terizidone	Cycloserine derivative	MDR, XDR	High	Non	Galietti et al., 1991
	Arabinogalactan	Ethambutol	Inhibiting arabinosyltransferase, arabinose acceptor	Active	Low	*embCAB* operon	Telenti et al., 1997; Wolucka, 2008
	Mycolic acid	Isoniazid	Activation katG enzyme and inhibits inhA gene	Active, latent	High	Mutations in *katG* and *inhA* genes	Vilche'ze and Jacobs, 2007; Riccardi et al., 2009
		Triclosan	Inhibits the inhA enzyme without activation katG	MDR	Low	–	Wang et al., 2004; Freundlich et al., 2009
		Pyridomycin	Inhibits the inhA enzyme	MDR, XDR	High	Mutations in *inha*	Hartkoorn et al., 2012
		Ethionamide	Inhibits InhA by enzyme ethA	MDR, XDR	High	Mutations in *inha*, *etha*	Wolff and Nguyen, 2012
		Prothionamide	Inhibits InhA by enzyme ethA	MDR, XDR	High	Mutations in *etha*	Wang et al., 2007
		Thiocarlide	Inhibiting synthesis of oleic acid	MDR, XDR	High	Mutations in *ethA*	Phetsuksiri et al., 2003
		Delamanid	Releasing Nitric oxide by Ddn enzyme	Active, latent, MDR, XDR	High	Non	Gler et al., 2012, Zhang et al., 2013
		SQ109	Membrane transporter *MmpL3*	Active, latent	High	Non	Owens et al., 2013
Protein synthesis inhibitor	Aminoglycosides	Streptomycin	Bind to 30S subunit of ribosome	MDR, XDR	High	Mutation in *rpsl*	Honort and Cole, 1994
		Amikacin	Bind to 30S subunit of ribosome	MDR, XDR	High	Mutation in *rrs*	Sowajassatakul et al., 2014
		Kanamycin	Bind to 30S subunit of ribosome	MDR, XDR	High	Mutation in *rrs*	Sowajassatakul et al., 2014
	Oxazolidone	Linezolid	Bind to 50S subunit of ribosome	MDR, XDR	High	Mutation in *G2576T*(23S)	Scheetz et al., 2008
		Sutezolid	Bind to 50S subunit of ribosome	MDR, XDR	High	Non	Zumla et al., 2015
	Peptidoglycan	Capreomycin	Peptidoglycan Breakdown	MDR, XDR	High	Mutation in *tlyA*	Chen et al., 2003
Nucleic acid inhibitor	Rifamycins	Rifampicin	RNA polymerase inhibitor	Active, latent	Low	Mutations in *rpoB* gene	Sensi, 1983; Telenti et al., 1993
		Rifapentine	RNA polymerase inhibitor (b-subunit)	Active, latent/HIV	High	Mutations in *rpoB* gene	Chan et al., 2014
		Rifabutin	RNA polymerase inhibitor (b-subunit)	Active, latent/HIV	High	Mutations in *rpoB* gene	Yan et al., 2015
		Rifalazil	RNA polymerase inhibitor (b-subunit)	Active, latent/HIV	High	Mutations in *rpoB* gene	Saribaş et al., 2003
	PAS	PAS	Folic acid synth inhibitor	MDR, XDR	High	Mutations in *thyA*	Patel et al., 2012
	Quinolones	Levofloxacin	DNA gyrase inhibitor	MDR, XDR	High	Mutations in *gyrA*	Pranger et al., 2011
		Moxifloxacin	DNA gyrase inhibitor	MDR, XDR	High	Mutations in *gyrA*	Pranger et al., 2011
New drugs		Bedaquiline	Inhibiting ATP synthase enzyme	Active, MDR, dorment,XDR	High	Mutations in *atpE* gene	Chan et al., 2013; Chahine et al., 2014
		Pyrazinamide	Interferes with binding to mRNA	Active,MDR	High	Mutations in *RpsA*, *pncA*	Zhang et al., 2003; Shi et al., 2011
		Clofazimine	Inhibits DNA replication	MDR, XDR/HIV	High	Mutations in *rv0678*	Arbiser and Moschella, 1995

PAS:para aminosalicylic acid.

Figure 2.17. First and second-line anti-tubercular (ATT) drugs.

Source: Al-Humadi HW, Al-Saigh RJ and Al-Humadi AW (2017) Addressing the Challenges of Tuberculosis: A Brief Historical Account. Front. Pharmacol. 8:689. doi: 10.3389/fphar.2017.00689

The development of multi-drug resistant tuberculosis (MDR-TB), fueled by target gene mutations and poor treatment compliance, endangers the effectiveness of these older drugs. Resistance typically develops when the long treatment duration, usually six months or longer, is cut short, with the survival of resistant subpopulations of bacteria. Therefore, public health practice puts its focus not only on the utilization of the first-line medicines but also on strict supervision of the treatment, such as directly observed treatment, short-course (DOTS) programs to monitor adherence. These treatments highlight the relationship between TB's pathogenesis, specifically the ability of the bacteria to endure and adapt, and the clinical need for effective treatment regimens with these first-line drugs (Al-Asady & Ali, 2023) (Figure 2.17).

2.5.2. Challenges in TB Treatment (e.g., Drug Resistance)

Treatment of tuberculosis has grown more complicated in the recent past, mainly because of drug-resistant strains. The MDR-TB and extensively drug-resistant tuberculosis (XDR-TB) have considerably weakened conventional treatment regimes, creating significant hurdles to successful control of the disease. The newer pharmacological compounds like bedaquiline and delamanid are notable developments, offering alternative options targeting resistant strains. Yet, their use has to be tightly controlled to avoid the quick development of additional resistance. Combination therapies have been shown in clinical trials to be promising, such as the BPaLM regimen, which combines bedaquiline, pretomanid, linezolid, and moxifloxacin, to better treat resistant cases. These advances notwithstanding, treatment complexity, side effects, and long duration persist as obstacles to patient compliance, fueling resistance growth. Continued international efforts at drug development, drug surveillance, and drug-taking strategies are still essential to surmount these therapeutic barriers to tuberculosis control (Shah & Shah, 2024). Compounding the challenge to controlling drug resistance is limited knowledge of the bacterium's pathogenesis in the human host, which inhibits the design of targeted interventions. The complex interaction between host immune responses and MTB makes the pathogen persistent and challenging to eradicate entirely. Recent efforts such as controlled human infection models (CHIM) seek to untangle the complex host-pathogen interactions, and in the process, open doors to new treatment and prevention options. While these models are technically and safety-wise challenging, genetically modified tuberculosis strain advances and live attenuated mycobacteria provide promising routes for encouraging new therapeutic gains. These models would expedite vaccine design and enhance drug efficacy testing by more closely simulating natural infection conditions and, in the long run, alleviating some of the basic impediments in TB treatment innovation due to inadequate pathogenesis know-how (Gordon et al., 2023). Besides pharmacological and biological problems, socio-economic reasons also play a significant role in causing problems in treating tuberculosis, particularly in areas with poor healthcare infrastructure. Long treatment regimens and side effects of second-line drugs usually lead to poor patient compliance, maximizing the risk of incomplete treatment and, as a consequence, secondary drug resistance emergence. Poor diagnostic facilities further delay proper treatment, fueling the bacterial survival and transmission process. Public health interventions aimed at these systemic challenges are imperative, such as the use of rapid diagnostic technologies, patient education, and community support schemes to improve adherence. Combination with innovative nanotechnologies and drug delivery systems is also under investigation for minimizing toxicity and enhancing drug availability, potentially shortening treatment duration and optimizing patient outcomes. The defeat of the multifactorial nature of TB treatment challenges calls for a multidisciplinary solution synthesizing scientific innovation and sound healthcare policy (Shah & Shah, 2024).

2.5.3. Public Health Strategies for TB Control

Successful control of tuberculosis (TB) in communities depends on early detection and focused intervention, which in turn is based on comprehension of the pathogenesis of the disease. Diagnostic methods play a crucial role in detecting both LTBI and active disease. The American Thoracic Society and CDC emphasize diagnostic methods using tuberculin skin tests (TSTs) and microbiologic testing to differentiate states of infection properly. These categories are crucial to implement proper treatment regimens, reducing the development of latent infection to active disease. Public health programs utilizing these diagnostic criteria improve case finding among high-risk groups, such as immunocompromised patients and those who are in close contact with active cases of TB. Accordingly, such frameworks not only simplify clinical management but also promote efficient public health interventions directed at decreasing transmission, thereby slowing down incidence rates and interrupting the chain of infection (American Thoracic Society Committee on Revision of Diagnostic Standards, 2025). Concurrently with diagnostic accuracy, the application of coordinated surveillance and control strategies is key to interrupting TB transmission. Lessons learned from the control of bovine tuberculosis in Swedish reindeer herds illuminate challenges and solutions that are also relevant to human TB control. Careful monitoring and testing, for example, tuberculin skin testing conducted by experienced staff—are required to find infected carriers and exclude outbreaks. Test administration variability can circumvent these efforts, highlighting the value of quality control and practitioner training to ensure accuracy. In addition, modeling infection spread to estimate and model approaches for evaluating intervention efficiency assists in planning sustainable control programs. They guide testing frequency decisions, isolation policies, and resource deployment in endemic populations. Therefore, complementing epidemiological knowledge with stringent testing facilities facilitates a holistic strategy for dealing with the prevalence of TB (Wahlström et al., 2004). A second pillar of TB public health policy is the integration of preventive therapy with community education and socioeconomic measures. Because tuberculosis pathogenesis includes a latent phase, prophylactic treatment of persons with latent infection is requisite to minimize progression to active disease. Educational campaigns enhance awareness of routes of transmission and symptoms, stimulating early seeking of health care and compliance with treatment. Social determinants, including overcrowding, malnutrition, and restricted access to health care, are further addressed, decreasing exposure to infection and stimulating generalized resilience to TB. Public health interventions that combine biomedical approaches with social support structures have been effective across diverse settings. These multi-component strategies recognize the complex interaction between the biology of the pathogen and the environment, which eventually seeks to reduce the burden of TB on global public health systems (Wahlström et al., 2004; American Thoracic Society Committee on Revision of Diagnostic Standards, 2025).

Summary

Deciphering the complex host immune response-MTB interplay is the key to the furtherance of tuberculosis science and improved patient outcomes. The pathogenesis of tuberculosis entails complex immune mechanisms that both contain and propagate the disease process. The development of high-throughput technologies, particularly transcriptomic profiling, has revealed more refined insights into the molecular signatures of various stages of tuberculosis infection. These have identified key mediators, for example, IL-32, that could potentially act as correlates of protection and guide future therapeutic and diagnostic approaches. Combining OMICS data with rigorously characterized clinical metadata is a promising path to deciphering the enigmatic correlates of protective immunity that are critical to the development of efficient vaccines and innovative treatment modalities (Deffur et al., 2015). In addition, the dualistic function of IFNs in tuberculosis pathogenesis highlights the importance of careful understanding in therapeutic targeting. Although these cytokines have established antiviral activities, their role in MTB infection is dualistic, with the potential to enhance bacterial growth and disease exacerbation in certain situations but with protective activities in others. This dichotomy highlights a key problem of tuberculosis research: identifying the context-dependent mechanisms through which immune reactions exacerbate or restrain pathology. Developments from transcriptional and experimental models have started to deconstruct these challenges, but a key necessity remains to define the specific immunological thresholds that turn protection into disease (Moreira-Teixeira et al., 2018). Such information would dramatically enhance the specificity of modulator interventions of host immunity. Tuberculosis pathogenesis is a complex biological process characterized by sophisticated interactions of host and pathogen that still puzzle scientific knowledge. The convergence of systems biology methods, including transcriptomics, with conventional immunological expertise provides unequaled opportunities to unravel the intrinsic mechanisms that control disease susceptibility and resistance. Future studies should emphasize establishing complete, multidimensional platforms for sharing data and meta-analyses to maximize the potential of current and future datasets. Through the lens of key correlates of protection and contextual functions of immune mediators, the science will move towards more accurate, personalized, and potent interventions to counter this chronic global health challenge (Deffur et al., 2015; Moreira-Teixeira et al., 2018).

The complex interaction between host genes and immune responses essentially defines the pathogenesis of tuberculosis (TB). Current research accentuates how genetic variants affect cytokine generation essential for the control of MTB infection. Genomic variations in *REL* and *BHLHE40* are now identified to modulate levels of IL-12 and IL-10, cytokines pivotal in the pro-inflammatory versus regulatory immune pathways balance. These genetic determinants are not only associated with the innate immune system but also influence adaptive immunity, as seen in varied T-cell responses to the BCG vaccine. These observations reinforce the understanding that genetic variation in an individual can determine susceptibility to TB and clinical status, which is very important in understanding the mechanisms of disease as well as therapeutic targets (Javeed et al., 2022). This enhanced comprehension interoperates molecular immunology and clinical epidemiology, enhancing the knowledge needed for more tailored interventions in TB treatment. In addition to genetic control, social determinants and system factors also have a complex impact on the transmission and control of tuberculosis, especially in times of public health emergency. Equity becomes a central principle for comprehending TB pathogenesis at the population level since socioeconomic inequalities disproportionately affect vulnerable populations. These differences tend to be compounded by poor data collection and a lack of disaggregated health surveillance, which impedes the detection and response to disease burden inequities. Finland's experience of the COVID-19 pandemic is a good example of how wide-ranging health registers can support equity-based interventions. However, there are wide gaps in data capture in those groups that are marginalized and excluded, including undocumented immigrants and racialized minorities, which could mirror gaps observed in TB control programs. Combining social epidemiological insights with preparedness in the health system is thus crucial for remedying both biological and societal determinants of TB pathogenesis. Synthesizing these points of importance discloses a complex recognition of tuberculosis pathogenesis involving molecular, immunological, and social aspects. At the molecular level, the discovery of SNPs that influence cytokine signaling pathways offers a basis for the explanation of individual susceptibility and immune dynamics of TB infection. At the same time, social and structural determinants identified by health system data underscore the need for equity-driven responses to prevent TB's toll, particularly on vulnerable populations. The coming together of these findings necessitates an integrated approach to TB research and intervention, which brings together genetic and immunological progress with strong, comprehensive public health approaches. This integration could maximize early diagnosis and individualized therapeutic interventions, and eventually reduce the inequalities fueling TB's longevity around the world (Javeed et al., 2022).

CLOSER LOOK

DISSEMINATION (MILIARY TB)

Miliary TB is an uncommon but aggressive presentation of disseminated TB that follows widespread hematogenous dissemination of MTB. The condition is so named based on the millet seed-like radiographic appearance of multiple tiny nodules on chest X-rays or CT scans. Miliary TB may involve several organs at once, including the lungs, liver, spleen, bone marrow, and CNS.

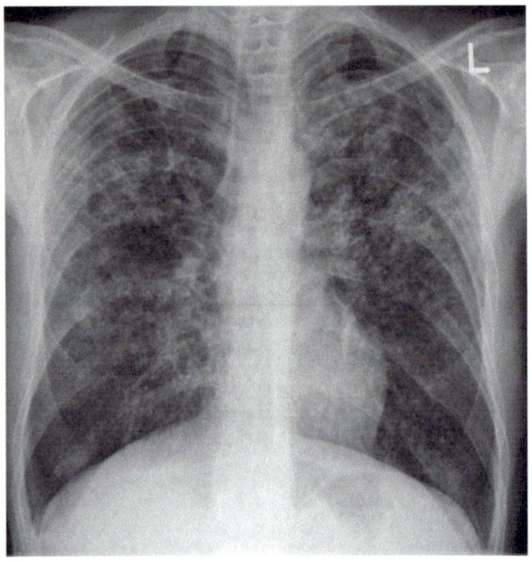

Source: By James Heilman, MD - Own work, CC BY-SA 4.0, https://commons.wikimedia.org/w/index.php?curid=49082178

The condition occurs when TB bacilli enter the bloodstream in increased numbers, usually as a result of the failure of the immune system to suppress a primary infection or the reactivation of a latent TB. Disseminated spreading causes a systemic infection and occurs most frequently among young children, older adults, and immunocompromised persons, for example, HIV/AIDS patients or those receiving immunosuppressive therapy. Clinically, miliary TB mimics non-specific symptoms like prolonged fever, night sweats, weight loss, and fatigue. Respiratory manifestations in the form of cough or dyspnea may also be seen. In severe disease, hepatosplenomegaly, lymphadenopathy, and organ dysfunction signs may manifest. Miliary TB is frequently under-diagnosed or diagnosed late because of its non-characteristic presentation. This results in high morbidity and mortality. Diagnosis is based on a blend of clinical suspicion, imaging (particularly chest radiography, presenting with miliary nodules), microbiological documentation (sputum or blood culture, PCR), and histopathology in cases of need. IGRAs and TSTs can aid the diagnosis but become negative in advanced disease because of anergy. Treatment consists of the routine four-drug anti-TB regimen (isoniazid, rifampicin, pyrazinamide, and ethambutol) for at least six months, with prolonged courses in extrapulmonary disease. Corticosteroids are employed in CNS involvement or severe inflammation. Miliary TB is an emergency condition that needs rapid diagnosis and treatment. Early identification and management are important to enhance the outcome of the patient and avert fatal complications.

References

1. Gardner, M. B., & Luciw, P. A. (2008). Macaque models of human infectious disease. *ILAR journal*, *49*(2), 220–255. https://doi.org/10.1093/ilar.49.2.220
2. Modlin R. L. (2012). Innate immunity: ignored for decades, but not forgotten. *The Journal of investigative dermatology*, *132*(3 Pt 2), 882–886. https://doi.org/10.1038/jid.2011.373
3. Gorna, A. E., Bowater, R. P., & Dziadek, J. (2010). DNA repair systems and the pathogenesis of Mycobacterium tuberculosis: varying activities at different stages of infection. *Clinical science (London, England : 1979)*, *119*(5), 187–202. https://doi.org/10.1042/CS20100041 (accessed on 10 May 2025).
4. Aryanpur, M., Mortaz, E., Masjedi, M. R., Tabarsi, P., Garssen, J., Adcock, I. M., Mozafarian, A., & Sharifi, H. (2016). Reduced Phagocytic Capacity of Blood Monocyte/Macrophages in Tuberculosis Patients Is Further Reduced by Smoking. *Iranian journal of allergy, asthma, and immunology*, *15*(3), 174–182. (accessed on 10 May 2025).
5. Al-Asady, I. N., & Ali, J. F. (2023). Review article: Virulence factors of *Mycobacterium tuberculosis*. https://core.ac.uk/download/597862363.pdf Al-Asady, I. N., & Ali, J. F. (2023). Review Article: Virulence Factors of Mycobacterium Tuberculosis. *Journal for Research in Applied Sciences and Biotechnology*, *2*(3), 221–237. https://doi.org/10.55544/jrasb.2.3.31 (accessed on 10 May 2025).
6. Alipoor, S. D., & Elieh-Ali-Komi, D. (2024). Significance of extracellular vesicles in orchestration of immune responses in *Mycobacterium tuberculosis* infection. *Frontiers in cellular and infection microbiology*, *14*, 1398077. https://doi.org/10.3389/fcimb.2024.1398077(accessed on 10 May 2025).
7. American Thoracic Society Committee on Revision of Diagnostic Standards. (2025). Diagnostic standards and classification of tuberculosis in adults and children. https://core.ac.uk/download/144158659.pdf (accessed on 10 May 2025).
8. Andersen, C. J. (2018). Impact of dietary cholesterol on the pathophysiology of infectious and autoimmune disease. https://core.ac.uk/download/268550158.pdf (accessed on 10 May 2025).
9. Apt, A., Götz, A., Zumla, A., Wolf, A. J., Alisaac, A., Howie, B., et al. (2015). Susceptibility to tuberculosis is associated with variants in the *ASAP1* gene encoding a regulator of dendritic cell migration. *Nature Genetics, 47*(5), 523–527. https://core.ac.uk/download/77018498.pdf (accessed on 10 May 2025).
10. Zumla, A., Atun, R., Maeurer, M., Mwaba, P., Ma, Z., O'Grady, J., Bates, M., Dheda, K., Hoelscher, M., & Grange, J. (2011). Viewpoint: Scientific dogmas, paradoxes and mysteries of latent Mycobacterium tuberculosis infection. *Tropical medicine & international health : TM & IH*, *16*(1), 79–83. https://doi.org/10.1111/j.1365-3156.2010.02665.x (accessed on 10 May 2025).
11. Olaleye, A., & Beke, A. (2018). Determinants of Survival of Patients with Tuberculosis in Developing Countries. InTech. doi: 10.5772/intechopen.75890 (accessed on 10 May 2025).
12. Hayward, S. E., Dowd, J. B., Fletcher, H., Nellums, L. B., Wurie, F., & Boccia, D. (2019). A systematic review of the impact of psychosocial factors on immunity: Implications for enhancing BCG response against tuberculosis. *SSM - population health*, *10*, 100522. https://doi.org/10.1016/j.ssmph.2019.100522 (accessed on 10 May 2025).

13. Li, M. S., Monahan, I. M., Waddell, S. J., Mangan, J. A., Martin, S. L., Everett, M. J., & Butcher, P. D. (2001). cDNA-RNA subtractive hybridization reveals increased expression of mycocerosic acid synthase in intracellular Mycobacterium bovis BCG. *Microbiology (Reading, England), 147*(Pt 8), 2293–2305. https://doi.org/10.1099/00221287-147-8-2293

14. Moreira-Teixeira, L., Tabone, O., Graham, C. M., Singhania, A., Stavropoulos, E., Redford, P. S., Chakravarty, P., Priestnall, S. L., Suarez-Bonnet, A., Herbert, E., Mayer-Barber, K. D., Sher, A., Fonseca, K. L., Sousa, J., Cá, B., Verma, R., Haldar, P., Saraiva, M., & O'Garra, A. (2020). Mouse transcriptome reveals potential signatures of protection and pathogenesis in human tuberculosis. *Nature immunology, 21*(4), 464–476. https://doi.org/10.1038/s41590-020-0610-z (accessed on 10 May 2025).

15. Cluj-Napoca, S. F., Robert, R., Van, E. B., Keskimäki, L. K., Tynkkynen, T., et al. (2023). Power and politics of health system data: How data shape responses and equity during pandemics. *The European Journal of Public Health, 33.* https://www.semanticscholar.org/paper/d6dd3f2ceeb49d92b596991dd84ceac0398d38d9 (accessed on 10 May 2025).

16. Colombo, M. I., Giai, C., & Zarelli, V. E. P. (2018). Interaction of *Mycobacterium tuberculosis* with the host cells: A focus in the molecular mechanism involved in trafficking and autophagy. SM Group-Open Access eBooks. Libro: Tuberculosis (pp. 1-16). SM Group-Open Access eBooks

17. ISBN: 978-1-944685-00-3. https://core.ac.uk/download/287883713.pdf (accessed on 10 May 2025).

18. Deffur, A., Wilkinson, R. J., & Coussens, A. K. (2015). Tricks to translating TB transcriptomics. *Annals of translational medicine, 3*(Suppl 1), S43. https://doi.org/10.3978/j.issn.2305-5839.2015.04.12 (accessed on 10 May 2025).

19. Cunha, S. S., Merle, C. S. C., & Rodrigues, L. C. (2010). BCG vaccination and leprosy protection: Review of current evidence and status of BCG in leprosy control. *Expert Review of Vaccines, 9*(2), 209–222. https://doi.org/10.1586/erv.09.161.

20. Dick, A. D., Forrester, J. V., & Kuffova, L. (2018). Autoimmunity, autoinflammation, and infection in uveitis. https://core.ac.uk/download/156963569.pdf (accessed on 10 May 2025).

21. Dorhoi, A., Fortin, A., Kahnert, A., Mantovani, A., Becker, A. M., Giagu, A., et al. (2013). Interferon regulatory factor 8-deficiency determines massive neutrophil recruitment but T cell defect in fast growing granulomas during tuberculosis. *PLoS ONE, 8*(5), e62751. https://core.ac.uk/download/11694401.pdf (accessed on 10 May 2025).

22. DuPont, M., Rousset, S., Manh, T. V., Monard, S. C., Pingris, K., Souriant, S., Vahlas, Z., et al. (2022). Dysregulation of the IFN-I signaling pathway by *Mycobacterium tuberculosis* leads to exacerbation of HIV-1 infection of macrophages. *Journal of Leukocyte Biology, 112*(6), 1329–1342. https://www.semanticscholar.org/paper/1acd3b895045d487ef4ce9dab73ab76af5d5f257 (accessed on 10 May 2025).

23. Gordon, D. E., Jang, G. M., Bouhaddou, M., Xu, J., Obernier, K., White, K. M., O'Meara, M. J., et al. (2020). A SARS-CoV-2 protein interaction map reveals targets for drug repurposing. *Nature, 583*(7816), 459–468. https://doi.org/10.1038/s41586-020-2286-9.

24. Gordon, S., Sichone, S., Chirwa, A., Hazenberg, P., Kafuko, Z., Ferreira, D., Flynn, J., et al. (2023). Practical considerations for a TB controlled human infection model (TB-CHIM); the case for TB-CHIM in Africa, a systematic review of the literature and report of 2 workshop

discussions in UK and Malawi. *Wellcome Open Research, 8*. https://www.semanticscholar.org/paper/c4a28dafe2c5afb9d9ca2908a7b41a9dd8244338 (accessed on 10 May 2025).

25. Hu, X., Li, J., Fu, M., Zhao, X., & Wang, W. (2021). The JAK/STAT signaling pathway: From bench to clinic. *Signal Transduction and Targeted Therapy, 6*, 402. https://doi.org/10.1038/s41392-021-00791-1.
26. Klionsky, D. J., Petroni, G., Amaravadi, R. K., Baehrecke, E. H., Ballabio, A., Boya, P., Bravo-San Pedro, J. M., et al. (2021). Autophagy in major human diseases. *The EMBO Journal, 40*(17), e108863. https://doi.org/10.15252/embj.2021108863.
27. Meunier, N. V., Sebulime, P., White, R. G., & Kock, R. (2017). Wildlife-livestock interactions and risk areas for cross-species spread of bovine tuberculosis. *The Onderstepoort journal of veterinary research*, *84*(1), e1–e10. https://doi.org/10.4102/ojvr.v84i1.1221 (accessed on 10 May 2025).
28. Lin, D., & Koskella, B. (2015). Friend and foe: factors influencing the movement of the bacterium Helicobacter pylori along the parasitism-mutualism continuum. *Evolutionary applications*, *8*(1), 9–22. https://doi.org/10.1111/eva.12231
29. Malefane, L., & Maarman, G. J. (2023). Post-tuberculosis lung disease and inflammatory role players: Can we characterize the myriad inflammatory pathways involved to gain a better understanding? *Chemico-Biological Interactions, 387*, 110817. https://doi.org/10.1016/j.cbi.2023.110817.
30. Moreira-Teixeira, L., Mayer-Barber, K., Sher, A., & O'Garra, A. (2018). Type I interferons in tuberculosis: Foe and occasionally friend. *The Journal of experimental medicine*, *215*(5), 1273–1285. https://doi.org/10.1084/jem.20180325
31. Napier, G., Campino, S., Merid, Y., Abebe, M., Woldeamanuel, Y., Aseffa, A., Hibberd, M. L., et al. (2020). Robust barcoding and identification of *Mycobacterium tuberculosis* lineages for epidemiological and clinical studies. *Genome Medicine, 12*, 114. https://doi.org/10.1186/s13073-020-00817-3.
32. Oo, N., & Agrawal, D. K. (2025). Epidemiology, pathogenesis, clinical manifestations, and management strategies of tuberculous meningitis. *Archives of Internal Medicine Research, 8*, 48–58. https://www.semanticscholar.org/paper/51053aee2b7ecda5285b076131a87f89c499453c (accessed on 10 May 2025).
33. Rahmanian, S. (2015). Outcomes of HIV-positive patients with renal insufficiency on treatment with HAART at Charlotte Maxeke Johannesburg Academic Hospital. https://core.ac.uk/download/188769812.pdf (accessed on 10 May 2025).
34. Shah AM, Shah SV. Recent advances in drug therapy for tuberculosis. Natl J Physiol Pharm Pharmacol. 2024; 14(5): 805-814. doi:10.5455/njppp.2024.14.04164202416042024
35. (accessed on 10 May 2025).
36. Shah, J. A., Warr, A., Graustein, A., Saha, A., Dunstan, S., Thuong, N., Thwaites, G., et al. (2022). REL and BHLHE40 variants are associated with IL-12 and IL-10 responses and tuberculosis risk. *The Journal of Immunology, 208*(6), 1352–1361. https://www.semanticscholar.org/paper/abacb1becd54a97243620b6e7e7f10bc40c03acd (accessed on 10 May 2025).
37. Shim, D., Kim, H., & Shin, S. J. (2020). *Mycobacterium tuberculosis* infection-driven foamy macrophages and their implications in tuberculosis control as targets for host-directed

therapy. *Frontiers in Immunology, 11*, 910. https://doi.org/10.3389/fimmu.2020.00910.

38. Stamp, J. T. (1952). Some aspects of the pathology and pathogenesis of bovine tuberculosis (and other published papers). https://core.ac.uk/download/429735295.pdf (accessed on 10 May 2025).

39. Xiang, Y., Ma, L., Wu, W., Liu, W., Li, Y., Zhu, X., Wang, Q., Ma, J., Cao, M., Wang, Q., Yao, X., Yang, L., Wubuli, A., Merle, C., Milligan, P., Mao, Y., Gu, J., & Xin, X. (2014). The incidence of liver injury in Uyghur patients treated for TB in Xinjiang Uyghur autonomous region, China, and its association with hepatic enzyme polymorphisms nat2, cyp2e1, gstm1 and gstt1. *PloS one, 9*(1), e85905. https://doi.org/10.1371/journal.pone.0085905 (accessed on 10 May 2025).

40. Vijaya, S., Admuthe, N., Sreenivas, A., Garg, H. G., Malar, S. E., V. S., Padghane, S., et al. (2023). Role of plant-based bioflavonoids in combating tuberculosis. *International Journal of Membrane Science and Technology.* https://www.semanticscholar.org/paper/c909e6925c01b3b219d3e225b67170fd649660f0 (accessed on 10 May 2025).

41. Wahlström, H. (2004). Bovine tuberculosis in Swedish farmed deer. https://core.ac.uk/download/11694788.pdf (accessed on 10 May 2025).

42. Yadav, S., & Rawal, G. (2024). Understanding the spectrum and management of post-tuberculosis lung disease: A comprehensive review. *Cures, 16.* https://www.semanticscholar.org/paper/15bed74bcdb4430b5cd3d0a7dfe76a4a23fd7994 (accessed on 10 May 2025).

43. Zhou, Y., Anthony, R. M., Wang, S., Xia, H., Ou, X., Zhao, B., Song, Y., et al. (2024). Understanding the epidemiology and pathogenesis of *Mycobacterium tuberculosis* with non-redundant pangenome and population genetics. *bioRxiv.* https://www.semanticscholar.org/paper/f80949da48afc4ed6c150d2c33d57c4e58ad9dab (accessed on 10 May 2025).

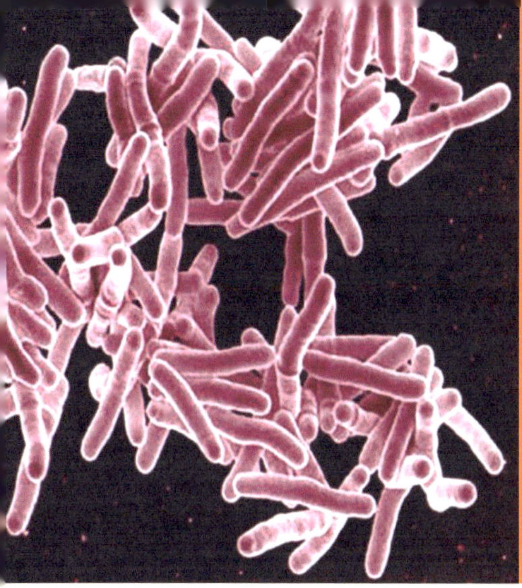

Chapter 3

DIAGNOSIS OF TUBERCULOSIS

Contents

Introduction

The burden of infectious diseases worldwide continues to pose an enduring challenge to public health systems, especially in low-resource settings. Of all these diseases, tuberculosis (TB) is noteworthy because of its complex pathogenesis and dynamic transmission. Even with progress in the field of medical science, the accurate and timely diagnosis of TB remains a serious barrier to controlling TB transmission. The challenge of diagnosis not only contributes to the delay in treatment but also enables continued transmission within communities, fueling the public health burden. This is compounded by the lack of quick, point-of-care diagnostic tests that are capable of detecting active infections with a high degree of certainty, which is an immense resource gap in TB control activities. Knowledge of the current situation regarding TB diagnostics is critical to help formulate effective methods for fighting the disease and its spread across the globe (McNerney et al., 2012). Proper diagnosis of tuberculosis depends on the possibility of detecting *Mycobacterium tuberculosis* (MTB) effectively and distinguishing it from nontuberculous mycobacterial (NTM) disease. Novel diagnostic strategies have opened up with advances in molecular and biochemical methods. One such promising approach includes the mycolic acid analysis, an important cell wall constituent of mycobacteria, by advanced mass spectrometry methods. By fingerprinting distinct fatty acid patterns characteristic of *Mtb*, scientists have shown the ability to detect the pathogen in a quick and highly specific manner. These diagnostic advances imply that the integration of highly advanced chemical profiling into clinical practice may abbreviate the duration of diagnosis, thereby facilitating more rapid treatment initiation and better patient outcomes (Szewczyk et al., 2013). Despite technological advancement, existing tuberculosis diagnostics are confronted with challenges that limit their widespread use, particularly in resource-limited settings where the tuberculosis burden is most significant. Traditional laboratory-based tests, although the gold standard, usually take long periods and several tests before making a definitive diagnosis, creating impediments to timely patient treatment. In addition, the expense, intricacy, and availability of new diagnostic equipment determine their feasible application in endemic areas. The search for rapid, point-of-care tests must also face operational and logistical limitations that come with the delivery of diagnostic services. Tackling these complex problems is essential to strengthening TB control programs and making advances in diagnosis pay dividends in the form of concrete public health gains (McNerney et al., 2012).

Importance of Early Diagnosis

The nuances of tuberculosis (TB) go beyond being an infectious disease, given that delays in diagnosis lead to serious complications that worsen patient outcomes. It is important for early detection not just for the purpose of starting treatment on time but also to avoid secondary conditions that exponentially increase morbidity and mortality. For instance, multi-drug resistant tuberculosis (MDR-TB) poses especially challenging problems with its lengthy treatment course and increased risk of serious complications like pulmonary thromboembolism (PTE). The recognition that PTE is a commonly under-recognized but potentially lethal complication highlights the importance of clinicians keeping a heightened state of alertness. Identifying early signs of tuberculosis, as well as its complications, enables timely therapeutic interventions and, thereby, minimizes risks that can significantly deteriorate patient prognoses. This observation indicates that early diagnosis is no longer a clinical mere formality, but a critical factor that can irrevocably determine survival and quality of life among TB patients (Marwah et al., 2023). In addition, the diagnostic process has significant implications in the pediatric population where manifestations of tuberculosis are less characteristic and harder to identify. In such cases, the challenge is compounded within this demographic due to variable symptomatology and possible overlap with other pediatric pathology, and consequently, sophisticated diagnostic skills and technologies are required. The cooperation among different medical departments, from child neurology to infectious disease experts, demonstrates the interdisciplinary effort involved in obtaining a correct and prompt diagnosis. This collaborative approach maximizes the likelihood of detecting TB early when irreversible and or disease progression are not yet possible. The use of expert professionals from different disciplines stresses that early diagnosis is not only dependent on technological interventions but also on extended clinical evaluation and interprofessional consultation, which are critical to limiting morbidity in at-risk groups (Fernández et al., 2023). Apart from clinical merit, early diagnosis of tuberculosis has greater public health benefits by limiting transmission in communities. Since TB is largely an infectious disease transmitted by airborne droplets, there is a risk of transmitting to close contacts and the general public with each delay in diagnosis and treatment. The capability to identify and confirm TB infections early allows for quick institution of isolation control and contact tracing, which are important in outbreak control. In addition, early treatment decreases bacterial loads in patients, lowering infectiousness and eliminating the potential for drug resistance through delayed or suboptimal therapy. Early diagnosis is therefore a double insurance policy: it enhances patient outcomes as well as plays a fulcrum role in breaking disease transmission chains, a key goal of global TB control programs. Its significance, therefore, cannot be overemphasized when developing strategies for successful TB control.

Overview of Diagnostic Methods

Correct diagnosis of tuberculosis (TB) is still a key problem because TB is a complex disease with heterogenous clinical presentations. Conventional diagnostic methods are largely dependent upon detecting the presence of MTB by sputum smear microscopy and culture, but they are often not very sensitive, particularly in extrapulmonary tuberculosis (EPTB). Moreover, immune-based tests like the tuberculin skin test (TST) and interferon-gamma release assays (IGRAs) can identify *Mtb* infection but are unable to differentiate latent infection from active disease, making clinical decision-making challenging. These shortcomings have evoked a demand for better diagnostic modalities with the capability to yield rapid, valid, and specific results, thus facilitating the timely initiation of treatment and improved patient outcomes. Improvements in molecular technologies, such as nucleic acid amplification tests (NAATs), are increasingly improving sensitivity and specificity, representing a major advancement in TB diagnosis (Huang et al., 2022). Imaging technologies also have an important role to play in the diagnosis and control of tuberculosis, specifically in detecting extrapulmonary manifestations where conventional microbiologic methods can fall short. Cardiovascular TB, while being uncommon, also poses diagnostic challenges that necessitate non-invasive and accurate imaging modalities. Cardiac magnetic resonance imaging (CMR) has become an essential modality with better tissue characterization and function measurement compared to echocardiography. By combining clinical data with refined radiological markers like late gadolinium enhancement and parametric imaging, CMR supports differentially diagnosing cardiac involvement related to TB, that is, tuberculous myocarditis and pericarditis. By being not only more accurate but also a step quicker and less invasive compared to biopsy, this multimodal technique makes for earlier, thereby more effective therapeutic interventions (Karuna et al., 2022).

Recent attempts to improve TB diagnostic techniques aim to use new technologies that yield more in-depth information on both pathogen detection and host immune response. New techniques such as flow cytometry and mass spectrometry are being tested to enhance the specificity and sensitivity of TB diagnostics, which could bypass the limitations of traditional tests. Further, artificial intelligence (AI)-driven algorithms and high-throughput sequencing have the potential to revolutionize TB diagnosis. These technologies will combine heterogeneous clinical, microbiological, and immunological information to produce precise diagnostic profiles. All these developments highlight the move towards personalized medicine in TB case management where diagnostic modalities are designed according to individual patient presentations and complexity of diseases." Through the optimization of traditional approaches in combination with new molecular technologies, the diagnostic landscape of tuberculosis is changing to decrease diagnostic delay and enhance clinical outcomes (Huang et al., 2022).

3.1. Historical Context of Tuberculosis Diagnosis

The journey to precise tuberculosis diagnosis has been influenced by centuries of unfolding medical knowledge and technological innovations. Tuberculosis is initially diagnosed based on its clinical presentation of chronic cough, weight loss, and night sweats, which sometimes results in incorrect diagnosis due to symptom overlap with other respiratory ailments. Identifying the *Tuberculosis bacillus* by Robert Koch in 1882 was a turning point, shifting diagnosis from symptom-based to bacteriological demonstration. Notwithstanding this advance, technical impediments to cultivating and identifying the bacteria hindered extensive diagnostic use. In the 20th century, the tuberculin skin test (TST) and chest radiography were developed, increasing sensitivity to diagnosis but with limitations to discriminate latent infection and active disease. Such past diagnostic techniques formed the basis of recognizing tuberculosis' clinical and microbiological complexity, highlighting the need for enhanced diagnostic methods and identifying ongoing obstacles in proper detection, particularly in settings where resources are limited (Huang et al., 2022) (Figure 3.1).

Concurrent with medical advancements, health systems organization and quality have traditionally affected tuberculosis case detection effectiveness. Prior to standardized procedures and strong health infrastructures, case detection was erratic, frequently handicapped by uneven expertise and restricted diagnostic facility access. As international health objectives changed towards the control of infectious diseases, the quality of health systems was critical to the management of tuberculosis. The capacity of health systems to provide competent and timely tuberculosis diagnosis indicates broader problems reported in the management of most diseases where deficits in quality of care constrain results. In the majority of low- and middle-income countries (LMICs) where there is a high tuberculosis burden, systemic deficiencies such as weak patient retention, limited integration across care platforms, and insufficient staff training exacerbate suboptimal diagnostic capacities. These system problems emphasize the interaction between historical diagnostic approaches and the quality of health systems, underlining the pressing necessity of health system improvement in combination with technological progress to enhance tuberculosis diagnosis effectiveness and equity (Margaret et al., 2018).

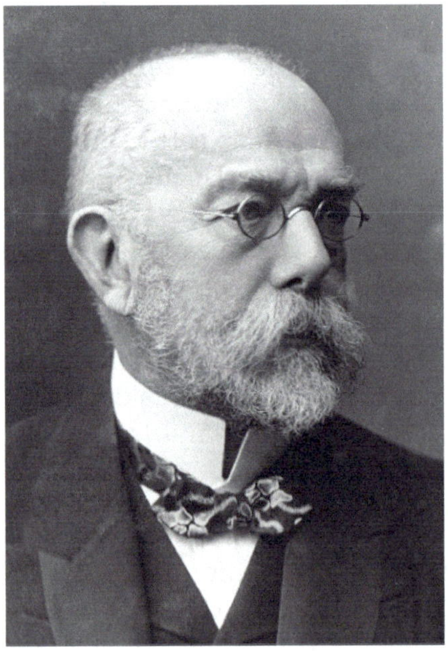

Figure 3.1. Robert Koch, a Prussian physician, discovered the cause of tuberculosis.

Source: Wikipedia. (n.d.). *Portrait of Robert Koch, who discovered Mycobacterium tuberculosis in 1882.* https://en.wikipedia.org/wiki/History_of_tuberculosis.

The changing historical context of tuberculosis diagnosis emphasizes the importance of incorporating new approaches to diagnosis within performing health systems to meet ongoing disease burdens. The limitations of conventional diagnostic methods, such as delayed results, poor sensitivity, and inability to differentiate between latent and active infections, have necessitated the introduction of molecular diagnostics and rapid tests that are supposed to provide earlier and more sensitive detection. However, their influence is very much contingent on the ability of health systems to apply these technologies optimally. Patterns from the past indicate that technological advancements are not enough without solid healthcare systems that guarantee accessibility, affordability, and quality of treatment across populations. It takes collective efforts in the areas of governance, workforce development, and patient participation guided by observations from successes and failures of the past in controlling tuberculosis. With the diagnosis of tuberculosis ongoing, integrating this historical context is necessary for the development of interventions that not only increase diagnostic effectiveness but also enhance health outcomes worldwide (Margaret et al., 2018).

3.1.1. Early Methods of Diagnosis

The success of tuberculosis control relies largely on the early detection of disease; however, the diagnostic pathway in most areas causes significant delays. Patients face extended periods between symptom development and initiation of proper treatment, a factor that makes disease management more difficult and increases transmission risk. Research has shown that patient-related delays, including the time to present to a healthcare provider, are more than those caused by healthcare providers. Socioeconomic factors like illiteracy, advanced age, and low income perpetuate these delays and generate a complex interweave of health-seeking behavior. For example, patients visit many family physicians and travel through several providers before the correct diagnosis is made, incurring huge amounts of out-of-pocket costs without receiving any timely therapeutic benefit. These delays highlight the necessity for strategies specifically designed to hasten early case detection to improve treatment outcomes, especially for resource-constrained settings (Bawankule et al., 2010). Current diagnostic methods mostly rely on clinical and radiological assessments for detecting tuberculosis in its initial phases. Chest X-rays have traditionally been used to detect suspicious pulmonary lesions suggestive of tuberculosis infection as an essential screening tool where there is a high prevalence. Sputum smear microscopy is also a cornerstone for early detection, with direct visualization of acid-fast bacilli (AFB). Even though they are commonly utilized, they are subjected to limitations in terms of sensitivity and specificity, tending to need adjunctive methods or multiple sampling for validation of diagnosis. Advances in technology have brought with them computer-aided diagnosis systems that increase the accuracy of image interpretation. Techniques like active contour models and feature extraction algorithms are used to better differentiate tuberculosis features in radiographic images. These initial diagnostic interventions are critical milestones toward timely treatment initiation, but their effectiveness is highly dependent on the presence of trained staff and diagnostic facilities (Beevi et al., 2023). The infusion of advanced computing methods into the early detection of tuberculosis holds the potential to mitigate some of the inherent difficulties with traditional practices. Deep learning technology, for instance, has shown significant promise in detecting tuberculosis-causing microbes with increased precision and efficiency. Through the utilization of large data sets of clinical imaging and lab information, such algorithms are capable of identifying subtle patterns difficult to discern on their own through human analysis. Therefore, deep learning makes it possible to recognize the disease rapidly, enhancing patient outcomes despite preventing complete mortality continuing to prove challenging. Such technologies are especially worth their while in environments where skilled radiologists and microbiologists are in short supply, allowing automated or semi-automated assessment processes to aid in decision-making. Although technological innovations cannot completely replace extensive healthcare services, they represent an impressive step toward the early diagnosis of tuberculosis, which can boost the chances of timely intervention and control (Beevi et al., 2023).

3.1.2. Evolution of Diagnostic Techniques

The process of attaining reliable tuberculosis diagnosis has been characterized by major milestones in clinical observation as well as laboratory techniques. The diagnosis initially depended largely on symptomatology supplemented with chest radiographs and microscopic examination of sputum smears. These traditional approaches, however, were hampered by low sensitivity and specificity and tended to result in delayed or missed diagnoses. The emergence of culture methods introduced a giant leap in diagnostic precision, but it took extended incubation periods, often weeks before the results could be established. This was crucial for tuberculosis control, and hence techniques to yield more swift and dependable diagnostics had to emerge. Subsequent innovations in immunodiagnostic tests then enabled clinicians to identify latent infection, even though there were still difficulties, particularly in immunocompromised individuals, where the body's immune responses can be aberrant or blunted (Mencarini et al., 2016). These nuances heightened the need for developing diagnostics that could effectively offer timely and accurate detection of *Mycobacterium tuberculosis* (MTB). Molecular methods have revolutionized the face of tuberculosis diagnosis, providing a combination of speed and sensitivity that was not hitherto available using conventional methods. Incorporating DNA amplification technologies like polymerase chain reaction (PCR) revolutionized the diagnosis of mycobacterial infections by detecting genetic material directly from clinical specimens. This strategy enhanced turnaround times considerably and raised diagnostic yield for smear-negative and extrapulmonary tuberculosis (EPTB) diseases. Novel molecular assays' specificity, however, is threatened by closely related mycobacteria, and target sequences were required to be optimized to prevent false positives. Studies with mycobacterial isolates illustrate the dangers of genetic similarity across species, highlighting the need for the establishment of diagnostic protocols that distinguish among the mycobacteria with greater accuracy (Englund et al., 2002). Ever since, the relentless development of molecular diagnostics has played a critical role in enhancing detecting tuberculosis in both clinical and subclinical scenarios. The shift to more advanced diagnostic modalities goes beyond detection to include the characterization of disease and discrimination from other granulomatous diseases. In patients with concurrent infections like HIV, for example, the process of diagnosis becomes even more complicated because overlapping clinical manifestations and immune changes obscure interpretation (Mencarini et al., 2016). Consequently, systematic workflows involving the exclusion of reactivation tuberculosis, other mycobacterial infections, and malignancies have become integral parts of current diagnostic protocols. Additionally, current emerging protocols now increasingly include preventive therapy decisions made on the basis of sophisticated immunological and molecular information, bridging diagnosis with patient care. This dynamic development parallels a larger movement in tuberculosis diagnosis—a continuous improvement focused on diminishing diagnostic uncertainty, enabling earlier treatment, and finally improving outcomes through precision medicine strategies (Figure 3.2).

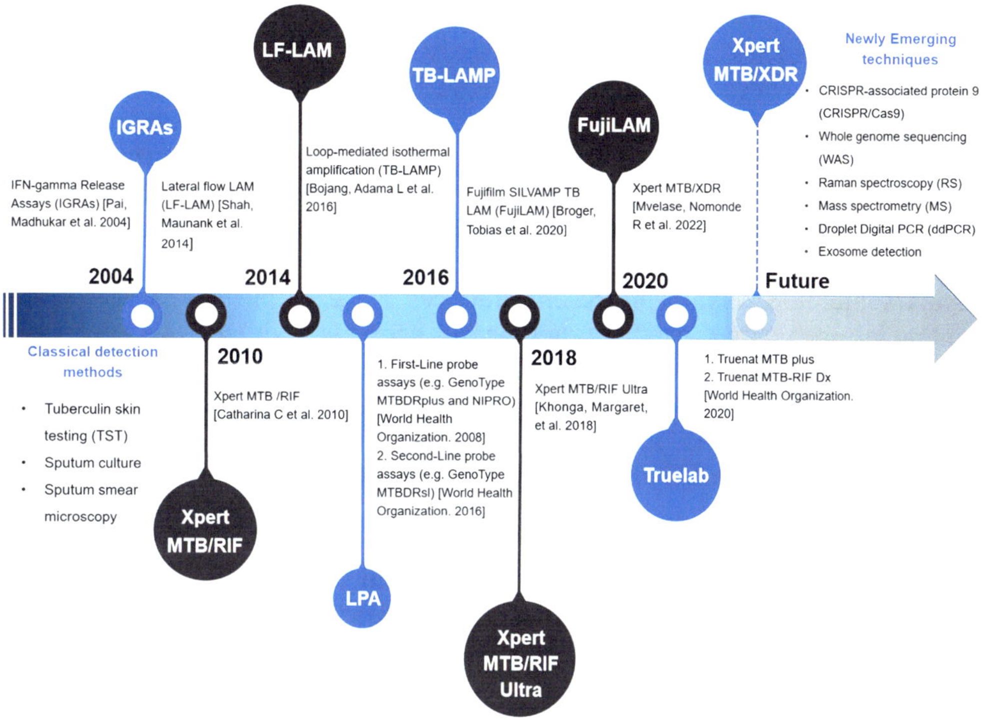

Figure 3.2. The timeline for the development of tuberculosis (TB) diagnosis.

Source: ResearchGate. (n.d.). *The timeline for the development of tuberculosis (TB) diagnosis: From classical methods to emerging technologies.* https://www.researchgate.net/publication/370711403/figure/fig2/AS:11431281255501960@1719421239354/The-timeline-for-the-development-of-tuberculosis-TB-diagnosis.png.

3.1.3. Impact of Historical Perspectives on Current Practices

The path of tuberculosis diagnosis mirrors a course influenced by historical advances in medical science and technology. Initial attempts at diagnosis were based mostly on clinical observation and crude microscopy, which were frequently stymied by an incomplete understanding of the pathogenesis of the disease. Progress came with improvements in bacteriology and immunology, which paved the way for more advanced diagnostic methods like sputum smear microscopy, culture, and eventually molecular tests. This development highlights a key shift away from subjective towards more objective, evidence-based strategies in healthcare. Additionally, historical insights highlight the significance of contextual determinants, such as social determinants and the capacity of the health system, that affect diagnostic habits today. By valuing these historical roots, today's health professionals are aware that increasing coverage alone is not enough; quality and accuracy of diagnosis need to be the priorities so that substantial health outcomes are gained, especially in resource-constrained environments (Margaret et al., 2018). Modern diagnostic practices for tuberculosis are also deeply shaped by historical experience about health system weaknesses and inequalities. The realization that suboptimal care is often delivered to vulnerable groups has motivated efforts toward incorporating equity into diagnostic approaches. Mismanagement of tuberculosis in vulnerable groups in the past underscores the importance of trustworthy, accessible, and patient-empowering diagnostic services. This has resulted in point-of-care testing and decentralized diagnostics models that aim to overcome accessibility, stigma, and untimely initiation of treatment. These contemporary methods indicate a shift away from centralized, inaccessible diagnostic systems towards systems that focus on resilience, efficiency, and user experience. Historical lessons therefore not only inform the technical provision of diagnosis but also shape more extensive health system reforms that need to be implemented to support equitable and quality tuberculosis care (Margaret et al., 2018). The impact of historical insights goes beyond tuberculosis to guide diagnostic innovation in other chronic conditions, illustrating how interdepartmental lessons inform present practices. For example, similarities in the diagnosis and management of problems caused by rheumatoid arthritis highlight the ongoing demand for increased specificity and timely diagnosis in diseases with complexity. Similarly, as tuberculosis control has developed with a focus on detecting pathogens and systemic insight, developments in autoimmune disease diagnosis place greater emphasis on stages of disease progression and treatment pathways tailored to the individual. These analogies promote an integrated response to diagnostic strategy grounded in pathogen biology and patient-centered practice. Therefore, historical context promotes a critical understanding that changing diagnostic paradigms need to integrate scientific solidity with responsive health system action, eventually improving disease detection and patient outcomes in various clinical settings (Figure 3.3).

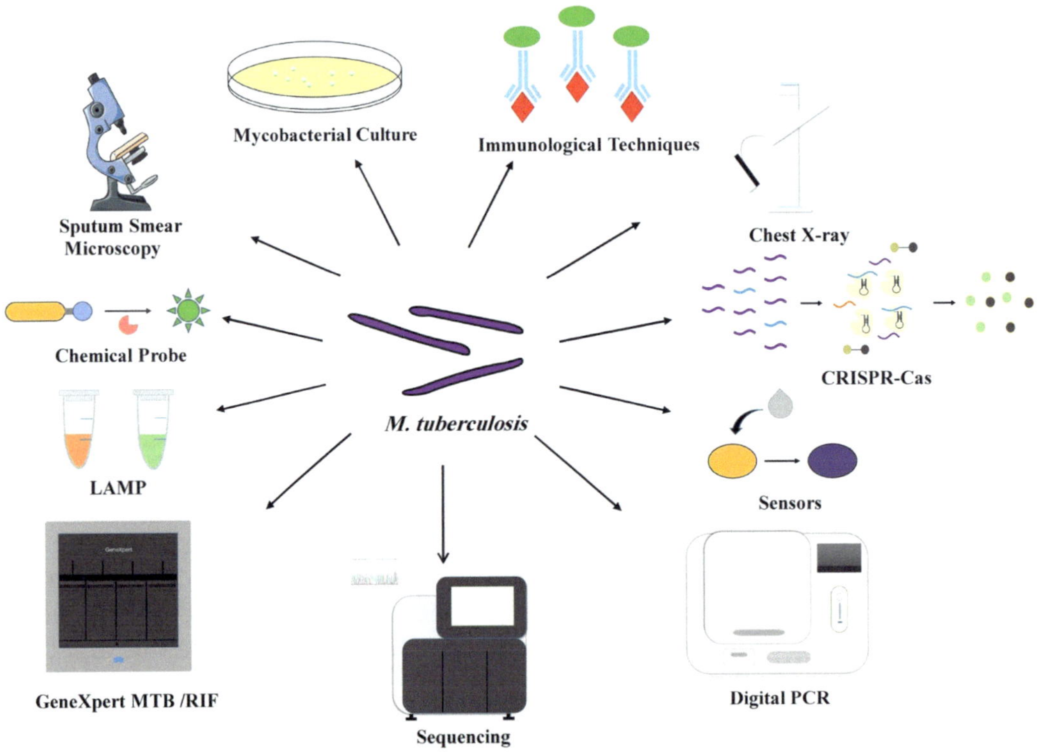

Figure 3.3. Conventional methods for diagnosis of TB.

Source: Dong B, He Z, Li Y, Xu X, Wang C and Zeng J (2022) Improved Conventional and New Approaches in the Diagnosis of Tuberculosis. Front. Microbiol. 13:924410. doi: 10.3389/fmicb.2022.924410

3.2. Symptoms of Tuberculosis

Clinical presentations of tuberculosis (TB) depend greatly on the location and course of infection. Pulmonary tuberculosis (PTB) is the most frequent manifestation, but extrapulmonary forms can confound the clinical presentation and may delay proper diagnosis. The presentations are usually nonspecific and include chronic cough, fever, night sweats, and unintentional weight loss, which are suggestive but not pathognomonic for TB. Abdominal pain and dysphagia can imply extrapulmonary involvement, especially in the gastrointestinal tract, a rare but reported presentation. Such heterogeneity requires an in-depth consideration of symptomatology to direct relevant diagnostic maneuvers. For example, gastric tuberculosis has been known to present as obstructive gastrointestinal disease, and thus histopathological confirmation becomes crucial to prevent such misinterpretation and start specific antitubercular therapy (ATT) promptly (Jain et al., 2024). Such symptom diversity makes it difficult for clinicians to make appropriate and timely diagnoses, highlighting the importance of an exhaustive clinical evaluation. Yet another difficulty in distinguishing between tuberculosis symptoms and other diseases and infections that share overlapping clinical features adds to the burden. In other instances, such similarities can result in a delay in treatment and complicate the patient's prognosis. The occurrence of systemic symptoms like recurring fever, malaise, and lymphadenopathy, in addition to the slow onset of respiratory symptoms, usually points clinicians toward the differential diagnosis of TB. Further, the diagnostic sophistication involves such populations and settings where co-infections or unusual pathogens affect symptom manifestation and intensity. Diagnostic instruments with increased sensitivity and specificity, similar to molecular methods employed in detecting pathogens, such as *Clostridium perfringens* in poultry, illustrate the urgent necessity for improved methods of TB diagnosis to support clinical evidence and minimize misdiagnosis occurrences (Stiwey et al., 2024). Integrative methods enhance detecting TB across varied clinical settings. Identifying the constellation of TB symptoms is essential for early diagnosis and treatment, particularly due to the disease's potential to present similarly to other conditions. Physicians need to be watchful for symptoms less typically seen with tuberculosis, that is, gastrointestinal obstruction symptoms, that can indicate extrapulmonary disease. Assessment of the fact that some presentations can challenge traditional respiratory presentations widens the diagnostic focus and invites the consideration of tuberculosis in the differential diagnosis, especially in high-incidence areas. Correlation of clinical, radiological, and histopathological data is necessary to establish the diagnosis and design appropriate treatment regimes. Early diagnosis on the basis of symptomatology not only enhances patient care but also limits transmission. Thus, a sophisticated understanding of tuberculosis signs in the diagnostic process still remains unavoidable (Jain et al., 2024).

3.2.1. Common Symptoms of Pulmonary Tuberculosis (PTB)

The clinical signs of PTB usually precede the definitive diagnosis and are important indicators for medical professionals. Of the frequent symptoms, a cough that persists for over two weeks is particularly noteworthy, usually with sputum production that can be purulent or contain blood. Fever is often described, although it may fluctuate in severity during the disease, and is usually associated with night sweats, which are typical of most mycobacterial infections. Fatigue and malaise can also occur, mirroring the systemic nature of the infection. Constitutional symptoms, although frequent in PTB, can also be shared with other respiratory diseases, making early diagnosis challenging and highlighting the severity of careful clinical evaluation in presumptive cases. Recognizing these symptoms assists in a reduced diagnostic pathway, particularly in high TB prevalence areas. The symptomatic presentation of PTB has shown variability based on age, immune status, and geographical location. For example, child patients have fewer characteristic symptoms than adults and present with less severe respiratory complaints and more systemic symptoms, including weight loss and failure to thrive. Based on clinical experience, the prevalence of classic symptoms of cough and fever in children, though frequent, is more frequently reduced in extra-pulmonary involvement, echoing the difficulties in diagnosis in this subgroup. This heterogeneity is an argument for the use of an integrated approach incorporating laboratory, radiologic, and epidemiologic information for a correct diagnosis. In addition, the worldwide burden of tuberculosis indicates a chronic prevalence of these kinds of symptoms among different populations, highlighting that symptom detection is still a pillar of premature tuberculosis control interventions (Spencer et al., 2018). Notwithstanding these typical symptoms, diagnosis is hindered by non-specificity in some clinical symptoms, as they are also present in other pulmonary conditions. Therefore, adjunctive diagnostic modalities like chest radiography, microscopy of sputum, and nucleic acid amplification tests (NAATs) are critical to establishing PTB diagnosis. However, initial symptom identification directs the urgency and intensity of subsequent investigations. Fever, cough, and weight loss tend to alert clinicians about tuberculosis, especially in regions where this disease is endemic or where high-risk groups present. The difficulty is in distinguishing PTB symptoms from other infections of the respiratory tract and chronic pulmonary disease, requiring thorough patient history-taking and cautious interpretation of clinical results (Spencer et al., 2018). Subsequently, knowledge about the typical symptomatology of PTB not only allows timely diagnosis but also guides public health measures and patient management strategies (Figure 3.4).

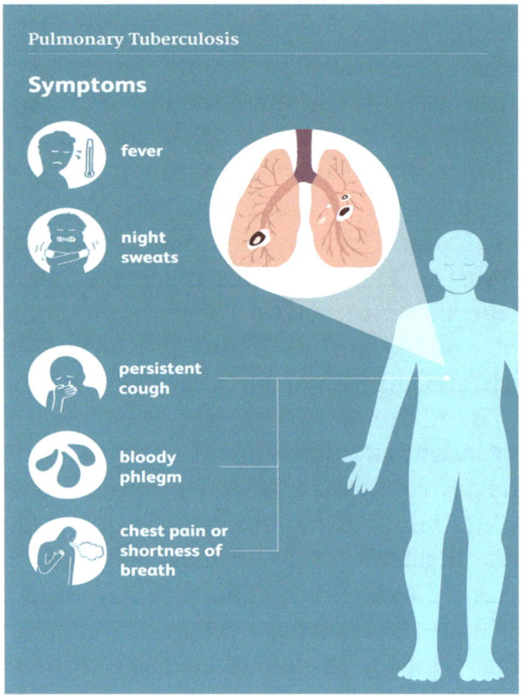

Figure 3.4. Pulmonary tuberculosis (PTB) symptoms.

Source: Verywell Health. (n.d.). *Symptoms of tuberculosis: Fever, night sweats, persistent cough, bloody phlegm, and chest pain or shortness of breath.* https://www.verywellhealth.com/thmb/jXXMDkR7r63zXJEvBzwx0Hi_-GQ=/700x0/filters:no_upscale():max_bytes(150000):strip_icc()/tuberculosis-symptoms1-5af07aed1d64040036a103cc.png.

3.2.2. Symptoms of Extrapulmonary Tuberculosis (EPTB)

EPTB is generally a diagnostic challenge because it has varied clinical presentation, which generally depends on the involved anatomical location. In contrast to PTB, in which respiratory findings are predominant, symptoms of EPTB are generally less obvious and could be difficult to distinguish from other chronic inflammatory or neoplastic diseases. For example, gastrointestinal tuberculosis may present by non-specific symptoms like abdominal pain, weight loss, and gastric outlet obstruction, which make it hard to be diagnosed early on and may result in extended diagnostic delays as well as inappropriate treatment as explained in current case analysis (Saha, 2024). Symptom recognition thus demands a high level of suspicion, particularly in high-endemicity regions or in immunocompromised patients. This emphasizes the importance of a thorough clinical assessment outside the respiratory system with the use of patient history in detail, including exposure risk and pertinent epidemiological factors. Symptomatology of EPTB is quite diverse depending on the organ system affected, with frequent involvement of signs referable to localized inflammation of the tissue and systemic disease. For instance, lymphadenitis in EPTB can manifest as painless lymph node swelling (LNs), whereas genitourinary tuberculosis can present with dysuria, hematuria, or pelvic pain. These presentations are often not accompanied by typical pulmonary symptoms such as chronic cough or hemoptysis, leading to the under-recognition of the disease (Singh et al., 2024).

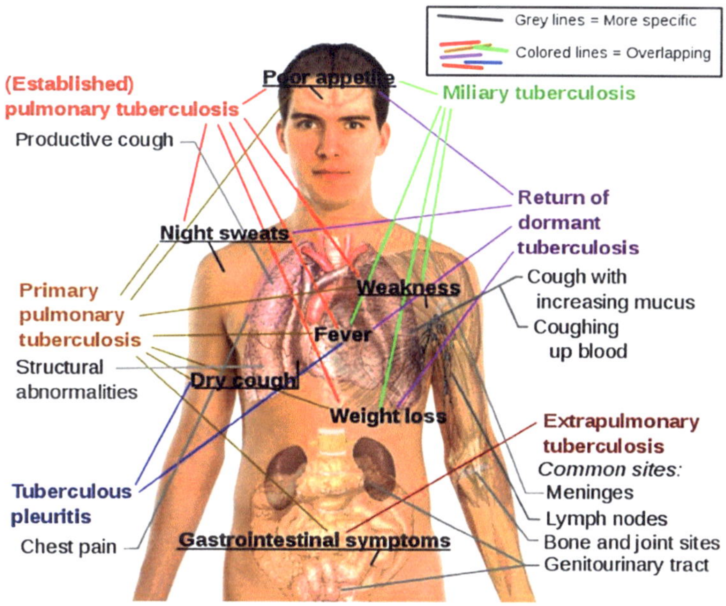

Figure 3.5. Extrapulmonary tuberculosis (EPTB) symptoms.

Source: Slideserve. (n.d.). *Symptoms of tuberculosis: Pulmonary, extrapulmonary, miliary, and dormant TB with associated clinical signs.* https://image3.slideserve.com/6879239/extrapulmonary-tb1-l.jpg.

Histopathological investigation with granulomatous inflammation, usually accompanied by caseous necrosis, along with Ziehl-Neelsen staining for AFB and molecular diagnostics like GeneXpert MTB, is instrumental in establishing a diagnosis when clinical symptoms tend to overlap with other chronic diseases. Therefore, a multi-modal diagnostic strategy is indispensable to properly decode the symptom profile and differentiate EPTB from other conditions. Untimely diagnosis associated with the atypical and frequently insidious presentation of symptoms in EPTB can have a profound effect on patient outcomes. The illness can occur in uncommon sites in the extrapulmonary locations like the pericardium, middle ear, and musculoskeletal system, in which symptoms are even less characteristic, such as chronic pain, effusions, or swelling. These can be conveniently mistaken for other diseases (Singh et al., 2024). This requires increased clinical alertness, especially in those with chronic, unexplained symptoms not responding to routine therapies. Following stepwise diagnostic algorithms from extensive clinical history, PTB exclusion, and then biopsy with histopathological and microbiological correlation has been recommended to avoid delays in diagnosis and ensure proper identification and treatment of EPTB (Saha, 2024) (Figure 3.5).

3.2.3. Importance of Symptom Recognition

Early detection of tuberculosis (TB) symptoms is important for preventing disease advancement and containing transmission within a community. Despite the widely recognized clinical presentations of TB, the main challenge lies in identifying cases with subtle or unusual symptoms, especially those with sputum culture-negative pulmonary TB. This paucibacillary presentation tends to have fewer symptoms and less severe radiographic findings than in culture-positive cases and hence is easily missed in clinical practice.

Not detecting these early forms of infection prevents the initiation of treatment, which increases the chances of developing active, communicable disease. Thus, sensitizing healthcare personnel to the varied symptomatology of TB results in earlier detection. Enhanced awareness of the early and fine TB symptoms would, in turn, decrease morbidity and break chains of transmission, highlighting symptom recognition as an integral part of successful TB control programs (Minh-Vu et al., 2019). The inherent flaws in the healthcare system further complicate TB diagnosis and symptom detection, particularly in LMICs where the burden is highest. Health systems commonly face problems like poor clinical assessment, misdiagnosis, and poor follow-up, which are added to delays in detecting TB symptoms and treatment. In addition, quality deficits entail too little focus on patient communication and trust, which can discourage honest symptom reporting by patients and effective symptom evaluation by providers. This interaction decreases diagnostic accuracy as well as the efficacy of care delivery. Efforts therefore to enhance health system quality, for example, increasing clinical competence, promoting respectful provider-patient relationships, and combining patient-centeredness—are crucial to enhance symptom recognition. Until these system issues are addressed, the potential of early symptom detection to enhance outcomes in TB will be largely unfulfilled (Margaret et al., 2018).

Beyond clinical and systemic concerns, detecting TB symptoms also need to be framed within more expansive public health paradigms to have maximum impact. For example, symptom-based screening is an inexpensive method to detect individuals in need of further diagnostic work-up, especially in resource-constrained settings. This approach is based primarily on the skill of health workers to identify early signs like chronic cough, weight loss, and radiographic features even when not clearly evident. Improved diagnostic facilities and biomarkers supplement symptom detection but cannot fulfill the role of the initial clinical judgment required to suspect TB. Capacity building by way of training programs, community awareness programs, and quality assurance strategies has to be the focus to develop symptom recognition skills. Giving precedence to this element in TB control strategies can dramatically cut back on underdiagnosis, enable prompt intervention, and eventually lower TB transmission and death rates (Margaret et al., 2018; Minh-Vu et al., 2019).

3.3. Diagnostic Tests for Tuberculosis

The difficulty of diagnosing tuberculosis (TB) in multi-ethnic populations, especially in poor-resource environments, has prompted great strides in diagnostic testing. New developments prioritize detecting either the pathogen itself or a host's individual immune response to MTB. Though classical microscopy and culture continue as the cornerstones, these new tests seek to be faster, more sensitive, and more specific. Most notably for pulmonary TB, the development of molecular tests and immunodiagnostic methods holds the promise of dramatic advances in early detection. This is essential not only to limit disease transmission but also to introduce treatment on a timely basis. In addition, these advances hold greater significance for pediatric tuberculosis diagnosis, when sample acquisition complications and uncharacteristic presentation complicate accurate detection.

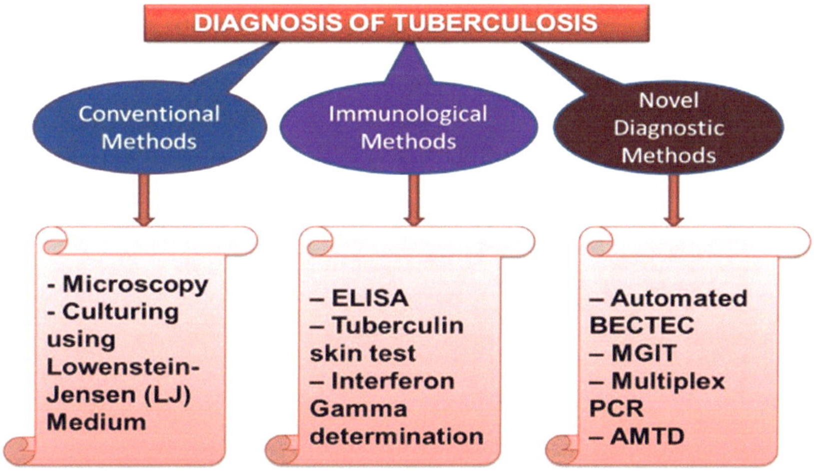

Figure 3.6. Different diagnostic methods of tuberculosis.

Source: Elsevier. (n.d.). *Diagnosis of tuberculosis: Comparison of conventional, immunological, and novel diagnostic methods*. https://ars.els-cdn.com/content/image/1-s2.0-S0009279721000338-gr2.jpg.

Enhancing clinical sample quality, in addition to including innovative diagnostic technologies, is the foundation of better TB diagnosis globally (Connell et al., 2011). No matter how advanced the diagnosis of PTB, EPTB, like colonic tuberculosis, tends to be evasive until invasive procedures such as surgery are undertaken. The nonspecific clinical presentation often imitates other gastrointestinal illness, leading to diagnostic delay and enhanced morbidity. Colonoscopy, made possible by fiberoptic technology, now makes it possible to directly visualize diseased colonic mucosa and immediately obtain samples for histopathological and microbiological evaluation. The immediate diagnostic return of the procedure helps differentiate TB from other chronic inflammatory or infectious conditions of the colon. Considering the common under-suspicion in the past before surgical exploration, increased clinical suspicion aided by aggressive utilization of high-yield diagnostic modalities is required. Prompt utilization of such modalities or initiating empirical anti-tuberculosis therapy can avoid delay-related complications (Sibuea et al., 2001). Molecular testing like NAATs and IGRAs has changed TB detection by targeting specific genetic material or immune responses. These methods offer rapid and accurate detection of Mycobacterium tuberculosis complex (MTBC) from different clinical specimens. Their cost-effectiveness and accessibility continue to be impediments in most high-burden nations. IGRAs identify latent tuberculosis infection (LTBI) by quantifying T-cell release of interferon-gamma (IFN-γ), but not active and latent disease, requiring conjunction with clinical and radiologic findings. In addition, new research targets enhancing sample processing methods, particularly from paucibacillary cases like pediatric or EPTB. The synergy of these new diagnostic methods and the conventional methods maximizes accuracy and facilitates early detection, ultimately minimizing transmission and maximizing patient outcomes (Connell et al., 2011) (Figure 3.6).

3.3.1. Tuberculin Skin Test (TST)

TB diagnosis requires accurate methods to identify latent infection, especially among high-risk groups. Traditionally, TST has been a mainstay in the screening for LTBI. The technique is done via the intradermal administration of purified protein derivative (PPD), with induration size measured after 48 to 72 hours. Although commonly utilized because of its availability and cheapness, the TST is problematic with regard to specificity, particularly in subjects vaccinated with Bacillus Calmette-Guérin (BCG) or with past exposure to nontuberculous mycobacteria (NTM). These phenomena can result in false-positive testing, making diagnosis more difficult as well as clinical decision-making afterward (Figure 3.7).

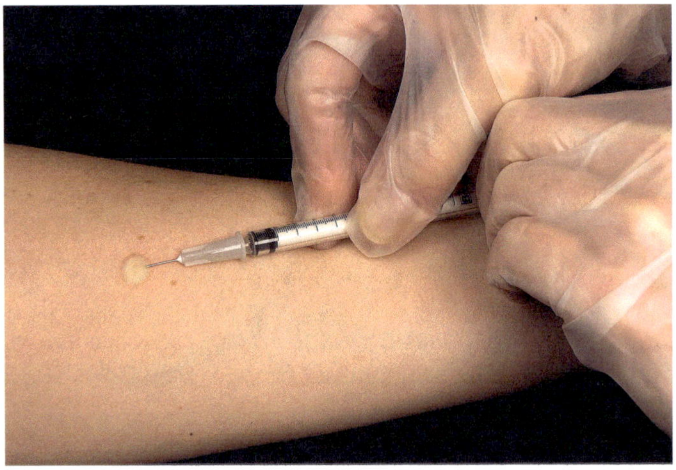

Figure 3.7. A TB skin test measures your immune system's response to a purified protein derivative (PPD) solution injected under your skin.

Source: By Greg Knobloch - This media comes from the Centers for Disease Control and Prevention's Public Health Image Library (PHIL), with identification number #6806.Note: Not all PHIL images are public domain; be sure to check copyright status and credit authors and content providers. العربية | Deutsch | English | македонски | slovenščina | +/−, Public Domain, https://commons.wikimedia.org/w/index.php?curid=848106

Despite these constraints, the TST continues to play a role in resource-constrained environments and is part of a stepwise diagnostic strategy to diagnose risk patients who would be treated prophylactically. The development of TB diagnosis has brought in IGRAs as substitutes for the TST with better specificity and reduced cross-reaction with BCG vaccination, but the TST still holds importance on account of operational and economic factors. Recent health economic analysis, for instance, on cost-effectiveness in pediatric settings, emphasizes the tension between TST and IGRA tests. For instance, findings from settings such as Colombia show that although the QuantiFERON (QFT) test can be cost-effective, the TST's cost-effectiveness and diagnostic accuracy sustain its use in initial screening protocols, particularly among immunocompetent children who have been exposed to active cases of TB (Navarro et al., 2025). These results highlight the continued utility of the TST and the value of strategic integration with newer modalities of testing in national programs of tuberculosis control. Though the TST has practical merits, interpretation must be well-appraised clinical context because of fluctuating sensitivity thresholds based on host immunity and a history of BCG vaccination. Furthermore, indeterminate or uncertain results from IGRAs highlight the importance of ancillary testing strategies. Investigation into combined methods, in which the TST is complemented by IGRA or other assays, seeks to improve diagnostic sensitivity and inform treatment choice effectively. A recent publication placed the TST in a diagnostic algorithm that prioritized QFT-Plus for standard screening but suggested reserve tests such as C-Respond T-SPOT.TB when indeterminate results are obtained, so as to maximize LTBI detection (Pagnoncelli et al., 2024). Such suggested strategies indicate continuous attempts to optimize cost, availability, and diagnostic accuracy so that the TST maintains an essential but subtle role in the diagnosis of tuberculosis (Figure 3.8).

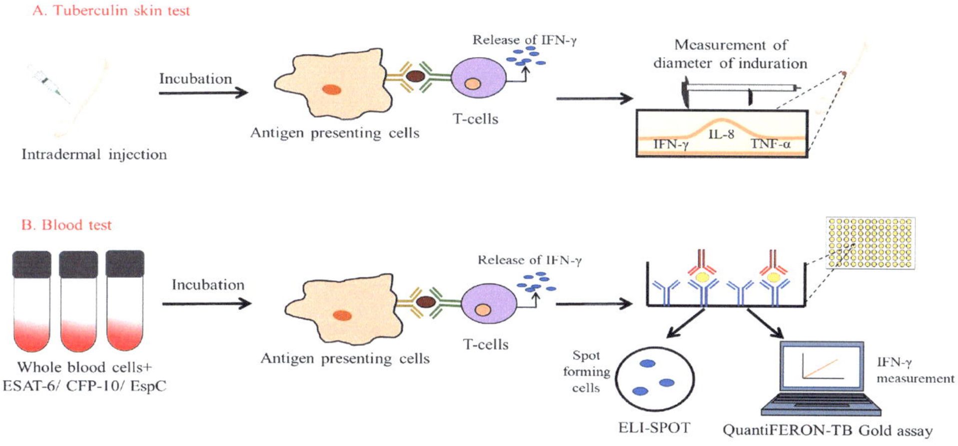

6

Figure 3.8. Detection of latent tuberculosis infection. (A) Tuberculin skin test; and (B) blood test.

Source: Elsevier. (n.d.). *Comparison of tuberculosis diagnostic tests: (A) Tuberculin skin test and (B) Interferon-gamma release assays (IGRAs).* https://ars.els-cdn.com/content/image/1-s2.0-S1472979223000380-gr6_lrg.jpg.

3.3.2. Interferon-Gamma Release Assays (IGRAs)

The diagnosis of tuberculosis has become much improved with the recent advances in immunological testing, specifically the establishment of IGRAs. These tests quantify the immune reaction to certain MTB antigens by measuring the release of IFN-γ from sensitized T-cells. In contrast to the conventional TST, which may give false results because of previous BCG vaccination or NTM exposure, IGRAs have greater specificity. Several commercial IGRAs, including QuantiFERON-TB Gold Plus (QFT-Plus) and recent updates like TBF-ELISA and TBF-FIA, have been investigated for their diagnostic performance. Comparative studies show sensitivity among the assays tends to be high overall but may slightly differ in specificity, thus emphasizing the need for proper selection of the most suitable test for various epidemiological conditions (Kutame et al., 2024). These data show the way that IGRAs add to enhanced diagnostic accuracy, particularly in the presence of extensive BCG vaccination in the population.

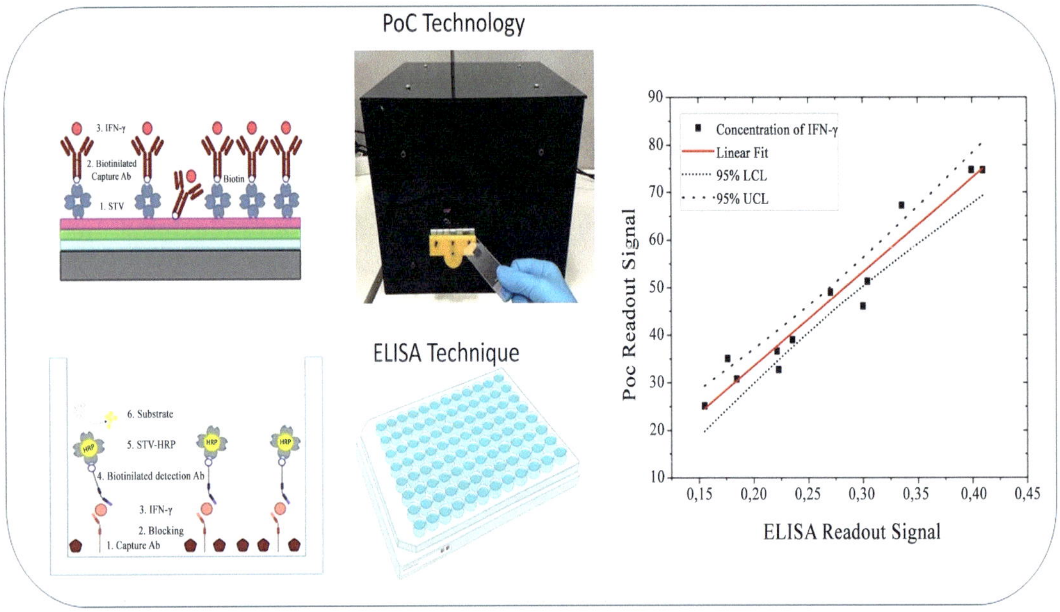

Figure 3.9. Steps of interferon-gamma release assay test (IGRA Test).

Source: Heras MFL, Ramirez Y, Fernández Martín C, L. Espinosa R, Lavín A, Holgado M. A Point-of-Care Based on Label-Free Interferometric Optical Detection Method to Evaluate Interferon Gamma (IFN-γ): A Correlation with the ELISA Technique. *Sensors*. 2020; 20(17):4776. https://doi.org/10.3390/s20174776

Assessment for the practical utility of IGRAs involves measurement of their predictive accuracy in various populations, especially those at risk of developing active disease from LTBI. In one study performed in an urban district with high-risk populations, IGRAs were used to diagnose LTBI among those with fibrotic lesions on chest radiographs, a finding commonly linked with increased risk of progression. The study found that during a median observation interval in excess of three years, the rate of annual incidence of active TB in these IGRA-positive subjects was 1.18 cases per 100 person-years. Interestingly, some patients reverted to active disease despite anti-TB treatment, indicating that although IGRAs are effective in screening for those at risk, ongoing follow-up and integrated management are still crucial (Komukai et al., 2023). This information highlights the value of IGRAs for the early detection and stratification of TB risk across different populations. Despite the benefits of IGRAs over TSTs, some limitations should be recognized in the framework of TB diagnosis. The variable sensitivity and specificity between assays highlight the requirement for thoughtful interpretation with concurrent clinical and epidemiological data. In addition, conditions of immunosuppression, HIV co-infection, and technical variation in assay performance may affect IGRA outcomes. The selection of an IGRA must not only be based on diagnostic performance but also on logistical factors such as cost, laboratory capacity, and patient population demographics. Recent studies indicate promising changes and newer modalities to enhance accuracy and applicability. Ongoing comparative research and convergence with other diagnostic modalities will further solidify the place of IGRAs in integrated tuberculosis control efforts (Kutame et al., 2024) (Figure 3.9).

3.3.3. Sputum Smear and Culture Tests

Timely and accurate diagnosis forms a foundation for the efficient treatment of tuberculosis (TB), and one of the oldest and most prevalent diagnostic methods is sputum-based testing. While imaging and molecular testing have made improvements, sputum smear microscopy continues to be heavily utilized, especially in resource-constrained settings, because it is inexpensive and simple. This technique entails staining sputum specimens and viewing them under a microscope to identify AFB, the characteristic of TB infection. Although rapid, however, sputum smear microscopy has poor sensitivity, particularly in the case of paucibacillary disease and patients co-infected with HIV, who have lower bacterial load. Thus, while sputum smear tests yield rapid and convenient preliminary proof of infection, their accuracy requires verification by more sensitive tests to minimize false-negative results and enhance patient treatment. Following up on smear microscopy, sputum culture tests provide better diagnostic specificity through the growth and identification of MTB in laboratory cultures. Culturing is still the gold standard for diagnosing TB due to its higher sensitivity and capacity to evaluate bacterial viability, which is very important for the evaluation of response to treatment and for detecting drug resistance.

Although culture techniques like the mycobacterial growth indicator tube (MGIT) and Löwenstein-Jensen (LJ) media are time-consuming, taking weeks to produce results and hence delaying clinical decision-making. In addition, culture accuracy is prone to contamination and technical restraints, particularly in specimens rich in competing flora. Research stresses that the combination of culture with microscopy maximizes diagnostic yield yet also indicates the requirement for other sample types or adjunct diagnostic tests to avoid these constraints and allow early detection (Rahane et al., 2024). Current advances in TB diagnosis have been directed at investigating the usefulness of molecular tests and surrogate specimens to circumvent the intrinsic limitations of sputum smear and culture testing. For example, stool specimens, examined using RNA-based tests like tuberculosis molecular bacterial load assay (TB-MBLA), show high sensitivity and specificity in identifying viable TB bacilli, especially in patients with limited or no sputum production. In comparison with traditional culture techniques, which are often plagued by contamination and reduced specificity because of the complex microbial environments, TB-MBLA provides quantification of bacterial load with higher diagnostic sensitivity. This development highlights the potential for non-sputum-based diagnostic strategies to complement historic sputum smear and culture testing, increasing case detection rates and valuable information about bacterial burden, ultimately guiding individualized treatment strategies (Musisi et al., 2022) (Figure 3.10).

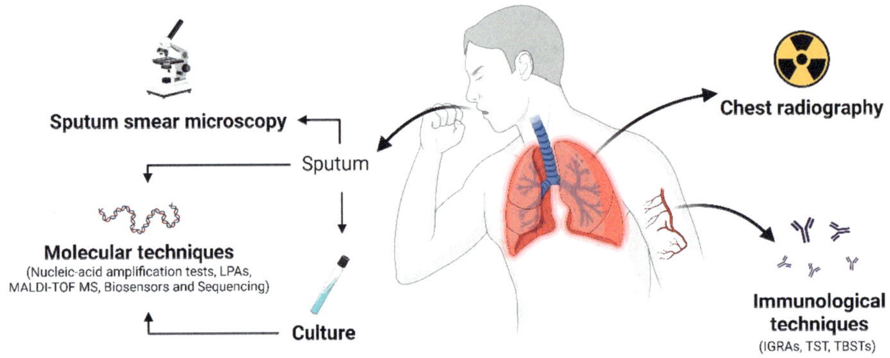

Figure 3.10. Illustration of relevant diagnostic techniques employed for pulmonary tuberculosis (PTB) diagnosis. Sputum is collected and examined under a microscope for *acid-fast bacilli* (AFB). Chest radiography assesses lung abnormalities such as infiltrates, cavities, or pleural effusions. Molecular techniques detect the genetic material of *MTBC* using methods like NAATs, LAMP, MALDI-TOF MS, biosensors, and sequencing.

Source: Bartolomeu-Gonçalves G, Souza JMd, Fernandes BT, Spoladori LFA, Correia GF, Castro IMd, Borges PHG, Silva-Rodrigues G, Tavares ER, Yamauchi LM, et al. Tuberculosis Diagnosis: Current, Ongoing, and Future Approaches. *Diseases*. 2024; 12(9):202. https://doi.org/10.3390/diseases12090202

3.4. Imaging Techniques in Diagnosis

Improved medical imaging has greatly improved the diagnosis of tuberculosis, particularly distinguishing it from other conditions with similar symptoms. Diagnosis of extrapulmonary types, including intestinal tuberculosis, requires an integrated diagnostic approach where imaging is a vital component in addition to clinical assessment and biopsy. Methods such as ultrasound, computed tomography (CT), and magnetic resonance imaging (MRI) are crucial in imaging involved tissues and in the direction of needle biopsies, which augment diagnostic accuracy. Imaging techniques can identify classic lesions, lymphadenopathy, and structural deformities that would otherwise be unrevealed by symptoms alone. Through the integration of precise imaging with microbiological and immunological examinations, diagnostic assurance is enhanced to facilitate early intervention. The multidimensional use of these technologies is ever more critical in countries with high tuberculosis incidence, particularly where co-infection with HIV complicates the clinical scenario and requires increased clinical alertness (Donoghue & Holton, 2009). Integrating imaging into tuberculosis treatment goes beyond simple identification, including comprehension of the disease's diverse presentations among patient groups. Adult and pediatric patients both exhibit overlapping yet unique imaging characteristics, necessitating clinicians to be skilled at reading these subtleties to prevent misdiagnosis. Pediatric cases, for instance, can have specific anatomical susceptibilities that affect imaging results. Radiologists and clinicians need to work closely to optimize imaging protocols that incorporate local epidemiological influences and patient-specific variables like HIV co-infection and drug resistance. Highlighting shared expertise guarantees precise detection and classification of tuberculosis lesions, particularly where radiological facilities are meager or radiologists are scarce. Such dynamic interaction of expert interpretation and applied technology becomes crucial to improving tuberculosis diagnosis and conforms with modern imaging classifications (Andronikou et al., 2009). Modern imaging techniques not only enhance initial diagnosis but also play a role in continuous patient monitoring and treatment efficacy evaluation. Serial imaging enables clinicians to monitor disease progression or regression and identify complications that can necessitate a change in therapeutic approach. High-resolution modalities enable identifying minor variations in lesion size, number, and features, which are essential in dealing with complicated presentations like multi-drug resistant tuberculosis (MDR-TB) or disseminated disease. Moreover, technological advances enable minimally invasive sampling procedures, which minimize patient risk and allow for earlier diagnosis. Despite these advantages, the impact of imaging in the diagnosis of tuberculosis also relies upon clinicians being aware of the heterogeneous presentation of the disease. Thus, greater educational input and uniform imaging protocols need to be applied to derive maximum benefit from these technologies across various healthcare environments (Donoghue & Holton, 2009).

3.4.1. Role of Chest X-Rays

The process of diagnosing lung infections demands equipment that is able to offer timely, accurate, and non-invasive monitoring of pulmonary illness. In this respect, chest X-rays are crucial as they allow clinicians to see the anatomy and pathological changes of the lungs that are characteristic of tuberculosis. In contrast to more invasive procedures, chest radiographs are able to provide evidence of patterns typical of PTB, for example, infiltrates, cavitations, or nodules, rapidly. Current advances in image recognition using artificial intelligence (AI) have continued to improve the accuracy of diagnosis of chest X-rays using convolutional neural networks to categorize images into categories such as tuberculosis with remarkable precision. The machine learning models like VGG19 have proved to have accuracy levels higher than 95%, highlighting the possibility of integrating chest X-rays with computational tools to enhance early TB diagnosis and enable timely initiation of treatment (Pratama et al., 2021). While molecular and microbiologic methods are still the standards of reference for tuberculosis diagnosis, the diagnostic value of chest X-rays holds especially in the case of smear-negative patients and HIV-infected patients where bacillary burden is commonly low. Recommendations set forth by the World Health Organization (WHO) highlight the role of chest radiography in diagnostic strategies to enhance detection and care of smear-negative PTB. In real-life contexts, chest X-rays assist clinicians in detecting suspicious lesions that call for additional microbiological investigation or empiric therapy, filling the gaps when sputum examinations don't yield decisive results. Operational effectiveness revealed by field trials also underscores the immediate screening and triage capability of chest X-rays, which had high compliance rates in low-resource settings, thus facilitating the diagnostic process for vulnerable groups (Koole et al., 2011). Though diagnostic, chest X-rays have limitations that justify careful interpretation, especially with regard to specificity and treatment decision implications. Though radiographs of the chest can reveal abnormalities consistent with tuberculosis, such observations are not pathognomonic and might overlap with other pulmonary processes, prompting further testing. Moreover, adherence to recommendations for ordering chest X-rays and treatment initiation may be variable, subject to healthcare infrastructure and delays in clinician judgment. Sensitivity and specificity values of approximately 60% and 80%, respectively, indicate that chest X-rays cannot be used as isolated diagnoses but in conjunction with a multidimensional strategy involving clinical assessment, microbiology, and imaging modalities. Therefore, although chest X-rays are still invaluable in the prompt detection of tuberculosis, their utility is maximized when implemented within inclusive diagnostic schemes (Koole et al., 2011) (Figure 3.11).

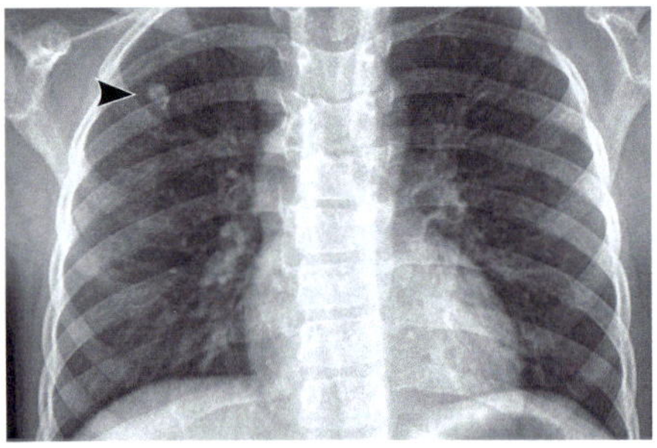

Figure 3.11. Chest X-ray for screening for tuberculosis.

Source: Radiology Assistant. (n.d.). *Chest X-ray showing calcification in the right lung suggestive of prior tuberculosis infection.* https://radiologyassistant.nl/assets/_1-calcification-right-lung-1.jpg.

3.4.2. Use of CT Scans

New imaging modalities have played a major role in the detection and diagnosis of lung diseases at an early stage. Of these, the CT scan produces high-definition images that detect fine abnormalities in lung tissue, allowing clinicians to detect typical findings of TB not seen on routine chest radiography. CT scans can outline the extent of active disease, depicting granulomas, cavitations, and lymphadenopathy, which are important for precise diagnosis and treatment planning. Also, CT imaging can identify sequelae of earlier TB infections, such as calcifications and fibrosis, that may complicate differential diagnosis in endemic regions. Nevertheless, the occurrence of such sequelae can lower the specificity of CT in differentiating active tuberculosis from other pulmonary conditions, which may require corroborative clinical and microbiological evaluation to ascertain accurate diagnosis (Kim et al., 2020). Therefore, CT scans are an important diagnostic adjunct in the complete assessment of tuberculosis. Through the development of machine learning and AI, CT imaging interpretation has become more accurate and effective in the diagnosis of lung infections, such as tuberculosis. Artificial intelligence programs learned through massive collections of lung CT scans develop high sensitivity in distinguishing TB from other infectious conditions, including viral and bacterial cases of pneumonia, by identifying unique radiographic patterns. These platforms minimize the dependence on subjective human judgment, which is time-consuming and susceptible to inter-observer variability, thus streamlining diagnostic processes in clinical practice. Current research shows that AI-aided CT analysis provides sensitivity and specificity levels of over 98% for pulmonary infections, while its utility in improving early diagnosis, particularly in resource-poor environments where skilled radiologists are not readily available, is also shown (Fu et al., 2020). The integration of AI-based CT interpretation complements conventional diagnostic practices to ensure timely and reliable diagnosis of tuberculosis for the management and control of patients. Even with the benefits that come with them, the application of CT scans in diagnosing tuberculosis has its pitfalls. In areas where TB prevalence is high, post-infectious changes present can result in false-positive findings, reducing the specificity of CT screening and making it difficult to differentiate between active disease and residual lung changes. This diagnostic uncertainty can lead to unwarranted treatments or additional invasive testing, which further emphasizes the necessity for standardized reporting systems like Lung CT Screening Reporting and Data System (Lung-RADS) to enhance interpretative consistency. Additionally, CT scans expose patients to ionizing radiation and are more expensive than other imaging modalities, which precludes their accessibility and regular use in most endemic regions. Balancing the advantages of CT imaging against such limitations calls for combined diagnostic strategies, integrating clinical assessment, microbiologic documentation, and radiologic information to maximize tuberculosis diagnosis accuracy and effectiveness (Kim et al., 2020) (Figure 3.12).

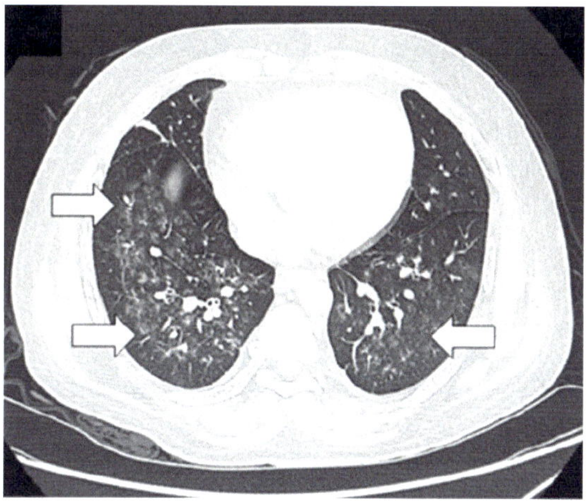

Figure 3.12. Pulmonary tuberculosis (PTB). High-resolution CT scan of lung window showing pulmonary tuberculosis in a case of cirrhosis. Centrilobular nodules are seen in both lungs with tree-in-bud appearance.

Source: ResearchGate. (n.d.). *Spectrum of imaging findings in pulmonary tuberculosis (TB): Axial computed tomography (CT) scan showing bilateral lung involvement.* https://www.researchgate.net/figure/Spectrum-of-imaging-findings-in-pulmonary-tuberculosis-TB-A-Axial-computed_fig1_271217961.

3.4.3. Limitations of Imaging Techniques

Medical imaging has certainly improved diagnostic capacity; yet, in the case of tuberculosis (TB), such methods are presented with significant challenges. Imaging modalities such as chest X-rays and CT scans tend to be nonspecific because radiographic findings of TB may be similar to other pulmonary conditions of malignancy or fungal disease. Also, imaging tends to show structural abnormalities instead of directly detecting the pathogen or the load of bacteria. This restriction makes not only early diagnosis but also assessment of treatment response challenging, particularly because heterogeneous tissue involvement and changing bacillary populations might not be consistent with visual changes. As a result, while imaging yields crucial morphological data, it is short of fully illustrating MTB dynamics in lesions, making the need for complementary diagnostic strategies reflecting active bacterial presence and host responses imperative (Bruyn et al., 2016). The imaging challenges are even higher in the diagnosis of EPTB, where lesions are usually less accessible and have lower concentrations of bacteria. In such instances, standard imaging methods may be able to identify granulomatous inflammation but may not be able to distinguish between TB and other etiologies of identical tissue changes. The problem is further increased by the heterogeneous distribution of bacteria in involved tissues, which can result in potentially incorrect or false-negative imaging findings. Pleural and vertebral TB, for example, can present different radiologic features, but their sensitivity is still inadequate to secure a diagnosis with certainty in the absence of supportive microbiological or histological proof. Additionally, imaging is not able to consistently evaluate bacterial load, which is essential in tracking treatment response and disease progression in EPTB, highlighting the deficiency inherent in only using radiologic assessment for diagnostic conclusions (Azarhoush et al., 2014). The other key limitation is the inability of imaging to be used as a consistent surrogate for therapeutic monitoring in managing tuberculosis. Radiographic changes are usually delayed relative to the microbiological response to therapy, making imaging less helpful in real-time measurement of disease resolution or risk of relapse. The slow therapy duration added to the complex pharmacodynamics of MTB subpopulations complicates the interpretation of imaging data even further. This lack of correlation between radiographic presentations and clinical results requires extra biomarkers or diagnostic methods capable of portraying the host-pathogen interactions more accurately. The creation of such modalities is a research focus to overcome the limitations of existing imaging tools, particularly in heterogeneous patient populations, such as drug-resistant strains or pediatric and extrapulmonary types of TB (Bruyn et al., 2016) (Figure 3.13).

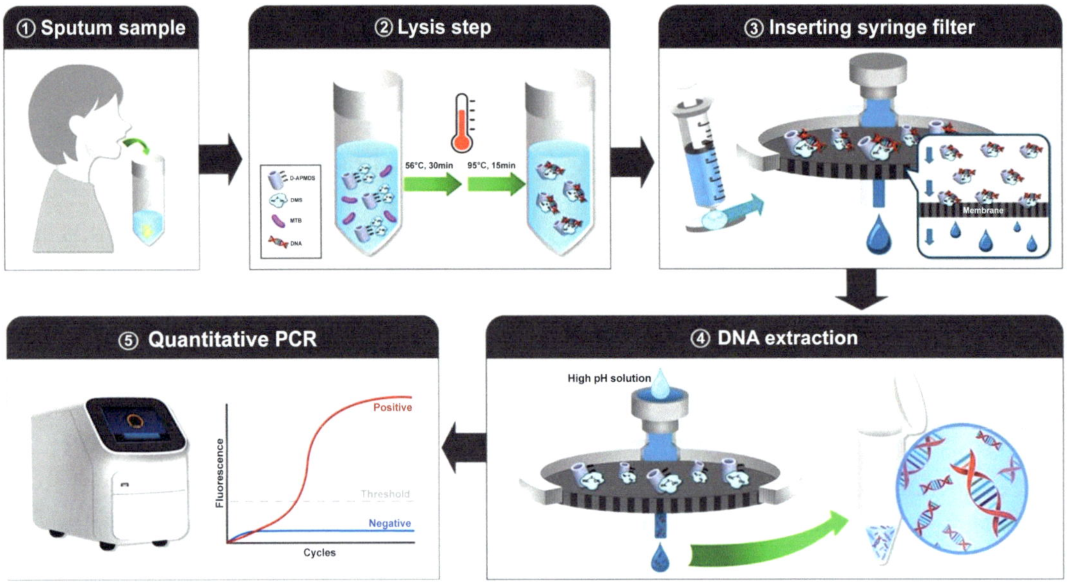

Figure 3.13. Detection of tuberculosis infection by biosensors.

Source: Lee HJ, Kim NH, Lee EH, Yoon YS, Jeong YJ, Lee BC, Koo B, Jang YO, Kim S-H, Kang YA, et al. Multicenter Testing of a Simple Molecular Diagnostic System for the Diagnosis of Mycobacterium Tuberculosis. *Biosensors*. 2023; 13(2):259. https://doi.org/10.3390/bios13020259

3.5. Challenges in Diagnosing Tuberculosis

Diagnosis of tuberculosis has advanced in great measures in recent years, but many challenges still hinder effective diagnosis. Undiagnosed TB cases account for a huge global burden, with almost a third of infections not being detected every year, mostly because of diagnostic unreliability and unavailability. Despite the increased sensitivity and specificity from newer methods like liquid culture, drug susceptibility testing (DST), and nucleic acid amplification, their use in resource-constrained and rural areas is limited by cost, infrastructural requirements, and expertise demands. This inequality fuels an important gap where the most disadvantaged populations are left behind, and transmission continues unabated. In addition, the changing threat of drug-resistant organisms calls for more advanced diagnostic tools that can perform rapid resistance profiling. While these advances have been made, there is still no ideal point-of-care triage test that is inexpensive, sensitive, and deployable in various environments, which emphasizes the urgency of further research and development to fill this diagnostic gap (Shrivas & Singh, 2025). The pathologic complexity of tuberculosis also underlies diagnostic challenges, especially in differentiating latent and active disease and to detect extrapulmonary forms. Traditional diagnostic techniques tend to use sputum samples, which can be absent or false negatives in certain patient groups, for example, children or immunocompromised patients. Radiological techniques, although common, have their own limitation with variability in interpretation and the risk of overlapping clinical presentations with other pulmonary conditions. Recent attempts at integrating AI using deep learning platforms hold the potential to improve diagnostic performance by computerizing image interpretation and capturing faint radiographic patterns consistent with TB. Such methods, such as convolutional neural networks with segmentation algorithms, have shown exceptional sensitivity and specificity in initial studies. These exciting technologies need to be validated across various clinical environments to guarantee robustness and generalizability across populations (Bhalerao, 2024). Another critical obstacle is the timely and thorough diagnosis of drug-resistant tuberculosis (DR-TB), hindering therapeutic approaches and compromising international health efforts.

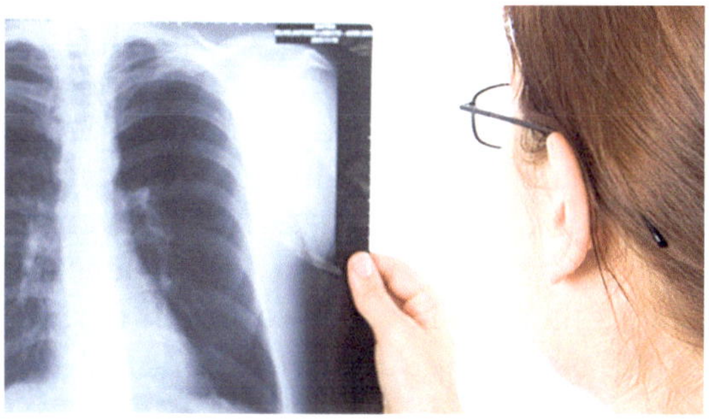

Source: Centers for Disease Control and Prevention (CDC). (n.d.). *Doctor viewing a chest X-ray for signs of tuberculosis.* https://www.cdc.gov/tb/media/images/Doctor_viewing_xray_1200x675.jpg.

Conventional culture and drug susceptibility testing, although regarded as gold standards, are prolonged and can cause undue delay in instituting proper treatment. Molecular methods like line probe assays (LPAs) provide quicker detection of resistance but are hampered by the availability of resources and technical sophistication, which limits their routine application. In addition, the co-existence of several resistance mechanisms necessitates multiplex diagnostic tools that can identify a wide range of mutations. Implementing such high-level diagnostic devices in national TB control programs necessitates transcending logistical barriers such as supply chain stability and health worker capacity. Countering these interrelated challenges requires a coordinated response that blends technical innovation and strengthening of the health system to enhance early diagnosis and efficient management of tuberculosis (Shrivas & Singh, 2025).

3.5.1. False Positives and Negatives

In the quest to enhance tuberculosis diagnosis, it is crucial to acknowledge the limitations imposed by false positives and false negatives that impact clinical outcomes as well as public health efforts. Conventional smear microscopy, widely practiced in most resource-constrained settings, tends to miss out due to a higher limit of detection since 5000 to 10,000 bacilli per milliliter of sputum is needed to result in a positive. This threshold leads to false negatives, that is, infected patients may remain undiagnosed and untreated, hence still spreading the disease. False positives, in contrast, may cause unnecessary treatment, loading patients with side effects and health systems with expenses. Current research emphasizes that more sensitive technologies such as GeneXpert MTB/RIF eliminate false negatives by identifying a minimum of 131 to 250 colony-forming units per milliliter, enhancing early case detection and treatment initiation enormously (Asare et al., 2024). This innovation highlights the significance of diagnostic precision in preventing tuberculosis transmission. Tuberculosis diagnosis complexity is further amplified when taking EPTB into perspective, where unusual clinical presentations tend to complicate timely detection. Diagnostic tests can produce different levels of false positive and false negative results based on sample type and technique. For example, AFB culture, the long-held gold standard, has high specificity but low sensitivity, producing numerous false negatives that cause prolonged therapy. In contrast, new technologies like TNS have excellent sensitivity and specificity, with lower false positive rates in a wide range of extrapulmonary samples. The capability of TNS to properly differentiate tuberculosis DNA from other mimicking infections reduces diagnostic uncertainty, ultimately leading to more accurate clinical choices (Yu et al., 2024). The results emphasize the delicate balance between sensitivity and specificity necessary to reduce diagnostic errors in extrapulmonary cases. The consequences of false positives and negatives reach beyond patient care into public health implications, notably in controlling tuberculosis spread. An underestimated rate of false negatives, as with less sensitive diagnostic methods, results in cases of untreated infection being a source for ongoing transmission chains. In contrast, false positives can result in the wastage of scarce resources and subjecting uninfected individuals to potentially toxic treatment schedules. As such, incorporating diagnostics such as GeneXpert and TNS, which have better sensitivity and specificity profiles, can help avoid such pitfalls. Their improved accuracy reduces both false positives and false negatives, facilitating early diagnosis and proper treatment while maintaining high healthcare efficiency. Such balance is crucial for enhanced tuberculosis control programs and mitigating the worldwide burden (Asare et al., 2024; Yu et al., 2024).

3.5.2. Co-Infection with Other Diseases

Co-infection is a major challenge in the diagnosis and treatment of tuberculosis, usually complicating clinical presentation and treatment approach. Patients with co-infection with tuberculosis and human immunodeficiency virus (HIV) are a classic example. HIV compromises the immune system, causing patients to become susceptible to many opportunistic infections, such as EPTB, which occurs with varied and unusual symptoms. As an example, co-infected individuals will experience pleural or pericardial effusions (PEs), presentations that can be confused with other pathologies. The overlap of clinical features in this case makes it challenging to diagnose, necessitating that medical professionals embrace multi-disciplinary strategies and use specialized diagnosis tools such as adenosine deaminase testing and mycobacterial cultures to diagnose tuberculosis in the face of co-infection. Early and correct diagnosis in these situations is very important to start adequate antiretroviral and anti-tuberculosis treatments simultaneously, which are extremely effective in enhancing patient outcomes (Hadiatma & Triyono, 2023). Placing another level of complexity, the recent outbreak of COVID-19 has introduced new diagnostic challenges for tuberculosis, particularly where both infections overlap. Because COVID-19 and tuberculosis have similar clinical presentations, such as fever, dry cough, and shortness of breath, the risk of misdiagnosis is higher when there are widespread viral outbreaks. This convergence threatens to cause delays in tuberculosis diagnosis that can result in cases left untreated and propagate public health conditions. Additionally, employing immunosuppressive agents in treating COVID-19 can compound underlying tuberculosis infections, and therefore, there is an urgent need for well-designed screening programs that detect co-infections early. This awareness allows for timely and individualized therapeutic interventions before the disease becomes severe and transmissible among vulnerable groups (Niazkar et al., 2022). These diagnostic challenges highlight the need for increased clinical vigilance and upgraded diagnostic infrastructure, particularly in settings of high burden. Co-infection with conditions like HIV or COVID-19 usually leads to unusual manifestations of tuberculosis that necessitate advanced radiological investigations, molecular diagnostics, and immunologic tests for proper detection. Comprehensively integrated healthcare services that address multiple infections at one time can optimize diagnostic procedures and enhance treatment protocols. In addition, educating healthcare providers in detecting possible co-infections and interpreting diagnostic results in this context is important to prevent missed or delayed tuberculosis diagnoses. With the changing healthcare landscape on a global scale, the interconnection of tuberculosis with other infectious diseases highlights the need for comprehensive diagnostic strategies to enhance patient outcomes as well as prevent transmission (Niazkar et al., 2022; Hadiatma & Triyono, 2023).

3.5.3. Socioeconomic Factors Affecting Diagnosis

The availability of healthcare facilities and environmental living conditions significantly impact the early diagnosis of tuberculosis, especially in places where socioeconomic inequalities are evident. People living in semiurban or slum areas tend to have cramped living spaces and insufficient sanitation facilities, conditions that enhance the spread of tuberculosis and hinder early detection. These conditions are usually characterized by low levels of awareness about the disease and therefore delayed consultation and diagnosis. For example, in New Delhi, a study found that most patients with TB resided in privately owned homes with inconsistent sanitary access where low to poor awareness levels were common, negatively affecting treatment compliance (Zaidi et al., 2024). The interaction between poor hygiene, starvation, and crowding creates an environment that is both a facilitator of disease transmission and diagnostic postponement, emphasizing the important role socioeconomic status takes in hindering prompt detection and successful intervention. Demographic factors like age, gender, and economic status also act as mediators of the course of tuberculosis diagnosis by affecting patient awareness and decision-making to seek healthcare. Middle-aged adults, especially those from lower socioeconomic classes, seem to be disproportionately impacted by the musculoskeletal presentation of tuberculosis that can escape early diagnosis based on nonspecific presenting symptoms. A study involving musculoskeletal TB patients revealed that most patients belonged to the upper-lower social class and presented nonspecific complaints that delayed the diagnostic workup (Babu et al., 2024). In addition, comorbidities such as diabetes among these groups may complicate clinical presentations, further hindering recognition. These observations underscore how social determinants, rather than just access, influence clinical outcomes by regulating disease visibility, healthcare use, and, in turn, diagnosis timing. The societal stigma of tuberculosis, rooted in socioeconomic determinants, is a critical contributor to diagnostic delay because it keeps patients from seeking care promptly. Social stigma usually results in inadequate patient education and resistance to symptom disclosure, further compounding disease progression and transmission among vulnerable populations. Besides physical obstacles like poverty and living conditions, psychological and social factors also impede successful patient involvement in diagnosis processes. Interventions for TB control must then go beyond clinical and laboratory diagnosis to confront socioeconomic determinants of health such as education at the community level and better living conditions, which are critical to improve health literacy and diminish stigma (Zaidi et al., 2024). Lacking such a comprehensive approach, the cycle of socioeconomic hardship fueling late diagnosis will continue, defeating tuberculosis elimination efforts in the world.

Summary

The ultimate culmination of tuberculosis diagnosis is dependent on correlating clinical, radiographic, and laboratory results to provide timely and accurate diagnosis. Despite the improvements made in molecular biology methods and immunological tests with respect to increasing the sensitivity of diagnosis, there remain challenges, especially where resources are low. The variety of symptoms presented by tuberculosis and other respiratory infections makes clinical evaluation challenging, thus complementing the use of diagnostic tools. Additionally, new challenges, including the interplay between tuberculosis and other infectious disorders like COVID-19, indicate that there is a need for holistic diagnostics, which can be responsive to co-morbidities and possible risk factors. By assessing diagnostic approaches stringently and refining them, healthcare systems can enhance case detection and curb the spread of tuberculosis and thus enable improved patient outcomes and public health control (Gao et al., 2020). Another essential aspect in the diagnosis of tuberculosis is the use of computer-aided methods that complement conventional imaging analysis to achieve greater precision and consistency. Deep learning architectures, especially convolutional neural networks, have shown promising performance in analyzing chest X-rays even when trained on small and biased datasets. Lung segmentation and advanced data augmentation techniques play important roles in enhancing the diagnostic accuracy by targeting analysis to the pertinent anatomical structure and reducing noise from irrelevant information. Despite issues like overfitting, these novel technologies are highly beneficial in resource-limited environments and augment human capability by optimizing the diagnostic process and speeding up clinical decision-making (Stirenko et al., 2018). Sustained development and testing of such AI instruments will play a key role in optimizing tuberculosis diagnosis worldwide. In reconciling the existing evidence and advances in technology, it is clear that the future of tuberculosis diagnosis lies in multifaceted strategies combining clinical expertise with novel methodologies. Guarantees of accuracy and accessibility of the diagnostic instruments require on-going research, particularly in heterogeneously diverse populations and different healthcare infrastructures. Moreover, the merging of data-driven approaches with traditional practices offers a route toward more accurate, fast, and non-invasive diagnosis. Such a paradigm shift can decrease the lag time to treatment initiation and decrease disease burden, especially in vulnerable populations with complicated health profiles. Finally, vigilance and cross-professional cooperation will be essential factors in optimizing diagnostic pathways and attaining improved control of tuberculosis globally (Stirenko et al., 2018; Gao et al., 2020).

Accurate diagnosis remains a cornerstone for the effective management of tuberculosis, necessitating a multifaceted approach that combines clinical, radiological, and laboratory data. The chief problem is to distinguish tuberculosis from other pulmonary diseases, especially malignancies whose presentation can be mimicked by tuberculosis. Such complexity calls for increased clinical acumen and employing differential diagnostic techniques to prevent misdiagnosis and mismanagement. Diagnostic advances have improved the accuracy of MTB identification, yet these need interpretation in the wider clinical setting. Dynamic observation combined with follow-up investigations is essential to validate the diagnosis and differentiate from other pathologies with similar signs or radiographic patterns, to provide timely and proper patient care (Manfredini et al., 2024). The heterogeneity of tuberculosis presentation further accentuates the necessity of inclusion of overall diagnostic criteria that consider etiology and pathophysiology as a whole. Important diagnostic highlights highlight the need for correlation of clinical presentation and symptoms with imaging and microbiological findings. This ensures optimization of tuberculosis identification accuracy and minimizes diagnostic errors that are commonly observed in everyday clinical practice because of overlapping between features of tuberculosis and other respiratory conditions. The understanding of tuberculosis's multifactorial origin educates further testing decisions and directs the use of appropriate treatment interventions. Additionally, evidence-based diagnosis system frameworks, in accordance with global standards, enhance clinicians' capacity to make context-specific interventions for each patient, advancing overall outcomes (Manfredini et al., 2024). In furthering tuberculosis diagnosis, multidisciplinary involvement and ongoing evaluation of diagnostic instruments are necessary. Adding further tests in case of doubt, even if there is bacterial excretion, avoids hasty conclusions and guarantees thorough patient assessment. It is essential because single results are not always indicators of active tuberculosis, particularly in the presence of oncological symptoms or unusual radiographic patterns. The focus on combining clinical awareness with instrumental findings underscores the appropriate balance between technology and medical judgment. By following these key points summarized above, medical professionals can improve the accuracy and trustworthiness of tuberculosis diagnosis, which plays an important role in disease control activities and patients' welfare (Elena, 2024).

CLOSER LOOK

INTERFERON-GAMMA RELEASE ASSAYS (IGRAS)

Interferon-gamma release assays (IGRAs) are the blood tests to detect latent MTB infection by the measurement of the immune response against TB-specific antigens. In contrast to the conventional TST, the IGRAs are more specific and are not influenced by previous BCG vaccination or most NTM and thus are useful tools in TB diagnosis, particularly among BCG-vaccinated individuals.

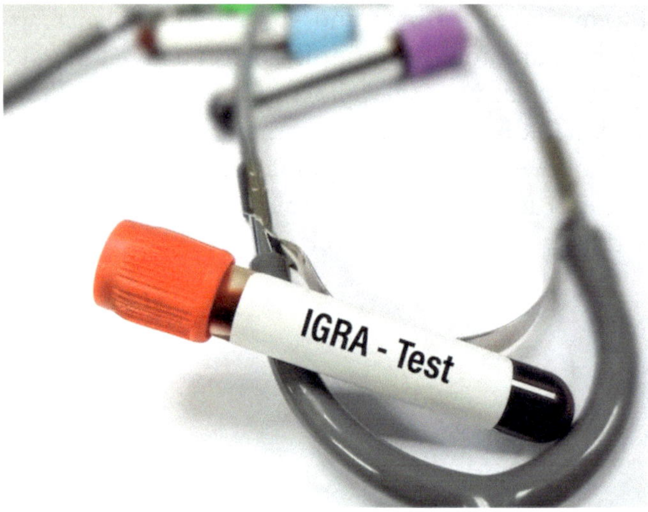

Source: Freepik. (n.d.). *Blood sample labeled IGRA (interferon-gamma release assay) test for tuberculosis diagnosis.* https://img.freepik.com/premium-photo/blood-sample-igra-interferon-gamma-release-assay-test-diagnosis-tuberculosis_595440-2399.jpg.

IGRAs function by quantifying the release of IFN-γ from antigen-stimulated sensitized T-cells to antigens like ESAT-6 and CFP-10, which are not found in BCG and most environmental mycobacteria. Two commercial IGRA tests widely available are QFT-Plus and T-SPOT.TB. In QFT-Plus, whole blood is stimulated with antigens specific for TB, and IFN-γ released is measured by an enzyme-linked immunosorbent assay (ELISA). In T-SPOT.TB, peripheral blood mononuclear cells (PBMCs) are isolated, are stimulated by TB antigens, and IFN-γ-secreting cells are quantitated using an ELISPOT method.

IGRAs are most commonly applied for the screening of LTBI, especially in high-risk groups like healthcare professionals, immunocompromised persons, and recent contacts of TB patients. Although very specific, IGRAs are not able to differentiate between latent TB disease and active TB disease. Hence, additional clinical assessment and testing should be done if active TB is suspected.

The benefits of IGRAs are the need for just one patient visit, objective laboratory-based findings, and little cross-reactivity. The disadvantages are the increased cost, the requirement for urgent blood sample processing, and decreased sensitivity in immunocompromised persons or very young children.

References

1. Connell, T. G., Zar, H. J., & Nicol, M. P. (2011). Advances in the diagnosis of pulmonary tuberculosis in HIV-infected and HIV-uninfected children. *The Journal of infectious diseases, 204 Suppl 4*(Suppl 4), S1151–S1158. https://doi.org/10.1093/infdis/jir413

2. O'Grady, Justina,b; Maeurer, Markusc; Mwaba, Peterb,d; Kapata, Nathanb,d; Bates, Matthewa,b; Hoelscher, Michaele; Zumla, Alimuddina,b. New and improved diagnostics for detection of drug-resistant pulmonary tuberculosis. Current Opinion in Pulmonary Medicine 17(3):p 134-141, May 2011. | DOI: 10.1097/MCP.0b013e3283452346 (accessed on 10 May 2025).

3. Andronikou, S., Vanhoenacker, F. M., & De Backer, A. I. (2009). Advances in imaging chest tuberculosis: blurring of differences between children and adults. *Clinics in chest medicine*, *30*(4), 717–viii. https://doi.org/10.1016/j.ccm.2009.08.022 (accessed on 10 May 2025).

4. Koole O, Thai S, Khun KE, Pe R, van Griensven J, Apers L, et al. (2011) Evaluation of the 2007 WHO Guideline to Improve the Diagnosis of Tuberculosis in Ambulatory HIV-Positive Adults. PLoS ONE 6(4): e18502. https://doi.org/10.1371/journal.pone.0018502 (accessed on 10 May 2025).

5. Asare, K. K., Azumah, D. E., Adu-Gyamfi, C. O., Opoku, Y., Adela, E. M., Afful, P., Abotsi, G. K., et al. (2024). Comparison of microscopic and Xpert MTB diagnoses of presumptive *Mycobacterium tuberculosis* infection: Retrospective analysis of routine diagnosis at Cape Coast Teaching Hospital. *BMC Infectious Diseases, 24*. https://www.semanticscholar.org/paper/b4f341ecf9e8c9f18f2bbafb66bea0dd33dc1d76 (accessed on 10 May 2025).

6. Azarhoush, R., Ghorbani, R., Kavian, F., & Nassaji, M. (2014). Acid fast staining in formalin-fixed tissue specimen of patients with extrapulmonary tuberculosis. *Journal of Infection and Public Health.* International Journal of Scientific and Research Publications, Volume 4, Issue 10, October 2014 1 ISSN 2250-3153 (accessed on 10 May 2025).

7. BABU, A., NAMBIKUTTY, A., VASUDEVAN, V., & V, M. C. (2024). CLINICAL PROFILE OF PATIENTS WITH MUSCULOSKELETAL TUBERCULOSIS VISITING A TERTIARY CARE CENTRE IN INDIA. *THE JOURNAL OF THE BULGARIAN ORTHOPAEDICS AND TRAUMA ASSOCIATION*, *61*(02), 79–88. https://doi.org/10.58542/jbota.v61i02.115 (accessed on 10 May 2025).

8. Mencarini, P., Bellagamba, R., Oliva, A., Ghirga, P., Giancola, M. L., Corpolongo, A., Ascoli Bartoli, T., De Nardo, P., Baiocchini, A., Del Nonno, F., Narciso, P., & Nicastri, E. (2016). Pulmonary tuberculosis followed by sarcoidosis in an HIV-infected patient: A case report and a simplified diagnostic flowchart for diagnosis and treatment of sarcoidosis. *Respiratory medicine case reports*, *19*, 150–154. https://doi.org/10.1016/j.rmcr.2016.09.006 (accessed on 10 May 2025).

9. Bawankule, S., Gaidhane, A., Khatib, N., & Quazi, Z. (2010). Delay in DOTS for new pulmonary tuberculosis patients from rural area of Wardha District, India. *Online Journal of Health and Allied Sciences.* https://core.ac.uk/download/pdf/87448.pdf (accessed on 10 May 2025).

10. G S, M. ., Beevi, L. ., Kumaran, J. C. ., G S, Y. ., & Shanmuganathan, M. (2023). A Enhanced Approach for Identification of Tuberculosis for Chest X-Ray Image using Machine Learning. *International Journal on Recent and Innovation Trends in Computing and Communication*, *11*(11s), 443–453. https://doi.org/10.17762/ijritcc.v11i11s.8173(accessed on 10 May 2025).

11. Bhalerao, R. (2024). Pulmonary tuberculosis detection from chest X-ray using deep learning. *International Journal of Scientific Research in Engineering and Management.* https://www.

semanticscholar.org/paper/7f7df2bf07636f722bee9adebb7344e69e68504a (accessed on 10 May 2025).

12. Andronikou, S., McHugh, K., Abdurahman, N., Khoury, B., Mngomezulu, V., Brant, W. E., Cowan, I., McCulloch, M., & Ford, N. (2011). Paediatric radiology seen from Africa. Part I: providing diagnostic imaging to a young population. *Pediatric radiology, 41*(7), 811–825. https://doi.org/10.1007/s00247-011-2081-8 (accessed on 10 May 2025).
13. Das, K. M., Al Mansoori, T., Alattar, Y. H., Gorkom, K., Shamisi, A., Melethil, A. P., & Alkoteesh, J. A. (2022). Tuberculosis of the heart: A diagnostic challenge. *Tomography, 8*, 1649–1665. https://doi.org/10.3390/tomography8040137.
14. Davuluri, M., & Novateur Publications. (2024). Novel device for enhancing tuberculosis diagnosis for faster, more accurate screening results. *International Journal of Innovations in Engineering Research and Technology*. https://www.semanticscholar.org/paper/d0017bffb9e759050d373f55bd6005b13119b881 (accessed on 10 May 2025).
15. Devrim, İ., Aktürk, H., Bayram, N., Apa, H., Tulumoğlu, Ş., Devrim, F., Erdem, T., et al. (2014). Differences between pediatric pulmonary and extra-pulmonary tuberculosis: A warning sign for the future. *Mediterranean Journal of Hematology and Infectious Diseases, 6*, e2014058. https://doi.org/10.4084/mjhid.2014.058.
16. Donoghue, H. D., & Holton, J. (2009). Intestinal tuberculosis. *Current opinion in infectious diseases, 22*(5), 490–496. https://doi.org/10.1097/QCO.0b013e3283306712(accessed on 10 May 2025).
17. Rockwood, N., du Bruyn, E., Morris, T., & Wilkinson, R. J. (2016). Assessment of treatment response in tuberculosis. *Expert review of respiratory medicine, 10*(6), 643–654. https://doi.org/10.1586/17476348.2016.1166960 (accessed on 10 May 2025).
18. Englund, S. (2002). *Molecular Biology Techniques as a Tool for Detection and Characterisation of Mycobacterium avium subsp. Paratuberculosis*. Acta Universitatis Agriculturae Sueciae. Veterinaria 2002, number: 123. Publisher: Swedish University of Agricultural Sciences. ISBN: 91-576-6366-1. https://core.ac.uk/download/11694594.pdf (accessed on 10 May 2025).
19. Faurholt-Jepsen D. (2013). The double burden. *Danish medical journal, 60*(7), B4673.(accessed on 10 May 2025).
20. Fernández Miaja, M., Alonso Álvarez, M. A., Concha Torre, A., Palacios Gutiérrez, J. J., González Sánchez, S., & Calle-Miguel, L. (2023). It looked like COVID-19, but it was not: The importance of an early diagnosis of disseminated tuberculosis. *The Pediatric Infectious Disease Journal, 42*, e181–e182. https://www.semanticscholar.org/paper/c524ba4365998b133622774fb0580b9c64008816 (accessed on 10 May 2025).
21. Fu, M., Yi, S., Zeng, Y., Ye, F., Li, Y., Dong, X., Ren, Y., et al. (2020). Deep learning-based recognizing COVID-19 and other common infectious diseases of the lung by chest CT scan images. *medRxiv*. https://doi.org/10.1101/2020.03.28.20046045.
22. Gao, Y., Liu, M., Chen, Y., Shi, S., Geng, J., & Tian, J. (2020). Association between tuberculosis and COVID-19 severity and mortality: A rapid systematic review and meta-analysis. *Journal of Medical Virology, 93*, 194–196. https://doi.org/10.1002/jmv.26311.
23. Guo, Q., Wang, Y., Xu, D., Nossent, J. C., Pavlos, N. J., & Xu, J. (2018). Rheumatoid arthritis: Pathological mechanisms and modern pharmacologic therapies. *Bone Research, 6*, Article 15. https://doi.org/10.1038/s41413-018-0016-9.

24. Hadiatma, F. N., & Triyono, E. (2023). A naive human immunodeficiency virus (HIV) patient with extrapulmonary tuberculosis manifestation: Diagnosis and management challenges. *Bali Medical Journal*. https://www.semanticscholar.org/paper/d88387c3cc322d94d5745f69a99c521c41eb6dcb (accessed on 10 May 2025).

25. McNerney, R., Maeurer, M., Abubakar, I., Marais, B., McHugh, T. D., Ford, N., Weyer, K., Lawn, S., Grobusch, M. P., Memish, Z., Squire, S. B., Pantaleo, G., Chakaya, J., Casenghi, M., Migliori, G. B., Mwaba, P., Zijenah, L., Hoelscher, M., Cox, H., Swaminathan, S., ... Zumla, A. (2012). Tuberculosis diagnostics and biomarkers: needs, challenges, recent advances, and opportunities. *The Journal of infectious diseases, 205 Suppl 2*, S147–S158. https://doi.org/10.1093/infdis/jir860(accessed on 10 May 2025).

26. Huang, Y., Ai, L., Wang, X., Sun, Z., & Wang, F. (2022). Review and updates on the diagnosis of tuberculosis. *Journal of Clinical Medicine, 11*, 5826. https://doi.org/10.3390/jcm11195826.

27. Jain, K., Hosur, N., Zaiba, Z., Shambhu, N., & Sai, P. K. (2024). Case study of rare diagnosis of tuberculosis in stomach. *International Journal of Scientific Research*. https://www.semanticscholar.org/paper/bbe2732d8dde11845c45a6f556dd771fbe152f20 (accessed on 10 May 2025).

28. James, S. L., Abate, D., Abate, K. H., Abay, S. M., Abbafati, C., Abbasi, N., Abbastabar, H., et al. (2018). Global, regional, and national incidence, prevalence, and years lived with disability for 354 diseases and injuries for 195 countries and territories, 1990–2017: A systematic analysis for the Global Burden of Disease Study 2017. *The Lancet, 392*, 1789–1858. https://doi.org/10.1016/s0140-6736(18)32279-7.

29. Szewczyk, R., Kowalski, K., Janiszewska-Drobinska, B., & Druszczyńska, M. (2013). Rapid method for Mycobacterium tuberculosis identification using electrospray ionization tandem mass spectrometry analysis of mycolic acids. *Diagnostic microbiology and infectious disease, 76*(3), 298–305. https://doi.org/10.1016/j.diagmicrobio.2013.03.025 (accessed on 10 May 2025).

30. Blount, R. J., Pascopella, L., Catanzaro, D. G., Barry, P. M., English, P. B., Segal, M. R., Flood, J., Meltzer, D., Jones, B., Balmes, J., & Nahid, P. (2017). Traffic-Related Air Pollution and All-Cause Mortality during Tuberculosis Treatment in California. *Environmental health perspectives, 125*(9), 097026. https://doi.org/10.1289/EHP1699

31. Kim, H., Kim, H. Y., Goo, J. M., & Kim, Y. (2020). Lung cancer CT screening and Lung-RADS in a tuberculosis-endemic country: The Korean Lung Cancer Screening Project (K-LUCAS). *Radiology, 296*, 181–188. https://doi.org/10.1148/radiol.2020192283.

32. Komukai, J., Matsumoto, K., Fukushima, W., & Kudoh, S. (2023). Pulmonary tuberculosis incidence among interferon-gamma release assays positive latent tuberculosis infection with fibrotic lesions in an urban vulnerable population of Osaka City, Japan, 2015–2021. *Japanese Journal of Infectious Diseases*. https://www.semanticscholar.org/paper/98a5ff9b6da8a4680f098f37f337657822063480 (accessed on 10 May 2025).

33. Korzh, E. V. (2024). Tuberculosis masks of lung cancer (differential diagnosis, clinical observations). *Clinical Review for General Practice*. https://www.semanticscholar.org/paper/f3317dabbfa4239abfef0bd471a852c081e54842 (accessed on 10 May 2025).

34. Kruk, M. E., Gage, A., Arsenault, C., Jordan, K., Leslie, H. H., Roder-DeWan, S., Adeyi, O., et al. (2018). High-quality health systems in the Sustainable Development Goals era: Time for a revolution. *The Lancet Global Health, 6*, e1196–e1252. https://doi.org/10.1016/s2214-109x(18)30386-3.

35. Kutame, R., Boateng, G., Adusi-Poku, Y., Sorvor, F., Antwi, L., Agyemang-Bioh, F., Ayensu, B., et al. (2024). Evaluation of diagnostic performance of three commercial interferon-gamma release assays for *Mycobacterium tuberculosis*. *Diagnostics, 14*. https://www.semanticscholar.org/paper/4f0860b49a0f71e50309b176819bd8359d5e7df0 (accessed on 10 May 2025).

36. Manfredini, D., Häggman-Henrikson, B., Al Jagshi, A., Baad-Hansen, L., Beecroft, E., Bijelic, T., Bracci, A., et al. (2024). Temporomandibular disorders: INfORM/IADR key points for good clinical practice based on standard of care. *Cranio: The Journal of Craniomandibular Practice.* https://www.semanticscholar.org/paper/6872d48a634f04904ee405af21357149df90a15f (accessed on 10 May 2025).

37. Marwah, V., Bhati, G., Chaudhary, R., & Sharma, A. (2023). Pulmonary thromboembolism in multidrug-resistant tuberculosis: A case series highlighting the importance of early diagnosis and management. *International Journal of Medical Students.* https://www.semanticscholar.org/paper/68715d0e627db1218c05707f82ea21f2062bea1c (accessed on 10 May 2025).

38. Musisi, E., Sessolo, A., Kaswabuli, S., Zawedde, J., Byanyima, P., Kasinga, S., Sanyu, I., et al. (2022). High *Mycobacterium tuberculosis* bacillary loads detected by tuberculosis molecular bacterial load assay in patient stool: A potential alternative for nonsputum diagnosis and treatment response monitoring of tuberculosis. *Microbiology Spectrum, 10*. https://www.semanticscholar.org/paper/0e2dbe067a2dfdbc976e2af347e3f6666e2a33ae (accessed on 10 May 2025).

39. National Center for HIV/AIDS, Viral Hepatitis, STD, and TB Prevention (U.S.), Division of Tuberculosis Elimination. (2025). *Latent Tuberculosis Infection: A Guide for Primary Health Care Providers.* https://core.ac.uk/download/144198509.pdf (accessed on 10 May 2025).

40. Navarro, C. E., Benjumea-Bedoya, D., Estupiñán-Bohorquez, A., & Florez, I. (2025). Cost-effectiveness analysis comparing QuantiFERON test and tuberculin skin test for the diagnosis of latent tuberculosis infection in immunocompetent children under 15 years of age in Colombia. *BMJ Open, 15*. https://www.semanticscholar.org/paper/1e9e291c21ee8a98eea1df7daf7f2b5fd9d4a226 (accessed on 10 May 2025).

41. Nguyen, M. V. H., Levy, N. S., Ahuja, S. D., Trieu, L., Proops, D., & Achkar, J. M. (2019). Factors associated with sputum culture-negative vs culture-positive diagnosis of pulmonary tuberculosis. *JAMA Network Open, 2*(7), e187617. https://doi.org/10.1001/jamanetworkopen.2018.7617.

42. Niazkar, H., Zibaee, B., Razavi, S. B., Ghanaeian, K., Talebzadeh, V., & Vosugh, N. H. (2022). Evaluation of tuberculosis infection in COVID-19 patients: A case of tuberculosis and COVID-19 co-infection. *The Egyptian Journal of Internal Medicine, 34*. https://www.semanticscholar.org/paper/02aa3f198103903792aa714d4e315994d9dacd86 (accessed on 10 May 2025).

43. Pagnoncelli, M., Arosio, M., Genovesi, A., Napolitano, G., & Farina, C. (2024). Performance of the T-SPOT.TB test in patients with indeterminate QuantiFERON-TB Gold Plus results: Proposal for an algorithm for the diagnosis of latent tuberculosis infection. *Le Infezioni in Medicina, 32*(4), 525–531. https://www.semanticscholar.org/paper/313cb322a94439f7b69f3611d9ba5f6645910ec9 (accessed on 10 May 2025).

44. Pratama, P. A. H., Sahay, A. S., Teguh, R., & Wilentine, et al. (2021). Deteksi COVID-19 berdasarkan hasil rontgen dada (chest X-ray) menggunakan Python. https://core.ac.uk/download/478782466.pdf (accessed on 10 May 2025).

45. Rahane, W., Shitole, S., Khanuja, A., Bedmutha, A., Samant, R., & Kurhade, M. (2024). Detection of tuberculosis using chest X-ray and hospital recommendation system. *2024 8th International*

Conference on Computing, Communication, Control and Automation (ICCUBEA). https://www.semanticscholar.org/paper/07687691b612ff57dc843153796ce21e706a8dc2 (accessed on 10 May 2025).

46. Rudd, K. E., Johnson, S. C., Agesa, K. M., Shackelford, K. A., Tsoi, D., Kievlan, D., Colombara, D. V., et al. (2020). Global, regional, and national sepsis incidence and mortality, 1990–2017: Analysis for the Global Burden of Disease Study. *The Lancet, 395*, 200–211. https://doi.org/10.1016/s0140-6736(19)32989-7.

47. Saha, S. (2024). Primary extrapulmonary tuberculosis diagnosis warrants extra-precautious pulmonary tuberculosis exclusion workup. *World Journal of Clinical Cases, 12*, 3295–3297. https://www.semanticscholar.org/paper/03c160ebe0d35fe6a34c95d2fb0d6c80d3ba8d5a (accessed on 10 May 2025).

48. Shrivas, A., & Singh, S. (2025). Tuberculosis Diagnosis and Management: Recent Advances. *Journal of global infectious diseases, 17*(1), 3–9. https://doi.org/10.4103/jgid.jgid_112_24(accessed on 10 May 2025).

49. Sibuea, T. P., Simadibrata, M., Syam, A. F., Yoewono, et al. (2001). Colonic tuberculosis and chronic diarrhea. https://media.neliti.com/media/publications/67638-EN-colonic-tuberculosis-and-chronic-diarrhe.pdf (accessed on 10 May 2025).

50. Singh, G. R., Sinha, A., Anushweta, Sharma, R., Saurabh, K., & Haldar, D. (2024). Rare extrapulmonary tuberculosis: Covert symptoms and diagnostic dilemma. *Nigerian Medical Journal: Journal of the Nigeria Medical Association, 65*, 92–100. https://www.semanticscholar.org/paper/8711f4129bbf9a75cca8eda6937d205643a84452 (accessed on 10 May 2025).

51. Song, J., Hwang, E. J., Yoon, S. H., Park, C. M., & Goo, J. M. (2025). Emerging Trends and Innovations in Radiologic Diagnosis of Thoracic Diseases. *Investigative radiology*, 10.1097/RLI.0000000000001179. Advance online publication. https://doi.org/10.1097/RLI.0000000000001179(accessed on 10 May 2025).

52. Stirenko, S., Kochura, Y., Alienin, O., Rokovyi, O., Gordienko, Y., Peng, G., & Zeng, W. (2018). Chest X-ray analysis of tuberculosis by deep learning with segmentation and augmentation. https://doi.org/10.1109/elnano.2018.8477564.

53. Lubna Stiwey, Wegdan Atiya, Weam Hamad (2024). Polymerase Chain Reaction (PCR) for the Diagnosis of Clostridium perfringens Infection in Poultry Molecular Analysis of the Relationship between Infection and Clinical Symptoms. SAR J Pathol Microbiol, 5(6), 214-217.(accessed on 10 May 2025).

54. Yu, G., Fang, L., Shen, Y., Zhong, F., & Xu, X. (2024). Targeted nanopore sequencing using clinical specimens for the rapid diagnosis of extrapulmonary tuberculosis. *BMC Infectious Diseases, 24.* https://www.semanticscholar.org/paper/324bbaaf2b155c05afd449ee4d6c604d1778fd7a (accessed on 10 May 2025).

55. Zaidi, I., Sarma, P., Khayyam, K., Ahmad, Q. T., Ramankutty, V., & Singh, G. (2024). Sociodemographic factors affecting knowledge levels of tuberculosis patients in New Delhi. *Journal of Family Medicine and Primary Care, 13*, 5152–5158. https://www.semanticscholar.org/paper/f233117c318cdd9360e283a4e8bc1d8669d9a772 (accessed on 10 May 2025).

56. Zwerling, A., Behr, M. A., Verma, A., Brewer, T. F., Menzies, D., & Pai, M. (2011). The BCG World Atlas: a database of global BCG vaccination policies and practices. *PLoS medicine, 8*(3), e1001012. https://doi.org/10.1371/journal.pmed.1001012

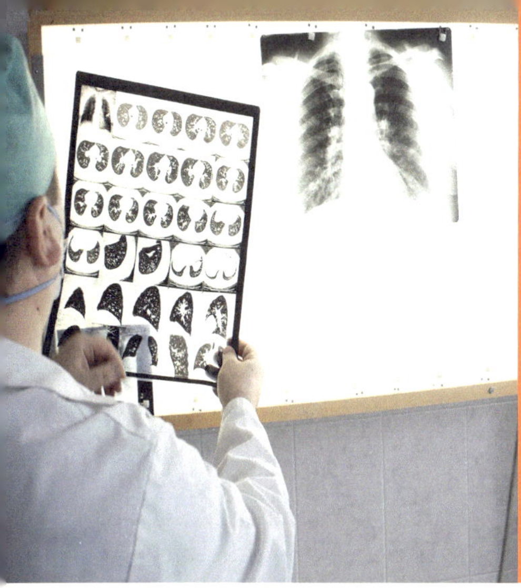

Chapter 4

CLINICAL MANIFESTATIONS OF PULMONARY TB

Contents

Introduction

The clinical presentation of pulmonary tuberculosis (PTB) is a persistent public health issue globally because of its varied and frequently non-specific presentation. Patients infected with *Mycobacterium tuberculosis* (MTB) can have a broad variety of presentations that are similar to other pulmonary conditions, making it difficult to diagnose on time and be treated. Symptoms such as cough, chest pain, and hemoptysis are frequent but overlap with other pulmonary diseases, presenting a diagnostic dilemma to clinicians. In addition, the disease's imitation of other pathologies like malignancies or autoimmune diseases creates layers of complexity in a clinical context, particularly in areas with high rates of TB. Knowledge of diverse clinical presentations is paramount for clinicians to institute proper investigations and prevent misdiagnosis that would delay effective therapy, consequently minimizing transmission and morbidity. PTB tends to be presented by insufficiently specific respiratory symptoms and therefore requires a complete differential diagnosis process. For example, hoarseness or laryngeal abnormalities may be inappropriately attributed to malignancies, as described in the situation where laryngeal TB can masquerade as neoplastic processes. This overlap emphasizes the need to combine clinical, radiological, and microbiological information to properly diagnose TB infection. New technologies, such as molecular methods, can identify even low quantities of MTB, allowing for earlier treatment even in the absence of traditional symptoms or radiographic evidence. This strategy improves patient outcomes by facilitating early initiation of anti-TB therapy and preventing such complications of late diagnosis as diffuse alveolar hemorrhage or granulomatous inflammation (Madolangan et al., 2024). The clinical presentation of pulmonary TB might also closely mimic autoimmune diseases or vasculitic disorders, further complicating clinical decision-making. For instance, GPA exacerbations present similar symptoms and radiographic features to pulmonary TB, such as productive cough, chest pain, and hemoptysis. Such overlap requires complete exclusion of TB before initiating immunosuppressive therapy to avoid worsening of infection with inappropriate treatment and to result in poor outcomes. Careful microbiological and histopathological studies are essential to differentiate these conditions, especially from areas of high TB burden. Diagnostic accuracy advancements via integrated clinical evaluation and laboratory examination guarantee that patients are prescribed individualized treatment regimes, demonstrating the intertwined nature of pulmonary TB's clinical presentation with varied disease processes (Perera et al., 2024).

Definition of Pulmonary Tuberculosis (PTB)

The complex interaction between infection and immune response is the basis of the disease that still poses a global health issue, especially in areas with high rates of incidence. PTB is a bacterial infection that is transmissible and occurs mostly in the lungs, caused by MTB. It appears once the bacteria, when inhaled into the respiratory system, avoid the initial defense mechanisms of the immune system, resulting in active infection or latency. The illness is defined by a spectrum of pulmonary diseases, such as inflammation, tissue necrosis, and cavitation, which individually add to the clinical presentation. Notably, PTB is not just an acute infectious disease but a chronic pulmonary disease that also affects respiratory function and overall health. Specifically, tuberculosis-associated pulmonary disease has been established as a major risk factor for chronic obstructive pulmonary disease (COPD), highlighting its wider effect on lung pathology and outcomes (Jiang et al., 2024). This association emphasizes the necessity of defining PTB not simply as infection but as encompassing its late sequelae. The assessment of PTB requires an understanding of its radiological and clinical heterogeneity.

The illness can have multiple findings like consolidation, cavitation, lymphadenopathy, and pleural effusions, which are representative of the underlying pathophysiologic processes and the stage of infection. Significantly, some of the fulminant presentations like miliary tuberculosis may advance to acute respiratory distress syndrome (ARDS), making it challenging for diagnosis and treatment. Radiographic imaging, such as chest X-rays and high-resolution computed tomography (HRCT), demonstrate typical patterns like nodules and consolidations that help identify the disease. For example, radiological findings such as the butterfly pattern of sparing lung apices and bases emphasize the unpredictable presentation of PTB. Moreover, endobronchial involvement can be identified by bronchoscopy, which is an immediate diagnostic technique. These varied manifestations call for an inclusive definition that encompasses both clinical symptoms and radiological findings to facilitate appropriate management (Malhotra et al., 2024).

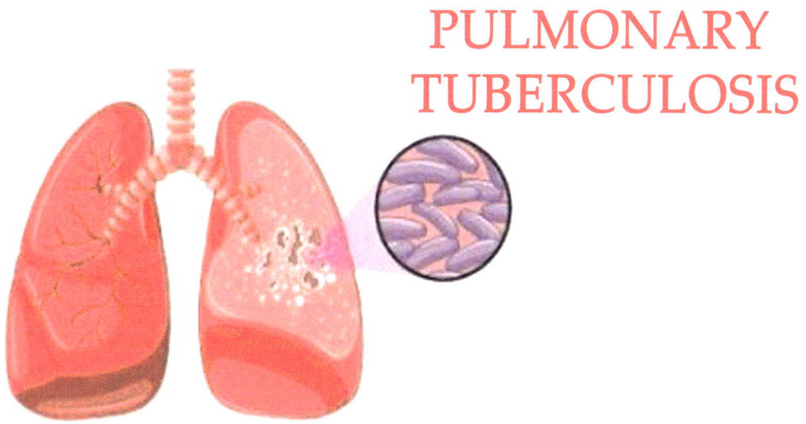

Source: YouTube. (n.d.). *Pulmonary tuberculosis: Illustration showing infected lungs and magnified view of Mycobacterium tuberculosis.* https://i.ytimg.com/vi/TV0CWoyKcSk/hqdefault.jpg.

The definition of PTB is also narrowed down by diagnostic criteria including clinical history, laboratory test results, and high-technology imaging. It goes beyond the simple identification of MTB to encompass consideration of sequelae of disease and possible overlap with other pulmonary diseases. Comprehensive assessment includes identifying active infection using microbiological examinations in conjunction with an evaluation of past tuberculosis evidence using radiological findings suggestive of fibrotic scarring or calcification. In addition, diagnostic approaches incorporate tests like interferon-gamma release assays (IGRAs) for identifying latent infection, particularly in unusual cases. The construct of COPD as a result of tuberculosis highlights the changing knowledge of PTB as a distinct pulmonary disease phenotype that needs to be addressed by specific therapeutic strategies and continuous clinical surveillance (Jiang et al., 2024). This integrated paradigm for the definition of PTB is critical to optimizing patient outcomes with accurate diagnosis and targeted clinical management.

Importance of Understanding Clinical Manifestations

Correct diagnosis of PTB is largely dependent on an in-depth knowledge of its clinical presentation. The range of symptoms, from chronic cough and hemoptysis to weight loss and night sweats, necessitates that clinicians be able to recognize these signs amidst a range of respiratory illnesses. Identifying these signs at an early stage not only makes treatment timely but also prevents disease progression and spread. Since pulmonary TB mainly involves the lungs, its presentation can simulate other conditions of the lungs, making it difficult to diagnose. TB is difficult to distinguish from nontuberculous mycobacterial (NTM) infections and other chronic lung diseases since there are usually overlapping clinical characteristics. Diagnosis in such cases mostly depends on an extensive understanding of clinical presentation and patient history, especially where a history of previous lung structural damage exists (Mortaz et al., 2017). Therefore, it is essential to understand the subtleties in symptomatology to guide proper diagnostic testing and enhance patient outcomes. In addition to diagnostic precision, knowledge regarding the clinical presentation of pulmonary TB is essential for developing effective treatment plans and public health interventions. Appearance of symptoms, including chronic cough and sputum, indicates the infectious stage of the disease, stressing the necessity for isolation and immediate treatment. Furthermore, diverse clinical presentations mirror variations in disease severity and host immune response, guiding therapeutic interventions. Evolution in research on mucosal immunity has shown that the immune environment of the respiratory tract plays a pivotal role in TB pathogenesis and containment (Mortaz et al., 2017). Thus, clinical presentations also offer clues to the underlying immunological mechanisms, guiding vaccine and new therapy development. A complete understanding of patterns of symptoms is required not just for the care of individual patients but also for the application of public health strategies designed to control the spread in high-transmission communities. Additionally, the combination of knowledge of clinical presentations with advancing scientific information maximizes the potential for better patient care and disease control. Pulmonary TB, which is commonly associated with immunosuppression and chronic lung disease, exhibits variable clinical manifestations that are influenced by complicated host-pathogen interactions (Mortaz et al., 2017). Characterizing such interactions helps in predicting disease complications and co-infections that are significant in prognosis and holistic treatment planning. Additionally, since new interventions like mucosal vaccines are being considered, identification of the mucosal immune responses associated with clinical symptoms can inform vaccine development strategies. Therefore, a complete understanding of clinical manifestations not only guarantees precise clinical assessment but also informs the development of novel strategies aimed at fighting TB at individual and population levels.

4.1. Epidemiology of Pulmonary TB

Worldwide pulmonary tuberculosis (PTB) prevalence shows a dynamic interplay of environmental, social, and biological determinants that shape disease distribution and outcome. In the past, the disease was strongly focused within low- and middle-income countries (LMICs), and urban crowding and reduced healthcare accessibility amplified risks for transmission elsewhere. The development of effective immunocompromised conditions, ongoingly fueled by HIV/AIDS, has profoundly reshaped epidemiological patterns by making it easier for people to fall ill. On the other hand, there is a growing body of evidence that structural lung diseases, including bronchiectasis and emphysema, also predispose to pulmonary infections, including those caused by *Mycobacterium tuberculosis* (MTB) and related species. The interplay between such predisposing factors shows the non-uniformity of TB epidemiology, where host susceptibility as well as bacterial factors are responsible for disease expression and transmission. Therefore, sound epidemiologic knowledge has to incorporate these risk factors into practical public health strategies and clinical practice. The comorbidity-pulmonary TB epidemiology relationship has attracted much interest, demonstrating complex clinical and prognostic correlates for the affected populations. For instance, the disease burden of diabetes mellitus (DM) in TB patients has been found to impact treatment outcomes and mortality. Findings have shown that although culture conversion rates may not be statistically different between diabetic and non-diabetic patients at the end of treatment, diabetes significantly increases the risk of TB early-related mortality, especially within 100 days of treatment. This enhanced mortality risk indicates diabetes might compromise host immune function or interfere with treatment effectiveness, complicating clinical management. In addition, the synergistic interaction between diabetes and HIV co-infection exacerbates mortality risk, highlighting the imperative of comprehensive care strategies addressing these intersecting pandemics to minimize TB complications (Faurholt-Jepsen et al., 2013).

Besides diabetes and structural lung conditions, nontuberculous mycobacteria (NTM) infection is an important epidemiological issue, tending to overlap with pulmonary TB from shared risk profiles and clinical syndromes. NTM species, which are ubiquitous in environmental reservoirs like soil and water, may lead to pulmonary disease characteristically in people who have some pre-existing lung destruction or impaired immune status. This overlap makes TB diagnosis and epidemiologic evaluation difficult because NTM infections can mimic or co-exist with *Mtb* infection. The new molecular diagnostic methods have improved the detection and discrimination of NTM from TB, but immunologic reactions to these pathogens are still poorly understood. Immunogenetic factors predisposing individuals to NTM infections may also similarly affect susceptibility to TB, implying convergent mechanisms in disease etiology and underlining the need to acknowledge these subtleties in TB epidemiology (Mortaz et al., 2017).

4.1.1. Global Prevalence and Incidence Rates

Comprehension of PTB distribution among varied populations is part of understanding its clinical burden. Even with improvements in public health, TB is a major issue, especially among low to middle-income nations where social determinants increase risks of transmission. Populations of children, for instance, show different prevalence based on immunological and environmental components. In a 10-year retrospective study at a referral hospital in Tehran, Iran, the total prevalence rate was estimated to be 56.6 per 1,00,000 admitted patients. The clinical presentation varied by age with disseminated TB being more prevalent in infants aged below one year, while pulmonary and extrapulmonary presentations were more or less evenly distributed in children above one year. These epidemiologic observations highlight the heterogeneity in TB morphologies and the imperative requirement for age-dependent diagnostic and management strategies (Movahedi et al., 2022). Incidence rates of tuberculosis worldwide correspond to complex relationships between host immunity, pathogen attributes, and environmental exposures. Although MTB continues to be the main causative agent of pulmonary TB, the rise in NTM infections, especially in the developed world, makes epidemiological evaluations challenging. For example, *Mycobacterium avium* complex (MAC) and *Mycobacterium abscessus* have been recognized as emerging pathogens with unique clinical presentations, largely infecting immunocompromised persons and persons with chronic diseases. Although the incidence of *Mtb* has decreased in certain high-income nations, the global mycobacterial lung disease burden remains, reflecting a transition in clinical epidemiology that stretches the conventional diagnostic and treatment models (To et al., 2020). This highlights the importance of strict surveillance for proper differentiation and management of pulmonary infections worldwide. Inequities in TB morbidity and mortality rates emphasize the need for more focused public health interventions in at-risk populations.

Evidence shows that children with comorbidities and disseminated tuberculosis have higher mortality, underscoring the importance of early detection and intervention strategies. The death rate of up to 10% in children admitted with TB confirms the serious consequences of late diagnosis and comorbidity. Incidence and prevalence variations worldwide emphasize the importance of effective screening, socio-economic development, and vaccine interventions to limit pulmonary TB's clinical burden. Ongoing endeavors to enhance epidemiological data gathering and aligning clinical presentation with demographic patterns are crucial for developing focused health policies globally (Movahedi et al., 2022) (Figure 4.1).

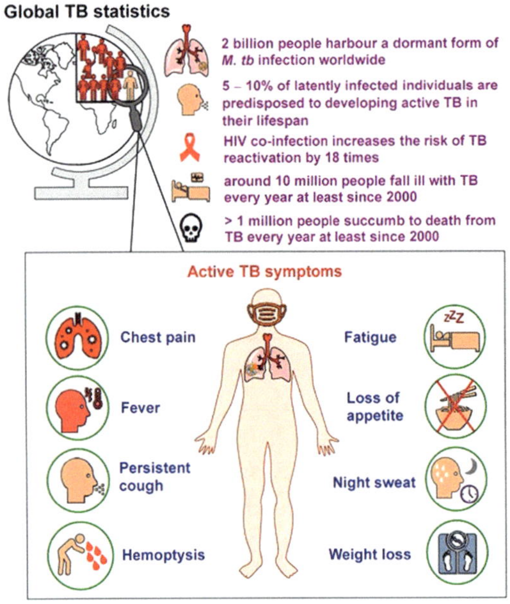

Figure 4.1. General TB statistics and main symptoms of pulmonary TB.

Source: Alsayed SSR, Gunosewoyo H. Tuberculosis: Pathogenesis, Current Treatment Regimens and New Drug Targets. *International Journal of Molecular Sciences*. 2023; 24(6):5202. https://doi.org/10.3390/ijms24065202

4.1.2. Risk Factors for Infection

The interaction among chronic diseases and infectious pathogens regularly complicates the clinical picture of PTB. Note particularly the strong role of DM in the susceptibility and development of tuberculosis infection. Evidence suggests that the co-morbid association of diabetes greatly increases the risk of active PTB, with diabetic patients showing threefold increased susceptibility compared to non-diabetic patients. This increased susceptibility is due to immune impairments resulting from hyperglycemia, weakening host defenses against MTB. Additionally, tuberculosis itself can further compromise glucose metabolism, establishing a twofold association that enhances both diseases. Epidemiological evidence from various parts of the world, including sub-Saharan Africa, attests to the need for understanding diabetes as a significant risk factor in tuberculosis cases, particularly in areas where both conditions have high prevalence. This double burden is particularly damaging to treatment outcomes and survival rates overall, and the need for an integrated disease management approach is emphasized by Faurholt-Jepsen (2013). Structural lung abnormalities are also an important predisposing condition to PTB. Parenchymal damage from previous infections or chronic lung conditions provides a substrate for mycobacterial colonization and persistence. Diseases like bronchiectasis, emphysema, and old tuberculosis lesions interfere with normal lung architecture and result in impaired mucociliary clearance and local immunity. These changes allow for infection establishment and persistence of MTB. Furthermore, NTM, sharing environmental niches with the bacilli of tuberculosis, takes advantage of similar weaknesses of structurally damaged lungs. The commutability of risk factors for PTB and NTM infection highlights the need for awareness and prevention of structural lung diseases as important determinants of risk of infection. The existence of co-morbid conditions that compromise pulmonary defenses requires careful clinical evaluation in patients with respiratory illness (Mortaz et al., 2017). Immunosuppression is another key risk factor affecting the clinical presentation and severity of PTB. Patients with damaged immune systems, secondary to HIV infection, immunosuppressive therapy, or genetic immunodeficiencies, become more prone to both primary infection and reactivation of latent tuberculosis. The defective immune response of the host to mount a proper defense permits uncontrolled mycobacterial growth, resulting in more widespread lung involvement and rapid disease progression. In addition, HIV coinfection often complicates the clinical presentation, as it not only accelerates tuberculosis risk but also alters the presentation of disease, tending to yield atypical radiographic and clinical presentations. It is important to comprehend the immunological status in identifying accurate diagnosis, prognosis, and appropriate treatment strategies in PTB, justifying detailed assessment of patients' immune function (Faurholt-Jepsen, 2013; Mortaz et al., 2017) (Figure 4.2).

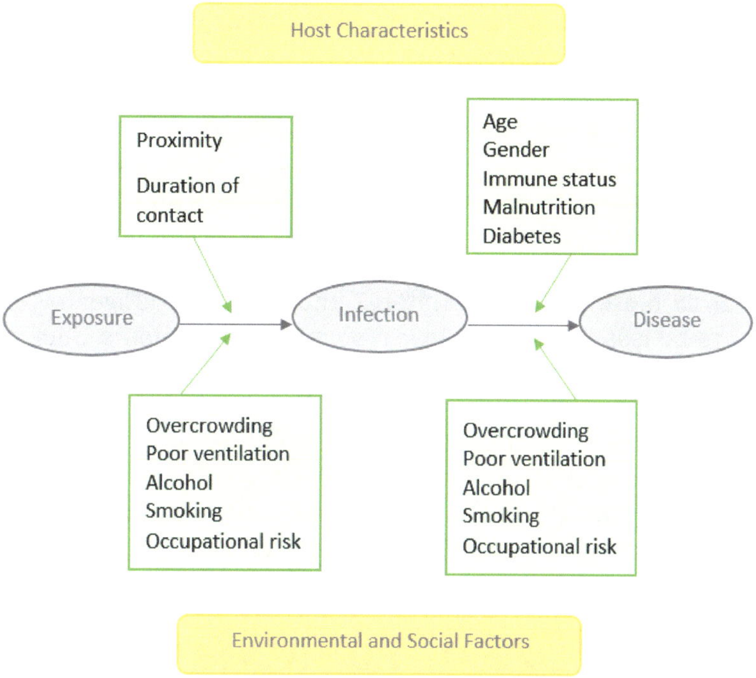

Figure 4.2. The risk factors for TB infection and disease.

Source: ResearchGate. (n.d.). *The risk factors for TB infection and disease: Host characteristics, exposure, and environmental and social factors.* https://www.researchgate.net/figure/The-risk-factors-for-TB-infection-and-disease-Adapted-from-Davies-2005_fig1_334142688.

4.1.3. Demographic Variations in Disease Presentation

Disease presentation variations commonly mirror quantitative differences in demographic parameters like age, gender, socioeconomic status, and geographic distribution. Clinically, in the setting of PTB, these quantitative variables have considerable impacts on symptoms, onset, and rate of progression. For example, the elderly patient is likely to present with less obvious or atypical respiratory symptoms secondary to immunosenescence, making early diagnosis more difficult. On the other hand, younger populations, especially those with healthy immune systems, may have more typical respiratory symptoms, such as chronic cough and hemoptysis. In addition, gender differences will impact symptom awareness and reporting, leading to possible delays in treatment. Socioeconomic conditions also come into play by influencing access to health care services and risk of exposure. Densely populated living arrangements, malnutrition, and restricted healthcare utilization, prevailing in low-income neighborhoods, contribute to disease severity and spread, further emphasizing the importance of demographic diversity in clinical evaluation and management guidelines. Lifestyle and environmental determinants, closely interlinked with demographic heterogeneity, add complexity to pulmonary TB clinical presentations. Urban versus rural residence also determines levels of exposure and quality of healthcare infrastructure, impacting disease detection and adherence to treatment. Also, comorbidities that are common among specific populations, for example, HIV coinfection in sub-Saharan Africa or diabetes mellitus in South Asia, modify the immune system, changing both the symptomatology and course of the disease. The interaction between these factors and the pathogenesis of TB necessitates specific diagnostic and therapeutic approaches. More recent research highlights the need for a multistakeholder response to managing immune-related complications in TB patients by acknowledging that the efficacy of treatment and side effects can differ by demographic factors (Bryan et al., 2021). Thus, an understanding of demographic and environmental determinants is called for to maximize pulmonary TB clinical outcomes and decrease the global disease burden. Antibiotic resistance is also an area in which demographic inequities impact pulmonary TB presentation and management. In developing countries, uncontrolled and widespread application of antibiotics in medical as well as veterinary applications has led to multi-drug resistant tuberculosis (MDR-TB) strains, making it difficult to treat. The resistant strains can manifest with unusual or more serious symptoms and can need longer or different therapeutic regimens, which tend to be less available in low-resource environments. Socioeconomic issues like inadequate sanitation, inadequate surveillance systems, and uncontrolled antibiotic prescription worsen these issues, especially in at-risk populations (Christy et al., 2018). Additionally, the spread of resistance via animal-source food items in some populations highlights the interrelatedness of social practices and infectious disease epidemiology. Management of these population differences calls for an organized public health response that combines antibiotic stewardship, education, and improved diagnostic capacity to check the effect of resistant pulmonary TB strains promptly.

4.2. Pathophysiology of Pulmonary TB

The complex interaction of the MTB *Bacillus* and the immune system of the host sets into motion the pathophysiological cascade resulting in PTB. The bacilli, on inhalation, are deposited in the alveoli and are phagocytosed by the alveolar macrophages. Instead of being eliminated, MTB can survive and multiply within these cells, avoiding immune defenses. This tenacity evokes a granulomatous inflammatory reaction with the recruitment of macrophages, T lymphocytes, and other cells of the immune system, which try to localize the infection. The formation of granulomas reflects the attempt of the host to localize the microbe but also causes tissue damage and necrosis at the center of the lesion, referred to as caseous necrosis. This localized damage undermines pulmonary architecture and forms the basis for most clinical presentations such as cough and hemoptysis, a manifestation of the ongoing tissue damage in the lungs. The chronic inflammation and immune-mediated tissue damage in PTB are responsible for causing progressive damage to the lungs, with the development of structural abnormalities. Pathological processes include vigorous immune activation with increased proteolytic enzyme activity, including matrix metalloproteinases, that break down components of extracellular matrix and destroy alveolar walls. Resultant cavitation and fibrosis become characteristics of severe disease, leading to airflow limitation and compromised gas exchange. In most instances, such fibrotic alterations are reflected in those seen in chronic obstructive pulmonary disease (COPD), underlining an overlapping pathophysiological substrate characterized by chronic inflammation and tissue remodeling (Choi, 2025). This reconstruction not only influences lung mechanics but makes patients prone to chronic respiratory manifestations and frequent infections, emphasizing the chronicity of PTB beyond the acute infection period. Chronic complications arising from PTB frequently take the form of post-tuberculosis lung disease (PTLD), a condition characterized by residual respiratory abnormality despite a microbiological cure (Yadav, 2024). The chronic residual lung injury includes fibrotic scarring, bronchiectasis, and airway obstruction and is all a result of the pathological events occurring during the phase of active infection. The chronic sequela reduces pulmonary function, which presents clinically as dyspnea, decreased tolerance to exercise, and chronic cough, complicating the management of clinical disease. Diagnostically, the clinical heterogeneity of the presentation tends to replicate other clinical chronic respiratory illnesses and requires extensive pulmonary function tests and imaging for determination of the extent of injury. Therapeutic strategies target the relief of symptoms and lung function preservation, necessitating multidisciplinary treatments that address both the immunopathogenic processes and structural lung changes generated by the tuberculosis infection (Figure 4.3).

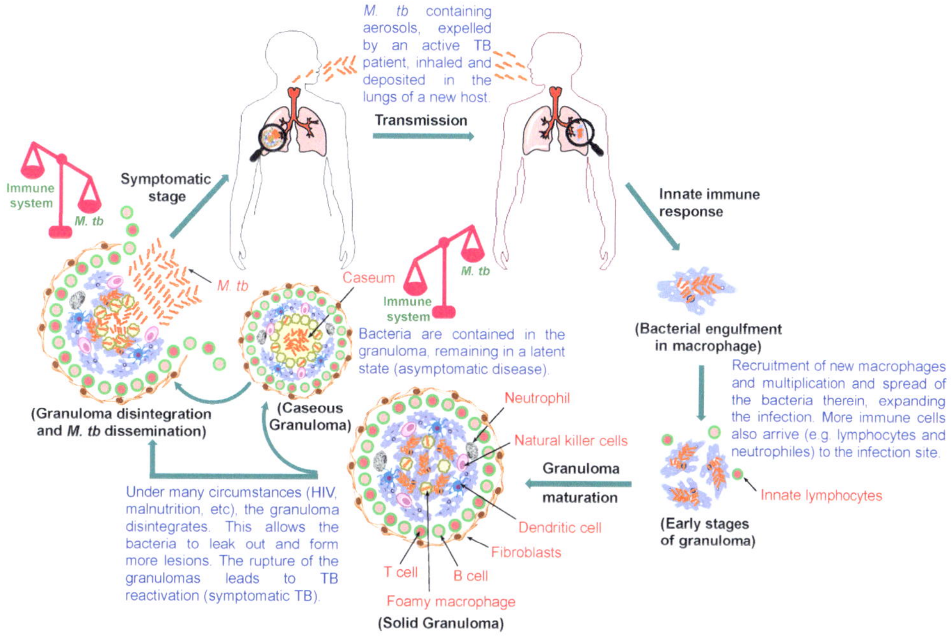

Figure 4.3. Pathophysiology of pulmonary tuberculosis (PTB).

Source: Alsayed SSR, Gunosewoyo H. Tuberculosis: Pathogenesis, Current Treatment Regimens and New Drug Targets. *International Journal of Molecular Sciences*. 2023; 24(6):5202. https://doi.org/10.3390/ijms24065202

4.2.1. Mechanism of Infection and Disease Progression

The interaction between host immune responses and *Mycobacterium tuberculosis* (*M. tuberculosis*/*Mtb*) is pivotal to the development of PTB, triggering a multifaceted cascade that determines disease progression. On inhalation, *Mtb* bacilli are deposited in the alveoli, where alveolar macrophages phagocytose them, trying to encapsulate the bacteria. The bacteria, however, have mechanisms to escape killing by blocking phagosome-lysosome fusion, enabling intracellular survival and growth. This avoidance provokes recruitment of other immune cells and granuloma formation, an organized structure that attempts to enclose the pathogen but also provides a niche for surviving bacilli. The ratio between immune control and bacterial growth determines whether the infection becomes latent or active disease with tissue damage and clinical manifestations. Interestingly, comorbid conditions like diabetes may influence the immune system, heightening vulnerability to active TB and remodeling the clinical course of the disease (Faurholt-Jepsen, 2013).

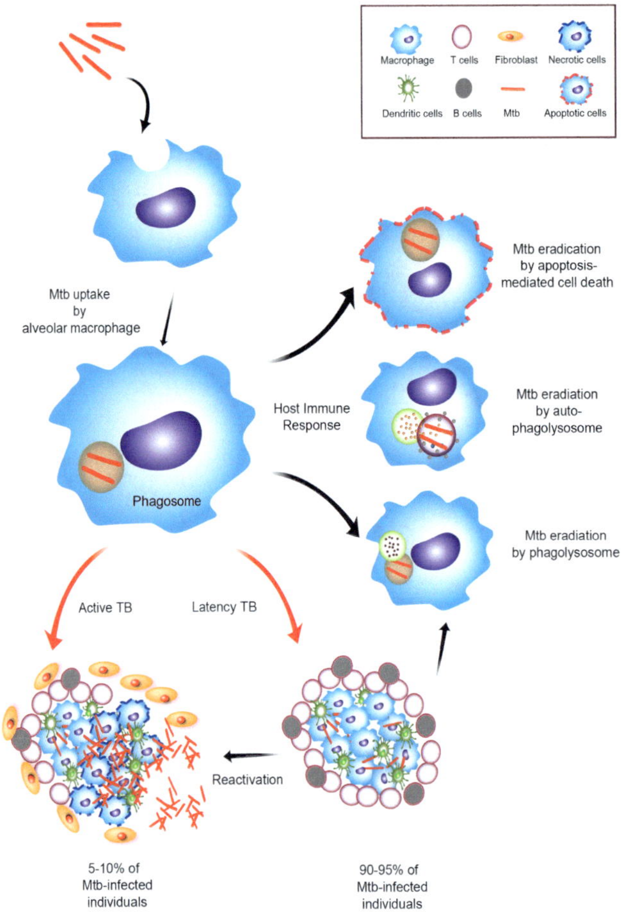

Figure 4.4. A schematic diagram of the host immune system against infection of *Mycobacterium tuberculosis* (*Mtb*). *Mtb* is inhaled by aerosols and transmitted to the lungs, where it is phagocytized by alveolar macrophages and eliminated via various mechanisms including apoptosis and autophagy.

Source: ResearchGate. (n.d.). *A schematic diagram of host immune system response against infection of Mycobacterium tuberculosis: Uptake, immune control, latency, and reactivation.* https://www.researchgate.net/publication/263741783/figure/fig1/AS:202810965663758@1425365310793/A-schematic-diagram-of-host-immune-system-against-infection-of-Mycobacterium-tuberculosis.png.

This interaction highlights the sophistication of pulmonary TB pathogenesis beyond simple microbial invasion. Host immune signaling networks also influence the outcome of *Mtb* infection, where type I interferons (IFNs) have a contentious role in disease progression. Although type I IFNs have antiviral activity and immunoregulatory roles, induction during *Mtb* infection paradoxically supportsthe survival of the bacteria and disease pathology. High type I IFN responses are linked with compromised host resistance, supporting bacterial growth and clinical deterioration. Experimental models and human studies propose type I IFNs dampen protective immunity, for example, Th1-driven macrophage activation, which results in reduced bacilli containment and enhanced lung tissue damage.

However, recent evidence has shown that context-dependent factors can also induce protective type I IFN effects against tuberculosis. Elucidation of these mechanistic subtleties is important for deconstructing the immunopathology of pulmonary TB and can potentially guide therapeutic approaches toward modulating host responses for better control of disease (Moreira-Teixeira et al., 2018). Apart from immunological influences, the metabolic interaction between tuberculosis and co-morbidity also plays an important role in shaping disease progression and clinical presentation. DM illustrates this interaction, in which hyperglycemia compromises innate and adaptive immune function, decreasing macrophage function and modifying cytokine patterns.

Diabetic patients thus have an increased risk of developing active tuberculosis from latent disease, with more severe clinical manifestations and worse outcomes upon treatment. The coexistence of diabetes and tuberculosis makes disease management difficult because metabolic derangement can delay bacterial elimination and enhance mortality during treatment. Additionally, the disease itself may interfere with glucose metabolism and lead to transient or permanent diabetic conditions, thus establishing a bidirectional disease relationship that contributes to increased disease burden in infected populations. This synergy underscores the need for combined diagnostic and therapeutic strategies that target both infections and metabolic disease to reduce the public health effect of PTB (Faurholt-Jepsen, 2013) (Figure 4.4).

4.2.2. Immune Response to Mycobacterium tuberculosis (MTB)

The early immune response to MTB is a multifaceted interaction between innate and adaptive immunity that determines the course and clinical presentation of pulmonary TB. Innate immune cells like macrophages in the early stages of infection try to hold back the pathogen, activating downstream T lymphocytes. Recent single-cell RNA sequencing analyses identified an increase in certain T-cell subsets after stimulation with *Mtb*-derived antigens; interestingly, $CD4^+$ T-cells and cytotoxic γδ T-cells have distinct phenotypic features reflecting distinct patterns of activation. The activated γδ T cells, as defined by CD16 and granzyme B expression, have cytotoxic functions that could play a role in limiting infection in the lung microenvironment. Additionally, cytokines such as IFN-γ and TNF-α are generated during the response, promoting macrophage activation and granuloma formation, whereas other cytokines, for example, IL-17, seem to be involved only marginally in this acute phase. The specific immune activation patterns encountered suggest targets for vaccine development and immunotherapeutic approaches targeting the enhancement of protective immunity in pulmonary TB (Felgueres et al., 2025). Exactly how *Mtb*-specific CD4+ Th1 cells drive disease outcomes is complex, an echo of the heterogeneity of pulmonary TB presentations. Although these Th1 cells play a pivotal role in the coordination of immune responses through IFN-γ release, their mere presence or polyfunctional cytokine patterns do not always follow disease severity or radiographic pathology. Comparative studies between patients with active TB and *Mtb*-exposed controls indicated that while polyfunctional Th1 cells amass in blood, their number does not correlate with the level of pulmonary destruction or bacterial burden. This indicates that even though they are critical in containing the infection, $CD4^+$ Th1 responses are not adequate to dictate clinical outcomes. Other immune parameters, such as the composition of leukocyte subsets, might have more determinative roles in the pathogenesis and progression of the disease (Panteleev et al., 2017). The general immune landscape of pulmonary TB is not only characterized by adaptive immunity but also by changes in innate immune cell populations that are strongly associated with clinical severity. Importantly, elevated numbers of band neutrophils and other granulocytic cells are positively correlated with more severe pulmonary tissue destruction and bacterial spread, as seen in radiographic scores. In contrast, depletion of circulating lymphocytes is linked with greater clinical disease, emphasizing the significance of immune cell number as well as function. These results point toward an aberrant hematopoietic response during TB infection, wherein granulocytic and lymphocytic lineage imbalances can directly worsen lung pathology. Grasping these systemic immunological changes provides vital insight into mechanisms underlying differential TB manifestations and highlights the imperative for therapeutic strategies targeting both immune activation and regulation (Panteleev et al., 2017) (Figure 4.5).

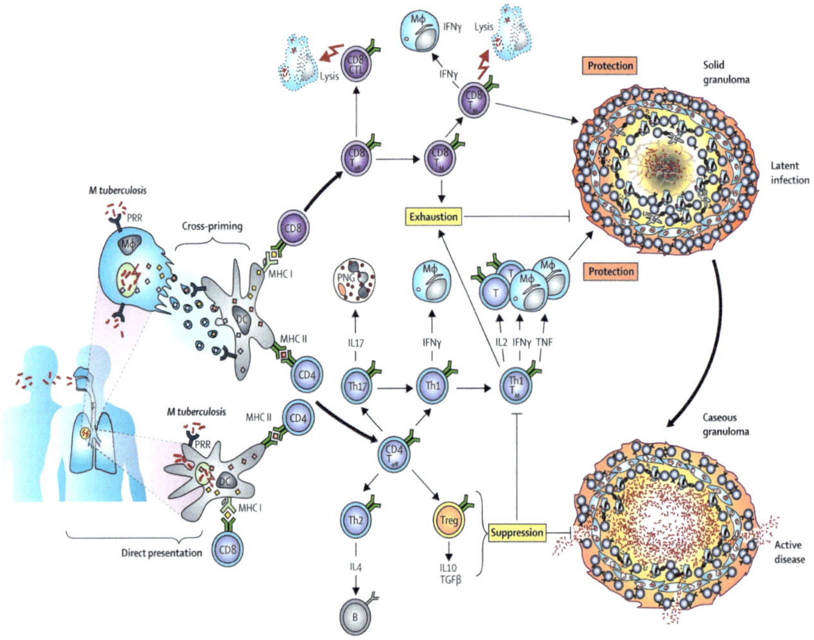

Figure 4.5. Immune response against *Mycobacterium tuberculosis*.

Source: ResearchGate. (n.d.). *Immune response against Mycobacterium tuberculosis: Antigen presentation, T cell differentiation, and granuloma outcomes.* https://www.researchgate.net/publication/339684225/figure/fig1/AS:865358722396162@1583329005997/mmune-response-against-Mycobacterium-tuberculosis.jpg.

4.2.3. Impact of Co-Morbidities on Disease Manifestation

The variability in PTB clinical presentations is largely determined by the occurrence of co-morbidities, which can modify disease susceptibility and progression. A very striking illustration is the interaction between TB and DM, which has become a major public health issue in endemic areas of infectious diseases and emergent chronic diseases. Epidemiological evidence has shown that diabetic patients have a significantly increased risk of acquiring active TB in comparison with non-diabetic populations. Diabetes-induced immune dysregulation can be held responsible for the increased susceptibility, which renders the host inefficient at containing mycobacterial infection. Further, shared epidemiology of TB and diabetes, particularly in urban and developing areas, makes disease control challenging and emphasizes the importance of integrated healthcare strategies. Diabetes-TB co-existence is not just a matter of co-existence, but also an inter-relationship impacting TB manifestations, responses to treatment, and outcomes (Faurholt-Jepsen, 2013). Although the immunological consequences of diabetes co-morbidity on susceptibility to TB are evident, its impact on disease pathogenesis and treatment response is also crucial. Clinical experience reveals that diabetic TB patients present with enhanced inflammatory processes and occasionally uncharacteristic symptom patterns like protracted fever. While diabetes is not seen to prolong sputum conversion times during anti-TB treatment, it is associated with a suboptimal course of recovery, with gradual weight increase and normalization of hemoglobin. All these considerations together point towards an impaired physiological recovery despite comparable bacteriological clearance rates. Interestingly, such co-morbidity is also associated with significantly elevated early mortality when undergoing TB treatment, especially in the initial phase, pointing to diabetes as a predictor of disease severity and prognosis of the patient. These findings further reinforce the importance of meticulous screening and treatment of diabetes among TB patients to enhance clinical outcomes (Faurholt-Jepsen, 2013). Apart from diabetes, other co-morbid diseases like HIV infection also complicate pulmonary TB presentation and prognosis. The synergistic action of co-infection with diabetes and HIV worsens mortality risks, with studies indicating a doubling of the risk of premature death in co-infected individuals compared to those without diabetes. The increased mortality cannot be entirely attributed to TB severity, indicating that immune suppression, metabolic stress, and potential drug interactions account for worse outcomes. Of note, this heightened early mortality highlights the imperative for more sophisticated clinical management strategies that take into account the interdependent pathophysiology of TB and its co-morbidities. Studies aimed at elucidating the mechanisms through which diabetes and other conditions influence TB treatment response may inform better therapeutic regimens and possibly make glycemic control a central element in TB care.

4.3. Common Clinical Symptoms

The presentation of PTB tends to be insidious, with initially nonspecific symptoms that may make early diagnosis challenging. Patients most commonly report having had a cough that has persisted for over two weeks, usually productive and possibly being associated with hemoptysis, which is an indicator of possible pulmonary parenchymal disease. Fever is also a common symptom, typically low-grade and experienced in the evening, and it is an expression of the systemic inflammatory response to MTB infection. Night sweats and unintentional weight loss also define the disease, the latter reflecting chronic disease and metabolic costs of the infectious process. Malaise and fatigue are frequently associated with these findings, impairing the patient's quality of life and functional ability. It is critical to appreciate this set of clinical manifestations since they reflect the body's defense reaction trying to keep the pathogen contained while respiratory tissues are subjected to progressive injury. Respiratory manifestations of pulmonary TB indicate localized tissue disease and can change over time in severity. Pleuritic or dull chest pain develops when the pleura is inflamed from the contiguous spread of infection. Dyspnea is less frequent but can occur in more advanced diseases, particularly if much lung tissue is involved or there are complications like pleural effusion or cavitary disease. The fact that sputum production, in quantity and consistency, is present suggests bronchial disease and the dissemination of mycobacterial organisms into the airways, thus risk for transmission. These respiratory findings, along with constitutional symptoms, predispose the clinician to suspect TB, particularly in endemic areas or risk groups.

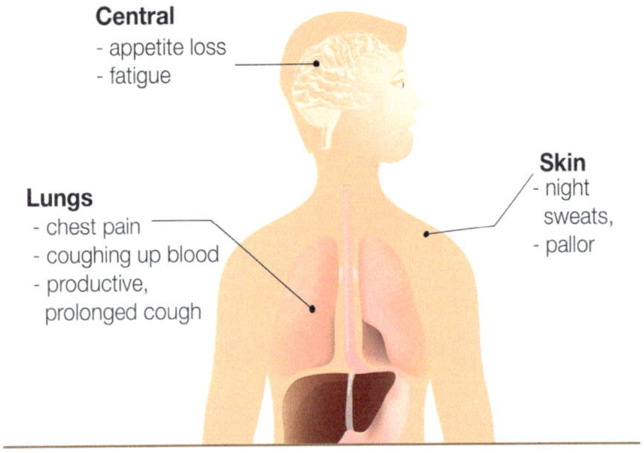

Figure 4.6. Main symptoms of pulmonary tuberculosis (PTB).

Source: Mahkota Medical Centre. (n.d.). *Symptoms of active tuberculosis (TB): Effects on lungs, central nervous system, and skin.* https://www.facebook.com/MahkotaMedical/photos/symptoms-of-active-tb-in-the-lungs-begin-gradually-and-develop-over-a-period-of-/10155790726750376/?_rdr.

Thus, identification and correlation of these presentations with diagnostic tests and epidemiological findings become paramount for early detection and control of the disease. Although PTB's presentation is mainly respiratory and systemic, presentation might sometimes overlap with presentations of other infective disorders, such as viral pneumonias, which need meticulous differential diagnosis. In contrast to some acute respiratory illnesses, which manifest with sudden onset and obvious systemic symptoms, TB symptoms generally develop insidiously, highlighting the difficulty of separating them from other chronic diseases. In addition, TB may in rare instances occur in extrapulmonary locations like the pericardium, where clinical presentations may consist of pericardial pain or constrictive physiology resulting in symptoms of heart failure (José et al., 2021). Clinical variability highlights the importance of a comprehensive clinical examination, encompassing imaging and investigations, to identify general TB manifestations and correctly differentiate them from other conditions, thus leading to appropriate therapeutic interventions (Figure 4.6).

4.3.1. Cough and Its Characteristics

Among the many symptoms noted in PTB, respiratory symptoms frequently give the earliest clinical lead towards diagnosis. Cough, especially, is an initial symptom calling for further evaluation, particularly in endemic areas. The quality of the cough of pulmonary TB is generally insidious, starting as a dry, nonproductive cough, thereafter evolving into a productive type with sputum expectoration. This sequence is a representation of the underlying pathophysiologic alterations as the infection progresses within the lung parenchyma, resulting in tissue necrosis and cavitation. Fever, weight loss, and night sweats are common accompaniments to the cough, highlighting the systemic nature of the disease. Cough can persist but be less severe in smear-negative TB, posing a challenge to early diagnosis. Research has shown that around 60% of smear-negative patients present with cough, making its diagnostic relevance present though with variable intensity and duration (Mohammed et al., 2024). This subtle variation in cough characteristics is vital for clinical suspicion and early diagnosis of pulmonary TB. Distinguishing cough characteristics of tuberculosis from other respiratory infections is clinically relevant due to the disease's infectious nature and global health burden. TB cough tends to be chronic, for more than two weeks, and may be accompanied by hemoptysis as cavitary lesions compromise blood vessels. Radiological correlations are supportive of these clinical observations, and cough severity tends to coincide with the extent of lesions and cavity formation. Advanced diagnostic tools like nanopore sequencing have further clarified the complex interaction of TB with co-infecting pathogens that can modify cough presentation. In mixed infections in patients with MTB and other respiratory pathogens, the cough could present with atypical characteristics because of these concomitant pathogens affecting airway inflammation and mucin secretion (Shu et al., 2024). An atypical or refractory cough should therefore raise the suspicion of TB co-infections or drug resistance, which in turn will inform more individualized diagnosis and treatment approaches. The course of cough over time in pulmonary TB also often mirrors the disease process with respect to treatment and course. Early symptoms can include a mild cough, progressing as the immune system fights the infection, further increasing bronchial secretions and inflammation. In other instances, underlying diseases such as DM can alter patterns of cough by affecting immune capacity and lung tissue integrity. Clinicians have noted that middle-aged male diabetes patients tend to present with more chronic cough accompanied by related lung consolidation and cavitary lesions (Mohammed et al., 2024). Further, nanopore sequencing diagnostics have shown that co-infections with *Candida albicans* and *Klebsiella pneumoniae* organisms complicate cough presentation, tending to delay symptoms and necessitating customized treatments (Shu et al., 2024). Thus, pulmonary TB cough is not just a symptom but an complex clinical sign encompassing host elements, stage of the disease, and microbial interactions, and is hence a mainstay of clinical evaluation and treatment (Figure 4.7).

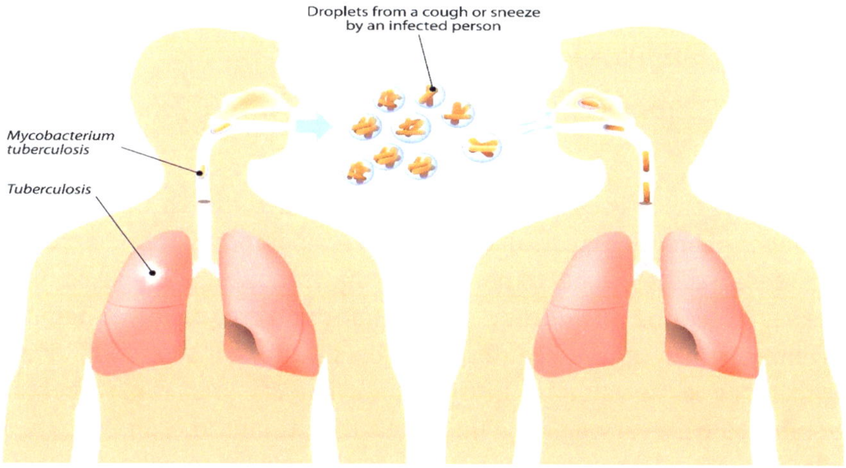

Figure 4.7. The cough in pulmonary TB.

Source: HealthXchange.sg. (n.d.). *Transmission of tuberculosis: Inhalation of Mycobacterium tuberculosis from droplets released by an infected person.* https://www.healthxchange.sg/sites/hexassets/Assets/heart-lungs/tuberculosis-types-symptoms-risks.jpg.

4.3.2. Hemoptysis: Causes and Implications

The observation of blood in the sputum indicates a complicated interaction of underlying pulmonary diseases, usually necessitating emergent clinical assessment for its potentially fatal connotations. In the scenario of PTB, hemoptysis is a serious sign representing the destructive inflammatory processes of MTB. Hemoptysis in TB Pathophysiologically results from erosion of bronchial arteries and cavitary lesions that violate vascular integrity.

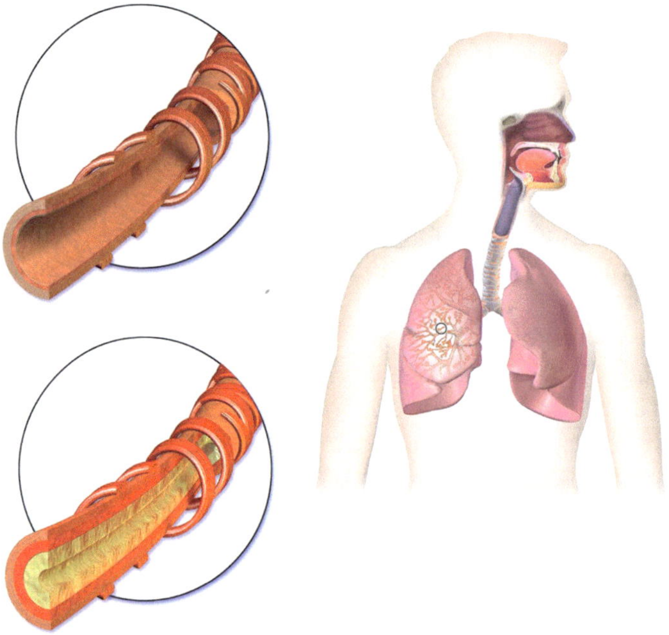

Figure 4.8. Hemoptysis (coughing up blood).

Source: By BruceBlaus - File:Bronchitis.png, CC BY-SA 4.0, https://commons.wikimedia.org/w/index.php?curid=56629686

These vascular disturbances cause bleeding in the airways, which may present to patients as streaks or large amounts of blood. Detection of hemoptysis is important in TB treatment since it not only signals active disease but also points to potential complications like fungal colonization of cavities or secondary bacterial infections. In addition, the amount and frequency of hemoptysis determine therapeutic management, such as the requirement for surgery or bronchial artery embolization, thus emphasizing the prognostic value of the symptom. The range of causes behind hemoptysis is larger than that of tuberculosis, varying from infectious to autoimmune, and thus renders diagnostic procedures difficult in practice. For example, NTM infections such as *Mycobacterium kansasii* can have comparable radiological and symptomatic manifestations like cavities and unilateral lung involvement, leading to hemoptysis with unique epidemiological associations (Matveychuk et al., 2012). Infectious causes tend to induce bronchiectasis or cavitary pulmonary disease, which compromises airway and vascular architecture. At the same time, systemic vasculitides like microscopic polyangiitis also present with alveolar hemorrhage and hemoptysis, often in the absence of renal disease, adding to the diagnostic dilemma (Singhvi et al., 2020). Subclassification of these conditions is critical in the planning of targeted therapy since hemoptysis is a reflection of underlying pathologies that need distinct medical or immunosuppressive treatment approaches, especially when it is a presenting clinical feature in pulmonary TB. The clinical significance of understanding hemoptysis within the context of pulmonary TB manifestations cannot be overemphasized, as it is a sign of severity and possible complications of the disease. Hemoptysis can precede the progression of disease such as cavity development or reactivation of infection, warranting urgent microbiological and radiographic evaluation to direct therapy. Apart from the control of infection, the symptom also requires attention to co-morbidities like chronic lung disease and vascular disease that enhance the risk of bleeding. Hemoptysis also affects patient morbidity and utilization of health resources since severe bleeding episodes may require intensive treatment. An assessment of the interaction between hemoptysis and pulmonary TB raises the significance of diligent clinical observation and the need to incorporate multidisciplinary strategies to optimize outcomes and minimize mortality related to this significant clinical presentation (Figure 4.8).

4.3.3. Chest Pain and Discomfort

Chest pain in PTB is typically a multifaceted clinical symptom deserving of careful assessment. The discomfort usually occurs as a result of pleural involvement, wherein the inflammatory process causes pleuritis, presenting with sharp, localized pain aggravated by respiratory motion such as cough or deep breathing. In contrast to chest pain related to the cardiovascular system, TB-related pain can be chronic and is frequently accompanied by systemic features like fever and nocturnal sweats. Furthermore, the nature and site of the pain can assist clinicians in distinguishing among other respiratory disorders. Assessment of these nuances is essential in early diagnosis and management as chest pain in pulmonary TB is not only attributed to lung parenchymal involvement but also may be caused by complications such as pleural effusion or empyema that need specific therapeutic interventions. This pain, thus, becomes an important clinical sign in the broader picture of TB infection. In others, discomfort in the chest associated with pulmonary TB is aggravated by immune-mediated reactions, affecting treatment decisions. Immune system inflammatory reactions can heighten pleural inflammation or even simulate other immune-related thoracic complications.

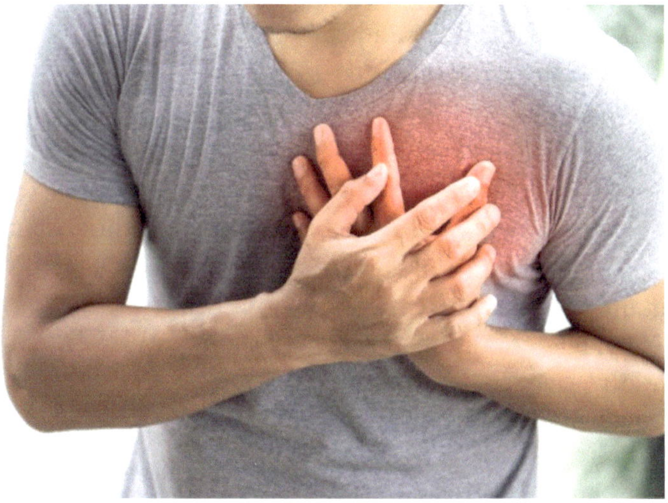

Source: PatientPop. (n.d.). *Individual clutching chest, indicating possible chest pain—a symptom associated with tuberculosis and other respiratory conditions.* https://sa1s3optim.patientpop.com/assets/images/provider/photos/2559345.jpg.

With the topicality of immune checkpoint inhibitors in treating oncologic and infectious disorders, knowledge of these immune-related adverse events (irAEs) is paramount. Consensus opinion dictates that management protocols for immune-related toxicities should be specific to severity, with corticosteroids as a key component to modulate inflammation.

Such immune-modulated chest pain in TB should be distinguished from infectious pathology to prevent delays or errors in treatment, highlighting the need for multidisciplinary treatment and monitoring during treatment (Bryan et al., 2021).

This interaction of infection and the immune response makes the clinical presentation challenging, making it difficult for simple diagnosis when chest pain is the chief complaint. The wider range of chest pain and distress in pulmonary infections reflects the necessity to take into account neurological and musculoskeletal causes in addition to primary pulmonary disease.

Infectious processes such as TB and other respiratory microorganisms may create a wide array of systemic symptoms affecting patient presentation. As noted in diseases such as Middle East respiratory syndrome, the complications of neuromuscular weakness and neuropathies can indirectly cause chest pain and simulate pulmonary symptoms (Jee-Kim et al., 2017).

Such possible overlap demands that clinicians evaluate chest pain within a broad clinical context encompassing infectious, immunologic, and neurologic conditions. The inability to understand these shared symptoms can have negative impacts on disease prognosis and treatment outcomes, underlining the interrelated nature of pulmonary TB's clinical manifestations.

4.4. Systemic Symptoms Associated with Pulmonary TB

Systemic manifestations of PTB tend to represent the body's systemic inflammatory response to the infection with MTB. The manifestations are headache, unexplained weight loss, persistent fever, night sweats, and weakness, which, though nonspecific, are important in clinical suspicion and diagnosis. Constitutional symptoms result from the host response, including cytokine release of pro-inflammatory substances that involve many organ systems outside the pulmonary site. Fever and night sweats, for example, are frequent early manifestations of active disease that frequently prompt patients to have medical evaluation. Dissemination or progression of TB as well as severity of disease are suggested by these systemic findings in addition to disease severity, and they require thorough clinical and radiological evaluation. Early diagnosis and treatment, enhanced patient outcomes, as well as decreased transmission risk, depend on recognizing these symptoms. In some instances, systemic manifestations of pulmonary TB can be complicated by conditions like vasculitis or immune disorders, which complicate diagnosis and treatment. For instance, cases have documented progressive pulmonary consolidations with cavity development alongside systemic vascular manifestations that mimic vasculitis, demonstrating the complexity of presentation (Patil et al., 2022).

This overlap highlights the importance of extensive diagnostic workup, such as microbiological, radiological, and immunological studies, to distinguish TB from other infectious or inflammatory illnesses. Also, complications like DVT may arise in patients on corticosteroids or with immobility for extended periods, further confusing the clinical profile and necessitating cautious prophylaxis (Patil et al., 2022). Such systemic involvement not only broadens the clinical presentation of pulmonary TB but also poses a challenge to conventional therapeutic practices, requiring multidisciplinary treatment. The application of immunomodulatory agents in tuberculotic-susceptible patients, most notably biologic drugs like interleukin-6 inhibitors, adds another layer to systemic presentations.

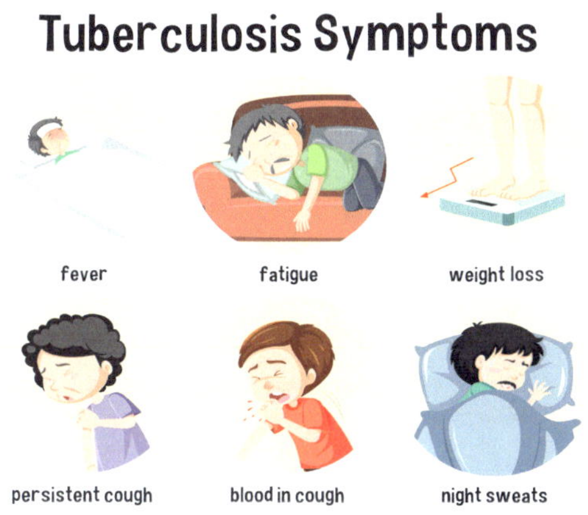

Figure 4.9. Systemic symptoms in pulmonary tuberculosis (PTB).

Source: Yashoda Healthcare. (2023). *Common symptoms of tuberculosis: Fever, fatigue, weight loss, persistent cough, blood in cough, and night sweats.* https://www.yashodahealthcare.com/blogs/wp-content/uploads/2023/04/Tuberculosis-scaled.jpg.

These drugs could modify host immune mechanisms and enhance reactivation of latent TB or primary infection, presenting initially with systemic manifestations such as fever and lymphadenopathy prior to pulmonary presentations. For example, in children treated with tocilizumab, systemic signs such as continued fever can antedate radiological evidence of PTB, highlighting the innocuity of systemic signs preceding overt pulmonary disease. This setting serves to emphasize the need for careful screening and monitoring for systemic presentation in at-risk groups receiving immunosuppressive treatment. Awareness of these systemic presentations is critical to enable early detection and prompt treatment of pulmonary TB, especially in immunocompromised hosts (Figure 4.9).

4.4.1. Fever and Night Sweats

Recurrent fever episodes typically herald the active immune response of the immune system to a covert infection, a key part of the clinical presentation of PTB. Fever in the case of TB presents as intermittent or continuous, usually with chills and malaise, and represents the host's systemic inflammatory response to MTB. Fever is a challenging symptom to diagnose because of its lack of specificity and a tendency to coexist with other infective or inflammatory conditions. The development of fever in TB indicates the pathogen's capacity to cause an immune cascade through cytokine release and activation of immune cells to contain the infection. Comprehension of the febrile reaction in pulmonary TB is thus essential, as not only does it assist in clinical suspicion but also acts as a marker for disease activity and disease progression, highlighting systemic participation over localized pulmonary inflammation (Wani et al., 2016).

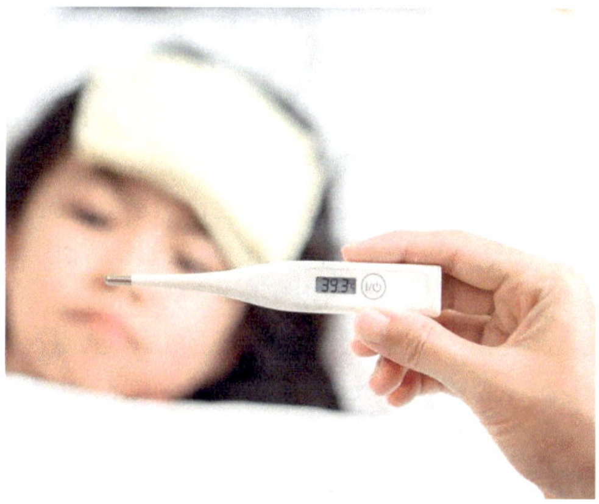

Source: Samarpan Physio Clinic. (2023). *Child with fever, showing thermometer reading 39.3°C—a common symptom of infectious diseases including tuberculosis.* https://samarpanphysioclinic.com/wp-content/uploads/2023/06/fever.webp.

Pacing closely interwoven with systemic symptomatology in pulmonary TB is the presence of night sweats, a hallmark feature that worsens patient distress and profoundly affects the quality of life. Night sweats are caused by body mechanisms ruled by fever rhythms and hypothalamic disturbances of thermoregulation, resulting in hyper-nocturnal sweating. This symptom continues to persist despite appropriate ambient temperature and tends to indicate continued immune stimulation and metabolic derangement concomitant with tuberculosis. Night sweats are therefore critical in the clinical setting since they often trigger medical assessment and are a signature symptom that, when coupled with fever and weight loss, raises the index of suspicion for TB. They also parallel disease severity and bacterial burden, indicating systemic infection burden (Wani et al., 2016). The diagnostic significance of fever and night sweats in pulmonary TB is underscored by situations where these two symptoms first resemble other disorders, making clinical judgment difficult. For example, gastrointestinal manifestations associated with TB can result in misdiagnosis because of coinciding symptoms like weight loss and abdominal pain, such as in patients first suspected of Crohn's disease before pulmonary TB was diagnosed radiologically and microbiologically. These situations highlight the importance of thorough evaluation when fever and night sweats present together with respiratory symptoms, supporting the use of imaging and microbiological diagnosis to prevent delay in treatment. Finally, awareness of these systemic presentations optimizes early diagnosis, directs therapy, and enhances patient outcomes in pulmonary TB.

4.4.2. Weight Loss and Anorexia

Inadvertent weight loss and anorexia are commonly encountered as nonspecific symptoms in PTB patients that may make the diagnosis more challenging. They occur due to the multifaceted interaction between systemic inflammation, metabolic changes, and direct action of mycobacterial infection. The protracted inflammatory condition caused by MTB causes the release of proinflammatory cytokines including tumor necrosis factor-alpha (TNF-α), which interferes with the normal appetite pattern and leads to muscle catabolism. As such, the affected patient tends to develop severe fatigue and nutritional losses, further complicating disease progression.

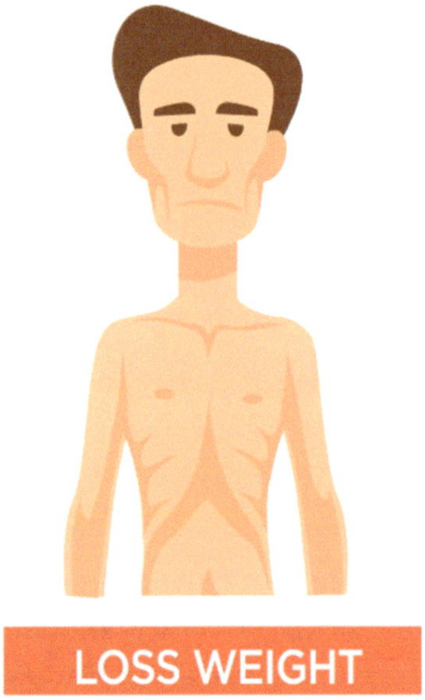

Source: VectorStock. (n.d.). *Weight loss as a symptom of tuberculosis: Illustration of an underweight man.* https://cdn.vectorstock.com/i/1000v/44/80/weight-loss-tuberculosis-symptom-man-vector-27104480.jpg.

Weight loss is not only a result of reduced caloric intake but also indicative of an underlying state of hypermetabolism. Physicians should take all these presentations into account as possible early warning signs of pulmonary TB, particularly in endemic areas or high-risk groups, to enable timely diagnosis and treatment. The diagnostic dilemma presented by weight loss and anorexia in pulmonary TB is highlighted by the common overlap with other granulomatous or systemic illnesses. As an example, GPA has several clinical characteristics common with TB, such as respiratory disease and systemic manifestations like weight loss and anorexia, as illustrated by case reports where misdiagnosis resulted in the use of inappropriate immunosuppressive treatment (Guruparan et al., 2024).

The additional complicating factor is the presence of positive anti-neutrophil cytoplasmic antibodies (ANCAs). In such a case, full clinical evaluation, backed by imaging and microbiological examinations, continues to be necessary to confidently assign the weight loss and anorexia to pulmonary TB and not to other concomitant pathologies. Identifying these concomitant and overlapping features is important to prevent delays in diagnosis and ensure the correct initiation of anti-tuberculous therapy. Nutritional intervention and assessment are most critical in the care of TB patients with severe weight loss and anorexia, as malnutrition directly compromises immune competence and negatively impacts clinical outcomes. While weight loss in pulmonary TB mimics other chronic respiratory illnesses like cystic fibrosis, where malnutrition is also a major characteristic (Guruparan et al., 2024), etiologies vary far more extensively. TB weight loss is largely caused by infection-related metabolic needs and suppression of appetite, whereas in cystic fibrosis, malabsorption and pancreatic insufficiency are major causes. Nutritional deficiencies in TB are treated with not only antitubercular therapy (ATT) but also specific diet support to correct energy balance and ensure recovery. Therefore, including nutritional assessment in routine clinical practice for treating TB maximizes treatment outcomes and alleviates morbidity related to cachexia and anorexia.

4.4.3. Fatigue and General Malaise

The systemic effect of PTB tends to go beyond regional respiratory symptoms and is characterized by non-specific symptoms of fatigue and malaise, which are added to the clinical syndrome. The patients also commonly complain of a generalized tiredness that is out of proportion to physical effort, emphasizing the disease's energy cost for the patient's whole metabolism. This lethargy is caused in part by the protracted inflammatory response induced by MTB, which initiates an immune cascade that generates cytokines that affect the central nervous system's (CNS) control of wakefulness and activity. Additionally, the metabolic requirements of the host are raised by prolonged infection, draining energy stores further.

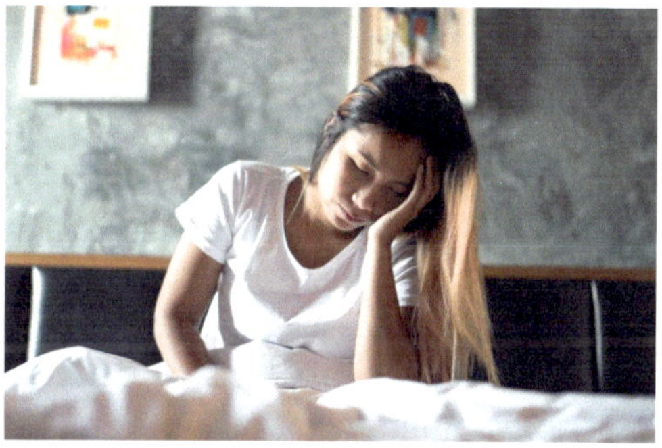

Source: Medical News Today. (n.d.). *Woman experiencing fatigue or malaise while lying in bed—common symptom in various infections including tuberculosis.* https://cdn-prod.medicalnewstoday.com/content/images/articles/327/327062/a-woman-lying-in-bed-and-feeling-unwell-because-of-malaise.jpg.

This nonspecific, generalized sense of sickness not only reduces quality of life but potentially also is a delaying factor in presentation to health care resources, thereby affecting early diagnosis and outcome of treatment necessary to contain disease severity and transmission rates. The gradual onset of malaise and fatigue in PTB patients is frequently difficult to distinguish from the nonspecific viral infections, potentially leading to misdiagnosis or delay in recognizing the inciting mycobacterial infection. Due to the non-specificity of these presentations, clinicians need to have a high level of suspicion, especially in patients with chronic systemic symptoms and risk factors such as being immunocompromised or history of exposure.

The persistence of fatigue in tuberculosis follows the pathogen's ability to cause a latent infection that reactivates intermittently and induces fluctuation of symptoms. In others, co-morbid conditions such as sarcoidosis or HIV complicate clinical evaluation, where a detailed diagnostic workup is needed to rule out overlapping syndromes before the initiation of therapeutic measures (Mencarini et al., 2016). This underscores the particular importance of a multidimensional evaluation strategy in capturing the entire clinical scope of PTB. In addition, fatigue and malaise are compounded by the metabolic and nutritional abnormalities often seen with tuberculosis. Weight loss, anorexia, and night sweats, commonly seen together with nonspecific malaise, represent the systemic state of catabolism evoked by the infection. These presentations are similar to those of extrapulmonary variants, including abdominal tuberculosis, where constitutional signs similarly compromise physical endurance and general health (Faurholt-Jepsen, 2013). Therapeutic treatment of tuberculosis can also create side effects that exacerbate fatigue, especially when hepatotoxicity or other treatment-related adverse effects arise with therapy. All of these clinical issues are addressed through a comprehensive approach that combines effective antimicrobial treatment with symptom management in an effort to optimize patient outcomes and prevent the incapacitating phenomenon of ongoing fatigue and malaise.

4.5. Diagnostic Approaches

Early and correct diagnosis is critical in the management of PTB, considering its enormous public health significance. A combination of clinical assessment and laboratory techniques is the cornerstone of existing diagnostic approaches. Sputum smear microscopy has been in use for decades to identify acid-fast bacilli (AFB), but its sensitivity is often poor in low bacterial load or HIV co-infection scenarios. The introduction of nucleic acid amplification tests (NAATs) like Xpert MTB/RIF has improved the accuracy of diagnosis by quickly identifying DNA of MTB and rifampicin resistance. This is not only a speedy way of diagnosing but also facilitates early detection of drug-resistant strains, which is essential in customizing effective treatment regimens. Despite these developments, clinical setting and history of the patient are still fundamental in the interpretation of test results, especially where co-morbid conditions such as diabetes affect disease occurrence and course (Faurholt-Jepsen, 2013). The difficulty of diagnosing tuberculosis in subjects with comorbid conditions underscores the importance of integrated diagnostic strategies. For example, DM is known to enhance susceptibility to active tuberculosis and complicate its clinical course. This co-morbid condition requires more sensitive and broad screening tests to detect tuberculosis among diabetic subjects effectively. Studies undertaken in sub-Saharan Africa highlight that traditional diagnostic methods might fail to detect the changed immune response observed with patients suffering from both diseases. Therefore, the combination of immunological and molecular assays can enhance detection rates and assist in distinguishing between latent and active tuberculosis. Including glycemic status and immune function is thus imperative in upgrading diagnostic protocols, ultimately leading to improved treatment results and survival rates in mixed disease groups

(Faurholt-Jepsen, 2013). In pediatric groups and extrapulmonary presentations, fine needle aspiration biopsy has become a crucial diagnostic intervention. Research comparing its use in the diagnosis of tuberculous lymphadenitis shows that the combination of cytological evaluation and molecular tests such as Xpert MTB/RIF increases diagnostic sensitivity and specificity. Although the conventional methods of AFB microscopy and culture are still useful, their fallibility among children and some forms of extrapulmonary tuberculosis makes it necessary to incorporate sophisticated molecular tools. The synergy of clinical evaluation, cytology, and NAATs allows for prompt, precise diagnosis, and timely intervention that minimizes disease morbidity. Continued research focuses on further validating these diagnostic algorithms, making them suitable for use in various, resource-poor environments with continued high tuberculosis burden.

4.5.1. Clinical Evaluation and History Taking

An exhaustive clinical assessment is the cornerstone in the identification and management of PTB, particularly due to the heterogeneity of its clinical presentation. Initial action begins with a thorough history, including the evaluation of symptoms like chronic cough, hemoptysis, fever, night sweats, and weight loss, which are characteristic features but often present subtly. It is important to ask about exposure risks such as exposure to known TB patients, past TB infection or treatment, and comorbid conditions such as HIV or diabetes that can affect disease progression. It is also important to assess the patient's socio-economic setting and place of residence to elicit factors predisposing to disease. Such an approach provides a focused physical examination with attention to respiratory findings such as crackles or decreased breath sounds. Adding radiological and laboratory results enhances this assessment, improves diagnostic sensitivity, and informs additional management interventions in suspected cases of pulmonary TB (Raghu et al., 2020). History taking for pulmonary TB is more than the general inquiry of symptoms. It includes a comprehensive examination of epidemiological factors and the patient's risk profile. Knowing the patient's geographic location, travel, and immunization status can provide vital information since the prevalence of TB differs widely geographically and by population. *Bacillus Calmette-Guérin* (BCG) immunization can alter clinical presentation or laboratory test results, which can affect interpretation. In addition, immunosuppressive therapy in the past or chronic conditions known to impair immune function is crucial, since they put patients at risk of more severe or unusual TB disease presentation. A detailed record of previous TB treatment, duration, and adherence assesses the risk for drug resistance, which is increasingly a concern worldwide. Such painstaking history-taking not only elucidates the probability of active disease but also assists in individualized plan management following trends of the day in epidemiology (Faurholt-Jepsen, 2013).

Clinical assessment of pulmonary TB also has to deal with differential diagnoses through insightful integration of history and clinical presentation. Since symptoms such as cough and weight loss are nonspecific, clinicians need to rule out other respiratory infections, cancers, or chronic pulmonary diseases, particularly in areas where there are competing disease burdens. The importance of the chronological evolution of symptoms and corresponding signs, such as lymphadenopathy or extrapulmonary disease, can be used for differentiation. Laboratory testing, such as sputum microscopy and molecular studies, is based on history and clinical suspicion formulated in the assessment phase. Particularly, the new paradigm of respiratory conditions, as marked by current pandemics and new pathogens, emphasizes the role of a thoughtful history and clinical assessment in preventing diagnostic overshadowing or delay. Piecing together all these factors is critical to constructing an integrated clinical image, fundamental to early diagnosis and efficient treatment of pulmonary TB (Figure 4.10).

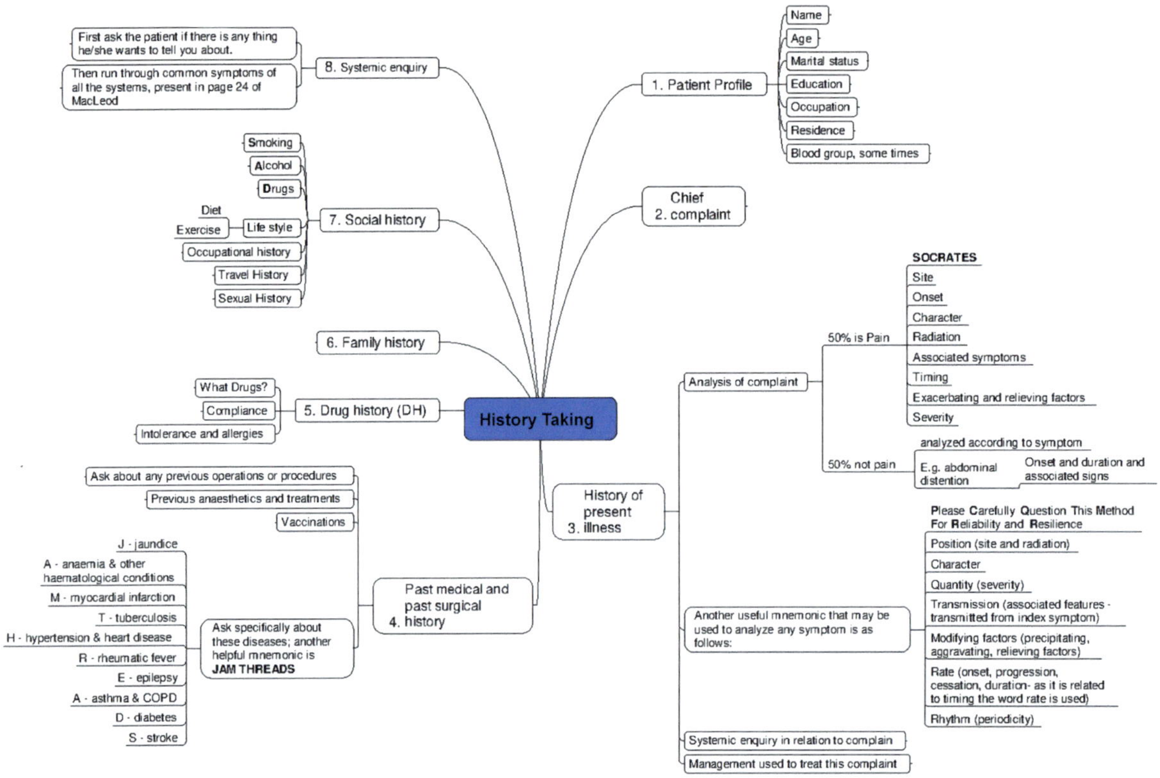

Figure 4.10. History taking.

Source: https://commons.wikimedia.org/wiki/File:History_Taking.pdf

4.5.2. Radiological Investigations: Chest X-Ray and CT Scan

Medical imaging advances have greatly improved pulmonary disease detection and assessment, especially tuberculosis (TB). Although clinical features of pulmonary TB may be nonspecific and variable at times, radiologic studies continue to play an important role in diagnosing the condition more definitively. Chest X-rays are a first-line, inexpensive imaging tool, offering critical information about lung parenchymal abnormalities like infiltrates, cavitations, and nodular lesions characteristic of active TB infection. Despite its common usage, the interpretation of chest radiographs needs specialized radiological knowledge to prevent misdiagnosis, particularly in low-resource settings where such skills may be lacking. Recent advancements in artificial intelligence (AI) hold the promise of solving this problem; for example, sophisticated deep learning algorithms can already correctly classify chest X-ray abnormalities with the same accuracy as experienced radiologists, potentially democratizing access to accurate diagnosis in those regions most encumbered by TB (Rajpurkar et al., 2018). This technological development highlights the changing role of the chest X-ray as an aid to clinical suspicion and a driver of further imaging decisions (Figure 4.11).

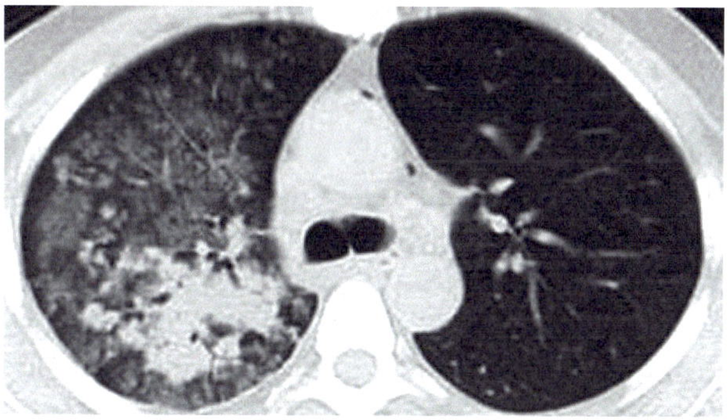

Figure 4.11. The radiological diagnosis of pulmonary tuberculosis (PTB).

Source: Radiology Key. (n.d.). *CT scan of lungs showing advanced pulmonary infection, indicative of tuberculosis.* https://radiologykey.com/wp-content/uploads/2016/09/A322239_1_En_8_Fig46_HTML.jpg.

Augmenting the chest X-ray, CT scans give a better visualization of pulmonary structures, which is important in determining how widespread and severe the tuberculosis is. High-resolution cross-sectional images given by CT imaging allow for the detection of subtle pathology like small nodules, tree-in-bud patterns signifying endobronchial dissemination, and mediastinal lymphadenopathy, which on plain radiographs cannot be detected. This precise anatomical information assists in the differential diagnosis of TB against other infectious and non-infectious lung illnesses, particularly in situations where clinical and traditional imaging results are indeterminate. In addition, CT scans can identify complications such as pleural effusions or bronchial stenosis, and guide proper therapeutic approaches. The sensitivity and specificity of CT in diagnosing active pulmonary TB reaffirm its crucial status as an adjunct diagnostic method, especially in complicated cases or treatment follow-up settings. In addition to pulmonary TB, radiological studies are equally important for detecting extrapulmonary involvement, which can have a major impact on treatment outcomes. Although CT and magnetic resonance imaging (MRI) of the brain are utilized more often in CNS TB, chest CT continues to be vital in detecting related thoracic pathologies as well as the extent of pulmonary involvement. In clinical assessment of suspected TB meningitis or disseminated disease, radiological evidence like meningeal enhancement or hydrocephalus supplements cerebrospinal fluid (CSF) examination in detecting complications like infarcts secondary to vasculitis (John, 2017). Thus, an integrated strategy involving clinical, radiological, and laboratory features maximizes diagnostic sensitivity and allows early treatment with anti-tubercular (ATT) therapy. The interaction between sophisticated imaging modalities and medical expertise therefore plays a central role in preventing TB morbidity and mortality globally.

4.5.3. Laboratory Tests: Sputum Smear and Culture

PTB diagnosis is largely dependent on the examination of sputum samples that give key information on the presence of MTB. Patients with pulmonary tuberculosis usually have sputum containing the bacilli, thus making sputum smear microscopy a primary laboratory test. This includes staining the sputum samples to identify AFB under the microscope. Sputum smear microscopy is appreciated for its fast turnaround and relative ease, enabling rapid diagnosis that is critical to the immediate initiation of treatment. Nevertheless, the sensitivity of the smear test could be affected by the amount of the bacterial load and the quality of the sputum specimen. Where sputum expectoration is challenging, sputum induction can be used, providing a less invasive and safer option compared to procedures such as fiberoptic bronchoscopy, improving the efficacy of sample collection (Farrugia et al., 2013). Apart from the immediate diagnosis offered by sputum smears, sputum sample culture is still the criterion standard for establishing pulmonary TB. Cultivation of the bacilli enables identifying live mycobacteria, which is a more sensitive method than smears. Though culture procedures take longer to incubate, typically several weeks, they are necessary for detecting low-density cases as well as carrying out drug susceptibility testing (DST). This is especially important for TB co-morbid conditions like diabetes, where the interaction between diseases may determine clinical outcomes and potentially slow down bacterial clearance. The culture method is therefore crucial for integrated patient management, allowing individualized therapeutic approaches to consider any drug resistance or disease complication (Faurholt-Jepsen, 2013). It also needs to be noted that laboratory analysis of sputum samples goes beyond diagnosis into the monitoring of disease progression and response to therapy in pulmonary TB. Serial smear and culture sputum examinations are part of monitoring the efficacy of therapy and detecting sputum conversion, which indicates a reduction in bacterial density. Research shows that although diabetes co-morbidity does not cause noteworthy delay in sputum conversion, it can affect other clinical parameters such as immune response and outcomes of treatment. Ongoing bacteriological monitoring using sputum examinations gives clinicians valuable information to modify treatment regimens accordingly and to recognize patients at increased risk of unfavorable outcomes, such as augmented mortality with co-morbid conditions. Hence, sputum smear and culture are still central to both the diagnosis and longitudinal care of pulmonary TB (Farrugia et al., 2013; Faurholt-Jepsen, 2013).

4.6. Complications of Pulmonary TB

The course of PTB tends to predispose patients to a variety of complications that markedly influence clinical outcomes. Of these, respiratory insufficiency and cavitary lesions are common, with cavities serving as a nidus for ongoing infection and additional tissue destruction. Such parenchymal structural damage predisposes patients to secondary infections, including bacterial or fungal causes. Of particular interest, in patients who are immunocompromised, particularly those with concomitant HIV infection, opportunistic pathogens such as disseminated histoplasmosis may occur, complicating or mimicking the clinical presentation of pulmonary TB. Such co-infections are liable to cloud the diagnosis and increase morbidity, presenting in a nonspecific manner as fever and weight loss that overlaps with TB presentation. The interplay of overlapping infections in complexity serves to highlight the necessity for increased clinical suspicion and individualized approaches to diagnosis in atypical or refractory cases (Arreola-Banda et al., 2024). Drug reactions to anti-tuberculars are another major cause of complications affecting both clinical courses as well as treatment compliance in pulmonary TB. Drug intolerance may manifest as a variety of toxic-allergic effects, not only compromising the patients' physiological stability but also limiting the efficacy of therapeutic regimens. Hepatic dysfunction is an arguable presentation, with increases in alanine aminotransferase (ALT) and aspartate aminotransferase (AST) levels indicating drug-induced hepatotoxicity. Immune dysregulation is paired with these toxic effects, with changes seen in T-lymphocyte subpopulations and natural killer (NK) cell function, which can reduce the host's capacity to effectively control the infection. These immunotoxicities have been addressed using adjunctive hepatoprotective therapies, which have shown the potential to lessen treatment-related adverse effects, thus allowing for more uniform and effective clinical management (Matvienko et al., 2023).

Parenchymal lesions
Thin walled cavity (Open negative syndrome)
Aspergilloma
End stage lung destruction
Scar carcinoma
Airway Lesions
Tuberculous Laryngitis
Bronchiectasis
Tracheobronchial stenosis
Anthracofibrosis
Broncholithiasis
Vascular Lesions
Rasmussen aneurysm
Pleural Lesions
Dry pleurisy
Pleural effusion
Empyema & Bronchopleural fistula
Pneumothorax
General Complications
Cor-pulmonale
Secondary amyloidosis
Chronic respiratory failure

Figure 4.12. Complications of pulmonary tuberculosis (PTB).

Source: Devi, P. S. (n.d.). *Complications of pulmonary tuberculosis, including parenchymal, airway, vascular, pleural lesions, and general complications.* https://www.semanticscholar.org/paper/Complications-of-Pulmonary-Tuberculosis-Devi/efc96b0dcaaff77831418b6daf8249d311e546c9/figure/0.

Given these multi-faceted complexities, PTB management requires an integrated strategy beyond MTB eradication. The co-existence of opportunistic diseases like histoplasmosis among immunocompromised subjects and drug toxicities demands thorough diagnostic evaluations and personalized treatment regimens. Initiation of diagnostic algorithms for co-infections at the earliest and vigilant follow-up of immunological and liver functions can anticipate life-threatening complications and enhance patient outcomes. In addition, treatment support of immune status and liver health, such as the application of probiotic-derived hepatoprotectors, has been associated with increased tolerance to treatment and reduced lengths of stay in the hospital. Identification and control of these complications are thus key to maximizing therapeutic benefits and minimizing mortality from PTB (Arreola-Banda et al., 2024; Matvienko et al., 2023) (Figure 4.12).

4.6.1. Development of Drug-Resistant Tuberculosis (DR-TB)

The development of drug-resistant TB (DR-TB) is an important complication in the clinical management of pulmonary TB, worsening diagnosis and treatment issues. Drug resistance is mainly due to genetic mutations in MTB, commonly promoted by suboptimal or inadequate antimicrobial treatment. DR-TB patients usually have more widespread manifestations of the disease, as evidenced by clinical research showing an increased incidence of comorbid diseases, including DM, which compromises immune function and allows the persistence of the pathogen. Significantly, CT scans show that DR-TB patients have more and larger pulmonary cavitations, greater calcification, and more extensive lung involvement. These extreme radiographic findings mirror both the virulent nature of resistant strains and the ineffectiveness of the host in suppressing the infection, demarcating the confluence of microbial adaptation and clinical severity (Wang et al., 2023). This trend highlights the imperative of early detection measures prioritizing resistant TB cases to prevent advancement and transmission. Pathophysiological alterations in drug-resistant pulmonary TB patients are not only reflected in radiological appearances but also in the hematological profile, which indicates systemic inflammatory and immune changes. Studies on MDR-TB show that as the severity of lung involvement becomes more extensive, there are significant alterations in blood indices. In particular, significant phagocytic neutrophil-stimulated leukocytosis and raised platelet counts reflect an active inflammatory response to contain extensive tissue damage. On the other hand, decreases in lymphocyte levels and mean platelet volume can indicate immune exhaustion or dysregulation, which may be responsible for the chronicity and severity of infection. These hematologic changes occur in concert with radiographic findings of lung injury such as pleural effusion, lobar collapse, and fibrotic scarring, demonstrating how drug resistance affects both localized pulmonary disease and distant hematologic derangements (Thungathurthi et al., 2022). Monitoring these clinical markers is critical for determining disease severity and individualizing treatment for resistant tuberculosis. The evolution of DR-TB radically transforms the clinical course and presentation of PTB, requiring more stringent diagnostic alertness as well as integrated patient care. Drug-resistant strains have the propensity to exhibit unusual and more severe presentations, such as bilateral multi-lobar pulmonary involvement and higher cavitary lesion burden. In contrast, drug-susceptible tuberculosis usually presents in more localized patterns. CT imaging is essential for capturing these variations, providing key information for identifying drug-resistant versus drug-susceptible tuberculosis (DS-TB), thus supporting early treatment. In addition, the presence of systemic disease conditions like diabetes worsens the clinical effect, most probably through compromised immunity and facilitating bacterial survival. Collectively, these observations highlight the delicate interplay between microbial resistance mechanisms, host elements, and disease manifestation, which altogether define the clinical scenario of pulmonary TB in the setting of rising drug resistance (Wang et al., 2023). This multifaceted nature highlights the necessity for combined diagnostic and therapeutic approaches to address resistant forms of tuberculosis.

4.6.2. Pleural Effusion and Other Respiratory Complications

The PTB condition is more than a primary infection, frequently accompanied by a series of pleural and respiratory complications obscuring clinical presentation and complicating diagnosis. Pleural effusion, the most common manifestation, is seen as fluid in the pleural space, usually an immune-mediated reaction to infection due to MTB. This exudation may occur in the form of either transudative or tuberculous exudative fluid accumulation, depending on tuberculosis-associated pleural effusions typically showing exudative properties as a consequence of the inflammatory reaction. The diagnosis of pleural effusion in TB patients is important to identify because not only does it indicate a disease state but also requires differentiated treatment approaches for the other underlying causes of pleural fluid formation. Identification of these respiratory complications is paramount in the complete evaluation of patients and emphasizes the subtle pathophysiology of pulmonary TB, particularly in geographic areas where TB is prevalent. Besides pleural effusion, other respiratory complications profoundly affect the clinical course of pulmonary TB, frequently exacerbating patient morbidity. Pulmonary edema, lobar pneumonia, and obstructive sleep apnea syndrome have been noted in TB patients, emphasizing the extensive pulmonary implications that can occur either as a direct result of the infection or secondary to co-morbid illnesses like chronic kidney disease (Pant et al., 2019). The interrelation of systemic disease and pulmonary complications requires multidisciplinary diagnosis and treatment strategies. For example, the pneumonia superimposed on tuberculous lung lesions complicates the outcome of treatment and can present as a mimic of TB exacerbation, highlighting the relevance of differential diagnosis. In addition, these respiratory complications can hinder pulmonary function and recovery delay, emphasizing being watchful in monitoring and management of these manifestations in TB care plans. Uncommon but clinically important is the association of pulmonary alveolar proteinosis (PAP) and tuberculosis, whose co-occurrence poses diagnostic dilemmas owing to common radiologic features of diffuse ground glass opacities and in the presence of calcified lesions along with pleural effusion (Fan et al., 2022). PAP in itself makes patients susceptible to secondary infections owing to the compromised function of alveolar macrophages, providing the niche for MTB to grow. This interaction requires increased clinical suspicion and a thorough diagnostic analysis to manage both conditions successfully. Interestingly, treatment of the mycobacterial infection in such a scenario with anti-tuberculosis drugs not only addresses the mycobacterial infection but can also improve underlying alveolar proteinosis, demonstrating the interplay between infectious and non-infectious pulmonary pathways in TB patients. Such a scenario underscores the need for individualized therapeutic strategies aimed at the multifactorial nature of pulmonary TB and its manifestations.

4.6.3. Extra-Pulmonary Manifestations

In addition to the classical pulmonary presentation, tuberculosis (TB) may also present in different extra-pulmonary forms, making diagnosis and treatment challenging. Manifestations arise when MTB spreads from the initial lung focus to other sites via lymphatic or hematogenous routes. Lymph nodes (LNs), pleura, bones, and the CNS are the most common extra-pulmonary sites. Involvement of the LNs, also called tuberculous lymphadenitis, usually presents as painless cervical swelling. Pleural TB can present with chest pain and effusion, which might masquerade as other respiratory disorders. Bone and joint TB, particularly Pott's disease of the spine, can present with structural deformities and neurological impairment. Because of the varied presentations, extra-pulmonary TB is often underdiagnosed when there are no classical respiratory symptoms. Clinicians should be aware of these varied presentations for proper clinical evaluation and early management of TB patients. Pediatric age groups exhibit specific susceptibility to extra-pulmonary manifestations, with TB meningitis and miliary TB more frequently noted in their severe forms. Hematogenous dissemination is more common in children younger than three years of age, resulting in disseminated organ involvement with significant effects on morbidity and mortality. Neurological TB involving meningitis may manifest insidiously with nonspecific signs and symptoms such as irritability, vomiting, and lethargy, making it challenging to achieve a prompt diagnosis. In addition, gastrointestinal TB or pericarditis can occur but usually go undetected with other childhood illnesses due to overlap. The nonspecific presentation in children and the frequent paucibacillary character of extra-pulmonary disease present diagnostic difficulties. Therefore, judicious clinical suspicion needs to be sustained, particularly in endemic regions or known contacts, to enable early detection and treatment of these potentially fatal forms. Histopathological and microbiological analyses continue to be crucial in the diagnosis of extra-pulmonary TB, but the sensitivity is site-specific. Diagnoses are often confirmed by samples such as LN biopsy, pleural fluid, or CSF. The paucibacillary status of most extra-pulmonary sites makes sputum tests often negative, and other diagnostic modalities need to be employed. Imaging methods like ultrasound, CT, and MRI help to detect lesions that are not accessible to routine examination. Treatment regimens usually replicate pulmonary TB regimens but have to take into account the site and extent of involvement. Irreversible tissue destruction may result from untreated or late diagnosis of extrapulmonary TB. Remarkably, co-infections like COVID-19 may mask clinical presentation or cause a delay in diagnosis, which necessitates detailed differential diagnosis of respiratory pathologies.

Summary

The intricacy of PTB clinical presentation highlights the significance of early and correct diagnosis in controlling the disease efficiently. Imaging methods, especially chest CT scans, yield key information about pathological alterations in the lungs, aiding differentiation of DR-TB from drug-sensitive ones on the basis of characteristic radiological findings. The coexistence of multiple cavities, thick-walled lesions, and widespread involvement of the lung are all high-level predictors of drug resistance, allowing for earlier recognition and best-practice treatment. These radiological markers not only add confidence to diagnoses but also allow for the customization of treatment approaches, which may lead to better patient outcomes. As a result, the integration of imaging findings with clinical presentation and laboratory results becomes an all-encompassing strategy for overcoming the pitfalls associated with pulmonary TB varied presentations, and hence minimizing morbidity and mortality related to the disease (Cheng et al., 2021). The complexity of tuberculosis goes beyond the involvement of the lungs, especially among susceptible groups like those with HIV (PLHIV), whose extrapulmonary presentations only add to clinical evaluation and management challenges. The challenge of accessing definitive microbiological or histopathological evidence in poor-resource settings compounds the need to trust clinical acumen and supportive diagnostic aids, potentially leading to a delay in initiating proper treatment. The increased mortality and loss to follow-up (LTFU) rates in patients with EPTB underscore the necessity of enhanced diagnostic function as well as integrated models of care for both TB and comorbid conditions such as HIV. Early antiretroviral therapy (ART) utilization serves to have a protective effect, emphasizing the need for inclusive management programs that cover both infectious diseases to improve survival rates in this population at risk (Arpagaus et al., 2020). The clinical presentation of PTB has a complexity that demands an assessment of diagnostic as well as therapeutic complexity. Improved imaging and molecular diagnostics have enhanced the capability to detect drug-resistant strains and extrapulmonary disease, but there remains a challenge, particularly in low-income settings and immunocompromised individuals. Strategies need to continue to develop affordable, quick, and precise diagnostics and effective treatment protocols to contain the disease burden. Generally, identifying typical clinical and radiological findings has a critical role to play in directing timely intervention, enhancing prognoses, and containing tuberculosis spread globally. Such holistic measures are critical in moving towards control of tuberculosis and ultimate elimination on a global scale (Arpagaus et al., 2020; Cheng et al., 2021).

The clinical presentation of PTB usually presents in a pattern of a constellation of signs and symptoms that represent the combination of both the direct effect of MTB infection and the host inflammatory response. Patients present with chronic cough, which might be productive, and sometimes hemoptysis. Constitutional signs and symptoms such as fever, night sweats, fatigue, and unintentional weight loss are commonly reported and represent systemic involvement. The progressive loss of lung parenchyma from granulomatous inflammation results in cavitation and fibrosis, causing respiratory impairment. These pathologic processes are indicative of important presentations such as chronic dyspnea and chronic respiratory infections. Moreover, increasing awareness of the overlap between pulmonary TB and COPD, among other respiratory conditions, has been observed, with post-TB lung damage being a major contributor to chronic airway obstruction and functional impairment (Choi, 2025). Assessment of the overlapping symptoms is needed to understand the clinical presentation to allow timely management and diagnosis. In addition to the classical pulmonary presentation, extrapulmonary manifestations usually complicate the TB clinical picture, thereby obscuring diagnostic clarity. Disseminated TB can involve multiple organs and cause nonspecific symptoms like malaise, anorexia, and weight loss, which are suggestive of other granulomatous conditions like GPA. This overlap is especially significant when there is the positivity of serologic markers like anti-neutrophil cytoplasmic antibodies (ANCAs), thus blurring differentiation from autoimmune vasculitis (Guruparan et al., 2024). The patient may present with lymphadenopathy and systemic inflammatory reactions, such as raised C-reactive protein and procalcitonin, suggesting bacterial infection instead of autoimmunity. Thus, the clinical presentation includes not only respiratory symptoms but systemic signs and organ-specific manifestations as well, which may complicate the clinical presentation and require comprehensive and multidisciplinary diagnostic evaluation for proper identification of TB. The other essential facet of pulmonary TB clinical manifestations is its long-term consequences, which contribute significantly to chronic pulmonary morbidity. Structural lung injury due to the infection causes chronic inflammation with increased matrix metalloproteinases and neutrophilic infiltration, inducing tissue destruction, fibrosis, and airway remodeling (Choi, 2025). Subsequent pathologies are bronchiectasis and chronic airflow obstruction with a COPD-like pattern; these abnormalities account for prolonged symptoms of dyspnea, chronic cough, and recurrent exacerbations despite microbiological cure. The presence of these residual changes highlights the necessity of proper management strategies that cover both active infection as well as its pulmonary sequelae. Identification of these persistent manifestations is crucial in complete care, as they have a notable influence on quality of life as well as respiratory status in TB survivors.

CLOSER LOOK

EXTRAPULMONARY SIGNS MIMICKING PULMONARY TB

Extrapulmonary tuberculosis (EPTB) arises when MTB infects the organs other than those in the lungs. Even if pulmonary TB is still the most prevalent type of the illness, extrapulmonary presentation often poses a diagnostic problem because of the non-specificity of symptoms. These extrapulmonary symptoms may present as other diseases, complicating the diagnosis and necessitating a high degree of suspicion, particularly in endemic regions. The most frequent extrapulmonary locations involved are the lymphatics, pleura, bones, and joints, CNS, genitourinary tract, and the gastrointestinal tract.

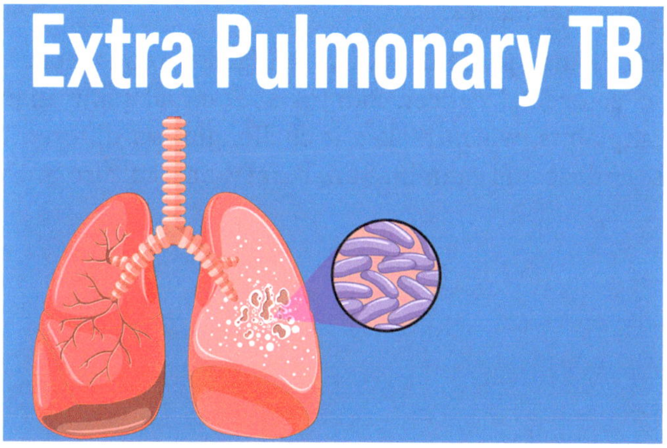

Source: StudyIQ. (2024). *Extra pulmonary TB.* https://www.studyiq.com/articles/wp-content/uploads/2024/05/16163915/Extra-Pulmonary-TB-blog.jpg.

One of the most common extrapulmonary manifestations of TB is lymphadenitis tuberculous, presenting as enlarged LNs, usually in the cervical area. The nodes are either firm or fluctuant, and while they are often tender, they are not necessarily always so. This presentation can readily be confused with other infections or even malignancies like lymphoma and thus proper diagnosis is crucial by biopsy or imaging tests.

Another frequent extrapulmonary presentation is pleural TB, in which the bacilli infect the pleura, the lung's covering membrane. Pleural TB usually manifests as dyspnea, cough, and pleuritic chest pain and may be misdiagnosed as a cause of pleuritis or pneumonia. It is typically accompanied by a pleural effusion, which can be visualized using imaging tests such as chest X-rays or CT scans. The clinical presentation may closely mimic other pulmonary conditions, such as malignancy or autoimmune illness, and therefore cause diagnostic confusion. The diagnosis is established by pleural fluid examination, with the demonstration of AFB or the presence of characteristic granulomas being diagnostic of TB.

Osteoarticular TB is the infection of bones and joints, particularly the spine (Pott's disease), hips, and knees. It usually presents with back pain or joint pain, and the symptoms might be insidious, mimicking diseases like rheumatoid arthritis or degenerative joint disease. Pott's disease, if not treated, can lead to catastrophic deformities and neurological impairment due to compression of the spinal cord, so early diagnosis is essential. If TB happens to occur in the CNS, it may lead to TBM, characterized by nonspecific manifestations like headache, fever, vomiting, and altered mental status.

These signs tend to be identical to those experienced with other forms of meningitis, such as viral or bacterial infections. Furthermore, tuberculomas, being masses of infected tissue in the brain, may present with focal neurological deficits, mimicking brain tumors or abscesses. Diagnosis of CNS TB is usually established by CSF examination and imaging methods.

Genitourinary TB may present symptoms like dysuria, hematuria, and lower abdominal pain, which may result in misdiagnosis as a urinary tract infection or even bladder cancer. The most frequently involved site is the kidneys, and in the absence of treatment, renal TB can result in chronic kidney disease and renal failure.

Lastly, gastrointestinal TB may present as various digestive conditions, including inflammatory bowel disease (IBD) and colorectal cancer. Painful abdominal pain, diarrhea, weight loss, and anorexia are frequent complaints, which makes it challenging to differentiate from other chronic gastrointestinal ailments. Endoscopic examination, biopsy, and culture to find MTB may be needed to diagnose it.

References

1. Singhvi, S. D., Singh, P., Khan, R., Patel, M., & Acharya, P. (2020). A case report of microscopic polyangiitis presenting as diffuse pulmonary symptoms with no renal involvement. *International Journal of Research in Medical Sciences*, *8*(4), 1578–1581. https://doi.org/10.18203/2320-6012.ijrms20201364 (accessed on 10 May 2025).
2. Mortaz, E., Moloudizargari, M., Varahram, M., Movassaghi, M., Garssen, J., Kazempour Dizagie, M., Mirsaeidi, M., & Adcock, I. M. (2018). What Immunological Defects Predispose to Non-tuberculosis Mycobacterial Infections?. *Iranian journal of allergy, asthma, and immunology*, *17*(2), 100–109. (accessed on 10 May 2025).
3. Faurholt-Jepsen, D., Range, N., PrayGod, G., Jeremiah, K., Faurholt-Jepsen, M., Aabye, M. G., Changalucha, J., Christensen, D. L., Grewal, H. M., Martinussen, T., Krarup, H., Witte, D. R., Andersen, A. B., & Friis, H. (2013). Diabetes is a strong predictor of mortality during tuberculosis treatment: a prospective cohort study among tuberculosis patients from Mwanza, Tanzania. *Tropical medicine & international health : TM & IH*, *18*(7), 822–829. https://doi.org/10.1111/tmi.12120 (accessed on 10 May 2025).
4. Arpagaus, A., Franzeck, F., Sikalengo, G., Ndege, R., Mnzava, D., Rohacek, M., Hella, J., et al. (2020). Extrapulmonary tuberculosis in HIV-infected patients in rural Tanzania: The prospective Kilombero and Ulanga antiretroviral cohort. *PLoS ONE*, *15*(2), e0229875. https://doi.org/10.1371/journal.pone.0229875.
5. Stylianou, E., Paul, M. J., Reljic, R., & McShane, H. (2019). Mucosal delivery of tuberculosis vaccines: a review of current approaches and challenges. *Expert review of vaccines*, *18*(12), 1271–1284. https://doi.org/10.1080/14760584.2019.1692657 (accessed on 10 May 2025).
6. Mencarini, P., Bellagamba, R., Oliva, A., Ghirga, P., Giancola, M. L., Corpolongo, A., Ascoli Bartoli, T., De Nardo, P., Baiocchini, A., Del Nonno, F., Narciso, P., & Nicastri, E. (2016). Pulmonary tuberculosis followed by sarcoidosis in an HIV-infected patient: A case report and a simplified diagnostic flowchart for diagnosis and treatment of sarcoidosis. *Respiratory medicine case reports*, *19*, 150–154. https://doi.org/10.1016/j.rmcr.2016.09.006(accessed on 10 May 2025).
7. Cheng, N., Wu, S., Luo, X., Xu, C., Lou, Q., Zhu, J., You, L., et al. (2021). A comparative study of chest computed tomography findings: 1030 cases of drug-sensitive tuberculosis versus 516 cases of drug-resistant tuberculosis. *Infection and Drug Resistance*, *14*, 1115–1128. https://doi.org/10.2147/IDR.S300754.
8. Choi, J. Y. (2025). Pathophysiology, clinical manifestation, and treatment of tuberculosis-associated chronic obstructive pulmonary disease: A narrative review. *The Ewha Medical Journal*. https://www.semanticscholar.org/paper/772382df5adcfe0a0e15e2ed4d3675301d467ec9 (accessed on 10 May 2025).
9. Rafael, M. A., Martins Figueiredo, L., Oliveira, A. M., Nuno Costa, M., Theias Manso, R., & Martins, A. (2020). Gastrointestinal Tuberculosis Mimicking Crohn's Disease. *GE Portuguese journal of gastroenterology*, *27*(4), 278–282. https://doi.org/10.1159/000504719 (accessed on 10 May 2025).
10. Bholla, M., Kapalata, N., Masika, E., Chande, H., Jugheli, L., Sasamalo, M., Glass, T. R., Beck, H. P., & Reither, K. (2016). Evaluation of Xpert® MTB/RIF and Ustar EasyNAT™ TB IAD for diagnosis of tuberculous lymphadenitis of children in Tanzania: a prospective descriptive

study. *BMC infectious diseases, 16*, 246. https://doi.org/10.1186/s12879-016-1578-z (accessed on 10 May 2025).

11. Fan, G., Huang, Y., Xue, F. H., & He, B. (2022). Complete remission of pulmonary alveolar proteinosis after anti-tuberculous chemotherapy: A case report. *The Journal of International Medical Research, 50*. https://www.semanticscholar.org/paper/044c3f21ba9d8d8c54c75eb49aa406e0f9e35991 (accessed on 10 May 2025).
12. Farrugia, B. (2013). *Tuberculosis in Malta: A Case for Sputum Induction*. https://core.ac.uk/download/46602348.pdf (accessed on 10 May 2025).
13. Faurholt-Jepsen D. (2013). The double burden. *Danish medical journal, 60*(7), B4673.(accessed on 10 May 2025).
14. Felgueres, M., Esteso, G., García-Jiménez, Á. F., Benguría, A., Vázquez, E., Aguiló, N., Puentes, E., et al. (2025). Cytolytic γδ T-cells and IFNγ-producing CD4-lymphocytes characterize the early response to MTBVAC tuberculosis vaccine. *NPJ Vaccines, 10*. https://www.semanticscholar.org/paper/06b4b9063a64184733c79da31d374e2a43f82e5b (accessed on 10 May 2025).
15. Matveychuk, A., Fuks, L., Priess, R., Hahim, I., & Shitrit, D. (2012). Clinical and radiological features of Mycobacterium kansasii and other NTM infections. *Respiratory medicine, 106*(10), 1472–1477. https://doi.org/10.1016/j.rmed.2012.06.023
16. Guruparan, T., Nasrin, T., Karki, P., Saito, R., Gul, Z., Goh, L., & Dulay, G. (2024). P20: Persistent anti-PR3 ANCA positivity in patient with extrapulmonary tuberculosis. *Rheumatology Advances in Practice, 8*. https://www.semanticscholar.org/paper/827dc3d89d56040ec3f9562e7596e4a46e173985 (accessed on 10 May 2025).
17. Ibrahim, M. A., & Shehta, M. (2024). Clinical, radiological varieties and diagnostic facilities of smear negative pulmonary tuberculosis in HIV uninfected patients: A retrospective analysis. *The Egyptian Journal of Chest Diseases and Tuberculosis, 73*, 23–29. https://www.semanticscholar.org/paper/439a29c4ad5a4ba7c00d70e109b236bef2ea2df0 (accessed on 10 May 2025).
18. Iskandar, A., Dwimartutie, N., Loho, T., Pitoyo, S., et al. (2006). *Abdominal Tuberculosis: Diagnostic and Management Problems*. https://media.neliti.com/media/publications/63512-EN-abdominal-tuberculosis-diagnostic-and-ma.pdf (accessed on 10 May 2025).
19. Jiang, Z., Dai, Y., Chang, J., Xiang, P., Liang, Z., Yin, Y., Shen, Y., et al. (2024). The clinical characteristics, treatment and prognosis of tuberculosis-associated chronic obstructive pulmonary disease: A protocol for a multicenter prospective cohort study in China. *International Journal of Chronic Obstructive Pulmonary Disease, 19*, 2097–2107. https://www.semanticscholar.org/paper/b693aa36557557d4cfac643371be09e96bc09c15 (accessed on 10 May 2025).
20. Kim, J. E., Heo, J. H., Kim, H. O., Song, S. H., Park, S. S., Park, T. H., Ahn, J. Y., et al. (2017). Neurological complications during treatment of Middle East respiratory syndrome. *Journal of Clinical Neurology, 13*, 227–227. https://doi.org/10.3988/jcn.2017.13.3.227.
21. Leonard, J. M. (2017). Central nervous system tuberculosis. *Microbiology Spectrum, 5*. https://doi.org/10.1128/microbiolspec.TNMI7-0044-2017.
22. López-López, J., Posada-Martínez, E. L., Saldarriaga, C., Wyss, F., Ponte-Negretti, C. I., Alexander, B., Miranda-Arboleda, A. F., et al. (2021). Tuberculosis and the heart. *Journal of the American Heart Association, 10*. https://doi.org/10.1161/JAHA.120.019435.
23. Madolangan, J., Fiqran, M., Affan, M., & Herman, B. (2024). A rare case of pulmonary tuberculosis

masquerading as laryngeal tuberculosis or malignant manifestation. *Jurnal Respirasi*. https://www.semanticscholar.org/paper/2faa7107b71ad3bcab6b2cfa86763aec18dd41c9 (accessed on 10 May 2025).

24. Malhotra, P., Unni, M., Vairagade, A., & Patil, S. (2024). Skin rash with acute respiratory distress syndrome in chronic miliary tuberculosis: The role of HRCT thorax and bronchoscopy as diagnostic tools. *The Journal of Association of Chest Physicians*. https://www.semanticscholar.org/paper/30e62daf9a4bedf9136f19de855362dacf5612ff (accessed on 10 May 2025).

25. Manyi-Loh, C. E., Mamphweli, S., Meyer, E. L., & Okoh, A. I. (2018). Antibiotic use in agriculture and its consequential resistance in environmental sources: Potential public health implications. *Molecules, 23*(4), 795. https://doi.org/10.3390/molecules23040795.

26. Matvienko, Y., Panasyukova, O., Rekalova, O., Zhadan, V., & Yasir, C. G. (2023). The use of natural hepatoprotector with immunomodulating properties in patients with pulmonary tuberculosis with various adverse reactions to antituberculosis drugs. *Asthma and Allergy*. https://www.semanticscholar.org/paper/1ac3aca57e602d1af21c91fede29bf59004e8796 (accessed on 10 May 2025).

27. Moreira-Teixeira, L., Mayer-Barber, K., Sher, A., & O'Garra, A. (2018). Type I interferons in tuberculosis: Foe and occasionally friend. *The Journal of experimental medicine, 215*(5), 1273–1285. https://doi.org/10.1084/jem.20180325Movahedi, Z., Mahmoudi, S., Banar, M., Pourakbari, B., Aziz-Ahari, A., Ramezani, A., & Mamishi, S. (2022). Pediatric tuberculosis in Iran: A review of 10-years study in an Iranian referral hospital. *Acta Bio Medica: Atenei Parmensis, 93*. https://www.semanticscholar.org/paper/49a057728bf12e403f827a573a052332b208e248 (accessed on 10 May 2025).

28. Pant, P., Baniya, S., & Jha, A. (2019). Prevalence of respiratory manifestations in chronic kidney diseases: A descriptive cross-sectional study in a tertiary care hospital of Nepal. *JNMA: Journal of the Nepal Medical Association, 57*, 80–83. https://www.semanticscholar.org/paper/1ea7fdddcd7b1bd9674cd8115b4b6316b88657fd (accessed on 10 May 2025).

29. Panteleev, A., Nikitina, I., Burmistrova, I., Kosmiadi, G., Radaeva, T., Amansahedov, R. B., Sadikov, P. V., et al. (2017). Severe tuberculosis in humans correlates best with neutrophil abundance and lymphocyte deficiency and does not correlate with antigen-specific CD4 T-cell response. *Frontiers in Immunology, 8*. https://www.semanticscholar.org/paper/0221993ba70af021bd65048178a9fd0a37ebe2a7 (accessed on 10 May 2025).

30. Patil, S., Toshniwal, S., & Gondhali, G. (2022). Cavitating lung disease is not always due to tuberculosis! Wegener's granulomatosis with mycetoma with deep vein thrombosis lower limb: Case report with review of literature. *Electronic Journal of General Medicine, 20*, em425. https://doi.org/10.29333/ejgm/12574.

31. Perera, T., Dissanayake, U., & Kowshika, S. (2024). A flare of granulomatosis with polyangiitis or reactivation of pulmonary tuberculosis? A diagnostic dilemma. *Anuradhapura Medical Journal*. https://www.semanticscholar.org/paper/33030767b84e95cfd547746680080229bdb0bcf3 (accessed on 10 May 2025).

32. Raghu, G., Rémy-Jardin, M., Ryerson, C. J., Myers, J. L., Kreuter, M., Vašáková, M., Bargagli, E., et al. (2020). Diagnosis of hypersensitivity pneumonitis in adults: An official ATS/JRS/ALAT clinical practice guideline. *American Journal of Respiratory and Critical Care Medicine, 202*(3), e36–e69. https://doi.org/10.1164/rccm.202005-2032ST.

33. Rajpurkar, P., Irvin, J., Ball, R. L., Zhu, K., Yang, B., Mehta, H., Duan, T., et al. (2018). Deep learning for chest radiograph diagnosis: A retrospective comparison of the CheXNeXt algorithm to practicing radiologists. *PLoS Medicine, 15*, e1002686. https://doi.org/10.1371/journal.pmed.1002686.

34. Schneider, B. J., Naidoo, J., Santomasso, B., Lacchetti, C., Adkins, S., Anadkat, M. J., Atkins, M. B., et al. (2021). Management of immune-related adverse events in patients treated with immune checkpoint inhibitor therapy: ASCO guideline update. *Journal of Clinical Oncology, 39*(36), 4073–4126. https://doi.org/10.1200/jco.21.01440.

35. Shu, W., Chen, W., Yao, L., Sun, M., Gao, M., Wan, Z., Xie, W., et al. (2024). A case series of co-infection in *Mycobacterium tuberculosis* and other pathogens: Insights from nanopore sequencing. *The Egyptian Journal of Bronchology*. https://www.semanticscholar.org/paper/f3ee75b1894f53540daeb0caf155a543aae81447 (accessed on 10 May 2025).

36. Thungathurthi, S., & Orsu, P. (2022). Radiological evidence in clinical prevalence of hematological changes in multidrug resistant pulmonary tuberculosis. *International Journal of Health Sciences*. https://www.semanticscholar.org/paper/1dc958006ca5db7746382cff9a67f36a9ba94937 (accessed on 10 May 2025).

37. To, K., Cao, R., Yegiazaryan, A., Owens, J., & Venketaraman, V. (2020). General overview of nontuberculous mycobacteria opportunistic pathogens: *Mycobacterium avium* and *Mycobacterium abscessus*. *Journal of Clinical Medicine, 9*. https://www.semanticscholar.org/paper/324ea6ebea9e2d35ac0011da8543e731b34dc295 (accessed on 10 May 2025).

38. Tu, Y. F., Chien, C. S., Yarmishyn, A. A., Lin, Y. Y., Luo, Y. H., Lin, Y. T., Lai, W. Y., et al. (2020). A review of SARS-CoV-2 and the ongoing clinical trials. *International Journal of Molecular Sciences, 21*, 2657. https://doi.org/10.3390/ijms21072657.

39. Velayati, A. A. (2016). Tuberculosis in children. *International Journal of Mycobacteriology, 5*(Suppl 1), S1–S2. https://doi.org/10.1016/j.ijmyco.2016.10.038.

40. Wang, T., Yang, Q., Gao, Y., Zhang, R., Zhou, C., Kong, W., Zhang, G., et al. (2023). Computed tomography manifestations in patients with rifampin primary drug-resistant tuberculosis in an infectious disease hospital in the Yi Autonomous Prefecture, China. *International Journal of General Medicine, 16*, 5109–5118. https://www.semanticscholar.org/paper/ce4bb06f64a38523ffac919a538218c9a72c5a17 (accessed on 10 May 2025).

41. Wani, & Serafino, R. L. (2016). Clinical manifestations of pulmonary and extra-pulmonary tuberculosis. https://core.ac.uk/download/478462642.pdf (accessed on 10 May 2025).

42. Wei, P. F. (2020). Diagnosis and treatment protocol for novel coronavirus pneumonia (Trial version 7). *Chinese Medical Journal, 133*, 1087–1095. https://doi.org/10.1097/CM9.0000000000000819.

43. Yadav S, Understanding the complexities of post-tuberculosis lung disease: Implications for global health. IP Indian J Immunol Respir Med 2024;9(1):1-2(accessed on 10 May 2025).

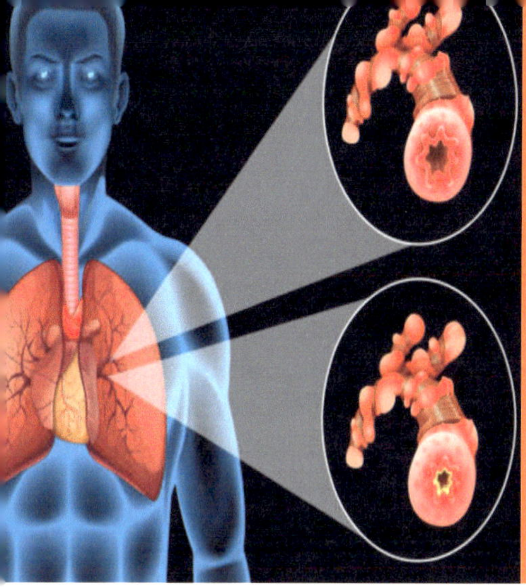

Chapter 5

EXTRAPULMONARY AND DISSEMINATED TB

Contents

Introduction

Tuberculosis (TB) remains a major global health issue, best known for its pulmonary form. The disease caused by *Mycobacterium tuberculosis* (MTB), though, is now not limited to the lungs; it may involve various systems of organs and thus lead to extrapulmonary tuberculosis (EPTB). While pulmonary TB presents with specific symptoms, EPTB usually has nonspecific symptoms, causing diagnosis and treatment delays. This type of TB includes a broad range of clinical syndromes, illustrating the pathogen's capacity to disseminate outside the respiratory system. Comprehending these differences is important, as EPTB represents a significant percentage of TB cases globally, specifically among vulnerable groups such as children and immunocompromised patients. Extrapolating extrapulmonary involvement demands increased clinical suspicion and vigilance, due to its diverse presentations and ability to cause severe complications. One significant drawback of EPTB is its insidious presentation and the variety of locations it can affect, making clinical detection more difficult. For instance, skeletal TB, which accounts for a small percentage of EPTB, affects the vertebrae but can also involve peripheral bones like those in the hands, primarily in young children. The presentation may be subtle, with nonspecific pain or swelling that may be confused with other pathologies, and therefore, delays diagnosis and treatment. The diagnostic challenges underscore the need for meticulous patient history and recognition of risk factors such as the absence of *Bacillus Calmette-Guérin* (BCG) vaccination and possible exposure to conventional practices that can mask clinical examination. Early detection and treatment can significantly alter the prognosis in such unusual cases of TB (Abdulrahman et al., 2025). The intricacy of EPTB is compounded in the setting of immunosuppression, including HIV/AIDS, where coinfection results in disseminated disease involving several organs at once. One such exceptional but important pattern is pancreatic tuberculosis, which in turn is mostly unveiled in extreme immunocompromised conditions and can be aggravated by immune reconstitution inflammatory syndrome (IRIS) after initiating antiretroviral treatment (ART). Such a vibrant interaction between HIV and MTB infections not only hinders the diagnostic and treatment approaches but also underscores the requirements for integrated strategies in care. The changing clinical scenario requires sharp observation of risk factors, pathophysiology, and possible complications of coinfection, to avoid morbidity and enhance outcomes in these immunocompromised patients (Akbar et al., 2024).

Overview of Extrapulmonary and Disseminated TB

The course of tuberculosis infection tends to extend beyond the pulmonary system, manifesting as extrapulmonary or disseminated tuberculosis, both complicating diagnosis and treatment. Whereas MTB infects lung tissue most predominantly initially, it can extend beyond through the hematogenous or lymphatic pathways, ultimately infecting multiple organs. The complicated interaction between the immune system and pathogen dictates this extrapulmonary dissemination, although the specific mechanisms are as yet incompletely outlined. Existing mathematical modeling techniques, for example, ordinary differential equations and agent-based models, are used to model within-host *Mtb* dynamics, yielding vital information on how dissemination takes place at both lung and extrapulmonary locations. These models explain how localized infection leads to extensive disease, providing invaluable insights into pathogen-host interactions and intervening points (Chakraborty et al., 2024). This interdisciplinary research is critical for the development of strategies specific to the wide-ranging clinical presentations of EPTB. Epidemiological data point to the differing clinical spectrum and risk factors for extrapulmonary and disseminated tuberculosis. In countries with high TB burden, extrapulmonary cases represent a considerable percentage of cases with frequently atypical symptoms presenting diagnostic difficulties. A North Indian retrospective study reported that although pulmonary TB was most common (77.7%), extrapulmonary and disseminated disease represented almost 22%, with uncommon presentations like fever of unknown origin and liver abscesses. These forms disproportionately affected groups with certain vulnerabilities, including those of lower socioeconomic status, malnourishment, and tobacco consumption, suggesting that socioeconomic and environmental conditions significantly affect disease expression. Additionally, the average age of patients presenting with unusual TB manifestations was greater than in typical cases, highlighting the imperative for heightened clinical watchfulness among diverse populations (Singh et al., 2022). Awareness of these epidemiological subtleties is critical for timely diagnosis and successful disease treatment. The clinical challenge of extrapulmonary and disseminated tuberculosis highlights the imperative for multifaceted diagnostic approaches and individualized treatment protocols. In contrast to pulmonary TB, which is favored by existing diagnostic standards, EPTB frequently evades early detection because of its protean presentation and varied organ involvement. Disseminated TB, indicating disseminated hematogenous spread, carries a very poor prognosis and necessitates thorough clinical assessment, including imaging and molecular diagnostic techniques. The presentation heterogeneity requires patients' immune status, nutritional status, and sociodemographic setting to be taken into consideration because they have a great impact on disease course and therapeutic response. Early detection and treatment are mandatory to decrease morbidity and mortality due to EPTB, and this is why clinicians must have a high index of suspicion, particularly in endemic areas. The combination of epidemiological information and immunopathological knowledge continues to guide specific interventions that improve patient care and control measures globally (Singh et al., 2022; Chakraborty et al., 2024).

Importance of Understanding Extrapulmonary Tuberculosis (EPTB)

The diversity of tuberculosis (TB) goes beyond its pulmonary form, frequently presenting multiple extrapulmonary locations that pose diagnostic and therapeutic dilemmas. Proper management of TB mandates that clinicians be aware of these multifaceted presentations since EPTB typically occurs in immunocompromised individuals who are also co-infected with HIV. The clinical and radiologic manifestations of EPTB may be non-specific or unusual, requiring a high level of suspicion and experience with sophisticated diagnostic techniques like molecular tests and cultures. This wide range of clinical presentations emphasizes the need for incorporating extrapulmonary factors into guidelines for management of TB so that it is diagnosed and treated promptly. Moreover, EPTB is of major morbidity and mortality concern, particularly in resource-constrained environments, where delays exacerbate poor outcomes, underscoring the need for increased awareness and specialized procedures (Bracchi et al., 2019). EPTB heterogeneity dictates careful comprehension of the pathogen's conduct in various anatomical niches. In contrast to pulmonary TB, extrapulmonary disease can affect the central nervous system (CNS), lymphatics, bones, or genitourinary system, each with specific clinical implications and treatment considerations. Diagnostic challenges are apparent since conventional methods like microscopy and radiography may not be adequate, necessitating dependency on sophisticated molecular tests like Xpert MTB/RIF assays. These strategies optimize early detection and allow for drug resistance identification, which is optimized in the therapy, particularly in drug-resistant and disseminated disease. Identification of the nuances of EPTB therefore allows maximum patient management, minimizing mortality and curtailing the transmission of resistant strains, particularly in populations with HIV co-infection, where immune suppression changes disease presentations considerably (Bracchi et al., 2019). Apart from clinical management, knowledge of EPTB has significant public health consequences. Transmission dynamics of TB are modified when extrapulmonary forms dominate, tending to signify reactivation or disseminated disease instead of direct contagion. Yet, missed diagnosis and inadequate treatment of these cases perpetuate continuing morbidity and possible community burden through undetected reservoirs. Incorporation of EPTB knowledge into health platforms facilitates extensive screening, including latent tuberculosis infection (LTBI) guidelines in at-risk populations. In addition, it emphasizes the necessity of multidisciplinary strategies with infectious disease clinicians, radiologists, and pathologists for tackling complexity in diagnosis. Finally, raising awareness and expanding research on EPTB strengthens TB control worldwide, indicating its pivotal position in the TB disease continuum (Bracchi et al., 2019).

5.1. Pathophysiology of Extrapulmonary Tuberculosis (EPTB)

The primary infection with *Mycobacterium tuberculosis* (MTB) is usually in the lung, but the spread of the bacteria to areas outside of the pulmonary system may lead to extrapulmonary tuberculosis (EPTB), a situation that makes diagnosis and treatment more complicated. Dissemination is viewed not as an unusual occurrence but as a basic process in all infections that enables *Mtb* to form secondary lesions at a different site. These extrapulmonary sites may harbor active or latent infections, complicating the immune response and clinical control.

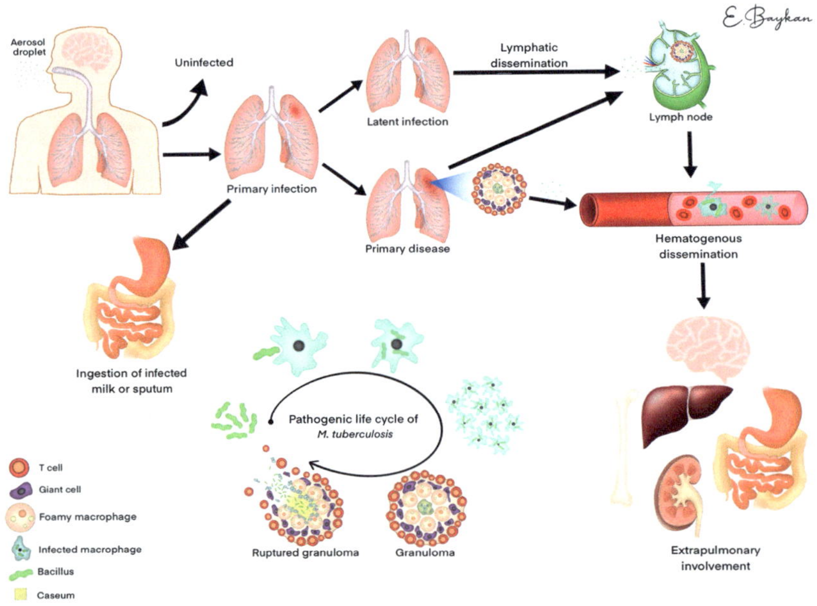

Figure 5.1. Pathogenic life cycle and extrapulmonary dissemination of *M. tuberculosis.*

Source: Kaur, H., & Sood, D. (2022). Pathogenic life cycle of *M. tuberculosis*. *Insights into Imaging*, *13*(1), Article 144.

The pathogen uses several virulence factors to aid its transport by the lymphatic and bloodstream systems to colonize extrapulmonary tissues. Although the precise mechanisms that enable *Mtb* dissemination are still only partially clear, various models derived from animal models and clinical experience have been put forward to explain the complex interplay between bacterial virulence determinants and host immune mechanisms in the process (Moule et al., 2020). After dissemination, *Mtb* is able to infect numerous extrapulmonary locations, the lymph nodes being the most frequently targeted. The pathophysiology is characterized by the development of granulomatous inflammation with necrotic lymph nodes (LNs), which are a characteristic of EPTB. These necrotic nodes and certain organ involvement, for example, in genitourinary, musculoskeletal, and central nervous systems

(CNSs), occur through unique pathological alterations that shape the clinical course and outcome of infection. Immunocompromised patients are most susceptible to disseminated TB with common involvement of the CNS, where infection causes severe complications. Conversely, immunocompetent patients can have long latency phases before developing renal or genitourinary presentations. The non-specificity of symptoms and imaging characteristics of various organ systems also hinders early detection and diagnosis of EPTB (Rodriguez-Takeuchi et al., 2019).

Musculoskeletal disease in EPTB demonstrates the relentless nature of bacterial spread and immune avoidance. Tuberculous spondylitis, the most common musculoskeletal presentation, is frequently diagnosed late based on non-specific clinical presentations and typically involves multiple vertebral bodies with resultant widespread paraspinal abscess formation. This indicates the pathogen's potential for invasiveness and persistence in bone and joint tissue, including the production of chronic synovitis and destructive lesions. In contrast to pulmonary TB, whose immune reaction is partially contained, EPTB lesions can grow extensively, leading to deformity and serious morbidity if left untreated. Articular illness, typically indicated by synovitis, ensues as the secondary musculoskeletal manifestation of TB infection. These presentations highlight the need for assessment of the unique pathophysiologic mechanisms allowing *Mtb* to survive and live in varied tissue environments outside the lung (Rodriguez-Takeuchi et al., 2019) (Figure 5.1).

5.1.1. Mechanism of TB Infection

The intricacy of tuberculosis infection is not just in its pulmonary presentation but also in its dissemination outside the lungs, making treatment and diagnosis more complex. The primary infection often starts when MTB bacilli are inhaled into the alveoli. Unlike previous presumptions that dissemination beyond the lungs was an uncommon occurrence, recent findings indicate that dissemination is a normal step in the infection process. This systemic dissemination leads to secondary lesions that can become latent or reactive, especially at extrapulmonary locations like LNs, pleura, or the CNS. Dissemination is the process where *Mtb* is transported via the lymphatic and circulatory systems, allowing extensive seeding of the bacterium. Notwithstanding great progress, the exact mechanisms of this dissemination are still partly explained, with research continuing to target the discovery of determining virulence factors allowing bacterial migration and survival beyond the pulmonary environment (Madeleine et al., 2020). It is important for infection mechanisms to be understood through early interaction between *Mtb* and host cells. In the past, the Trojan Horse model characterized infected alveolar macrophages as carriers that allowed the transit of the bacteria across the alveolar barrier. However, newer studies show a different pathway by invasion of alveolar epithelial cells. The bacterium within these cells assumes a strongly replicative and invasive form, which helps it to more effectively invade the alveolar epithelium and gain systemic circulation. This accommodation demonstrates the bacterium's phenotypic flexibility in infection. In addition, once the bacteria have reached extrapulmonary locations, a decrease in this invasive phenotype is observed, indicating a strategic regulation of virulence according to niche-specific environments. Together, these results add to the knowledge of the host-pathogen relationship, highlighting the intricacy of *Mtb* dissemination early during infection (Michelle et al., 2019). This shift of *Mtb* from a latent state within the sputum to a highly virulent phenotype in host tissues is indicative of an elaborate infection process. Such dynamic accommodation allows the initial establishment and secondary systemic dissemination of bacteria prior to the effective response of the host's cell-mediated immunity. Non-phagocytic alveolar epithelial cell involvement in bacterial invasion is similar to processes seen in other Gram-positive pathogens, where synergistic adhesins, toxins, and enzymes join forces to traverse mucosal barriers. This synergy facilitates immune early detection evasion by the bacteria and facilitates dissemination to extrapulmonary locations. More understanding of these molecular interactions holds the promise to reveal new targets for therapeutic intervention, perhaps refocusing on preventing infection establishment and dissemination. Such integration could have a major impact on vaccine design and lead to decreasing both active and latent tuberculosis burdens (Michelle et al., 2019).

5.1.2. Immune Response to Extrapulmonary Tuberculosis (EPTB)

The intricacy of tuberculosis infection goes beyond the pulmonary setting, since MTB commonly disseminates to extrapulmonary locations where immune reactions vary profoundly. In EPTB, immune recognition is challenged by a paucibacillary setting, rendering the diagnosis of *Mtb* less accessible and less apparent than in pulmonary infections. This finesse leads to non-specific clinical findings and interferes with prompt diagnosis, highlighting the immune system's sophisticated role in suppressing infection from a variety of anatomical sites. In particular, the immune cells within extrapulmonary tissues have to traverse separate microenvironments where granuloma development, a characteristic of TB immunity, tends to be variable in form and cellularity. This heterogeneity is a result of a balance between pathogen control and tissue integrity determined by spatially localized cytokine production and immune cell recruitment. The immune response depends both on innate and adaptive elements, which work together to contain bacilli but also potentially compromise collateral damage to tissues, an important factor in the management of ETB's variable presentations (Tuang et al., 2020). Newer immunological knowledge highlights the function of particular subsets of T cells in facilitating protection against TB, especially in extrapulmonary and disseminated disease. Vγ2Vδ2 T cells are a distinctive population in primates, mounting strong Th1-like immunity essential for efficient control of MTB outside the lungs. Immunization approaches using attenuated HMBPP-secreting bacterial vectors to target these cells have produced encouraging decreases in bacterial spread to extrapulmonary tissues and lowered pathology. These Vγ2Vδ2 tissue-resident T cells are responsible for producing important effector factors such as interferon-gamma (IFN-γ) and perforin, which enable intracellular killing of pathogens and restrict mycobacterial growth in extrapulmonary environments. Furthermore, triggering of Vγ2Vδ2 T cells seems to augment overall adaptive immunity by enhancing $CD4^+$ and $CD8^+$ T cell expansion, reflecting a synergistic network responsible for durable immunity against EPTB (Shen et al., 2019). Knowledge of the immune response to EPTB is important for tailoring diagnosis and therapy, in view of the disease's protean character and sometimes severe manifestations. The capacity of the immune system to create granulomas, accumulate macrophages, and mobilize T cells determines the course of infection or its limitation in extrapulmonary tissues. Yet, the difficulty in diagnosing ETB arises from immune-mediated regulation that restricts bacillary load, making it hard to obtain culture-positive samples and prompting dependency on histopathological and immunological findings. Improved immunodiagnostic methods for detecting antigen-specific T cell responses or interferon-gamma release assays (IGRAs) may enhance sensitivity for identifying ETB. Second, therapeutic approaches that promote protective T cell subset function, including that of Vγ2Vδ2 T cells, are promising for improved control of dissemination. Synthesis of immunological insight and clinical assessment is central to surpassing diagnostic and treatment challenges posed by EPTB's multifaceted presentation (Shen et al., 2019; Tuang et al., 2020) (Figure 5.2).

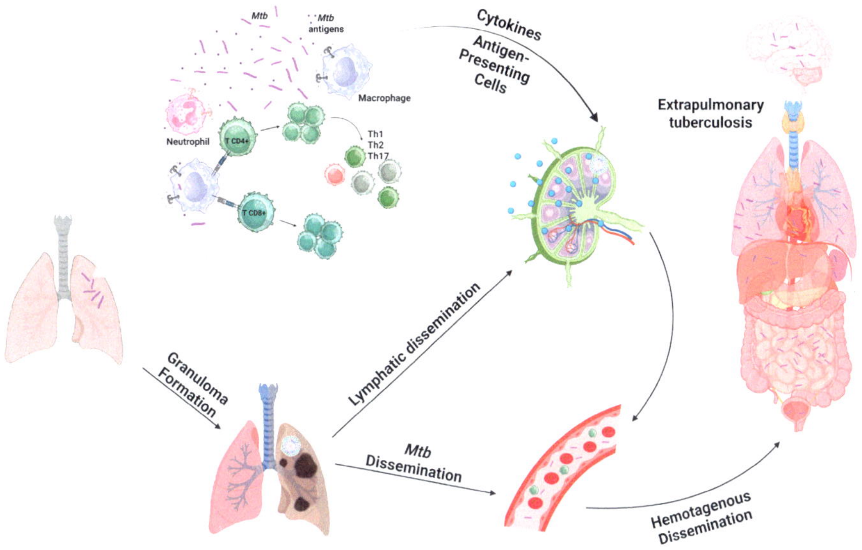

Figure 5.2. *Mycobacterium tuberculosis* (*Mtb*) infection begins with the recognition and internalization of bacteria by alveolar macrophages, allowing replication and establishment of infection. The immune response involves the secretion of cytokines and chemokines, recruitment of phagocytes, and activation of adaptive immunity, particularly $CD4^+$ and $CD8^+$ T cells.

Source: Rahman, M. M., Mendy, S., Leong, K. W., & Kang, S. W. (2023). Extrapulmonary tuberculosis dissemination mechanism. *International Journal of Molecular Sciences, 24*(11), Article 11385.

5.1.3. Differences Between Pulmonary and Extrapulmonary Tuberculosis (EPTB)

The clinical presentation of tuberculosis (TB) is quite different based on whether the disease is localized within the lungs or present in other organ systems. Pulmonary TB is confined mainly to the lungs and has classical symptoms of chronic cough, hemoptysis, and pleuritic chest pain. EPTB, on the other hand, occurs extrapulmonary and involves the LNs, pleura, bones, CNS, or genitourinary tract. These variations in clinical presentation are important for diagnosis and management since EPTB frequently has nonspecific presentations that can obscure and delay detection. Additionally, although pulmonary TB is more infectious as a result of aerosolization of the bacilli, EPTB is usually non-infectious, which indicates its focal pathology. The immune response in EPTB is also different, with granulomatous inflammation in tissues, reflecting a different pathological spectrum relative to EPTB and pulmonary TB (Yang et al., 2025). Diagnostic difficulties further reflect the differences between pulmonary and EPTB. Diagnosis of pulmonary TB primarily depends on sputum smear microscopy, culture, and molecular tests with relatively high sensitivity and specificity. Conversely, the diagnosis of EPTB is more challenging because of the paucibacillary character of the condition and the fact that representative tissue or fluid samples are hard to obtain. Methods such as biopsy, fine-needle aspiration, and imaging are used often, but these procedures might be invasive and non-diagnostic. Moreover, extrapulmonary involvement might need other diagnostic algorithms, incorporating biochemical markers and histopathological analysis. These diagnostic subtleties are significant as EPTB is usually characterized by the need for individualized strategies to confirm infection and rule out other differential diagnoses, highlighting the importance of increased clinical suspicion in unusual presentations (Gopalaswamy et al., 2020). Therapeutic distinctions also show significant variations between pulmonary and EPTB, affecting the duration of treatment and monitoring practices. Although the anti-TB drug regimen is generally the same for both presentations, EPTB tends to require long courses of treatment, especially when the CNS or bones are involved, to achieve bacteriolysis and avoid relapse. Penetration of drugs into infected extrapulmonary sites can be unpredictable, requiring judicious choice and modification of the therapy. Additionally, EPTB is more likely to be seen in immunocompromised individuals, including recipients of solid organ transplants who are at increased susceptibility with more severe clinical courses and the risk of drug toxicity (Yang et al., 2025). This calls for the adoption of a multidisciplinary approach for the best outcomes in EPTB as opposed to the pulmonary form (Figure 5.3).

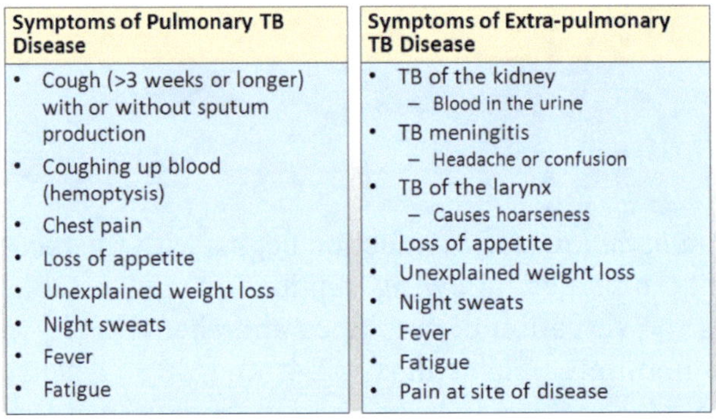

Figure 5.3. Pulmonary and extrapulmonary tuberculosis (EPTB).

Source: SlidePlayer. (n.d.). *Pulmonary versus extrapulmonary.* https://slideplayer.com/slide/6257518/21/images/29/Pulmonary+vs.+Extrapulmonary.jpg.

5.2. Common Sites of Extrapulmonary Tuberculosis (EPTB)

EPTB occurs in a wide variety of anatomical locations, an expression of the pathogen's capacity to spread from the lungs. Lymphatic disease is especially common, manifesting as tuberculous lymphadenitis, which tends to involve cervical LNs and manifests as painless swelling. Pleural TB is also widespread, occurring as a consequence of pleural infection with effusion and chest pain and being a notoriously difficult diagnosis due to its overlap with pulmonary TB syndrome. The CNS is also an important location, with TB meningitis being a serious threat, particularly in younger age groups where it can lead to significant morbidity and mortality. These locations demonstrate the intricacy of EPTB diagnosis and highlight regional epidemiological trends, as noted in pediatric populations where disseminated TB, TB lymphadenitis, pleural TB, and TB meningitis all contribute to a large disease burden (Wang et al., 2024). Knowledge of these frequent sites is important for prompt intervention and control measures. The pattern of EPTB is demographic and geographic, dependent on age and immunocompetence among patients (Figure 5.4).

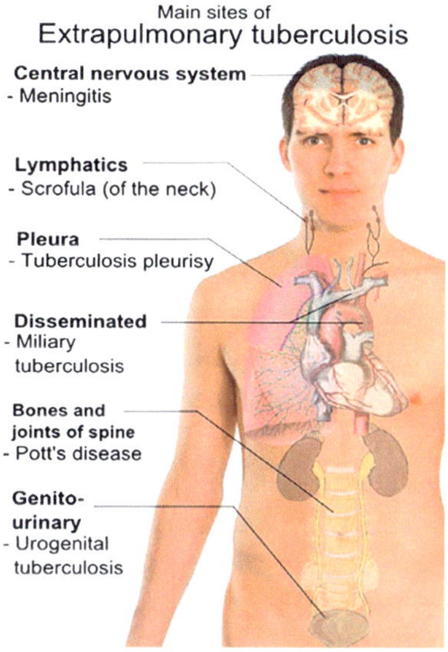

Figure 5.4. Main site of extrapulmonary tuberculosis (EPTB).

Source: Medizzy. (n.d.). *Extrapulmonary tuberculosis sites in the human body.* https://cdn.medizzy.com/Fu4m41HU0HOiptE8iW40AVi3zZk=/680x1034/img/posts/16ce3264-8021-409e-8e32-648021409e6c.

Pediatric patients, for instance, show a frequent presence of TB meningitis and disseminated TB in the youngest age groups, which mirrors immature immune defenses that allow for the spread of microorganisms beyond pulmonary tissue. Pleural TB is more often seen in older children and adults, which implies an age-related preference for certain extrapulmonary locations. Moreover, regional and ethnic determinants influence disease presentation; in Southwest China, regional populations like Tibetans have demonstrated a rising trend of pediatric EPTB, which underscores the necessity of culturally appropriate public health interventions. These epidemiological differences underpin the heterogeneous nature of EPTB and reinforce the value of local data to inform clinical suspicion and management (Wang et al., 2024). Although the emphasis on EPTB remains in its typical locations, successful treatment regimens today supplement such knowledge with better cure rates, even in complicated disseminated or drug-resistant cases. Some of the recent developments in drug therapy, specifically all-oral treatments like BPaLM/BPaL, have been highly efficacious in various manifestations of TB, including extrapulmonary and multi-drug-resistant types. These treatments are shorter and better tolerated, targeting both pulmonary and extrapulmonary disease domains. Treatment duration and complications are decreased. The introduction of such regimens into routine healthcare facilities in high DR-TB prevalence settings highlights the promise of treating TB-EPTB comprehensively within the public sector (Figure 5.5), enhancing TB control prognosis and minimizing transmission risks. Combining knowledge of frequent extrapulmonary sites with successful therapeutic approaches is therefore paramount for the global TB control agenda.

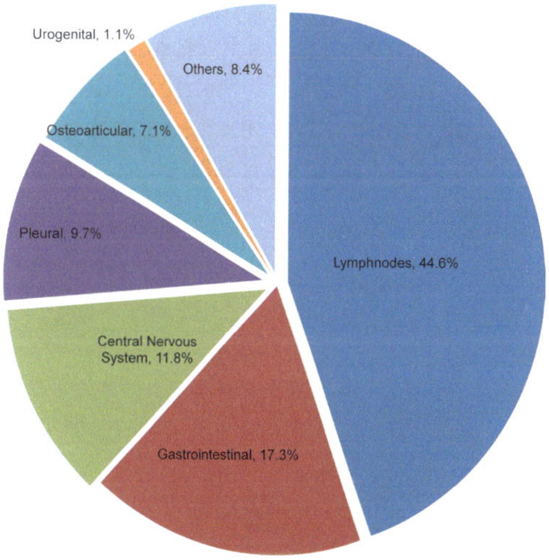

Figure 5.5. Distribution pattern of extra-pulmonary infection sites among 381 patients during 2009–2010.

Source: ResearchGate. (n.d.). *Distribution pattern of extra-pulmonary infection sites among 381 patients during the study period.* https://www.researchgate.net/figure/Distribution-pattern-of-extra-pulmonary-infection-sites-among-381-patients-during_fig3_272082307.

5.2.1. Lymphatic System

The complex interaction of MTB with the host immune system plays a pivotal role in establishing the dissemination of tuberculosis outside the pulmonary system. After inhalation, *Mtb* is engulfed by alveolar macrophages, triggering a cascade of immunity that often results in the development of granulomas, mainly in the lymphatic tissues. The granulomas are a protective wall, encapsulating infection but are also sites where extrapulmonary dissemination can gain a foothold. The lymphoid system, made up of a vast network of LNs and vessels, serves not only as a pathway for the trafficking of immune cells but also as a possible reservoir for the bacilli, which allows dissemination. The central position of the lymphatic systems in immune surveillance and response makes the role it plays in extrapulmonary and disseminated TB indicative of the complexity of the disease and presents diagnostic and treatment challenges. This involvement is usually identified using sophisticated imaging modalities like PET/CT, which may detect metabolically active lymphadenopathy beyond the radiographic limits (Katal et al., 2020).

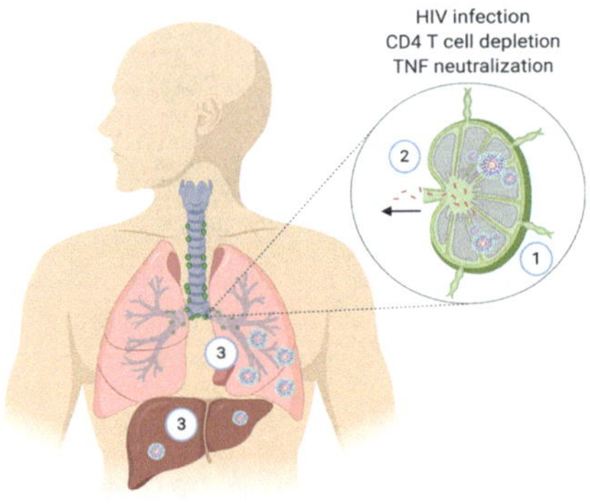

Figure 5.6. Latent TB reactivation can start in the lymph nodes (LNs).

Source: PLOS Pathogens. (n.d.). *HIV-related mechanisms of TB granuloma disruption and dissemination.* https://journals.plos.org/plospathogens/article/figures?id=10.1371/journal.ppat.1008632.

Delineating the patterns of lymphatic involvement in EPTB is important to arrive at a correct diagnosis and treatment intervention. Mycobacterial infections are often characterized by lymphadenitis with caseating granulomas, and the commonly involved areas are cervical, mediastinal, and abdominal LNs. The lymphatic spread of TB may imitate other infectious and neoplastic diseases, making clinical evaluation challenging. Diagnostic imaging like FDG-PET/CT has become critical in outlining active lymphatic disease by detecting increased metabolic activity related to infection and inflammation.

This imaging not only helps in detecting the degree of extrapulmonary dissemination but also in assessing therapeutic response. Interestingly, whereas pulmonary TB characteristically manifests with focal lung disease, disseminated disease generally includes generalized lymphatic involvement, which mirrors the pathogen's spread through lymphatic pathways (Katal et al., 2020). Pivotal to the effective management of EPTB is an understanding of these mechanisms within the lymphatic network. Host immune status decisively determines lymphatic TB manifestation, especially in comparing MTB with nontuberculous mycobacterial (NTM) infection. In immunocompromised hosts, for example, HIV-infected subjects, the lymphatic tissues usually become a site of widespread mycobacterial growth, seen as generalized lymphadenopathy and disseminated infection. In contrast to MTB, which typically causes miliary pulmonary infection with concurrent lymphatic disease, NTM more frequently results in extrapulmonary lymphatic infections with or without accompanying bronchiectasis or other focal immune dysfunctions. Treatment strategies must consider these distinctions, as NTM infections demonstrate variable drug susceptibilities and may require prolonged antimicrobial regimens or surgical intervention. The lymphatic system's role as a dissemination pathway highlights its importance not only in the immune response but also as a target for diagnostic evaluation and therapeutic monitoring in both TB and NTM diseases (Figure 5.6).

5.2.2. Central Nervous System (CNS)

The rich CNS vascular and lymphatic networks predispose the CNS to MTB hematogenous spread, causing a catastrophic form of EPTB. CNS tuberculosis exists predominantly in its tuberculous meningitis (TBM) form and carries high morbidity and mortality, particularly for immunocompromised patients like those with HIV/AIDS. Early suspicion by the clinician is paramount since the presentation is often subtle and non-specific in the initial stages and tends to mimic other neurological disorders. Diagnostic difficulty is also increased by the inability to obtain cerebrospinal fluid (CSF) specimens for direct microbiological confirmation. Nevertheless, the availability of nucleic acid amplification tests (NAATs), specifically the Xpert MTB/RIF assay, has enhanced diagnostic precision by identifying MTB and rifampicin resistance promptly, thus facilitating timely initiation of effective therapy (Chewe et al., 2020). This technology is critical in the management of CNS TB, where delayed diagnosis may lead to irreversible neurological sequelae. Management of CNS in disseminated TB is an integrative approach considering the limitation of drug entry into the brain by the blood-brain barrier and the requirement of extended therapy. The World Health Organization (WHO) and national guidelines recommend the use of multidrug regimens with core drugs that are able to achieve therapeutic levels in the CNS. Bedaquiline and linezolid, for example, have proved effective as part of extended therapy in DR-TB of the CNS, resulting in considerable clinical improvement in rifampicin-resistant strain patients (Chewe et al., 2020). Corticosteroids are frequently advised as an adjunct to decrease CNS inflammation, alleviate neurological complications, and enhance survival rates, though their administration should be closely monitored considering possible side effects. The intricacy of this treatment highlights the need for skilled clinical expertise and multidisciplinary management to maximize outcomes in patients with CNS EPTB. Despite technical improvements in diagnostics and therapeutics, there are gaps in standardized recommendations specifically incorporating CNS TB in the larger context of extrapulmonary and disseminated manifestations. While there are national efforts, like the Indian EPTB guidelines, that offer specific suggestions regarding diagnostic approaches, adjunct corticosteroid treatment, and duration of treatment, these underscore the lack of high-quality evidence from randomized controlled trials for CNS involvement.

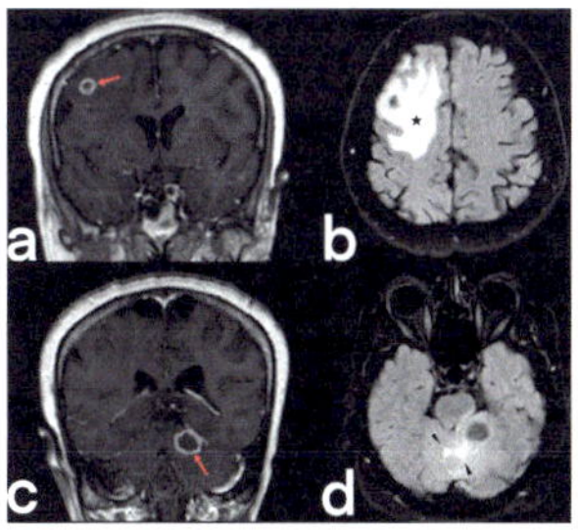

Figure 5.7. MR images of a 63-year-old female with central nervous system (CNS) TB. Focal lesions (arrows) with rim-like enhancement are seen (tuberculoma) on contrast-enhanced coronal T1-weighted images (a and c). Perilesional increased signals (asterisk and arrowheads) due to vasogenic edema are noted on axial FLAIR images (b and d).

Source: SpringerOpen. (2022). *Figure 4. MRI features of intracranial tuberculosis.* https://insightsimaging.springeropen.com/articles/10.1186/s13244-022-01172-0/figures/4.

This deficit necessitates the use of consensus-based clinical practice recommendations and the consequent need for targeted research to determine best management practices. Increased awareness, early diagnosis with molecular methods, and evidence-based treatment protocols are needed to tackle the high mortality of CNS TB. In addition, implementing these strategies in resource-constrained settings is a critical challenge, highlighting the need for strengthening healthcare systems to enhance patient outcomes in disseminated tuberculosis (Figure 5.7).

5.2.3. Skeletal System

The complex relationship between tuberculosis and the skeletal system unearths significant clinical insights in EPTB. Although the lungs remain the major site of MTB infection, the pathogen may seed hematogenously, infecting the skeleton. The spine is the most common skeletal location affected in TB, typically presenting as Pott's disease, which results in vertebral destruction, deformity, and neurological impairment. This condition continues to be a diagnostic dilemma because of its subtle onset and nonspecific presentation, often leading to delayed therapy. Sustained skeletal TB is especially a cause for concern in children, where delayed diagnosis leads to permanent impairment, emphasizing the necessity for expert care in these susceptible groups (Lehlogonolo et al., 2022). Prompt detection and multidisciplinary care are necessary to avoid complications that are irreversible and maximize outcomes. Bone in TB extension usually goes beyond the spine to involve large weight-bearing joints like the hips and knees, where the infection incites chronic osteomyelitis or arthritis. Pathogenesis includes the spread of bacilli through the bloodstream or lymphatics from a primary site, which causes granulomatous inflammation within bone tissue. This can result in progressive bone and cartilage destruction with resultant major morbidity from pain, joint dysfunction, and deformity. With disseminated TB, an immunosuppression-affected, more serious presentation, skeletal TB might occur along with other extrapulmonary involvement, making diagnosis and treatment more challenging. Since skeletal TB can be imitated by malignancies or other inflammatory conditions, diagnostic confirmation with imaging and biopsy is still not replaceable (Lehlogonolo et al., 2022). Treating skeletal TB comes with special therapeutic challenges in terms of managing pulmonary disease because of the anatomy and physiology of bone. Long-course antibiotic treatment continues to form the cornerstone of therapy and frequently entails intensive anti-tubercular (ATT) therapy over a period of 9 to 12 months. Surgical treatment can be indicated in instances with significant deformities, abscesses, or neurological impairment.

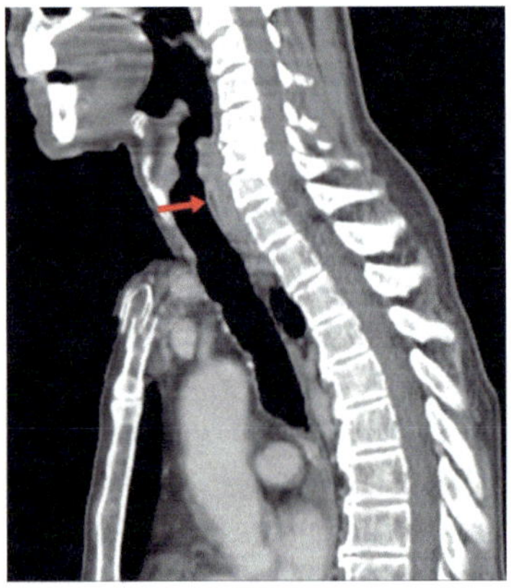

Figure 5.8. A 68-year-old-male. Sagittal reformatted contrast-enhanced CT image reveals an increased thickness of the larynx's posterior wall (arrow). Sternum fracture is also noted in the manubrium.

Source: Hayashi, Y., Noda, Y., Sato, M., Fujii, S., & Shinohara, T. (2022). Cervical esophageal perforation: Multidetector CT findings. *Insights into Imaging, 13*(1), 1–14.

Prevention measures in endemic regions also have to deal with the late identification of skeletal involvement, particularly among immunocompromised patients where dissemination risk is higher. Observations from other infectious diseases causing bone disease, like coccidioidomycosis, accentuate the need for early and correct diagnosis to avoid dissemination and maximize drug treatment regimens. Generally, a clear assessment of skeletal involvement in EPTB is important for the enhancement of long-term patient results (Figure 5.8).

5.3. Risk Factors for Extrapulmonary Tuberculosis (EPTB)

A number of host-related determinants play a significant role in the risk of developing EPTB, especially its disseminated forms. Age proves to be an important determinant, with older persons aged 45 years and older having an increased predisposition to some EPTB manifestations like bone and joint involvement. Nutritional status, that is a body mass index (BMI) of less than 18.5 kg/m^2, is always linked to enhanced risk at multiple extrapulmonary locations, highlighting the contribution of malnutrition towards weakening immune defenses. Furthermore, immunosuppressive therapy aimed at controlling other diseases markedly increases the risk of extrapulmonary dissemination, demonstrating the host immunity compromise that allows for MTB dissemination outside pulmonary boundaries (Huang et al., 2024). These risks together underscore the importance of focused screening and preventive interventions in populations with these attributes to reduce extrapulmonary disease burden. Apart from host characteristics, underlying comorbidities play an important role in EPTB's risk profile. End-stage renal disease (ESRD) patients have a strong predilection for disseminated TB, probably because chronic immune impairment inherent in renal failure exists. Furthermore, EPTB may variably present, depending on gender differences, with female patients showing higher incidence rates of involvement of lymphatics, peritoneum, and intestines. Such findings indicate that immunopathological responses and hormonal or genetic determinants may be responsible for such variability. During adolescence, especially among adolescents residing in high TB burden countries like Indonesia, latent infection leading to disseminated or spinal TB is uncommon but is modulated by nutritional and immunologic status. The complex interaction between comorbid conditions and demographic considerations requires the attention of clinicians to improve early detection and individualized treatment strategies (Huang et al., 2024).

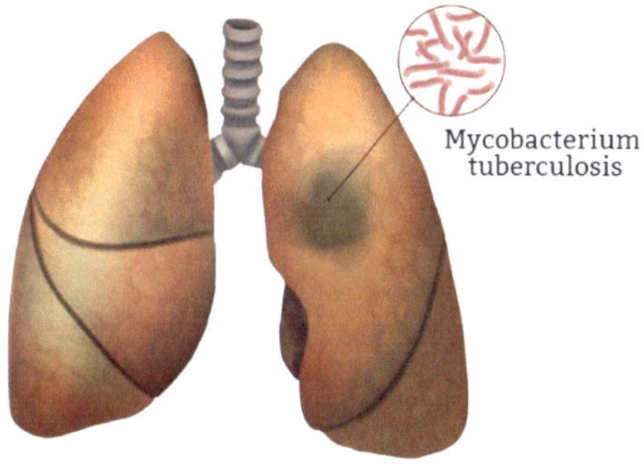

Figure 5.9. Causes of extrapulmonary tuberculosis (EPTB).

Source: Medindia. (n.d.). *Causes of extra-pulmonary TB.* https://images.medindia.net/patientinfo/950_400/causes-of-extra-pulmonary-tb.jpg.

The interaction of these risk factors also affects prognosis and clinical management of extrapulmonary and disseminated TB. Low BMI not only makes one more prone to more widespread disease but also is associated with increased mortality on follow-up, perhaps as a result of compromised systemic defense and delayed response to treatment. Patients on immunosuppressive therapy or with ESRD have compounded difficulties, such as vulnerability to cavities in pulmonary tissue and meningeal TB, which add to the complexity of outcomes. In young age groups, the intensity of spinal TB is related to the number of vertebrae affected and deformities, which underscores the clinical consequences of late diagnosis in at-risk populations. Identifying such risk factors is crucial to planning effective clinical management strategies and preventive measures in the long run, with a view to controlling mortality and morbidity due to EPTB (Huang et al., 2024) (Figure 5.9).

5.3.1. Immunocompromised Conditions

The complex interaction between host immunity and mycobacterial infections plays a critical role in the clinical presentation and severity of tuberculosis. Patients with weakened immune defenses, whether caused by primary diseases or iatrogenic factors, exhibit an increased susceptibility to extrapulmonary and disseminated forms of tuberculosis. Cellular immunity, more specifically mediated by T-lymphocytes, is responsible for containing mycobacterial growth; therefore, any disease that compromises this activity promotes bacillary dissemination beyond the initial pulmonary focus.

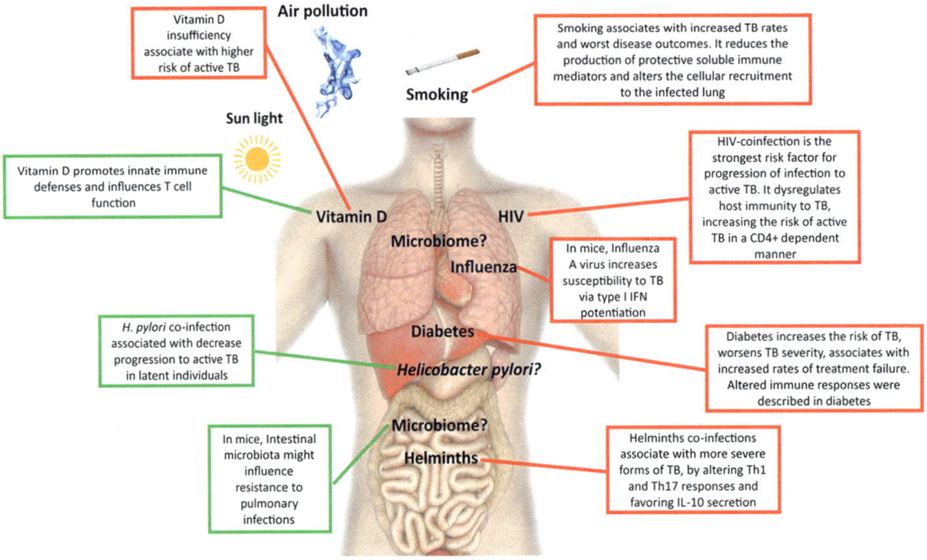

Figure 5.10. Extrinsic factors associated with active tuberculosis (TB). This figure depicts extrinsic factors associated with protection from active TB (green) or susceptibility/increased risk (red) for active TB development.

Source: Bastos HN, Osório NS, Gagneux S, Comas I and Saraiva M (2018) The Troika Host–Pathogen–Extrinsic Factors in Tuberculosis: Modulating Inflammation and Clinical Outcomes. Front. Immunol. 8:1948. doi: 10.3389/fimmu.2017.01948

Human immunodeficiency virus (HIV) infection, the world's pre-eminent cause of immunosuppression, suppresses $CD4^+$ T cell numbers, creating the environment that is permissive for both pulmonary and EPTB. Additionally, chemotherapy and post-transplant immunosuppressive therapy are also immunosuppressive conditions that add to the risk of dissemination through weakening host mechanisms of immune control (Sharma et al., 2020). Such an immunocompromised environment makes diagnosis and treatment challenging promptly, thereby causing heightened morbidity and mortality. Apart from HIV-associated immunosuppression, congenital immune deficiencies and acquired disorders such as malnutrition are major players in the pathogenesis of disseminated tuberculosis.

Congenital immune defects involving cellular immunity predispose the body's inability to effectively defend against the dissemination of MTB. Malnutrition also impairs several immune functions such as macrophage activity and cytokine production, which are critical in the containment of mycobacteria. Beyond tuberculosis caused by *Mtb*, NTM can also precipitate diseases predominantly in immunocompromised hosts. These environmental mycobacteria rarely cause infection in immunocompetent individuals but demonstrate pathogenic potential when cellular immunity is impaired, leading to localized or even disseminated disease manifestations that can mimic tuberculosis (Cantres-Fonseca et al., 2019).

Understanding these immunocompromised conditions is crucial for clinicians to consider atypical presentations and initiate appropriate diagnostic evaluations. Diagnostic difficulty is accentuated in immunocompromised hosts because extrapulmonary and disseminated tuberculosis have a non-specific and variable presentation. Immunosuppression modifies the normal immune response, often with unusual radiological and histopathological features that make differential diagnosis challenging. Additionally, the similarity in the presentation of *Mtb* with opportunistic infections such as those caused by NTM makes accurate laboratory confirmation even more important. Advances in molecular diagnostics have enhanced species-level identification, which is crucial for targeted therapy in immunocompromised patients, due to the variable drug susceptibility patterns of mycobacterial species (Sharma et al., 2020). As immunosuppression elevates disease severity and extends treatment duration, optimal detection and individualized management guidelines are necessary to enhance outcomes and restrict the morbidity related to these severe infectious syndromes (Cantres-Fonseca et al., 2019) (Figure 5.10).

5.3.2. Geographic and Environmental Factors

The spread and virulence of extrapulmonary and disseminated tuberculosis (TB) are inextricably linked to geographic and environmental settings, modulating transmission patterns and disease pathology. Some localities with the endemic burden of TB frequently overlap with socio-environmental stressors including crowded living environments, poor ventilation systems, and inadequate access to healthcare services, all of which play a role in enhancing exposure and compromised immune function. In addition, physical environmental factors including climate, pollution, and altitude are critical in influencing host susceptibility. For example, domestic air pollution caused by the combustion of biomass fuels in poorly ventilated domestic structures increases respiratory susceptibility, possibly contributing to *Mtb* spread outside the lung system. All these complexities highlight the need for holistic public health interventions that reduce environmental risks and take geographic specificities into account to prevent EPTB. It is important to grasp these subtleties to customize interventions in high-risk geographies where environmental risks and social determinants overlap to further fuel TB pathology (Bonnet et al., 2025). Microbial genetic diversity, dictated by geographic locale, adds complexity to the extrapulmonary and disseminated TB landscape. Extensive dissemination of multi-drug resistant (MDR) *Mtb* strains across some parts of the world is illustrative of this complexity. Particularly, the MDR B0/W148 clone, which is common throughout Russia and Europe, shows genetic adaptations that are responsible for its evolutionary success, although its direct association with increased virulence is still under study. Transcriptional regulators including WhiB6 and KdpDE show mutations that modify the gene expression of the pathogen, influencing cellular functions that could potentially affect persistence and dissemination in varied environmental settings.

Although these mutations are not necessarily virulence-increasing in animal models, their existence in geographically clustered strains indicates selective environmental pressures that allow clones to survive and transmit. Such results highlight the importance of geographic and environmental variables, as well as microbial genetics, in determining the epidemiology and clinical presentation of extrapulmonary and disseminated TB (Bonnet et al., 2025). The interaction of environmental exposures with host factors in various geographic locations further adjusts the risk and manifestation of EPTB. In countries such as Nepal, longitudinal cohort studies underscore how air pollution, especially by indoor biomass smoke, affects lung development and function early in life and may predispose individuals to severe and extrapulmonary TB disease later in life. Altitude and climatic variability within geographic areas add another level of complexity through effects on immune function and TB pathogenesis. These environmental stressors, along with socioeconomic inequality that restricts access to diagnosis and treatment, add to not just the burden of TB but to its spread beyond the pulmonary cavity. Incorporating environmental health into TB control programs will be essential to resolving the geographic heterogeneity of extrapulmonary and disseminated TB and enhancing results in at-risk populations (Kurmi et al., 2024)

5.3.3. Socioeconomic Status

Health outcome disparities are typically intrinsically tied to socioeconomic status, especially for infectious diseases such as extrapulmonary and disseminated TB. People of lower socioeconomic status commonly experience living situations that enhance their susceptibility, including crowding, inadequate ventilation, and compromised access to healthcare resources. These structural and environmental drivers not only add to enhanced MTB exposure but also to delayed diagnosis and treatment initiation. In such environments, the danger of TB spreading outside the lungs is increased, since immune response could be impaired by malnutrition and chronic stress, both associated with socioeconomic disadvantage. Understanding this convergence is key to dealing with the wider epidemiology of extrapulmonary and disseminated TB, noting that health interventions alone are not enough without intervention into underlying social determinants. Good access to healthcare is a significant factor that is determined by socioeconomic status, defining disease course in extrapulmonary and disseminated TB infections. Economically disadvantaged groups may face impediments like transportation fees, poor health insurance plans, and sparse coverage of specialist medical care required for optimal TB management. These create suboptimal patient compliance with treatment and incomplete follow-up, enhancing the risk of untreatable disseminated infections. Moreover, health infrastructure in underprivileged regions can be devoid of the diagnostic equipment to identify extrapulmonary involvement early on, adding to the complexity of clinical outcomes. Thus, socioeconomic conditions indirectly influence TB prognosis by way of systemic healthcare disparities, emphasizing policy interventions that improve both healthcare provision and social equity to fight the disease effectively. The wider social context influenced by socioeconomic status also determines individuals' vulnerability to advanced forms of TB, such as extrapulmonary and disseminated disease. Poverty-related chronic conditions like HIV infection and malnutrition compromise cellular immunity, making patients susceptible to greater mycobacterial dissemination. In addition, cultural and educational inequalities influence awareness and health-seeking behavior, frequently leading to late presentations to health facilities at advanced stages of the disease. These multifaceted layers are added upon in vulnerable populations, where non-clinical stressors exacerbate risk. Intervening with socioeconomic determinants thus demands multi-pronged approaches including educational interventions, nutrition assistance, and poverty alleviation. Such holistic intervention is crucial to mitigating the public health burden of extrapulmonary and disseminated TB, mirroring approaches in other emerging infectious diseases where socioeconomic status plays a central role in driving disease dynamics (Chris et al., 2021; Nancy, 2022).

5.4. Clinical Manifestations of Extrapulmonary Tuberculosis (EPTB)

The nature of tuberculosis is more complex than just pulmonary involvement since extrapulmonary manifestations pose distinct diagnostic challenges given the varied clinical presentations. EPTB patients tend to present with nonspecific signs and symptoms like intermittent fever, weight loss, and localized swelling or masses, which can easily be confused with other illnesses. Massive splenomegaly in immunocompetent patients is an uncommon presentation but is reported to be one of the manifestations of disseminated TB, underlining the potential of the disease to involve solid organs outside the lungs. Imaging techniques such as contrast-enhanced computed tomography (CT) tend to give decisive pointers by uncovering typical patterns, but diagnostic confirmation can remain elusive unless there is high clinical suspicion and therapeutic trials. Identification of these unusual signs is crucial for early diagnosis and treatment, as evidenced by presentations that improved dramatically following ATT, emphasizing the importance of including TB in differential diagnoses even in unexpected clinical settings (Das et al., 2025). Besides the involvement of solid organs, EPTB may present with crippling musculoskeletal manifestations, especially TB spondylitis, involving vertebral bodies and leading to a spectrum of neurological deficits. This presentation of TB occurs commonly in an insidious manner with manifestations of back pain, spinal deformities, and in severe cases, paraplegia, or urinary retention secondary to compression of the spinal cord. Clinical variation in these presentations usually leads to delayed diagnosis, particularly if classical pulmonary symptoms are not present. Integrated management approaches using long-term anti-tuberculous regimens and surgery have shown better results. Prognostic factors are patient age, the severity of spinal deformity, and general health, including nutrition. These results highlight the heterogeneity of manifestations of EPTB and the necessity of individualized treatment plans (Handryastuti et al., 2024). Clinical presentation of EPTB requires attention to subtle and varied symptomatology to avoid misdiagnosis and late intervention. Though pulmonary TB is the most well-known type, the infection is often found in extrapulmonary locations like LNs, pleura, abdomen, and CNS and may present with complex variable symptoms. Abdominal distention with no pulmonary disease, or neurological impairment due to TB spine, points to the occult nature of the disseminated disease. Early diagnosis is often based on a multidisciplinary strategy that includes clinical judgment, imaging, and in some cases empirical treatment. Increased clinician awareness of such unusual presentations is critical, as early diagnosis and treatment directly affect patient outcomes and minimize morbidity resulting from TB's extrapulmonary dissemination (Handryastuti et al., 2024; Das et al., 2025).

5.4.1. Symptoms Based on Affected Organs

The expression of tuberculosis outside the pulmonary system is characterized by an ever-varying array of symptoms, which are mostly dependent on the organs affected. If the abdominal area is involved in EPTB, the symptoms can be quite elusive and multiplex, making diagnosis challenging. For example, when the lymphatic system and peritoneum are involved, it usually causes nonspecific clinical manifestations like abdominal distension, pain, and fever. These signs do not clearly suggest tuberculosis and clinical assessment becomes difficult, as abdominal TB is often due to lympho-hematogenous spread from an initial focus. The ileocecal area, mesenteric LNs, and peritoneum are also frequent sites of involvement, each with a variety of complaints ranging from localized pain to generalized signs of infection. The polymorphic presentation of such symptoms highlights the requirement for thorough diagnostic strategies to determine extrapulmonary involvement correctly (Nikolaeva, 2021). When the liver and spleen are involved in disseminated tuberculosis, symptoms tend to mirror systemic disease with organ-specific failure. Patients present with clinical manifestations such as hepatosplenomegaly, fatigue, loss of weight, and low-grade fever, which represent the immune reaction and local tissue injury. These expressions are frequently associated with laboratory nonspecific abnormalities complicating clinical suspicion without specific imaging and histopathologic demonstration. Symptom overlap with other chronic infectious or inflammatory conditions makes modalities such as ultrasonography or CT necessary to identify characteristic organomegaly or lesions. This underlines the difficulty in differentiating disseminated TB from other systemic diseases and the need to correlate clinical presentations with radiological and microbiological findings to inform effective management (Nikolaeva, 2021). Besides the abdominal and reticuloendothelial systems, EPTB can affect other organs, each with unique patterns of symptoms. For instance, tuberculous lymphadenitis presents as painless peripherally located LN swelling, and TB meningitis as headache, stiff neck, and neurologic impairment. Skeletal TB presents as localized bone pain and swelling, with occasional limitation of movement, depending on the location. Since these symptoms are extremely variable depending on the organ system involved, clinicians need to have a high level of suspicion, particularly in those with risk factors like HIV infection or immunosuppression. Prompt identification of these organ-specific presentations is essential since delayed diagnosis can result in serious morbidity. This symptom complex requires a multidisciplinary approach to patient assessment, using clinical acumen in conjunction with diagnostic testing to establish EPTB (Figure 5.11).

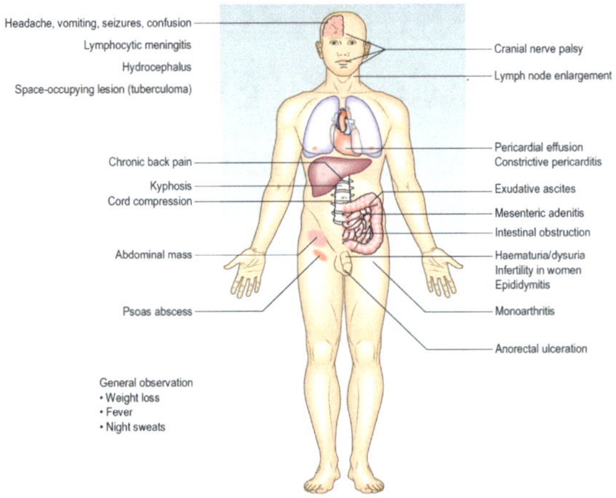

Figure 5.11. Symptoms of extrapulmonary tuberculosis (EPTB) depend on affected site.

Source: Southeastern National Tuberculosis Center. (n.d.). *Extrapulmonary TB: Signs and symptoms by site of disease.* https://sntc.medicine.ufl.edu/files/onthefly/content/ExtrapulmonaryTB.pdf.

5.4.2. Diagnostic Challenges

Extrapulmonary and disseminated tuberculosis (TB) often present diagnostic challenges due to their nonspecific clinical features and the variability in affected organ systems. Unlike pulmonary TB, where sputum analysis can confirm diagnosis, EPTB frequently lacks easily accessible sites for specimen collection. For instance, genitourinary TB can mimic other infectious or neoplastic conditions, making clinical suspicion essential but insufficient without corroborative evidence. Imaging modalities like high-resolution ultrasonography and CT yield useful anatomical and pathological information but have to be correlated with biochemical and cytological investigations to make a firm diagnosis. The tubercular epididymitis case highlights the necessity of combining multiple diagnostic modalities because routine urine cultures can be negative in the presence of active infection. Aspiration cytology with subsequent acid-fast bacilli (AFB) detection or histopathological analysis remains key to preventing misdiagnosis and delayed treatment in cases of disseminated TB (Kumar et al., 2025). The wide range of manifestations of EPTB tends to overlap with other infections, making the diagnosis even more challenging. Immunocompromised individuals, who are at higher risk for both TB and opportunistic infections, pose even more layers of complexity. Distinguishing TB from fungal diseases, like *Scedosporium* spp. infections, largely depend on newer diagnostic methods such as molecular testing or special staining techniques. The fact that extrapulmonary dissemination of some pathogens in immunocompetent hosts is exceedingly rare underscores the need for robust diagnostic approaches such as polymerase chain reaction (PCR) sequencing when standard cultures are negative. This technique guarantees precise identification of the causative organism, which is most critical for proper therapy direction and better patient outcomes in overlapping presentation cases (Berger et al., 2025). Radiological imaging continues to be the gold standard in detecting localized and disseminated EPTB, but they are not likely to offer pathognomonic characteristics. The challenge of diagnosis is compounded by the common requirement to distinguish TB from malignancies and other granulomatous diseases, particularly when imaging shows masses, calcifications, or abscesses. High-resolution imaging improves visualization of complications like sinus tracts or fistulous communications but cannot substitute for microbiological or histological proof. Therefore, a multidisciplinary approach that integrates clinical evaluation, imaging, cytology, and microbiological methods is required to surmount diagnostic uncertainties. Early and correct diagnosis decreases morbidity related to disseminated TB and facilitates focused interventions consistent with the disease's frequently stealthy course (Kumar et al., 2025).

5.4.3. Importance of Early Detection

The variability and complexity of extrapulmonary and disseminated tuberculosis tend to create diagnostic difficulties that may lead to delays in treatment. Patients can present with atypical presentations or nonspecific symptoms, which resemble other diseases, making clinical recognition difficult. Delays can actually considerably exacerbate patient outcomes since untreated tuberculosis can further disseminate and produce serious complications. Early diagnosis thus becomes critical to prevent the advancement of the disease and allow for the timely institution of proper ATT. Clinical acumen coupled with newer diagnostic methods can raise the prospect of detection of the disease early. Reportedly observed cases among elderly patients with extensive involvement highlight the importance of expeditious diagnostic avenues to avoid mortality and morbidity due to these advanced forms of tuberculosis (Liu et al., 2024). Early detection therefore not only enhances prognosis but also minimizes the impact on healthcare resources by avoiding widespread disease complications. In addition, the overlap of tuberculosis with other chronic illnesses like diabetes mellitus (DM) further adds complexity to the clinical picture and increases the importance of early detection. DM makes patients susceptible to a greater prevalence of pulmonary as well as EPTB, including disseminated variants, due to compromised immune function. Studies have shown a strong correlation between compromised glycemic control and vulnerability to tuberculosis lesions, highlighting the importance of metabolic control in disease development. Screening for tuberculosis on a routine basis has been suggested in diabetic patients to prevent risk and ensure early diagnosis, which is critical to avoiding severe complications and enhancing overall treatment success. These results underscore the necessity of incorporating tuberculosis screening procedures into diabetic care protocols, which address the two-fold public health issues inherent in tuberculosis and diabetes (Tiwari et al., 2024). Early detection in such high-risk groups becomes essential to halting disease progression and ensuring improved rates of recovery. Beyond clinical and epidemiological contexts, early identification of extrapulmonary and disseminated tuberculosis has a crucial role to play in public health containment efforts. Tuberculosis is a major infectious cause of morbidity worldwide, with a high prevalence in resource-constrained environments where delays in diagnosis are the norm. Disseminated tuberculosis, because it involves systemic disease, not only poses individual health risks but also poses transmission risks due to the delay in initiating therapy. Early detection and full treatment minimize the period of infectiousness and the emergence of drug-resistant strains, ultimately improving community health outcomes. In addition, awareness of the variability of presentations associated with extrapulmonary involvement leads to early intervention and individualized treatment strategies. Early detection in this case is a cornerstone for minimizing mortality, curtailing disease transmission, and alleviating the economic burden on health systems grappling with tuberculosis control (Liu et al., 2024). Therefore, emphasizing timely diagnosis becomes essential in the control of this multifaceted type of tuberculosis.

5.5. Diagnostic Methods for Extrapulmonary Tuberculosis (EPTB)

The reasons for the complexity of diagnosing EPTB include its wide range of clinical presentations and the challenge of coming up with appropriate specimens for laboratory analysis. Conventional diagnostic methods, including sputum smear microscopy and chest X-ray, are of limited value considering that EPTB also affects sites other than the lungs, including LNs, pleura, bone, or abdominal organs. In patients with concomitant disease such as DM, TB risk is heightened, while clinical signs are often masked by other conditions, further making diagnosis difficult. Diagnostic radiology and biopsy tissue histopathology continue to play an essential role in identifying lesions typical of TB. Further, microbiological culture techniques, which are the gold standard, are cumbersome and can delay the initiation of treatment, making it imperative for the establishment and implementation of quicker diagnostic approaches to enhance patient outcomes (Tiwari et al., 2024). Molecular diagnostic strategies have transformed identifying EPTB, especially the application of NAATs such as the Xpert MTB/RIF assay. This test permits the quick detection of MTB DNA and rifampicin resistance in clinical samples, especially useful in extrapulmonary locations where sample bacterial counts tend to be low. Pediatric studies have shown moderate sensitivity and specificity of Xpert MTB/RIF in the diagnosis of EPTB with differing detection rates based on the site of infection. For example, LN and neurological TB were more sensitive in the assay than pleural or abdominal TB. Nonetheless, the concordance of the assay with culture is moderate, and it can produce false negatives, particularly in DR-TB, highlighting the imperative of complementary diagnostic strategies (Shah et al., 2023). Maximization of EPTB diagnosis is imperative with the high morbidity that accrues with delayed or missed detection. Though molecular assays yield quick results, their sensitivity may be determined by the anatomical location, bacillary load, and existence of drug resistance. Therefore, combining clinical inspection, radiologic imaging, histopathology, and molecular and culture-based microbiological tests constitute the foundation for an overall diagnostic approach. For diabetic patients, in whom presentation of TB could be unusual or exacerbated, normal screening and diligent surveillance can lead to early detection and avert dissemination. The continuing challenge is to fine-tune these diagnostic modalities for greater precision and less turnaround time, thereby enhancing the management of EPTB and decreasing public health burdens (Shah et al., 2023; Tiwari et al., 2024) (Figure 5.12).

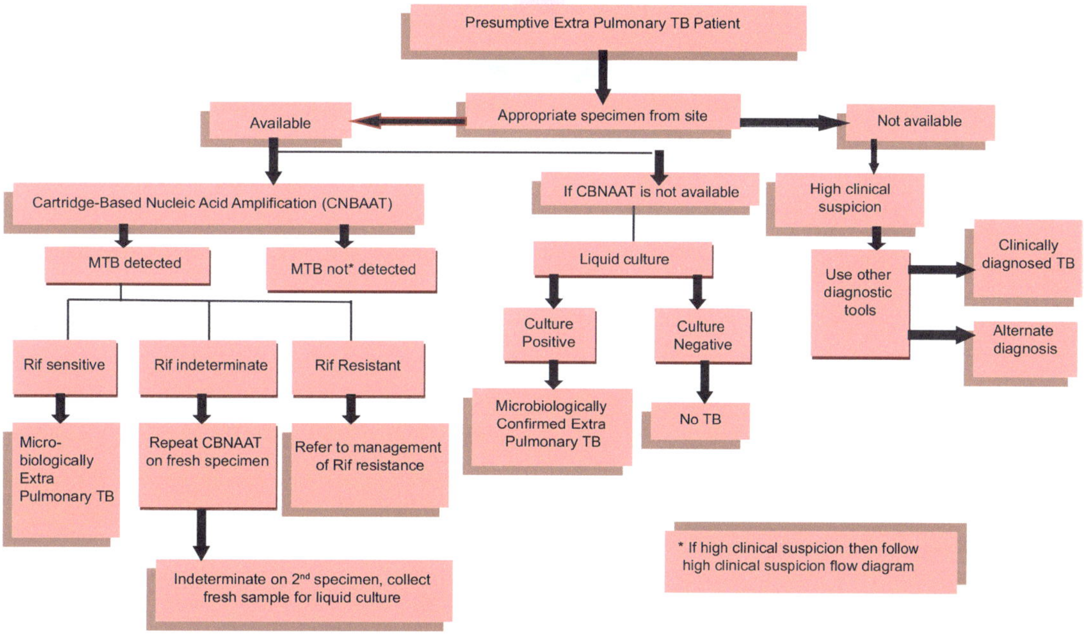

Figure 5.12. Diagnostic algorithm for extrapulmonary tuberculosis (EPTB) under the revised national tuberculosis control program (RNTCP).

Source: ResearchGate. (n.d.). *Diagnostic algorithm for extrapulmonary tuberculosis under the revised national guidelines.* https://www.researchgate.net/figure/Diagnostic-algorithm-for-extrapulmonary-tuberculosis-under-the-revised-national_fig2_320883110.

5.5.1. Imaging Techniques

Technological advances in imaging have dramatically increased diagnostic sensitivity and management of tuberculosis, especially in the extrapulmonary and disseminated presentations where clinical findings can be evanescent or nonspecific. Ordinary chest roentgenography is still a first-line modality, particularly for initial screening and assessment of pulmonary disease. Yet its failure to characterize sensitively or specifically, particularly for extrapulmonary disease, calls for more advanced modalities. CT offers better anatomical resolution, which allows for detecting nodules, lymphadenopathy, cavitations, and active or latent tuberculosis patterns. In disseminated tuberculosis, CT helps in detecting multisystem involvement and the planning of biopsy sites. These benefits notwithstanding, CT scan mainly provide structural assessment and not adequately define disease activity. Combining metabolic imaging methods enhances this gap by exhibiting tissue-level pathophysiological processes, thereby enhancing early detection and treatment monitoring in complex TB cases (Katal et al., 2020).

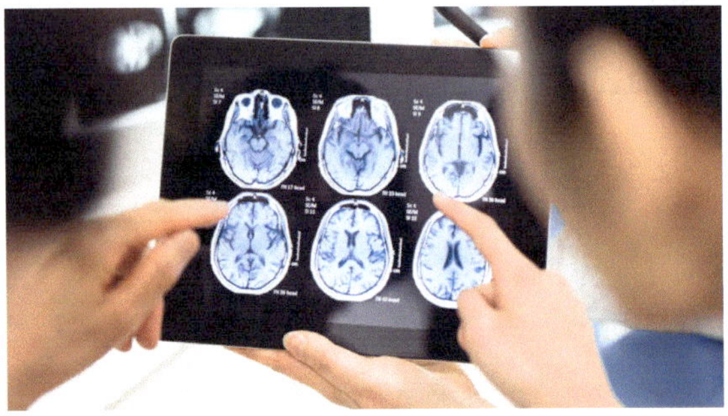

Source: Psych Central. (n.d.). *Types of brain imaging techniques.* https://psychcentral.com/lib/types-of-brain-imaging-techniques.

Molecular imaging, specifically fluorodeoxyglucose-positron emission tomography with computed tomography (FDG-PET/CT), has become a seminal diagnostic modality in evaluating both pulmonary and EPTB. FDG-PET/CT takes advantage of the heightened glycolytic metabolism of inflammatory cells in tuberculous granulomas, resulting in vigorous FDG uptake distinguishing active disease locations with exquisite sensitivity. This modality is superior in discerning occult extrapulmonary disease, commonly underappreciated by conventional imaging, thus offering thorough mapping of the burden of disease. In addition, since FDG-PET/CT combines metabolic and anatomical information, it allows for distinction between infection activity and fibrotic changes following treatment. This is necessary for making individualized treatment regimens and preventing over-treatment. While not generally applied for primary diagnosis because of cost and availability, FDG-PET/CT provides critical information in complex disseminated TB, allowing accurate staging of the disease and assessment of response (Arun et al., 2017). Although they have advantages, imaging methods in tuberculosis diagnosis are not free from challenges, particularly distinguishing TB from other infections, malignancies, or inflammatory processes based on overlapping radiological features. FDG-PET/CT, being sensitive, may show increased uptake in nontuberculous infections or inflammatory diseases, thus reducing specificity. Furthermore, morphological changes like cavities or nodules observed in CT can persist even after microbial clearance, making it difficult to assess response to treatment. Therefore, multidisciplinary strategies involving imaging, microbiologic assays, and clinical acumen continue to be essential. Future studies seek to advance imaging biomarkers and create new tracers to improve specificity for MTB. This new frontier has the potential to maximize diagnostic precision and therapeutic monitoring of extrapulmonary and disseminated TB, ultimately enhancing patient care through earlier detection and tailored management plans (Arun et al., 2017; Katal et al., 2020) (Figure 5.13).

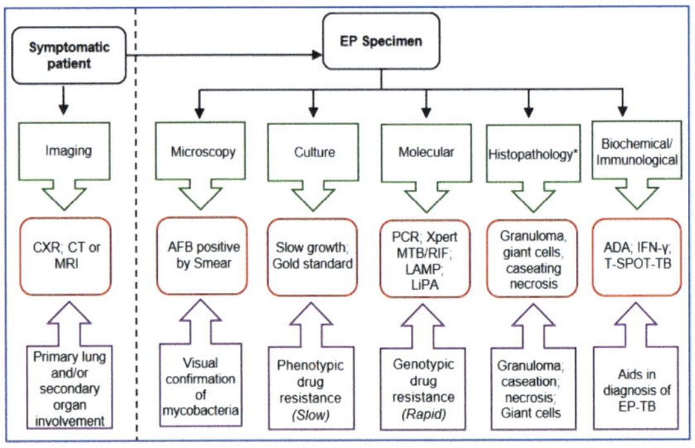

Figure 5.13. Flowchart showing a panel of diagnostic tests for EPTB due to *M. tuberculosis* complex organisms.

Source: Gopalaswamy R, Dusthackeer VNA, Kannayan S, Subbian S. Extrapulmonary Tuberculosis—An Update on the Diagnosis, Treatment and Drug Resistance. *Journal of Respiration*. 2021; 1(2):141-164. https://doi.org/10.3390/jor1020015

5.5.2. Laboratory Tests

The extrapulmonary and disseminated forms of tuberculosis pose a formidable challenge to diagnosis because the disease frequently has insidious and nonspecific presentations. Laboratory investigation holds a central role in overcoming these challenges, as the common clinical tests may be insensitive or nonspecific. The histopathological study continues, nonetheless, to be a gold standard in establishing tuberculosis, especially where biopsies show chronic granulomatous inflammation, caseating necrosis, and the presence of Langhans giant cells. For instance, in genital tuberculosis, granulomatous inflammation on biopsies presents irrefutable evidence of focal disease despite negative tumor markers, and this speaks to the importance of tissue studies (Lima et al., 2024). Equally, AFB staining is necessary to identify mycobacteria in tissue or fluid specimens, further supporting the diagnosis. These laboratory methods not only verify detecting MTB but also distinguish TB from other granulomatous or neoplastic diseases, an important step for the initiation of the right therapy. Apart from histopathology and microscopy, imaging and laboratory findings supplement the process of diagnosis in cases of EPTB. Radiologic investigations like CT scans help in detecting soft tissue and bone involvement, especially in musculoskeletal tuberculosis, where changes in bony density can be seen without apparent destructive lesions at first (Lesmana et al., 2023). Lab blood work commonly shows nonspecific inflammatory markers like increased erythrocyte sedimentation rate (ESR) and anemia, which, while not specific, confirm clinical suspicion. Culture of MTB from aspirate or biopsy continues to be the gold standard for diagnosis but is often hampered by low yield and long incubation periods. Therefore, an integration of thorough histological examination, microbiological investigations, and imaging contributes to a more accurate diagnosis, allowing prompt treatment of this severe, frequently under-recognized variant of tuberculosis. Notwithstanding progress, the diagnosis of extrapulmonary and disseminated TB continues to be hindered by limitations, requiring an integrated strategy in laboratory testing. Failure to find direct contact history or positive purified protein derivative (PPD) tests in certain patients reinforces the poor sensitivity of immunologic assays in these types of TB (Lima et al., 2024). As a result, molecular diagnostic methods, including NAATs, have appeared to be effective tools that can improve rates of detection, particularly when other methods prove unfruitful.

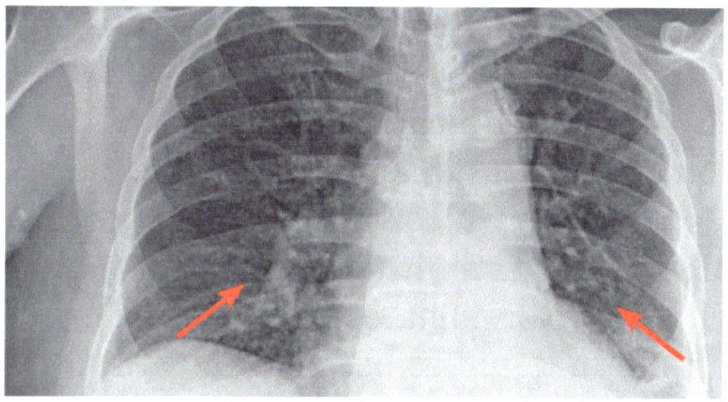

Figure 5.14. Chest radiography showed patchy left basilar consolidation with subtle, diffuse interstitial opacities (arrows) throughout both lungs.

Source: Cleveland Clinic Journal of Medicine. (n.d.). *Chest X-ray showing pulmonary abnormalities.* https://external-content.duckduckgo.com/iu/?u=https%3A%2F%2Fwww.ccjm.org%2Fcontent%2Fccjom%2F87%2F10%2F590%2FF1.large.jpg&f=1&nofb=1&ipt=dcb5601174c25dd4c114ab4297b2fb6041ee9683622769b8fafcb33591a8bd1e.

Nevertheless, access to these molecular tests can be inhibited in poor-resource settings. With the protean presentation of EPTB and the likelihood of delayed diagnosis, the assumption on the part of clinicians on the combined use of histopathology, acid-fast staining, culture, imaging, and, more recently, molecular diagnostics is paramount to lower morbidity and enhance patient outcomes. This multidisciplinary laboratory approach is critical in tailoring effective therapeutic interventions and preventing disease progression and complications (Figure 5.14).

5.5.3. Biopsy Procedures

Accurate diagnosis of disseminated and extrapulmonary tuberculosis (TB) usually depends on the accuracy of tissue sampling and thus indispensable biopsy procedures in clinical practice. When patients come with unusual symptoms like localized swelling or neurological impairment, routine microbiological methods will not yield conclusive evidence of MTB infection. In these situations, biopsy of involved tissues such as LNs, bone marrow, or epididymal accumulations allows for direct histopathological assessment for AFB and granulomatous inflammation. For example, in genitourinary TB, high-frequency ultrasonography targets epididymal lesions for aspiration, allowing cytological and culture confirmation without surgical invasion. This strategy enhances diagnostic accuracy by validating clinical and radiological findings with pathological findings, which is essential to initiate targeted antitubercular therapy (ATT) and prevent misdiagnosis with other granulomatous conditions or malignancies (Kumar et al., 2025). Therefore, biopsies are a cornerstone in the diagnosis of non-pulmonary TB manifestations, highlighting their clinical value. Difficulty with biopsy procedures in EPTB is usually encountered because of the heterogeneous nature of the sites of lesions and the paucibacillary nature of the illness. In CNS TB and spinal intramedullary manifestations, tissue biopsy samples are especially challenging to obtain because of anatomical and safety issues. Bone marrow biopsy proves to be a useful diagnostic tool in suspected disseminated TB, particularly when standard tests such as cartridge-based nucleic acid amplification test (CBNAAT) give negative results. Granulomas identified on bone marrow biopsy, along with AFB detection on staining, are key evidence for tuberculosis in the absence of microbiological proof in the fluid samples (Figure 5.15).

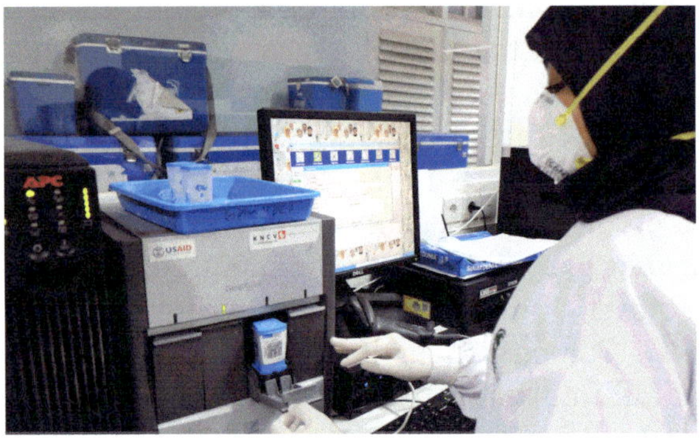

Figure 5.15. Cartridge-based nucleic acid amplification test (CBNAAT).

Source: https://commons.wikimedia.org/wiki/File:Mendeteksi_Tuberkulosis_dengan_GenExpert_%2828275748402%29.gif

Such invasive sampling makes up for the low sensitivity of noninvasive diagnostic techniques, especially in those with neurological complications such as longitudinally extensive transverse myelitis (LETM). Biopsy procedures, therefore, not only establish the diagnosis but also inform therapeutic choices in complicated EPTB (Diggikar et al., 2024). Due to the variability of clinical presentations and the diagnostic hurdles in disseminated TB, biopsy methods should be chosen with care and supplemented by imaging techniques. Methods like fine-needle aspiration cytology, core needle biopsy, or excisional biopsy are selected depending on lesion access, patient health, and suspected organ involvement. Radiologically guided approaches like high-resolution ultrasonography or CT improve biopsy accuracy by marking lesions and sparing surrounding critical structures. Histopathology, AFB staining, culture, and molecular studies are components of post-biopsy examination, greatly boosting diagnostic yield. Early acquisition of tissue samples accelerates the identification of TB etiology and facilitation of timely initiation or modification of ATT. Biopsy results also guide prognosis and potential drug resistance, crucial in treatment-refractory scenarios. Incorporating biopsy procedures into a multidisciplinary setup thus maximizes the management of extrapulmonary and disseminated tuberculosis (Diggikar et al., 2024; Kumar et al., 2025).

5.6. Treatment Options for Extrapulmonary Tuberculosis (EPTB)

Management of EPTB demands a strategy that considers the special challenges of its multiple anatomical locations and pathophysiology. In contrast to pulmonary TB, where sputum examination can frequently dictate treatment, EPTB often requires invasive diagnostic tests to establish infection, for example, biopsies or fluid sampling from the site of involvement. After diagnosis, the standard regimen of anti-tuberculous treatment as in pulmonary TB is usually used, consisting of an intensive course of four drugs, rifampicin, isoniazid, pyrazinamide (PZA), and ethambutol, for two months and a continuation phase of rifampicin and isoniazid for four months. Duration and intensity of treatment can be modified according to individual clinical situations, for instance, the CNS involvement, where prolonged therapy for a duration of up to 12 months is sometimes advised despite a lack of evidence to support extended duration. Special care must be exercised for monitoring drug interactions and side effects, especially in HIV-co-infected patients, to maintain treatment efficacy (Bracchi et al., 2019). Effective therapy of EPTB is also accompanied by adjunctive treatments that are specific to the organ system involved and the extent of involvement. Corticosteroids, for example, are routinely advised for TB meningitis and pericarditis to prevent inflammatory damage mediated by the immune response to MTB. These drugs can abate morbidity and mortality through the regulation of excessive inflammation, especially in critical locations like the CNS.

Furthermore, treating drug-resistant strains of EPTB needs serious thought, with frequently individualized regimens through phenotypic and genotypic drug susceptibility testing (DST) being used. The emergent rise in multi-drug resistant (MDR) and extensively drug-resistant (XDR) TB adds further complexity to the treatment process, highlighting the necessity of collaborative care strategies under the guidance of TB specialists. Therapeutic choices need to weigh efficacy, possible toxicity, and drug-drug interactions, particularly in the setting of concomitant antiretroviral therapy (ART) for HIV-positive patients (Bracchi et al., 2019). Recent evidence has demonstrated clinical heterogeneity of TB illness beyond traditional dichotomy of latent or active pulmonary disease, identifying a continuum with extrapulmonary forms.

This developing conceptual model implies that therapeutic regimens will need to be adaptive to the variable metabolic activity of bacteria and host immune status in EPTB. Current practice guidelines are largely based on research into pulmonary TB; nonetheless, there is growing emphasis on understanding how therapeutic approaches might be maximized for extrapulmonary disease states as well as incipient or subclinical ones. Such knowledge provides avenues to pre-empt disease progression and spread and to personalize treatment duration and intensity to the patient's disease spectrum. This subtle knowledge is crucial for the design of new diagnostics and therapies for enhancing extrapulmonary and disseminated TB outcomes (Figure 5.16).

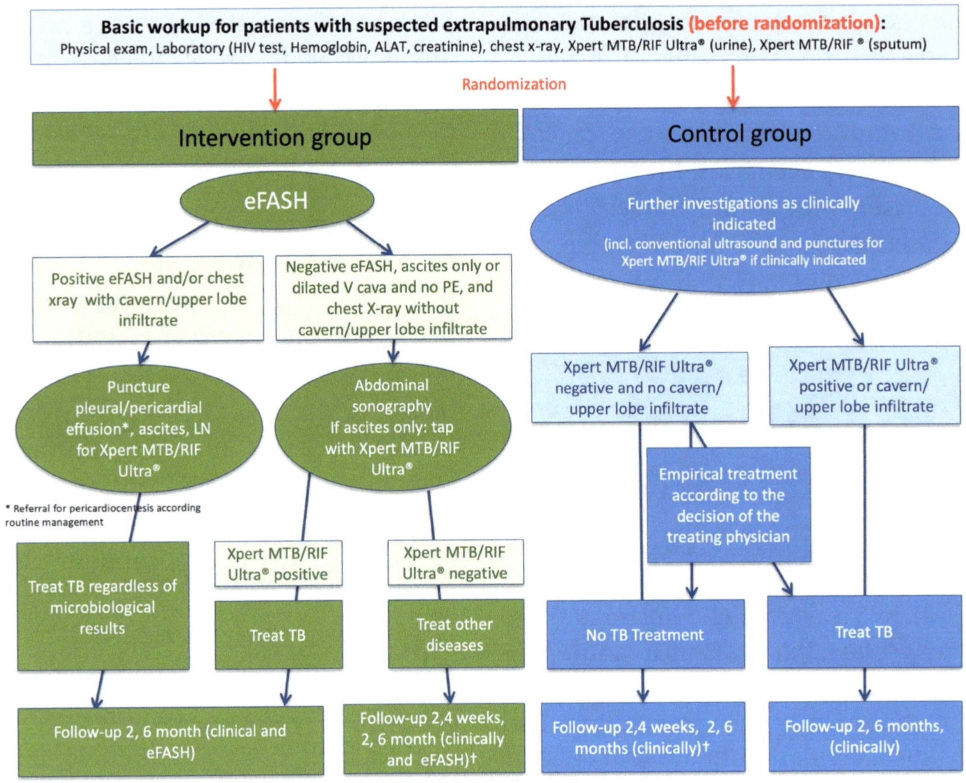

Figure 5.16. Algorithm for management of intervention group and control group. [LN: Lymph node; TB: Tuberculosis; eFASH: Extended focused assessment with sonography for HIV and tuberculosis; and PE: Pericardial effusion].

Source: Ndege, R., Ngome, O., Bani, F. *et al.* Ultrasound in managing extrapulmonary tuberculosis: a randomized controlled two-center study. *BMC Infect Dis* **20**, 349 (2020). https://doi.org/10.1186/s12879-020-05073-9

5.6.1. Pharmacological Interventions

Advances in the pharmacotherapy of extrapulmonary and disseminated tuberculosis (TB) have highlighted the pressing need for efficacious therapy regimens, especially with the rise of drug-resistant strains across the world. The complex characteristics of EPTB demand customized therapy regimens that not only target bacterial clearance but also counteract unfavorable treatment outcomes. Current treatment regimens commonly employ first-line drugs like isoniazid, rifampicin, and ethambutol; however, the increased prevalence of multi-drug-resistant tuberculosis (MDR-TB) has initiated the move towards newer drugs. Amongst them, bedaquiline has come into the spotlight with its established cost-effectiveness and treatment success rates, particularly when combined with multidrug regimens. Interestingly, the use of bedaquiline has been found to increase sputum culture conversion rates and reduce treatment length, aspects critical to controlling disseminated infections. Despite drug cost and access difficulties, pharmacological advancement remains at the forefront of combating TB's worldwide burden and patient prognosis (Nagar et al., 2024). Gastrointestinal symptoms' diagnosis complexity has a bearing on the following pharmacological intervention measures. Comprehensive diagnostic evaluations—usually consisting of imaging and histopathological examinations—guide the selection and duration of treatment but are limited by the subtlety of presentations of symptoms and the common need to rule out pulmonary TB or atypical mycobacterial infection. Diagnosis is often made late or inappropriately, emphasizing the need for a stepwise and careful evaluation process. Additionally, clinicians should take into account the underlying conditions like HIV infection that add complexity to both diagnosis and drug response, hence affecting the pharmacological efficacy. Attaining optimal ATT in such situations requires not only precise identification of MTB but also an integrated strategy in patient history and risk factors to provide focused pharmacological management (Saha, 2024). Regimen duration and cost factors greatly affect pharmacological management decisions for extrapulmonary and disseminated TB. Briefer regimens using new agents, even if more costly in the short term, have been seen to be more cost-effective overall when considering increased adherence and fewer side effects. Ethambutol, a long-time mainstay of TB therapy, is now less economical in comparison with newer drugs such as bedaquiline and delamanid, which have better efficacy profiles. Treatment delivery expenses, resistance patterns in drugs, and patient compliance rates all confer pharmacological regimen success and sustainability. They demonstrate the imperative for sustained pharmaceutical development against resistance mechanisms within budgetary restraints. Emerging development must consolidate such drivers of cost-effectiveness to steer therapeutic regimens and maximize results for patients suffering from disseminated EPTB (Nagar et al., 2024).

5.6.2. Duration of Treatment

Extrapulmonary and disseminated tuberculosis (TB) pose different challenges in management compared to pulmonary TB, particularly in the treatment period. In contrast to pulmonary TB, in which a generic six-month treatment is adequate in the majority of cases, extrapulmonary types usually require prolonged treatment based on the location and severity of infection. This is partly caused by challenges in attaining sufficient drug levels in extrapulmonary tissues and relapse should therapy be stopped prematurely. Other than this, disseminated TB, which involves numerous organ systems, needs long-term treatment to guarantee the complete destruction of MTB. The initial intensive period, typically with four drugs, is followed by a continuation phase that can be longer than six months depending on clinical response, radiological improvement, and microbiological status. All such tailoring of the duration of treatment highlights the role of intensive patient monitoring to maximize results while reducing the risk of adverse effects. The complexity of extended ATT for extrapulmonary and disseminated TB also introduces issues of drug toxicity and patient compliance. For example, ethambutol, an essential drug of ATT, can be given for more than eight months in certain treatment regimens, and there is concern regarding ethambutol-induced optic neuropathy (EtON). Not everyone who takes it develops this side effect, and genetic research indicates a mitochondrial predisposition to involve the oxidative phosphorylation pathway as the etiology of susceptibility. Identification of patients at increased risk via genetic screening would make it possible for clinicians to individualize treatment regimens, perhaps reducing ethambutol duration or replacing other agents in an attempt to reduce visual complications. This is part of a larger movement towards personalized medicine in treating TB, weighing the effective duration of treatment against the potential for severe adverse reactions (Kaur et al., 2022). Adding to treatment duration choices in extrapulmonary and disseminated TB are comorbid conditions including DM, which have profound impacts on disease course and therapeutic outcomes. Diabetic individuals have a greater prevalence of tuberculous lesions, with poor glucose control and longer disease duration having a relationship with risk increase as well as more complex clinical syndromes. These variables tend to prompt extended treatment durations to attain resolution of disease and avert relapse. Routine screening and combined management of TB among diabetic patients are necessary to avert the double burden of both diseases. Therefore, ATT duration in these individuals must be well thought out, taking into consideration metabolic control and the higher risk of extrapulmonary disease, with treatment completions being sufficient to avert the increased risk (Tiwari et al., 2024).

5.6.3. Management of Drug-Resistant Tuberculosis (DR-TB)

Successful management of drug-resistant tuberculosis (DR-TB) requires an all-encompassing strategy that is beyond the routine therapeutic schedules, particularly for extrapulmonary and disseminated presentations. Patients who carry multi-drug-resistant organisms are prone to treatment failure and higher mortality, highlighting the need for individualized interventions. Increased DR-TB management complexity is added by the common occurrence of comorbid conditions, including DM, that further accelerate disease progression and complicate treatment adherence. Recent case reports emphasize the possibility of disseminated MDR-TB, affecting varied anatomical locations such as LNs and lungs, highlighting the absolute necessity for strict screening procedures. Early detection of drug resistance via contemporary diagnostic methods can guide regimen modifications, enabling more effective treatment outcomes. This is especially important since EPTB presentations often escape early identification, thus leading to delayed critical interventions (Dadra et al., 2020). Diagnostic complexities also complicate the management of drug-resistant extrapulmonary and disseminated TB. Conventional chest radiographs can be ineffective in demonstrating characteristic signs of disseminated disease, requiring the use of sophisticated imaging methods like high-resolution CT and magnetic resonance imaging (MRI) to define the distribution of organ involvement. Supplemental diagnostic methods like histopathology and rapid culture methods aid in establishing MTB infection and detection of resistant organisms. Even with the existence of new diagnostic tests, the inefficiencies of point-of-care use and biomarker identification hold back early detection and timely therapeutic decision-making. Therefore, clinicians are required to keep a high suspicion index, especially when faced with unusual presentation or immunocompromised patients, to initiate proper antitubercular treatment regimens effectively and reduce the risks of morbidity and mortality (Ray et al., 2013). Treatment plans for drug-resistant EPTB involve careful weighing of drug activity, possible toxicities, and individual patient factors like coinfection with HIV and immunosuppression. First-line drugs against tuberculosis are active against sensitive strains but less so in multi-drug-resistant strains, where second-line drugs with longer regimens and increased risk of adverse effects are necessary. The lack of randomized controlled trials comparing optimal regimens and duration of treatment for drug-resistant disseminated TB adds to therapeutic uncertainty. The presence of drug-induced hepatotoxicity and drug-drug interactions poses important clinical dilemmas, particularly in populations with HIV/TB coinfection. Adjunctive therapy with corticosteroids is an area with continued investigation to establish its place in enhancing treatment outcomes. Therefore, tailored treatment regimens based on susceptibility testing and overall clinical evaluation are critical to effectively managing this multifaceted disease process (Ray et al., 2013).

SUMMARY

The complex problems presented by extrapulmonary and disseminated tuberculosis highlight the need for improved diagnostic and treatment regimes. Current research reveals that success rates for treatment, although high, invariably remain below national standards, a reflection of ongoing shortcomings in case management and patient follow-up. Most particularly, variables including age structure and the extrapulmonary course of TB directly impact outcomes in a manner reflecting the complexity of treating this condition in heterogeneous populations. These data underscore the importance of making TB control programs more responsive to these variables to optimize adherence and monitoring protocols. The need to improve healthcare infrastructure and resource deployment is apparent to attain maximum treatment success, considering the increased risk factor posed by extrapulmonary manifestations (Nurfeta et al., 2024). Such a policy can result in tighter control over TB, ultimately diminishing incidence and transmission rates. Additionally, patients' quality of life during pre-treatment and post-treatment provides valuable information regarding the overall consequence of EPTB outside of clinical success. Patient-reported outcome measures identify lasting health disparities associated with the variable presentations of EPTB, emphasizing that this presentation of the disease cannot be treated as a monolithic condition. While substantial recovery following treatment in both physical and psychological realms has been reported, residual impairment exists, notably in certain presentations such as lymphadenitis. Such inequities indicate that interventions need to be holistic and patient-focused with an integration of medical and socioeconomic factors. Meeting these complex needs via specialized health care might improve long-term outcomes and decrease disease burden (Hassan et al., 2024). An overall strategy of this sort is needed to assist patients' overall welfare and to enhance the responsiveness of healthcare systems to such a difficult disease spectrum. In conclusion, the care of extrapulmonary and disseminated tuberculosis requires a multifaceted approach based on focused treatment protocols and patient-focused care models. Understanding the specific clinical and social determinants of treatment success enables more targeted public health initiatives to bridge prevailing gaps. Coordination of sophisticated diagnostics, stringent follow-up, and comprehensive patient care, such as psychological and socioeconomic, will be crucial in further improving outcomes. The findings emphasize the importance of long-term dedication to context-specific interventions at institutional and community levels to surpass and fulfill existing standards in TB control. Ultimately, these all-encompassing initiatives will promote better treatment compliance, decrease disease transmission, and improve the quality of life in affected populations, a key milestone toward controlling this multifaceted and widespread public health issue (Hassan et al., 2024; Nurfeta et al., 2024).

Knowledge of the complexity of extrapulmonary and disseminated tuberculosis (TB) necessitates the assessment of its varied clinical presentations outside the pulmonary system. Though pulmonary TB is still the most prevalent type, EPTB affects locations like LNs, pleura, bones, and the CNS, making diagnosis and treatment relatively more complicated. Disseminated TB, with infection occurring throughout the body with the involvement of multiple organs, usually happens in immunocompromised patients or in those with late diagnosis. Early diagnosis is important because of the high morbidity and mortality of these types. The interaction between viral infections and TB, particularly in syndemic situations such as HIV, also adds to complexity, affecting both immune response and clinical course. The latest studies highlight the pressing need for better diagnostic measures and specific therapeutics, emphasizing that the treatment method cannot be universal but needs to take the involved organ systems and patient immunological status into account (Ong et al., 2020). The immunological pattern in extrapulmonary and disseminated TB is highly variable, determining the course of disease and responsiveness to treatment. *Bacillus Calmette-Guérin* (BCG) immunization, though the only vaccine currently available against TB, provides imperfect protection, especially against extrapulmonary forms. Emerging evidence emphasizes the role of both cell-mediated and humoral immunity in the control of TB, which is sometimes neglected. Antibody responses, which were previously underestimated, can apparently fulfill a dual function in modulating the infection and therapeutic responsiveness. This immunological sophistication calls for an increased understanding of the host-pathogen relationships, particularly when trying to develop improved vaccines and immunotherapies. Adapting vaccination strategy to boost specific B cell and antibody responses in addition to conventional T cell immunity could yield a broader defensive mechanism against the dissemination of TB (Tanner et al., 2019). In conclusion, extrapulmonary and disseminated tuberculosis represents a great challenge for diagnosis, treatment, and prevention. Their clinical variability requires a multidisciplinary intervention, considering immune status, infection site, and possible co-morbid viral infections. The insufficiently effective current vaccines and detection methods reveal a significant flaw in TB control efforts. Expanding knowledge of the immunological subtleties and epidemiological interactions will be crucial to formulating new interventions. Adopting a personalized treatment approach and synthesizing new vaccine research could dramatically enhance outcomes for patients suffering from these types of TB. Finally, these important points are addressed by providing a foundation for alleviating the burden of global extrapulmonary and disseminated tuberculosis (Tanner et al., 2019; Ong et al., 2020).

CLOSER LOOK

EXTRAPULMONARY TUBERCULOSIS (EPTB): CENTRAL NERVOUS SYSTEM (CNS) INVOLVEMENT

Extrapulmonary tuberculosis (TB) with central nervous system (CNS) involvement is a dangerous and life-threatening disease. The most frequent types of CNS involvement are TBM and tuberculomas, and they may be associated with a variety of nonspecific symptoms, so diagnosis might be difficult. The CNS is involved when MTB, the etiological agent of TB, disseminates from other sites in the body, including the lungs or LNs, into the bloodstream or the lymphatic system. In immunocompromised patients, including HIV/AIDS patients, CNS involvement is more likely to occur.

TBM is the most frequent type of CNS TB and characteristically presents with insidious onset of symptoms. Initial symptoms are usually headache, fever, and malaise, and may be attributable to other causes of meningitis or viral infections. With progression, nausea, vomiting, neck stiffness, and change in mental status may occur. In advanced stages, neurological impairment happens quickly, resulting in coma or death if not treated. Children, and especially those below the age of five, are highly susceptible to TBM, and the outlook may be grim without immediate diagnosis and treatment.

TBM can only be diagnosed if one has a high suspicion and usually requires the analysis of CSF. CSF usually presents with pleocytosis, decreased glucose, and increased protein levels. In some cases, AFB may be seen in CSF by smear microscopy or PCR, though not always diagnostic. MRI or CT scans of the brain may demonstrate inflammation, hydrocephalus, or other structural abnormalities.

Tuberculomas are focal granulomatous masses that may develop in the brain following MTB infection. Tuberculomas usually present with neurological abnormalities like seizures, focal weakness, or sensory impairment, based on the site of the mass. Tuberculomas can mimic brain tumors on imaging and therefore be misdiagnosed. Biopsy or stereotactic surgery could be necessary for diagnosis. Tuberculomas may produce extensive neurological destruction unless treated early, especially if they result in increased intracranial pressure or brainstem involvement.

In TBM as well as tuberculomas, prompt treatment with a regimen of antitubercular drugs (e.g., rifampicin, isoniazid, pyrazinamide, and ethambutol) is essential to avoid permanent damage and optimize the outcome for the patient. Corticosteroids can also be employed in certain patients to diminish inflammation and decrease the occurrence of complications like cerebral edema. CNS TB continues to be a leading cause of morbidity and mortality, but prompt diagnosis and treatment can result in successful outcomes in most individuals.

REFERENCES

1. Akbar, N., & Mariuz, P. (2024). Disseminated TB With IRIS Presenting as a Pancreatic Mass in Newly Diagnosed HIV: A Case Report. *Open forum infectious diseases, 12*(1), ofae746. https://doi.org/10.1093/ofid/ofae746(accessed on 10 May 2025).
2. AlGhazi, A. N., AlZahrani, M. H., Almutiri, W. A., & Alzoum, N. M. (2025). Disseminated tuberculosis presenting as finger swelling in a 2-year-old: A case report of TB osteomyelitis. *Case Reports in Plastic Surgery & Hand Surgery, 12.* https://www.semanticscholar.org/paper/5044dd06792459173d4511e137246e9a8038ff7a (accessed on 10 May 2025).
3. Amit Kumar Tiwari, Gautam Kumar Sandilya, Supriya Kumari, Kaushal Kishore(2024). Incidence of various tuberculous lesions in Indian patients with diabetes mellitus: A cross-sectional study. *International Journal of Medical and Biomedical Studies.* International Journal of Pharmaceutical and Clinical Research 2024; 16(5); 2831-2834. https://www.semanticscholar.org/paper/20959c39f5d8185b0a6b52f84f39f0d6fc73aed9 (accessed on 10 May 2025).
4. Berger, Steven MD; Se, Bobby MD; Delman, Mark MD. Hematogenous Dissemination of Scedosporiosis in an Immunocompetent Patient. Infectious Diseases in Clinical Practice 33(2):e1442, March 2025. | DOI: 10.1097/IPC.0000000000001442(accessed on 10 May 2025).
5. Bonnet, I., Orgeur, M., Brossier, F., Sayes, F., Frigui, W., Madacki, J., Varet, H., Chauffour, A., Aubry, A., Veziris, N., Sougakoff, W., Brosch, R., & Tournebize, R. (2025). Evaluation of the role of *whiB6* and *kdpDE* in the dominant multidrug-resistant clone *Mycobacterium tuberculosis* B0/W148. *Microbiology spectrum*, e0322424. Advance online publication. https://doi.org/10.1128/spectrum.03224-24(accessed on 10 May 2025).
6. Bracchi, M., van Halsema, C., Post, F. A., Awosusi, F., Barbour, A., Messenger, S., Coyne, K., et al. (2019). British HIV Association guidelines for the management of tuberculosis in adults living with HIV 2019. *HIV Medicine, 20.* https://doi.org/10.1111/hiv.12748.
7. Cantres-Fonseca, O., Rodríguez-Cintrón, W., Del Olmo-Arroyo, F., & Baez-Corujo, S. (2019). Extra pulmonary tuberculosis: An overview. *IntechOpen eBooks.* https://doi.org/10.5772/intechopen.81322.
8. Chakraborty, D., Batabyal, S., & Ganusov, V. V. (2024). A brief overview of mathematical modeling of the within-host dynamics of *Mycobacterium tuberculosis. Frontiers in Applied Mathematics and Statistics, 10.* https://www.semanticscholar.org/paper/5deaca0459ef94cab0136b8466c60879b816f643 (accessed on 10 May 2025).
9. Chewe, W., Chansa, A., Lungu, P., & Liusha, N. (2020). Extrapulmonary drug-resistant tuberculosis in Zambia: Case reports on the first two recorded cases. *Medical Journal of Zambia, 47*, 154–159. https://doi.org/10.55320/mjz.47.2.104.
10. Crouser, E. D., Maier, L. A., Wilson, K. C., Bonham, C. A., Morgenthau, A. S., Patterson, K., Abston, E., et al. (2020). Diagnosis and detection of sarcoidosis: An official American Thoracic Society clinical practice guideline. *American Journal of Respiratory and Critical Care Medicine, 201*, e26–e51. https://doi.org/10.1164/rccm.202002-0251st.
11. Crum, N. F. (2022). Coccidioidomycosis: A contemporary review. *Infectious Diseases and Therapy, 11*, 713–742. https://doi.org/10.1007/s40121-022-00606-y.
12. Dadra, R., Kajal, N., Malhotra, B., Pandiyaraj, P., Kaur, L., & Kaur, G. (2020). Disseminated multidrug-resistant tuberculosis in a young patient: A rare case report. *The Journal of*

Association of Chest Physicians, 8, 26–29. https://www.semanticscholar.org/paper/0c07644f2918e13399ac427a38eb86c7993483da (accessed on 10 May 2025).

13. Das, D., Mittal, R., Singh, A., & Bairwa, M. (2025). A rare case of massive splenomegaly in an immunocompetent adult: An unusual manifestation of tuberculosis. *International Journal of Scientific Research*. https://www.semanticscholar.org/paper/e5eb88b26152436ea3e2d382d11b51b242050493 (accessed on 10 May 2025).
14. Diggikar, P., Reddy, H., Mundada, M., Biju, A., & Yekkaluru, S. (2024). Disseminated tuberculosis presenting as transverse myelitis with bone marrow involvement: A rare case of pyrexia of unknown origin. *Journal of Clinical and Diagnostic Research*. https://doi.org/10.7860/JCDR/2024/74352.20192. https://www.semanticscholar.org/paper/5f4f7787f78f487d6d3f74596e179d2f0a44c259 (accessed on 10 May 2025).
15. Drain, P. K., Bajema, K. L., Dowdy, D. W., Dheda, K., Naidoo, K., Schumacher, S. G., Ma, S., et al. (2018). Incipient and subclinical tuberculosis: A clinical review of early stages and progression of infection. *Clinical Microbiology Reviews, 31*. https://doi.org/10.1128/cmr.00021-18.
16. Eldin, C., Melenotte, C., Mediannikov, O., Ghigo, É., Million, M., Edouard, S., Mège, J. L., et al. (2016). From Q fever to *Coxiella burnetii* infection: A paradigm change. *Clinical Microbiology Reviews, 30*, 115–190. https://doi.org/10.1128/cmr.00045-16.
17. Falzon, D., Schünemann, H. J., Harausz, E., González-Angulo, L., Lienhardt, C., Jaramillo, E., & Weyer, K. (2017). World Health Organization treatment guidelines for drug-resistant tuberculosis, 2016 update. *European Respiratory Journal, 49*, 1602308. https://doi.org/10.1183/13993003.02308-2016.
18. Gopalaswamy, R., Shanmugam, S., Mondal, R., & Subbian, S. (2020). Of tuberculosis and non-tuberculous mycobacterial infections–A comparative analysis of epidemiology, diagnosis and treatment. *Journal of Biomedical Science, 27*. https://www.semanticscholar.org/paper/099fb4667a9864709af9d5dc4f722730ab05537c (accessed on 10 May 2025).
19. Handryastuti, S., Kaswandani, N., Hendriarto, A., Tobing, S. D., Pebriansyah, & Rafli, A. (2024). Clinical manifestations and prognosis of tuberculous spondylitis in an adolescent with disseminated tuberculosis: A case report. *Paediatrica Indonesiana*. https://www.semanticscholar.org/paper/e11287dfda2c47194a3948a89e7fbe4405daf6f4 (accessed on 10 May 2025).
20. Hassan, S., Purohit, M., Kanthali, M., Yaesoubi, R., Jain, S., & Mustafa, T. (2024). Health-related quality of life among extrapulmonary tuberculosis patients and inequalities by disease manifestations: A longitudinal study analyzing the impact of TB treatment. *Quality of Life Research, 34*, 683–700. https://www.semanticscholar.org/paper/52cb29f7757e5d0b6c5d260409439898b757b054 (accessed on 10 May 2025).
21. Huang, W., Fei, Z. T., Yan, B., Liu, X., Liu, P., Xia, L., Liu, H. R., et al. (2024). Risk factors for disseminated tuberculosis and associated survival in adults without human immunodeficiency virus. *Open Forum Infectious Diseases, 12*. https://www.semanticscholar.org/paper/86c4d6afb7d5c3be753c3f6782ce1bd84aafc46c (accessed on 10 May 2025).
22. Katal, S., Amini, H., & Gholamrezanezhad, A. (2020). PET in the diagnostic management of infectious/inflammatory pulmonary pathologies: A revisit in the era of COVID-19. *Nuclear Medicine Communications, 42*, 3–8. https://doi.org/10.1097/mnm.0000000000001299 (accessed on 10 May 2025).

23. Kaur, P., Singh, S., Kaur, K., Mahesh, K., Tigari, B., Sehgal, V., Takkar, A., et al. (2022). The genetics of ethambutol-induced optic neuropathy: A narrative review. *Neuro-Ophthalmology, 46*, 304–313. https://www.semanticscholar.org/paper/dae500c219ca8b323042af4b9534e63a483ff6a2 (accessed on 10 May 2025).

24. Khan, M. A., Ismail, A., Ghafoor, A., Khan, N., Muzaffar, N., Zafar, F., Gupta, A., et al. (2024). Experience of piloting BPaLM/BPaL for DR-TB care at selected sites in Pakistan. *IJTLD Open, 1*, 508–515. https://www.semanticscholar.org/paper/11c1cd349ec418c5789fa19e9aeea5706ba6a4e4 (accessed on 10 May 2025).

25. Kumar, Vishal; Swain, Basanta Manjari; Panda, Sangram; Mohanty, Sudhanshu Sekhar. Epididymo-orchitis with epididymal abscess in a patient with disseminated tuberculosis. Journal of Integrative Medicine and Research 2(2):p 105-108, Apr–Jun 2024. | DOI: 10.4103/jimr.jimr_53_23(accessed on 10 May 2025).

26. Kurmi, O., Chaudhary, N., Delanerolle, G., Bolton, C., Pant, P., Regmi, P., Gautam, S., et al. (2024). Nepal Family Cohort study: A study protocol. *BMJ Open, 14*. https://www.semanticscholar.org/paper/6f57a0c6bbcc5f0213e10dd0b35aeb8e792516f7 (accessed on 10 May 2025).

27. Lesmana, A., Dewanti, H. R. ., Angin, L. B. P. ., Muzakky, M. I. ., Hayon, S. G. V. ., Sholihah, M. M. ., & Hanif, M. I. . (2023). Tuberculosis Mimicking-Musculoskeletal Tumor of The Hand: An Uncommon Case of Extrapulmonary Tuberculosis. *(JOINTS) Journal Orthopaedi and Traumatology Surabaya, 12*(2), 77–82. https://doi.org/10.20473/joints.v12i2.2023.77-82 (accessed on 10 May 2025).

28. V F N Lima, V L Feitosa, D J Haddad, J B Dettoni, C F Borges, (PM-02) GENITOURINARY TUBERCULOSIS IN MALE PATIENTS: A CASE SERIES FROM A FEDERAL UNIVERSITY HOSPITAL, *The Journal of Sexual Medicine*, Volume 21, Issue Supplement_3, April 2024, qdae018.034, https://doi.org/10.1093/jsxmed/qdae018.034(accessed on 10 May 2025).

29. Liu, H., Huang, X., & Jiao, Y. (2024). Disseminated tuberculosis complicated by intramuscular abscesses, meningoencephalitis, and hemophagocytic lymphohistiocytosis: A case report. *BMC Infectious Diseases, 24*. https://www.semanticscholar.org/paper/05c96dab09a7ddd25aea4c8bc190b519477b3094 (accessed on 10 May 2025).

30. Maphalle, L. N. F., Michniak-Kohn, B., Ogunrombi, M. O., & Adeleke, O. A. (2022). Pediatric tuberculosis management: A global challenge or breakthrough? *Children, 9*, 1120. https://doi.org/10.3390/children9081120.

31. Moule, M. G., & Cirillo, J. (2020). *Mycobacterium tuberculosis* dissemination plays a critical role in pathogenesis. *Frontiers in Cellular and Infection Microbiology, 10*. https://www.semanticscholar.org/paper/cc2c2ef12959cf7b3ae69ade69687ecb1dbb771d (accessed on 10 May 2025).

32. Nachiappan, A. C., Rahbar, K., Shi, X., Guy, E., Mortani Barbosa, E. J., Shroff, G. S., Ocazionez, D., et al. (2017). Pulmonary tuberculosis: Role of radiology in diagnosis and management. *Radiographics, 37*, 52–72. https://doi.org/10.1148/rg.2017160032.

33. Nagar, S., Nicholls, D., & Dawoud, D. (2024). A systematic review of economic evaluations of pharmacological treatments for active tuberculosis. *Frontiers in Public Health, 12*, Article 1201512. https://www.semanticscholar.org/paper/dbb5f738d109a619b1c59d61460bb68fcc0bdb76 (accessed on 10 May 2025).

34. Nurfeta, R., Ababiya, T., Woldeamanuele, N., Ababiya, R., Deregasso, B., Tema, L., Hailu, S., et al. (2024). Tuberculosis treatment outcomes and associated factors at Zewditu Memorial Hospital, Ethiopia. *International Journal of Infectious Diseases and Therapy*. https://www.semanticscholar.org/paper/d87805cf18a78a44ce9cd38d40f59bd94f37022c (accessed on 10 May 2025).

35. Ong, C., Migliori, G. B., Raviglione, M., Macgregor-Skinner, G., Sotgiu, G., Alffenaar, J. W. C., Tiberi, S., et al. (2020). Epidemic and pandemic viral infections: Impact on tuberculosis and the lung. *European Respiratory Journal, 56*, 2001727. https://doi.org/10.1183/13993003.01727-2020.

36. Pang, Y., An, J., Shu, W., Huo, F., Chu, N., Gao, M., Qin, S., et al. (2019). Epidemiology of extrapulmonary tuberculosis among inpatients, China, 2008–2017. *Emerging Infectious Diseases, 25*, 457–464. https://doi.org/10.3201/eid2503.180572.

37. Ray, S., Talukdar, A., Kundu, S., Khanra, D., & Sonthalia, N. (2013). Diagnosis and management of miliary tuberculosis: Current state and future perspectives. *Therapeutics and Clinical Risk Management, 9*, 9–26. https://www.semanticscholar.org/paper/3906b62193498bd0f1a767c5b030e0cf0e9843c9 (accessed on 10 May 2025).

38. Rodriguez-Takeuchi, S., Renjifo, M., & Medina, F. (2019). Extrapulmonary tuberculosis: Pathophysiology and imaging findings. *Radiographics: A Review Publication of the Radiological Society of North America, Inc., 39*(7), 2023–2037. https://www.semanticscholar.org/paper/6395ce78407598cb7b5ec02901ccbc436cc040ec (accessed on 10 May 2025).

39. Ryndak, M. B., & Laal, S. (2019). *Mycobacterium tuberculosis* primary infection and dissemination: A critical role for alveolar epithelial cells. *Frontiers in Cellular and Infection Microbiology, 9*. https://doi.org/10.3389/fcimb.2019.00299.

40. Saha, S. (2024). Primary extrapulmonary tuberculosis diagnosis warrants extra-precautious pulmonary tuberculosis exclusion workup. *World Journal of Clinical Cases, 12*, 3295–3297. https://www.semanticscholar.org/paper/03c160ebe0d35fe6a34c95d2fb0d6c80d3ba8d5a (accessed on 10 May 2025).

41. Shah, I., Bhamre, R., & Shetty, N. (2023). Accuracy of Xpert® MTB/RIF in diagnosing extrapulmonary tuberculosis in Indian children. *The National Medical Journal of India, 35*(6), 334–337. https://www.semanticscholar.org/paper/a2dd4adb83b0327c612d94ad387b30f2e1fb2337 (accessed on 10 May 2025).

42. Sharma, S. K., & Upadhyay, V. (2020). Epidemiology, diagnosis, and treatment of non-tuberculous mycobacterial diseases. *The Indian Journal of Medical Research, 152*, 185–226. https://doi.org/10.4103/ijmr.ijmr_902_20.

43. Sharma, S. K., Ryan, H., Khaparde, S. D., Sachdeva, K. S., Singh, A. D., Mohan, A., Sarin, R., et al. (2017). Index-TB guidelines. *The Indian Journal of Medical Research, 145*, 448–463. https://doi.org/10.4103/ijmr.ijmr_1950_16.

44. Shen, L., Frencher, J. T., Huang, D., Wang, W., Yang, E., Chen, C. Y., Zhang, Z., et al. (2019). Immunization of Vγ2Vδ2 T cells programs sustained effector memory responses that control tuberculosis in nonhuman primates. *Proceedings of the National Academy of Sciences of the United States of America, 116*, 6371–6378. https://www.semanticscholar.org/paper/f2936b5aa29f69b806d819fa535c5f456683c778 (accessed on 10 May 2025).

45. Singh, J., Dinkar, A., & Gupta, P. (2022). Uncommon manifestations in tuberculosis: An expanding clinical spectrum from North India. *International Journal of Mycobacteriology, 11*,

30–37. https://www.semanticscholar.org/paper/765e8b0f6afb449a803e63dab7a1551acf12553f (accessed on 10 May 2025).

46. Tanner, R., Villarreal-Ramos, B., Vordermeier, H. M., & McShane, H. (2019). The humoral immune response to BCG vaccination. *Frontiers in Immunology, 10*, Article 1317. https://doi.org/10.3389/fimmu.2019.01317.

47. Tiwari, D., & Martineau, A. R. (2022). Inflammation-mediated tissue damage in pulmonary tuberculosis and host-directed therapeutic strategies. *Seminars in Immunology, 65*, 101672. https://doi.org/10.1016/j.smim.2022.101672.

48. Triggle, C. R., Bansal, D., Ding, H., Islam, M. M., Farag, E., Hadi, H. A., & Sultan, A. A. (2021). A comprehensive review of viral characteristics, transmission, pathophysiology, immune response, and management of SARS-CoV-2 and COVID-19 as a basis for controlling the pandemic. *Frontiers in Immunology, 12*. https://doi.org/10.3389/fimmu.2021.631139.

49. Tuang, G. J., Muhammad, A., & Zahedi, F. (2020). Master of many faces: Extrapulmonary tuberculosis in the eyes of otolaryngologists. *Postgraduate Medical Journal, 98*, 311–312. https://www.semanticscholar.org/paper/ff3dffb0b2be574f12c5a23ad9544371c8b018ac (accessed on 10 May 2025).

50. Wang, D. M., Wang, C., An, Q., Yang, Q., & Liao, Y. (2024). Clinical characteristic, common sites, and geographical distribution of pediatric tuberculosis patients in Southwest China. *Frontiers in pediatrics, 12*, 1327648. https://doi.org/10.3389/fped.2024.1327648 (accessed on 10 May 2025).

51. Weerasuriya, C. K., Clark, R. A., White, R. G., & Harris, R. C. (2020). New tuberculosis vaccines: Advances in clinical development and modelling. *Journal of Internal Medicine, 288*, 661–681. https://doi.org/10.1111/joim.13197.

52. Yang, J., Ko, J., Cho, S. Y., Kang, C., Chung, D., Peck, K., Rhu, J., et al. (2025). P-2315. Clinical outcome of rifabutin-based treatment for pulmonary tuberculosis in solid organ transplant recipients. *Open Forum Infectious Diseases, 12*. https://www.semanticscholar.org/paper/3138faca82650776fb889a8acf9ef916422ff78a (accessed on 10 May 2025).

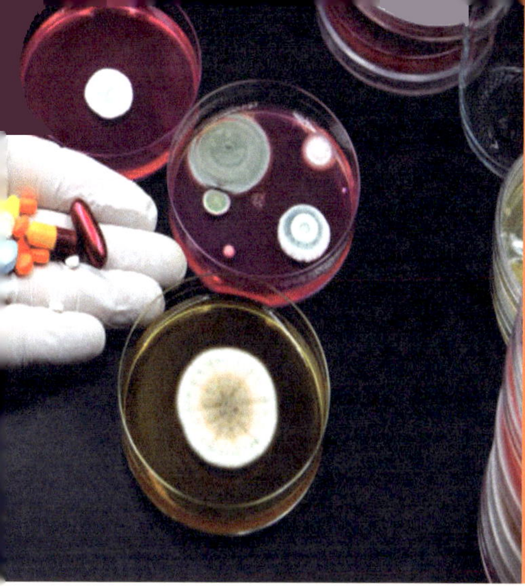

Chapter 6

DRUG-SUSCEPTIBLE TB TREATMENT

Contents

Introduction

Tuberculosis (TB) remains the world's oldest infectious disease, posing serious public health issues, particularly in high-burden nations. Despite advances in the field of medical science, the prevalence of TB continues to be alarming as many cases remain undiagnosed or untreated, with ongoing transmission and complications. In nations such as Sierra Leone, the disease burden of tuberculosis is particularly high, with a reported incidence rate of 286 per 1,00,000 population in 2023. Efforts to increase the treatment coverage and case notification have been relatively successful since there is quite a big gap between the treated and diagnosed cases. This disparity underscores the dire necessity of prioritizing drug-susceptible tuberculosis (DS-TB) treatment strategies to minimize mortality and disease transmission, particularly since backslides in DS-TB management could amplify the spread of drug-resistant strains (Koroma et al., 2025). Complicating control of TB is its overlap with socioeconomic determinants such as undernutrition, which severely affects outcomes. Undernutrition in patients with tuberculosis (PWTB) exposes them to a higher risk of treatment failure, relapse, and mortality. Nutritional intervention is a vital adjunct to drug therapy in averting these adverse outcomes. Although randomized controlled trials with conclusive evidence on macronutrient supplementation are lacking due to ethical issues, observational studies such as a comparison of neighboring countries yield valuable information. For instance, comparing treatment outcomes among resource-constrained states with and without nutrition support programs provides insight into the possible advantages of nutrition interventions in DS-TB care, emphasizing an interlinked strategy beyond antibiotics (Cintron et al., 2025). The recent global COVID-19 pandemic has further added to the complexity of TB care by interrupting healthcare services and restricted access to care. During this time, the identification and treatment of cases of DS-TB were hindered, which might have led to an increase in cases of drug-resistant tuberculosis (DR-TB) in addition to the drop-in successful cure rates. Sierra Leonean data show this pattern in a wide drop in treatment completion rates during the pandemic followed by a return to normal after the pandemic. These results highlight the susceptibility of TB treatment programs to public health crises and the need for resilient health systems that can support essential services. An understanding of these dynamics is critical to inform effective strategies to sustain and enhance DS-TB treatment outcomes under different circumstances (Koroma et al., 2025).

Overview of Drug-Susceptible TB

The international health environment is still facing the endemic danger of infectious diseases, of which tuberculosis (TB) is a major burden, especially in resource-constrained environments. DS-TB, due to susceptible strains of *Mycobacterium tuberculosis* (MTB) to first-line drugs, is the source of most of the TB disease around the world. Treatment for this type consists of a uniform regimen that includes isoniazid, rifampicin, pyrazinamide, and ethambutol (HRZE), which, if followed strictly, provides excellent cure rates. DS-TB is very important to understand because it constitutes the root from which drug-resistant strains develop, making clinical situations complicated and mortality risk high. The efficiency of treatment initiatives is highly reliant on early diagnosis, sufficient drug availability, patient adherence, and healthcare infrastructure. Despite the progress, challenges such as antimicrobial resistance (AMR) continue to frustrate these endeavors by increasing mortality and prolonging disease duration, calling for integrated measures that are applicable to diverse demographic and geographic settings (Dartois & Rubin, 2022). The epidemiology of DS-TB indicates that it remains a treatable disease, a stark contrast from multi-drug resistant and extensively drug-resistant (XDR) forms. Nevertheless, the persistence of drug-susceptible strains necessitates sustained public health attention, especially because of inequality in the delivery of healthcare across regions. Animal populations, for example, Asian and African elephants, to which MTB could potentially be transmitted, represent the zoonotic interface and reservoirs that may ensure persistence and transmission of DS-TB strains. Non-human host treatment has similar challenges to those of human medicine, such as side effects and compliance problems, which, if poorly managed, can lead to microbial resistance. This emphasizes the complex ecological and biological dynamics of TB infections in animals, supporting the importance of comprehensive human-animal health methods for TB control (Kay et al., 2019). DS-TB management calls for a multi-dimensional strategy that brings together diagnostic precision, drug compliance, and surveillance for adverse drug reactions (ADRs). The routine six-month treatment course is usually adequate; however, variability in medication intake or inadequate healthcare systems can lead to complications. The international burden of AMR brings into focus the danger presented by lax DS-TB treatment, which could promote resistant pathogen strain development and the overall disease burden. These processes emphasize strengthening healthcare delivery and diagnostic networks, particularly in high-risk areas, to reverse the velocity of treatment failure and prevent resistance emergence. Policymakers must consider local health capacities and pathogen types to optimize intervention effectiveness and reduce TB-related morbidity and mortality worldwide (Dartois & Rubin, 2022).

Importance of Effective Treatment

The triumph in treating DS-TB is heavily dependent on the performance of the therapeutic regimen, underlining the complex challenges in TB management in the world. Delayed or inappropriate treatment not only extends disease but also jeopardizes the development of drug resistance, which tremendously complicates treatment outcomes. The multi-drug-resistant tuberculosis (MDR-TB) literature highlights the system problems underlying treatment effectiveness, including weak healthcare infrastructure and poor case detection, which are most directly applicable to DS-TB too. Overcoming these systemic impediments is key to facilitating early diagnosis and treatment compliance, both of which are necessary for avoiding resistance development. Better diagnostic tests and combined therapeutic regimens can increase patient outcomes and prevent transmission, supporting the need for an integrated approach to TB control (Jeffry et al., 2025). Increased duration of treatment and complexity of regimen contribute to higher difficulty in maintaining patient compliance, which is an important determinant of resistance development in TB treatment. The emergence of heteroresistance; where drug-susceptible and resistant strains of bacteria inhabit the same host—raises drastic diagnostic and therapeutic challenges. Studies on the resistance to bedaquiline in MDR-TB populations highlight how even in TB-endemic areas, resistance may emerge without prior exposure to this lifesaving drug, pointing to existing problems in treatment strategies and detection capacity. These results emphasize the value of accuracy in treatment regimens and the necessity of extensive diagnostics to recognize developing resistance in good time. Successful treatment will thus have to adapt with advances in molecular diagnostics to accurately distinguish between susceptible and resistant bacterial populations for best practice (Rashid et al., 2025). Adequate treatment of DS-TB is not just an issue of individual patient health but also a pillar of public health policy to regulate TB transmission worldwide. Inadequate treatment protocols threaten to extend infectiousness, enhance community transmission, and promote resistant strain development. Literature highlights multi-pronged solutions incorporating international cooperation and financial support to enhance diagnostic accuracy and treatment availability. Introduction of new therapy strategies with firm support from robust health systems can shorten treatment duration and facilitate adherence, ultimately improving patient outcomes. The importance of successful treatment, therefore, is due to its capacity to avert resistance, enhance cure, and shorten TB's broader social burden, emphasizing the need for continuous research and system strengthening (Jeffry et al., 2025).

6.1. Epidemiology of Drug-Susceptible TB

Global TB epidemiology's landscape provides valuable insights into drug-susceptible tuberculosis (DS-TB) distribution and population dynamics, especially among vulnerable populations. Pediatric populations are used to represent this vulnerability since a recent study conducted in Kazakhstan showed that children and adolescents form a high percentage of TB cases, of which 76% are considered DS-TB. The study reported a declining trend in TB notification between 2018 and 2020 that was eventually stabilized through the following years, demonstrating the fluctuating pattern of TB incidence despite ongoing public health efforts. Adolescents aged 15–17 years had higher odds of unsuccessful treatment outcomes, which could potentially have an impact on disease transmission and resistance patterns. This information highlights the need for age-targeted public health interventions and improved diagnostic methods to deal effectively with the burden of DS-TB among young people and maintain treatment effectiveness in this group (Prikhodchenko et al., 2025). Current epidemiological studies demonstrate that DS-TB resistance patterns are affected by subtle molecular and social determinants. For example, the development of isoniazid-resistant but rifampin-susceptible TB (Hr-TB) defies classical assumptions regarding DS-TB's susceptibility pattern. In Haiti, a prevalence of 7.7% Hr-TB among pulmonary TB patients was detected, with adolescents less than 20 years being significantly more at risk. Molecular analysis also proved that such isoniazid-resistant strains are not only transmitted in community settings but not solely through household contacts, representing a complex pattern of disease transmission complicating treatment regimens and control strategies. These results call for re-examination of epidemiological surveillance practices and focused interventions designed to break chains of transmission, especially in younger groups at risk for these resistant yet otherwise drug-susceptible strains (Walsh et al., 2024). The epidemiology of DS-TB also needs to consider geographic and demographic diversity that modulates disease occurrence and treatment responses. The patterns of variation seen in pediatric and adolescent cases of TB, as well as the localized molecular epidemiology of resistance mutations, represent a dynamic public health problem involving both biological and socioeconomic elements. The integration of national databases, combined with sophisticated molecular diagnostic techniques, has enabled greater characterization of these patterns, enabling better public health intervention to respond to changing trends in epidemiology. Therefore, attempts to manage DS-TB need to focus on intensified surveillance, age-adapted treatment protocols, and increased community-based interventions taking into account transmission risk beyond the household setting, in order to maximize outcomes and minimize disease burden (; Walsh et al., 2024; Prikhodchenko et al., 2025).

6.1.1. Global Prevalence and Incidence Rates

The global health ecosystem is constantly being defined by infectious illnesses, with tuberculosis (TB) also being one of the top causes of morbidity and death globally. The incidence of DS-TB is particularly a result of complex relationships between economic conditions, access to healthcare, and epidemiologic patterns. Current information suggests that in 2021, the age-standardized incidence rate (ASIR) for HIV-related DS-TB was about 11.59 per 1,00,000 population across the world. This statistic highlights the endemic nature of TB in the setting of HIV co-infection, making diagnosis and treatment even more complex. In addition, the total mortality rate attributed to HIV-DS-TB averaged around 2.22 per 1,00,000 in the same year, highlighting the importance of strong public health measures. These figures bring to the foreground the urgency to strengthen global TB control activities to combat primary infection as well as co-infection patterns effectively (Zhang et al., 2024). Trend analysis in epidemiology demonstrates heterogeneity in TB prevalence and incidence across geographic and demographic variations. With treatment practices enhanced by advances in protocols, outcomes for drug-susceptible TB have been better, but the rates of incidence are still inequitably distributed with increased burdens in low-resource environments. This inequality is usually compounded by antimicrobial resistance (AMR), which makes it harder to treat and compels global health priorities. In 2019, bacterial AMR was linked to almost 5 million global deaths, with the prevalence of resistant infections such as TB strains well illustrated. While DS-TB is significantly different from forms resistant to it, the interrelationship of AMR and TB epidemiology dictates the constant observation of resistance patterns as well as incidence rates for real-time guidance of tailored treatment protocols as well as policy-making (Dartois & Rubin, 2022). The endemicity of DS-TB in most areas reflects major challenges to disease management and control efforts. Immunocompromised individuals, especially those who are co-infected with HIV, account for a large portion of the worldwide TB disease burden and reflect the complexity of sustaining reduction in incidence rates. Strengthening health infrastructures, such as improved diagnostic capabilities and treatment access, continues to be central to interrupting TB transmission and disease progression. The age-standardized rate of new TB cases and TB deaths further highlights the importance of integrating public health education with clinical treatment to reduce new infections and deaths. Addressing these epidemiological problems by means of multi-pronged approaches may further enhance the effectiveness of DS-TB treatment internationally (Zhang et al., 2024).

6.1.2. High-Risk Populations

The battle against tuberculosis (TB) is still a daunting one because of the complex cross-talk between the pathogen and potential susceptible hosts in various populations. Of these, hosts with weakened immune systems, including those infected with HIV, are especially at risk of progressing to active TB disease following infection. The increased risk among such groups arises because the immune system fails to contain latent tuberculosis infection (LTBI) sufficiently, resulting in disease progression. Pregnant women also constitute a specific high-risk population, in which the interaction between pregnancy-induced immunological alterations and TB infection challenges prevention and treatment uniquely. Interventions to enhance outcomes among such groups have involved the use of specific tuberculosis preventive treatment (TPT) regimens, whose safety and efficacy across all ages and risk profiles are increasingly being acknowledged (Chihota et al., 2024). These approaches highlight the need for interventions adapted to the particular vulnerabilities of high-risk populations to limit the spread of DS-TB. Geographic and socio-behavioral considerations also add to the vulnerability of particular groups to DS-TB. For example, populations in high TB-burden areas have a risk amplified by extensive transmission and restricted access to health care services. In populations such as Uganda's Karamoja region, where poor nutrition and nomadic lifestyles dominate, treatment success rates for DS-TB are poor. According to a retrospective study, treatment success was significantly decreased by high-risk factors including age, HIV-positivity, and undernutrition, highlighting the interaction between social determinants and outcomes of TB treatment (Opito et al., 2024). These findings highlight the need for integrated care mechanisms that address nutritional care and HIV control at the same time in TB treatment services. Addressing these interconnected factors is key to improving therapeutic outcome and reducing TB morbidity among high-risk groups. Identification and control of high-risk groups are key in advancing the worldwide vision of halting the TB epidemic. Effective TB control means scaling up preventive treatment and ensuring universal access to care for groups at risk of adverse outcomes. Advances notwithstanding, there are still gaps in the provision of TPT among vulnerable populations like children, pregnant women, and household members of infectious TB cases. Context-specific delivery models with integrated social support, accelerated diagnostics, and harmonized treatment regimens have the potential to overcome implementation bottlenecks (Chihota et al., 2024). In addition, improving risk stratification instruments can improve early detection of the most likely to advance to active TB so that timely intervention becomes feasible. In the end, ongoing dedication to TB care equity and creative programmatic approaches are critical to ending the transmission cycle and maximizing high-risk populations' access to optimal DS-TB treatment.

6.1.3. Impact of Socioeconomic Factors

The DS-TB disease burden is unfairly shouldered by groups subject to socioeconomic adversity, in which poverty, undernutrition, and poor living conditions undermine susceptibility to infection and access to effective therapy. In overcrowded and poorly ventilated settings, transmission likelihoods are elevated, thereby increasing tuberculosis incidence. Further, limited economic resources frequently hamper patients' access to timely diagnosis and completion of required antimicrobial therapy. This is further compounded by the multifaceted nature of antibiotic stewardship needed to counteract resistant strains, with drug interruptions as a result of economic hardship playing a crucial role in treatment failure as well as the development of multi-drug-resistant tuberculosis (MDR-TB) (Uddin et al., 2021). Thus, socioeconomic determinants do not only affect initial susceptibility to TB but also affect continued treatment success, and hence the importance of integrated social support measures in addition to medical intervention to enhance overall health outcomes. Disparities in healthcare infrastructure further amplify the role of socioeconomic status in DS-TB management. In most high-burden settings, public health systems are plagued by underfunding, leading to constrained access to diagnostic technologies and weak drug supply chains. These systemic constraints have the greatest impact on marginalized populations, in which access to reliable and effective TB care is compounded by geographic and economic access barriers. The global TB report underscores that despite advances in treatment options, the slow progress in TB control reflects persistent social inequities that underlie the disease's epidemiology (Chakaya et al., 2021). These disparities require policy interventions focusing on increasing equitable access to healthcare, enhancing nutritional care, and tackling social determinants of TB causal factors like undernutrition and household air pollution exposure, which are major drivers of TB prevalence and unsuccessful treatment in poorer socioeconomically disadvantaged groups. Chronic social determinants like unemployment, poor education level, and comorbid chronic conditions like diabetes add to the DS-TB treatment adherence and success problems. These conditions not only increase the risk of infection but also hinder the capacity of patients to adhere to the stringent and extended antibiotic regimens needed to guarantee the total elimination of *Mycobacterium tuberculosis* (MTB). The interaction between socioeconomic position and treatment outcomes is important; for example, those with stable incomes and social support are likely to receive regular healthcare and follow treatment guidelines, minimizing the potential for relapse and resistance development (Uddin et al., 2021). In addition, incorporating socioeconomic factors into TB programs would enhance patient retention and cure rates, given that comprehensive solutions for poverty and hunger in addition to clinical treatment are requisite to achieving global TB elimination targets set by health leaders (Chakaya et al., 2021).

6.2. Pathophysiology of TB

The multifaceted interactions between MTB and the host immune system are the basis of tuberculosis pathophysiology and play a very important role in determining outcomes of therapy. The bacilli target alveolar macrophages after inhalation, which triggers a local immune response that produces granulomas—organized groups of cells that try to encapsulate the infection. *Mtb*, though, can remain within granulomas in a latent form, dodging immune elimination and exhibiting phenotypic drug resistance. This dormant infection is a therapeutic challenge because the metabolic dormancy of bacteria lowers susceptibility to the usual anti-tubercular (ATT) drugs, requiring longer treatment courses to completely eliminate them. Knowledge of these long-term bacterial populations is important for maximizing DS-TB treatment because it indicates the necessity of regimens that penetrate granulomatous lesions and be effective against both actively dividing and resting bacilli. Complicating the management of DS-TB is the emergent understanding of biofilm-like forms that *Mtb* can assume within the host.

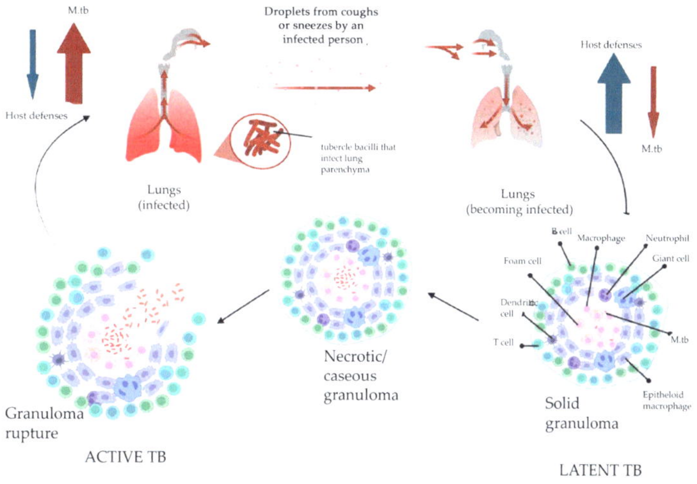

Figure 6.1. Schematic representation of tuberculosis pathogenesis. Infection with *Mycobacterium tuberculosis* occurs when aerosol droplets containing tubercle bacilli from an actively infected person reach the alveoli of an uninfected contact.

Source: Mancuso G, Midiri A, De Gaetano S, Ponzo E, Biondo C. Tackling Drug-Resistant Tuberculosis: New Challenges from the Old Pathogen *Mycobacterium tuberculosis*. *Microorganisms*. 2023; 11(9):2277. https://doi.org/10.3390/microorganisms11092277

Biofilms are organized groups of cells trapped within extracellular matrices that present physical and chemical barriers to the penetration of antibiotics, leading to phenotypic drug resistance. Development of such biofilms in combination with bacterial persistence strategies like metabolic adaptations to stationary phases and phenotypic switching prolong the time needed to effectively clear TB infection. Such bacterial subpopulations have also changed antibiotic susceptibility profiles, necessitating protracted and combination therapies capable of reaching the heterogeneous bacterial populations within the host. Augmenting our knowledge of these biofilm-related states may lead to adjunctive therapies against recalcitrant bacilli, thus enhancing treatment outcomes and the duration of treatment (Kaur et al., 2022). Apart from bacterial elements, host hereditary vulnerability also plays a role in TB pathophysiology and the ensuing treatment outcomes. For example, mitochondrial genetics' role in contributing to oxidative damage in the course of ATT illustrates the host-bacterial interaction. A few patients on routine regimens, especially with long-term use of ethambutol, experience optic neuropathy associated with mitochondrial dysfunction. Such toxicity indicates that the efficacy and safety of treatment are not entirely drug susceptibility profile-related but also host-biologically variable. Identification of genetic predispositions may assist in modifying drug regimens to ensure an optimal balance between efficacy and toxicity and guide clinical decisions in treating DS-TB. Thus, incorporating knowledge from mitochondrial genetics into the knowledge of TB pathophysiology can not only maximize therapeutic benefits but also reduce the complications of treatment (Kaur et al., 2022) (Figure 6.1).

6.2.1. Mechanism of Infection

The pathogenesis of tuberculosis begins when MTB bacilli are inhaled and reach the alveoli of the lungs, where they encounter resident macrophages. These immune cells attempt to phagocytose and contain the bacteria; however, *Mtb* possesses multiple virulence factors that allow it to evade destruction. The bacilli can inhibit phagosome-lysosome fusion, enabling intracellular survival and replication. This primary infection tends to become latent because the host immune response limits the spread within granulomatous lesions. Knowledge of this initial interaction between the pathogen and the host immune system is key to optimizing treatment timing and type of DS-TB. Interventions are directed at both actively growing bacteria and those in a resting form within granulomas, highlighting the importance of extended multidrug regimens that take into account the complex microbial microenvironment within the lungs (Ang et al., 2024). After the initial immune response, the mode of infection changes based on host immunity and bacterial determinants. Where immunological control is lost, the bacteria spread and result in productive pulmonary disease with tissue necrosis and cavitation. Not only do such pathological alterations worsen symptoms but enhance infectiousness, leading to airborne transmission. Treating DS-TB must thus target various growth phases of the bacteria and metabolic forms to avoid failure of treatment and resistance emergence. Recent progress emphasizes the value of prompt diagnosis and drug-susceptibility testing that consider the infections dynamic nature, enabling individualized pharmacologic regimens that maximize therapeutic activity while minimizing toxicity (Ang et al., 2024).

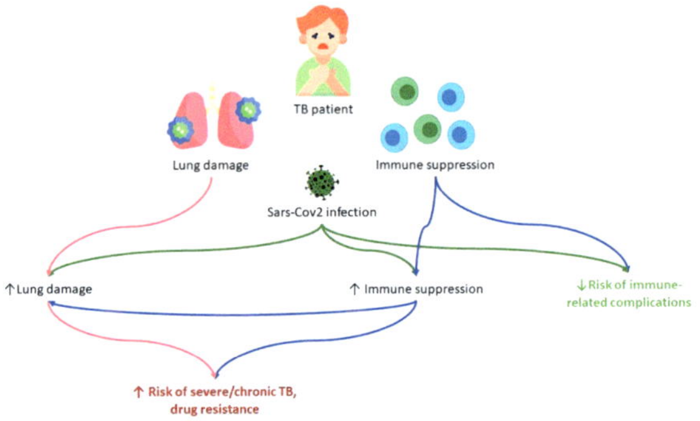

Figure 6.2. The supposed mechanisms of SARS-CoV-2 infection influence on tuberculosis infection. Tuberculosis infection contributes either lung damage and general immune suppression, which is enforced by SARS-CoV-2 infection and predisposes to the development of severe/chronic tuberculosis with drug resistance.

Source: Starshinova AA, Kudryavtsev I, Malkova A, Zinchenko U, Karev V, Kudlay D, Glushkova A, Starshinova AY, Dominguez J, Villar-Hernández R, et al. Molecular and Cellular Mechanisms of *M. tuberculosis* and SARS-CoV-2 Infections—Unexpected Similarities of Pathogenesis and What to Expect from Co-Infection. International Journal of Molecular Sciences. 2022; 23(4):2235. https://doi.org/10.3390/ijms23042235

Further, household contact studies in high-burden settings also shed light on how the infections spread at the population level. Contact with infected cases often leads to latent or active TB in close contacts, and so early diagnosis and preventive treatment are crucial. Immunodiagnostic methods like interferon-gamma release assays (IGRAs) identify infection prior to clinical disease, and intervention can be initiated in time. The latent bacteria remain in a resting form, which can be reactivated particularly if immunity declines. DS-TB regimens capitalize on multi-drug combinations to clear both replicating and non-replicating bacilli, reducing the risk of relapse. The addition of a test-and-treat approach for contacts further strengthens control by cutting off transmission at its source, illustrating how knowledge of infection mechanisms translates into public health and clinical management interventions (Figure 6.2).

6.2.2. Immune Response to TB Bacteria

The multifaceted interaction between MTB and the host immune response is the key to the development and management of DS-TB. During infection, the bacteria are phagocytosed by alveolar macrophages, which trigger a complex cascade of immune events. The macrophages try to harbor the pathogen in granulomas, specialized structures that are intended to localize and limit bacterial expansion. Nonetheless, the virulence of TB bacteria can interfere with usual cellular functions by inhibiting key bacterial enzymes like 4-hydroxy-tetrahydrodipicolinate reductase (DapB), which is vital for ensuring bacterial cell wall stability. Inhibition of DapB would compromise the bacterial defenses and increase susceptibility to immune clearance and treatment with antibiotics. Such molecular therapies highlight the synergy between host immunity mechanisms and pharmacological interventions in combating TB bacteria (Ang et al., 2024). This combined strategy is an example of how impairing bacterial metabolism not only suppresses bacterial growth but also supports immune function in eliminating the infection. Cellular bioenergetics are critical to controlling the immune response during TB infection, especially in blood lymphocytes and monocytes. The metabolic wellness of these immune cells determines their ability to effectively respond to the pathogen. During DS-TB infection, oxidative phosphorylation and glycolytic function in such cells are severely compromised early, limiting their capacity to respond optimally. Successful treatment of TB, however, is accompanied by gradual normalization of bioenergetic metrics such as spare respiratory capacity and maximal rates of respiration, which map to enhanced immune cell function. Restoration of these metabolic processes is essential for coordinating optimal immune responses, dampening inflammation, and minimizing tissue destruction. Therefore, treatment regimens for TB not only need to aim for bacterial killing but also assist the metabolic robustness of immune cells (Bridgette et al., 2024). Coordination of immune response is further intensified by sophisticated cytokine signaling networks that enable interaction among immune cells throughout the process of TB treatment. With the progression of treatment, a very synchronized network is realized, indicating improved immune regulation and control of infection-induced inflammation. This restoration of immunometabolic homeostasis at the system level is crucial for avoiding bacterial reactivation and facilitating healing. The coordination between bioenergetic recovery and cytokine signaling proposes potential therapeutic targets focused on enhancing immune strength with minimal collateral tissue damage. Therefore, knowledge of immune cell metabolism and signaling pathways and their modulation might complement conventional DS-TB treatment approaches, potentially hastening patient cure and long-term outcomes. These observations highlight the need for incorporating immunometabolic support into holistic TB treatment strategies (Bridgette et al., 2024) (Figure 6.3).

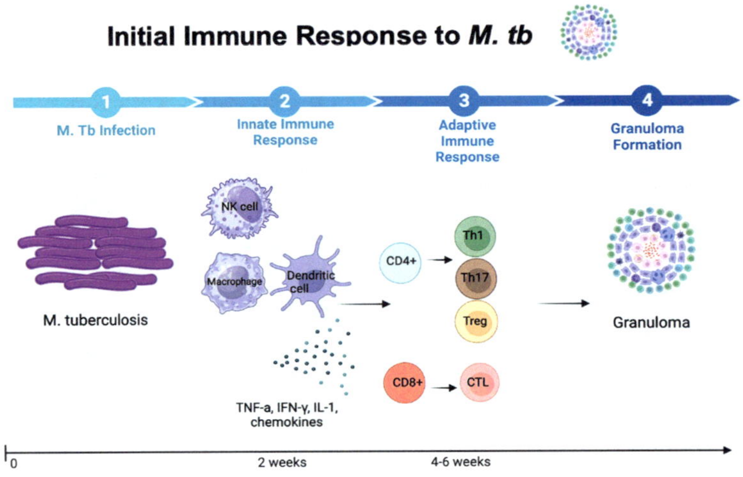

Figure 6.3. Schematic representation of three modes of interaction of the tubercle *Bacillus* with a macrophage. Panel A: The macrophage kills the organism. Panel B: The organism kills the macrophage. Panel C: The organism takes up residence in the macrophage and establishes chronic infection, where both the tubercle *Bacillus* and macrophage can survive together in a tenuous chronic infection.

Source: Hosseinian K, Gerami A, Bral M, Venketaraman V. *Mycobacterium tuberculosis*–Human Immunodeficiency Virus Infection and the Role of T Cells in Protection. Vaccines. 2024; 12(7):730. https://doi.org/10.3390/vaccines12070730

6.2.3. Progression from Latent to Active TB

The shift from latent to active tuberculosis (TB) is a pivotal point in the natural history of disease, profoundly shaping treatment strategies for DS-TB. In the latent phase, MTB is dormant in the host, regulated by a functioning immune response, making the subject non-contagious and frequently asymptomatic. Disrupting this balance through factors undermining immunity, like HIV infection, can lead to bacterial re-activation and resultant active disease. This risk of reactivation adds to the necessity of detecting LTBI among at-risk populations and starting preventive therapy to prevent advancement. Complicating this situation is co-infection with HIV, which heightens the struggle for TB control through interactions between antiretroviral and anti-TB medication as well as possible onset of immune reconstitution inflammatory syndrome (IRIS), an immune reconstitution phenomenon that paradoxically complicates patient outcomes during treatment (Jadhav et al., 2024). Comprehension of these dynamics is critical to maximizing DS-TB treatment and minimizing morbidity and mortality. Developments in immunomodulatory therapies have introduced another level of complexity to TB control and the risk of latent to active disease progression. Interfering agents with immunological signaling pathways, especially tumor necrosis factor (TNF) inhibitors, have been shown to increase the risk of reactivation of latent TB, and thus careful screening and prophylaxis must be initiated prior to starting such therapies. On the other hand, there is new evidence that newer biologics against pathways like IL-17 and IL-23 are less likely to cause reactivation of TB, leading to a reconsideration of blanket preventive treatment policies for all immunomodulators (Torres et al., 2024) (Figure 6.4).

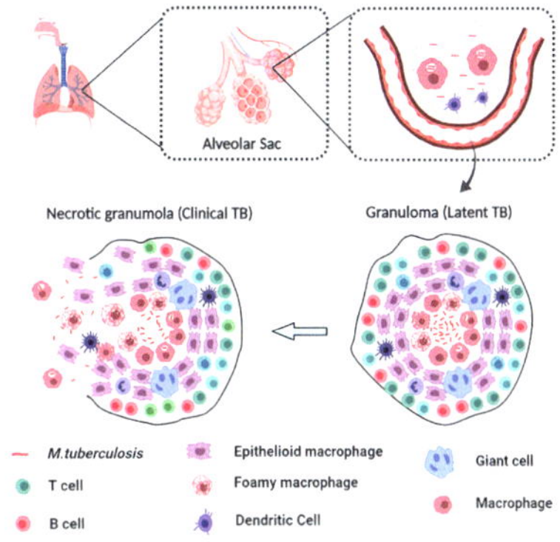

Figure 6.4. TB pathogenesis and progression of latent TB to clinical TB.

Source: ResearchGate. (n.d.). *TB pathogenesis and progression from latent to clinical tuberculosis.* https://www.researchgate.net/figure/TB-pathogenesis-and-progression-of-latent-TB-to-clinical-TB_fig1_359123555.

This subtle assessment encourages individualized risk evaluation in patients undergoing such treatments, weighing the advantages of immune modulation against the possibility of promoting TB reactivation. These concepts are critical to informing DS-TB treatment guidelines, especially for immunosuppressed individuals.

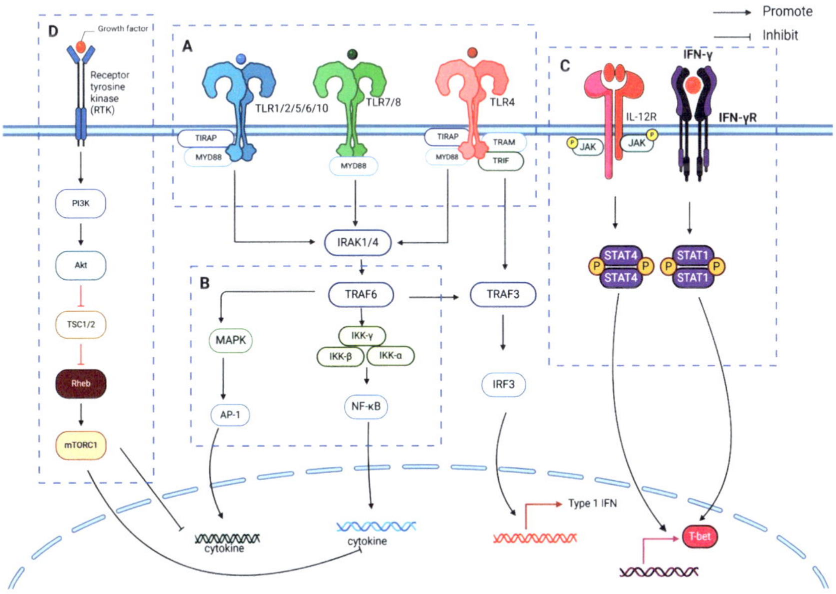

Figure 6.5. Schematic representation of the IL-12/IFN-γ pathway illustrating various activation pathways associated with the killing of intracellular bacterial organisms such as *M. tuberculosis* (*Mtb*) and Salmonella.

Source: Wang H, Ruan G, Li Y, Liu X. The Role and Potential Application of IL-12 in the Immune Regulation of Tuberculosis. International Journal of Molecular Sciences. 2025; 26(7):3106. https://doi.org/10.3390/ijms26073106

Even with these clinical developments, the development of latent to active TB is still a major public health issue, particularly among high HIV prevalence settings. The two-way interaction between HIV and TB enhances the severity of disease and complicates therapy, leading to increased mortality levels worldwide. Besides immunosuppression-induced activation, diagnostic gaps and treatment deficiencies of LTBI significantly account for transmission and relapse. In addition, the emergence of DR-TB strains makes it more challenging, with an accentuation on not just therapeutic treatments for DS-TB but also overall strategies for co-infection and management of latent disease (Jadhav et al., 2024). Ongoing research and clinical guidelines with revisions need to focus on early intervention and integration into care services to reduce the development from latent to active TB, finally to enhance patient outcomes and stem the tide of the global burden of TB (Figure 6.5).

6.3. Standard Treatment Regimens

Treating DS-TB has also seen major improvements due to changing clinical evidence and advances in technology. Treatment regimens are mainly driven by the need to balance safety, efficacy, and patient compliance, with recent revisions focusing on shorter regimens that improve patients' compliance without affecting outcomes. Singapore's National TB Programs (NTPs) multidisciplinary panel reviewed existing international and local guidelines to revise clinical management practice. These initiatives included recent trial results, allowing for implementing streamlined regimens that shorten treatment duration with retention of efficacy in curing DS-TB infection and disease. Moreover, including new diagnostic modalities like next-generation sequencing (NGS) for drug susceptibility testing (DST) guides the choice of regimen to allow for accurate and individualized treatment strategies. These adjustments embody a blend of clinical severity and practicality towards enhancing patient outcomes across various healthcare environments (Ang et al., 2024). Children and youths constitute a special group within the context of DS-TB management, requiring specialized therapeutic regimens that take into consideration differences in development and physiology. Internationally accepted clinical practices place significant emphasis on weight-based dosing and early therapy initiation, especially in fulminant conditions like TB meningitis and disseminated disease. Individualized treatment regimens are stressed to ensure proper drug exposure with minimal risk of resistance development or subtherapeutic response. In addition, increasing consensus points toward the necessity for community-based support for treatment and age-targeted care to maximize adherence and clinical outcomes. These strategies reflect a holistic model in which the standard regimens are modified to suit the individual pediatric populations in light of the fact that successful TB control goes beyond the realm of pharmacology to include psychosocial support and surveillance (Chiang et al., 2023). Standard DS-TB treatment regimens typically include an intensive phase that is followed by a continuation phase, conventionally using a combination of first-line anti-TB medications like isoniazid, rifampicin, pyrazinamide, and ethambutol (HRZE). More recently, clinical guidelines have supported shorter treatment regimens grounded on evidence from more recent trials that preserve therapeutic efficacy while diminishing patient load and healthcare expenditure. Shorter regimens also facilitate more effective resource use, vital in endemic settings where the disease burden is still significant. Supplementing drug-based approaches, the revised managements incorporate newer technologies such as artificial intelligence (AI) computer-aided radiological screening and video-observed therapy to improve diagnosis accuracy and treatment adherence, respectively. All these components collectively create an integrated and dynamic strategy for standard regimens of treatment, paramount in the attainment of long-term control of DS-TB (Ang et al., 2024).

6.3.1. First-Line Anti-TB Medications

Successful control of DS-TB depends significantly on an established regimen of first-line anti-TB drugs, which have proven successful in MTB eradication. The drugs are usually HRZE and are the foundation of routine TB treatment because of their strong bactericidal and sterilizing action.

Their administration is phased strategically, commencing with an intensive phase to quickly decrease the bacterial burden, followed by a continuation phase to kill any remaining bacilli and forestall relapse. Nevertheless, the clinical value of these drugs is frequently threatened by adverse drug reactions (ADRs), which can impair treatment effectiveness and compliance. A cohort in the Philippines has had an ADR incidence near 9% with skin reactions and hepatitis being frequent presentations. Among these drugs, rifampicin is most often implicated, emphasizing the importance of close monitoring during treatment (Jorge et al., 2024).

These results emphasize the fine balance between therapeutic effectiveness and drug tolerability in TB treatment. Adjunctive issues in the administration of first-line anti-TB agents involve their safety profile, particularly in exposed groups such as children with manifestations of extrapulmonary tuberculosis (EPTB) including tuberculous meningitis (TBM). Studies have compared combined regimens that include conventional first-line drugs in combination with other antimicrobials for differences in efficacy as well as adverse effects. In a comparative study, the conventional four-drug HRZE regimen was evaluated in comparison with the combination including linezolid (HRZEL) in pediatric TBM cases. Although clinical, including cerebrospinal fluid (CSF) improvement and microbiological clearance, outcomes did not vary significantly, hematologic and gastrointestinal adverse effects occurred more frequently under the HRZEL regimen, necessitating frequent changes in treatment (Ai et al., 2024).

This finding highlights the utmost significance of balancing the merits of intensified regimens with increased risk of toxicity in treating complicated cases as part of the overall first-line treatment strategy. Knowledge of the pharmacological properties and limitations of first-line anti-TB drugs is essential to maximize DS-TB treatment regimens. These drugs not only act against fast-growing bacilli but also exhibit mycobactericidal activity against semi-dormant cells and are, therefore, crucial for preventing relapse of the disease. However, first-line agents' tendency to cause ADRs that need effective patient monitoring to guarantee treatment completion and avoid drug resistance generation. Harmonization of clinical information from geographically and demographically different backgrounds identifies uniformity in patterns of ADRs, supporting international use of standard regimens as well as promoting local caution.

Moreover, new drugs or drug combinations, regardless of their potential to improve therapeutic effects, need to be thoroughly examined for safety profiles in order to avoid compromising treatment compliance (Ai et al., 2024; Jorge et al., 2024). As a result, initial anti-TB drug regimens continue to form the foundation of DS-TB treatment, supported by evidence-based practices aiming to optimize both efficacy and tolerability (Figure 6.6).

Drug classification	Drugs	Route of administration	Dosage form	Half-life (Hours)	Bioavailability (Percentage)
First-line drugs	Isoniazid	Oral	Tablet	1–4 h	78 – 93%
	Rifampicin	Oral	Tablet	2–5 h	71–87%
	Pyrazinamide	Oral	Tablet	9–10 h	–10 h
	Ethambutol	Oral	Tablet	3–4 h	82–87%
Second-line drugs	Streptomycin	*i.m*	Powder for solution for injection	2– 4 h	84–88%
	Amikacin	*i.m., i.v*	Solution for injection, powder for injection	2–3 h	95.2%
	Kanamycin	*i.m., i.v*	Solution for injection, powder for injection	4–6 h	very low
	Ofloxacin	Oral, *i.v*	Tablet, infusion	5–8 h	85–95%
	Levofloxacin	Oral, *i.v*	Tablet, powder for injection, oral solution	4–7 h	80–100%
	Moxifloxacin	Oral, *i.v*	Tablet, infusion	12–14 h	90%
	Ciprofloxacin	Oral, *i.v*	Tablet, infusion	4 h	70–80%
	Clarithromycin	Oral	Tablet, granules for oral suspension	2 h	55%
	Cycloserine	Oral	Capsule	16–20 h	80%
	Para-amino salicylic acid	Oral	Delayed-release granules	1 h	20%
	Clofazimine	Oral	Soft-gel capsule	10 days	68 – 95%
	Capreomycin	*i.m., i.v*	Powder for injection	4.8 ± 1 h	59%
	Ethionamide	Oral	Tablet	2–3 h	90–100%
	Prothionamide	Oral	Tablet	1.5–2 h	33%
	Terizidone	Oral	Capsule	5.27–17.8 h	100%
	Rifabutin	Oral	Tablet	ablett	20%
	Linezolid	oral, *i.v*	Tablet, infusion	5–7 h	100%
	Bedaquiline	Oral	Tablet	164 days	Unknown
	Pretomanid	Oral	Tablet	ableta	ablet

Figure 6.6. WHO recommended doses of the first line anti-TB drugs.

Source: Nair, A., Greeny, A., Nandan, A. *et al.* Advanced drug delivery and therapeutic strategies for tuberculosis treatment. *J Nanobiotechnol* **21**, 414 (2023). https://doi.org/10.1186/s12951-023-02156-y

This table includes all the first-line and second-line ATDs and their pharmacokinetic parameters. As per WHO guidelines, the standard 6-month regimen for the treatment of drug-susceptible

TB includes daily administration of isoniazid (H), rifampicin (R), pyrazinamide (Z), and ethambutol (E) for two months, followed by daily administration of isoniazid and rifampicin for an additional four months; 2HRZE/4HR. There is a new recommendation for the treatment of people aged 12 years or older with drug-susceptible pulmonary TB that they may receive a 4 month regimen of isoniazid (H), rifapentine (P), moxifloxacin (M), and pyrazinamide (Z); 2HPMZ/2HPM. Second-line drugs are used when treatment with first-line drugs fails or in the presence of multidrug-resistant TB (MDR-TB). Levofloxacin, moxifloxacin, clofazimine, linezolid, bedaquiline and pretomanid are the prominent drugs under drug-resistant TB treatment regimens. *i.m.* intramuscular, *i.v.* intravenous

6.3.2. Duration of Treatment

Successful treatment of DS-TB involves following a precisely measured duration of therapy, striking a balance between pathogen clearance and patient compliance and toxicity. The typical treatment period is six months, with a combination of antibiotics aimed at full clearance of bacteria and minimizing relapse. The duration is determined from clinical trials showing best outcomes, but longer or shorter durations can be undertaken based on the patient's clinical outcome and comorbid conditions. The presence of factors such as co-infection with HIV, malnutrition, or depression may complicate the treatment process, potentially affecting adherence and response to therapy. For instance, depression, prevalent in more than half of certain DS-TB patient populations, can indirectly influence treatment length by affecting patients' ability to comply fully with the regimen, ultimately impacting cure rates and morbidity (Olarewaju et al., 2025). These psychosocial parameters underscore the need for tailoring treatment duration while conforming to standardized schemes. New studies concerning genetic and transcriptomic patterns of MTB strains are important in providing insights into variables likely to extend the treatment duration beyond the standard six months. Comparative genomic analysis has shown certain types of genetic mutations such as non-synonymous single-nucleotide polymorphisms in the *pe_pgrs9* and *ppe34* genes that occur only in cases of prolonged treatment. In addition, these isolates demonstrate differential expression of genes, including enhanced expression of virulence-related proteins and downregulation of ribosomal protein expression, that may aid in persistence and resistance to antibiotic attack (Ko et al., 2024). Such molecular changes may fuel extended infections, requiring prolonged therapy to totally eliminate. This new evidence indicates that the best treatment duration for DS-TB is not strictly based on clinical factors but also at the level of the bacterial genome and transcriptome, making it crucial to study further in order to customize treatment durations appropriately.

The complexities of treatment duration need to be explored to maximize DS-TB management while ensuring minimized risks for under- and overtreatment. Variations from the routine six-month duration are at times required when slower clinical or microbiological responses among patients may result from host factors like immunocompetence or bacterial factors like those elucidated by genomic heterogeneity (Ko et al., 2024; Olarewaju et al., 2025). Long-term treatment is at risk of enhanced toxicity, patient exhaustion, and cost burden, justifying the requirement for appropriate biomarkers to foretell those likely to gain from brevity or extended periods of treatment. On the other hand, drug withdrawal too early may result in relapse and drug resistance. Accordingly, whereas the six-month timeframe continues as the basis of therapy, current research combining clinical, psychosocial, and molecular information holds the potential to optimize treatment durations, enhancing outcomes and maintaining antibiotic effectiveness against varied patient and pathogen variables (Figure 6.7).

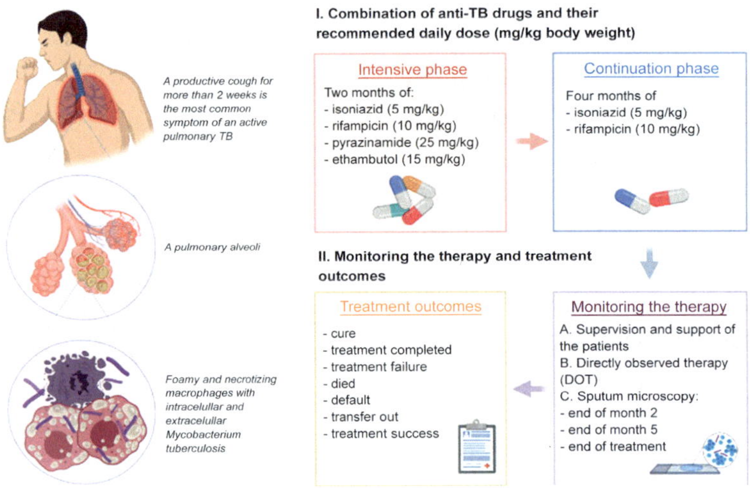

Figure 6.7. Chemotherapy for drug-susceptible tuberculosis (DS-TB).

Source: Springer Nature. (n.d.). *Anti-TB drug regimen, treatment monitoring, and outcomes.* https://media.springernature.com/lw685/springer-static/image/chp%3A10.1007%2F978-3-031-15955-8_13/MediaObjects/497831_1_En_13_Fig2_HTML.png.

6.3.3. Importance of Adherence to Treatment

Effective control of DS-TB relies heavily on adherence of patients to ongoing treatment regimens. Disruptions or early termination of treatment can lead to bacterial persistence or recurrence, which can make a potentially curable infection turn into a more lethal, drug-resistant strain. Complexity of treatment, which usually incorporates multiple drugs spanning many months, requires strict adherence to prevent suboptimal drug levels that do not eliminate MTB effectively. This threat emphasizes the necessity of strong patient education and systemic support to promote uninterrupted medication taking. In addition, the global tuberculosis burden continues to be significant with high rates of incidence focusing in resource-poor settings where impediments to adherence like stigma, economic challenge, and restricted healthcare access exist. Promoting adherence is therefore not only a matter of clinical necessity but also a public health needs to prevent transmission and meet goals defined by tuberculosis control programs globally (Chakaya et al., 2021). The implications of non-adherence go beyond the determinants of individual health and represent serious challenges to public health structures. If patients fail to finish their complete regimen of DS-TB treatment, the risk of MDR-TB development is greatly enhanced, making it difficult to manage future therapy and overloading healthcare systems with more costly, longer, and more toxic treatment options. In this regard, adherence promotes individual cure as well as community health by avoiding the development of resistance strains. Development in treatment regimens, such as shorter and better-tolerated ones, is aimed at mitigating compliance problems, but global strategies encompassing therapeutic drug monitoring (TDM), counseling of the patient, and ongoing follow-up continue to be essential. Adherence emphasis is in line with the objectives of the World Health Organization (WHO) and national policies to enhance cure rates and overall TB morbidity and mortality (Nahid et al., 2019). Maintaining adherence to DS-TB treatment also has psychological and socioeconomic aspects that need to be addressed by health programs. Patients are frequently confronted with side effects, socioeconomic stressors, and practical difficulties that compromise their ability to sustain prolonged therapy. Adopting community-based support systems, direct observed therapy (DOT), and social rewards has been demonstrated to improve adherence, minimize treatment default, and assure improved health outcomes.

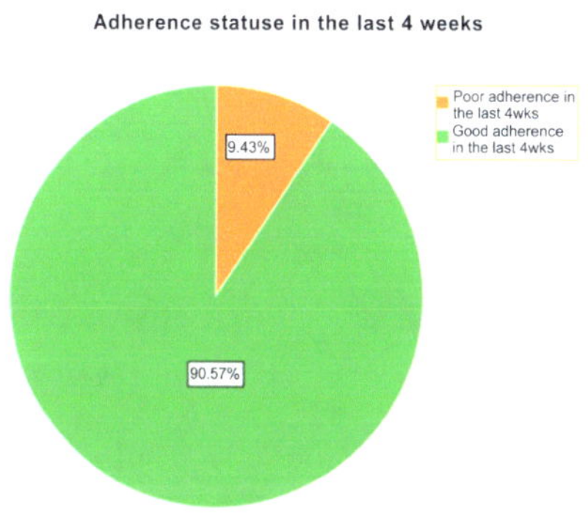

Figure 6.8. Factors identified by patients as affecting adherence to TB therapy.

Source: Gebremariam, R.B., Wolde, M. & Beyene, A. Determinants of adherence to anti-TB treatment and associated factors among adult TB patients in Gondar city administration, Northwest, Ethiopia: based on health belief model perspective. *J Health Popul Nutr* **40**, 49 (2021). https://doi.org/10.1186/s41043-021-00275-6

Realizing that adherence is a dynamic process that is affected by individual, social, and structural factors is necessary when designing patient-centered interventions. Bolstering adherence ultimately leads to ending the cycle of infection and re-infection, ultimately aligning with global efforts towards tuberculosis elimination. Prioritizing compliance therefore represents an all-encompassing strategy, unifying clinical effectiveness with sociocultural factors essential to the success of DS-TB treatment (Chakaya et al., 2021; Nahid et al., 2019) (Figure 6.8).

6.4. Challenges in Treatment

Successful DS-TB treatment demands strict patient compliance with comparatively long courses of medication, frequently spanning six months. Yet one of the key challenges facing DS-TB management is sustaining high cure rates with treatment in the face of obstacles including ADRs and socioeconomic factors. For instance, research shows that side effects of antitubercular drugs can decrease patients' compliance with treatment, thus raising the chances of treatment failure or loss to follow-up (LTFU). Additionally, mental health status upon initiation of treatment is also important in determining outcomes; non-depressed persons are likely to have successful treatment outcomes. These issues mandate integrated patient management approaches that extend beyond treatment alone and include psychosocial support for the purpose of enhancing compliance and preventing adverse effects, hence promoting greater overall treatment effectiveness (Djochie et al., 2025). Alongside patient-related characteristics, clinical markers like baseline body weight and weight increase over the course of therapy have been recognized as significant predictors of outcomes for DS-TB. Those who gain 3 kilograms or more during treatment have considerably higher proportions of good outcomes, indicating that nutritional status has an important impact on recovery. Low body weight at treatment initiation is associated with a greater risk of poor outcomes, which supports the importance of nutritional interventions within TB care programs. To address such challenges includes ensuring consistent observation of patients' physical well-being and supportive care that promotes good nutritional intake. Such complex measures are central to addressing biological and treatment-related barriers to suboptimal outcomes in DS-TB therapy (Djochie et al., 2025). Although DS-TB treatment itself poses significant challenges, the larger context of TB treatment programs must also take into account the increasing danger of drug-resistant strains. MDR-TB places further demand on healthcare systems, with longer, more costly, and less successful treatment regimens. The continued poor outcome in high-burden countries highlights systemic issues, such as weak healthcare infrastructure and limited access to early diagnostics and treatments. These challenges indirectly affect DS-TB management, as scarcity issues may limit the availability of comprehensive care and patient follow-up. In addition, initial treatment weight is a still pivotal factor predicting treatment response, emphasizing the interdependence of clinical and systemic issues. Interdisciplinary therapeutic strategies and tailored care models are acutely needed to manage these overlapping issues and enhance outcomes in both drug-susceptible and DR-TB patients.

6.4.1. Drug Resistance and Its Implications

Successful treatment of tuberculosis relies on proper drug susceptibility determination, but drug resistance makes it difficult to the point of significantly threatening the efficacy of those efforts. Resistance to the first-line drugs rifampicin and isoniazid not only erodes standard regimens but also requires implementing more complicated, longer, and frequently more toxic regimens. In countries such as Korea, improvements in molecular drug susceptibility testing (mDST) have facilitated higher rates of detection of resistant strains, allowing for more targeted interventions. Disagreements between molecular and phenotypic drug susceptibility tests can introduce uncertainties in clinical decision-making, resulting in non-adherence to guideline-recommended regimens for MDR-TB. Education of health workers to properly interpret discordant results is important since inappropriate selection of treatment due to such discordance is responsible for continuous transmission and exacerbation of drug resistance (Shin et al., 2024). Adapting treatment regimens to drug susceptibility patterns continues to be important in addressing DR-TB adequately without compromising the effectiveness of DS-TB treatment. The public health impact of DR-TB strains goes beyond individual patient outcomes, largely impacting tuberculosis control worldwide. In settings like Zambia, research shows that a significant percentage of cases of tuberculosis, about 35%, are resistant to critical drugs like rifampicin and isoniazid.

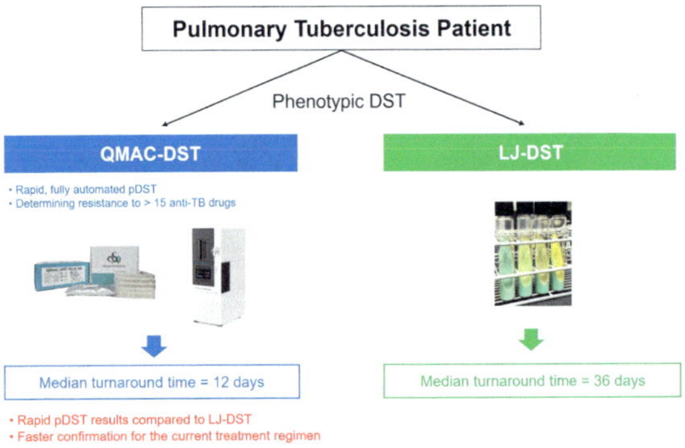

Figure 6.9. Drug resistance in pulmonary tuberculosis (PTB) patients.

Source: Kwak N, Lee S, Kim S, Song E, Yim J-J, Shim TS, Jeon D, Jhun BW, Seok K-H, Kim S, et al. QMAC-DST for Rapid Detection of Drug Resistance in Pulmonary Tuberculosis Patients: A Multicenter Pre–Post Comparative Study. Journal of Clinical Medicine. 2024; 13(10):2941. https://doi.org/10.3390/jcm13102941

The prevalence of MDR-TB, in this case, among patients with past treatment failure or LTFU, highlights systemic issues of treatment compliance and monitoring. These drug-resistant infections require increased laboratory monitoring and early detection to reduce morbidity and mortality. Additionally, the correlation between unrecognized HIV status and higher risk of isoniazid mono-resistance portends the complexities in treating co-infections that further complicate the treatment regimen. These are critical issues to address for the maintenance of gains in tuberculosis control and the effectiveness of DS-TB treatment regimens (Kangongwe et al., 2024) (Figure 6.9).

The consequences of drug resistance call for an overall response that incorporates diagnostic, treatment, and public health approaches. Failure to adhere appropriately to drug regimens and consistent diagnostic tools allows resistant organisms to grow, undermining the effectiveness of routine TB therapy and threatening global elimination efforts. The added complexity of molecular and phenotypic test variability calls for health system capacity investment and algorithm development to improve treatment accuracy. In addition, surveillance systems have to be strengthened to detect emerging resistance patterns early and update treatment recommendations accordingly. This is not only useful in containing the transmission of resistant TB strains but also helps to conserve the efficacy of available drugs, which continue to be effective for most drug-susceptible patients. Finally, the fight against drug resistance is critical to preserving the effectiveness of DS-TB treatment and enhancing patient results globally (Kangongwe et al., 2024; Shin et al., 2024).

6.4.2. Side Effects of TB Medications

The availability of first-line antitubercular therapy represented a major milestone in the fight against DS-TB, but these drugs come with their own set of complications. These regimens commonly incorporate HRZE, each of which carries with it a unique set of adverse effects. Although these drugs are needed to cure TB, their side effects can be mild or severe and may impact patient compliance and overall treatment outcome. As an example, isoniazid is notorious for hepatotoxicity, which requires close monitoring of liver function during therapy. At the same time, rifampicin can induce flu-like reactions and, less commonly, hepatotoxic effects. The wide range of side effects attributed to drugs for TB emphasizes the importance of close clinical monitoring and patient counseling to ensure that the therapeutic benefits will be greater than the risks. Adverse effect monitoring and management are essential to maximize therapeutic effectiveness and reduce treatment breaks (Muteeb et al., 2023). Neurological and gastrointestinal side effects commonly complicate treating DS-TB and present in diverse clinical patterns requiring early intervention. Peripheral neuropathy has a strong link with the use of isoniazid, due to the drug's interference with vitamin B_6 metabolism; pyridoxine supplementation is a universal preventative measure. Furthermore, pyrazinamide (PZA), while highly effective, is significantly associated with arthropathy and hyperuricemia, potentially worsening gout in predisposed persons. Nausea, vomiting, and abdominal pain commonly follow the intake of many TB drugs and affect patients' health-related quality of life as well as possibly interfere with adherence. These side effects not only depict the complexness of TB pharmacotherapy but also indicate the need for customized patient management plans to counteract adverse outcomes and ensure sustained treatment efficiency (Uddin et al., 2021). Along with acute physiological effects, there are long-term ocular and renal side effects to be considered with TB treatment using regular drugs. Ethambutol, the most important ingredient in most regimens, has a hazard associated with optic neuritis, which presents as visual impairment and can result in permanent loss of vision if undetected until late. Ophthalmologic examination is thus advisable to observe and detect visual function changes. Rifampicin is guilty of precipitating acute kidney injury (AKI) in occasional cases, underlining the need to have renal function tests during treatment. The task of weighing successful bacterial eradication against the control of such potentially dangerous side effects is further complicated by the growing resistance to drugs, which requires continuing research into alternative safer and more effective treatments. Knowledge of such side effects in the context of antitubercular therapy (ATT) continues to be important as the health community works to increase treatment compliance and patient outcomes (Muteeb et al., 2023; Uddin et al., 2021) (Figure 6.10).

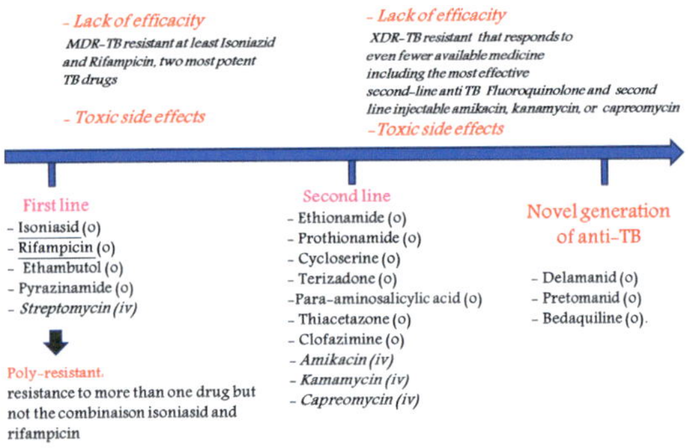

Figure 6.10. Common side effects of TB drugs.

Source: Mignani S, Tripathi RP, Chen L, Caminade A-M, Shi X, Majoral J-P. New Ways to Treat Tuberculosis Using Dendrimers as Nanocarriers. Pharmaceutics. 2018; 10(3):105. https://doi.org/10.3390/pharmaceutics10030105

6.4.3. Barriers to Accessing Treatment

Adherence to treatment for DS-TB is often undermined by systemic barriers in healthcare infrastructure. In most areas, poor access to key diagnostic equipment like functional X-ray machines inhibits effective monitoring of disease, causing delays in timely interventions. Furthermore, shortages in specialized healthcare staff, such as psychologists and nutritionists, detract from the provision of complete care appropriate to patient needs. Facility-based DOT, though designed to promote compliance, can inadvertently impose logistical challenges to patients, especially adolescents who have educational and social responsibilities. This set of barriers leads to treatment interruption and unfavorable outcomes, even with access to free TB treatment and readily accessible health centers. Such complex challenges need to be addressed by augmenting the accessibility, acceptability, and appropriateness of TB care so that it can better serve vulnerable groups with distinctive needs (Arango et al., 2025). Aggravating infrastructure problems are socioeconomic determinants that enhance barriers to regular treatment adherence. The long treatment course of DS-TB therapy frequently conflicts with patients constrained financial resources and work-related obligations, and thereby results in the omission of doses or premature cessation of treatment. Innovative adherence-support technologies, like computerized adherence tools such as clever pillboxes and medication labels, have proved promising in mitigating some of these burdens by offering daily reminders and lowering the number of in-person encounters. These digital interventions also build stronger patient-provider relationships, ultimately leading to improved treatment engagement. Nevertheless, their potential is limited by issues including variability in access to cellphones, dependence on electricity for device operation, and network connectivity problems; issues especially common in low-resource environments (Gon et al., 2024). In addition to logistical and technical challenges, psychosocial factors pose important but frequently underappreciated impediments to DS-TB treatment access. Stigma against TB may discourage patients from initiating or continuing treatment, while insufficient emotional and educational support aggravates feelings of isolation during treatment. Adolescents in particular illustrate an urgent need for adolescent-centered services that foster trust and decrease treatment anxiety. Without adequate counseling and empowerment by healthcare providers, patients feel unsupported, which raises the risk of disengagement from care. Therefore, interventions that combine psychological care with medical treatment must be implemented to enhance adherence and outcomes of treatment. Priorities should be placed on enhancing the patient experience through the elimination of both emotional and practical barriers in order to overcome ingrained barriers to effective TB treatment (Arango et al., 2025).

6.5. Monitoring and Follow-Up

Optimal management of DS-TB transcends the treatment initiation to include strict monitoring and follow-up procedures. These are essential to guarantee that patients stick to prescribed regimens and to detect early arising complications or drug resistance. Adherence is particularly important owing to the protracted therapy and complexity of multi-drug regimens, which may result in serious difficulties with patient compliance. Monitoring involves frequent clinical evaluations, laboratory examinations, and sputum cultures to monitor microbiological responses and identify potential ADRs. How crucial it is to incorporate molecular diagnostic tools early in treatment cannot be overemphasized since these resources facilitate guiding pathogen identification and monitoring drug susceptibility, thereby optimizing treatment more appropriately. These overall surveillances enable preventing treatment failure and transmission and development of resistant strains (Bracchi et al., 2019; Dartois & Rubin, 2022). The follow-up process is marked by ongoing assessment through clinical, radiological, and laboratory examination, focusing on therapeutic effectiveness and patient safety. For example, interval chest radiographs and sputum examinations are important indicators of validating disease resolution or detecting relapse. Of similar significance is drug-related toxicity monitoring that, if undetected, can lead to premature withdrawal of treatment and exacerbation of disease. Liver function tests are used routinely because of the hepatotoxicity of first-line anti-TB drugs such as isoniazid and rifampicin, and counseling on adherence reinforces patient interaction. In addition, the overlap of TB and HIV co-infection requires highly specialized follow-up regimens taking into account changes in immune status and the risk of IRIS, highlighting the importance of a multidisciplinary team with infectious disease and HIV specialists (Bracchi et al., 2019). Follow-up on a long-term basis also supports public health's overall goal of minimizing TB spread and AMR formation. With systematic reporting and data collection, public health authorities and healthcare providers can track epidemiologic trends and resistance patterns, allowing for evidence-based policy making. Standardized monitoring protocols guarantee patient care consistency and improve outcome data reliability, as well as the ability to detect gaps in healthcare provision, especially in resource-limited settings where disease burden is most significant (Dartois & Rubin, 2022). Finally, the optimization of monitoring and follow-up strategies benefits not just the patient level but also international efforts in countering the increasing danger of DR-TB by accelerating investments in microbiology laboratory infrastructure and education to maximize diagnostic and monitoring potentials (Bracchi et al., 2019; Dartois & Rubin, 2022).

6.5.1. Importance of Regular Follow-Up Appointments

Successful management of DS-TB is greatly dependent on regular monitoring to monitor adherence to treatment regimens. Disruptions or alterations in therapy may result in suboptimal control, so it goes to relapse or progresses to DR-TB types. Routine follow-up visits allow direct healthcare provider-patient interactions, allowing for early detection of ADRs, therapeutic response evaluation, and reinforcement of medication adherence. By making these follow-up appointments, clinicians are able to modify treatment regimens as needed and continue education, which is important considering the extended length of TB treatment. It is a mistake not to keep these scheduled visits, as this jeopardizes not just individual patient health decline but also exacerbates the likelihood of ongoing spread in the community, thereby defeating public health measures. The necessity for such systematic follow-up is highlighted by the necessity to pre-empt antibiotic resistance, a worldwide increasing issue threatening the efficacy of treatment (Yamin et al., 2023). In addition, the overlap of TB treatment with general infectious disease management indicates the need for periodic patient assessments. The current COVID-19 pandemic has uncovered weaknesses in TB control programs, specifically caused by interrupted health services as well as compromised patient mobility. Regular follow-up visits are vital checkpoints to counteract these interruptions by maintaining uninterrupted treatment regardless of outside factors. These check-ups allow practitioners to screen for possible co-infections and treat comorbid conditions that can complicate treatment outcomes. In addition, quick diagnostic equipment employed in assessments allows verification of treatment outcomes or early detection of complications, enabling appropriate adjustments. The double burden of TB and COVID-19 highlighted that ongoing monitoring of TB patients is critical to enhancing individual outcomes and decreasing mortality rates related to these respiratory illnesses (Cioboat et al., 2023). Finally, routine follow-up visits are crucial in enhancing patients' quality of life during the long process of DS-TB treatment. Apart from clinical assessment, such sessions provide psychological support by resolving issues and removing fear about chronic illness management. They also serve as a forum for counseling about lifestyle changes, dietary advice, and infection control measures that are necessary for complete recuperation. Regular follow-ups reinforce trust and rapport between healthcare providers and patients and improve communication, making treatment adherence more probable. This holistic approach not only aids physical health but also counteracts stigma and social exclusion commonly faced by TB patients. Maintaining strict adherence to planned visits is therefore of critical importance to ensuring the efficacy of DS-TB treatment protocols and public health objectives.

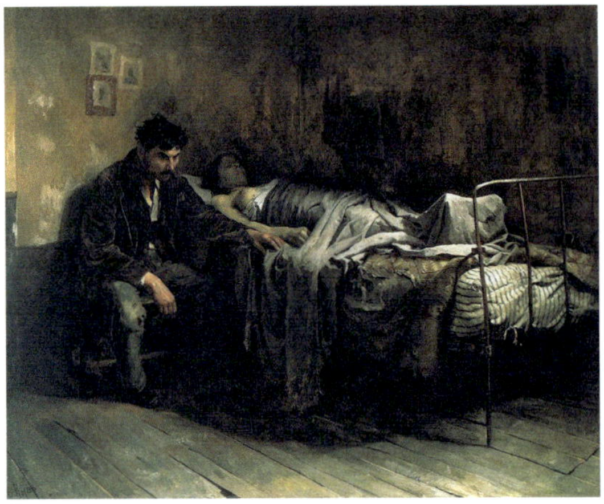

Source: By Cristóbal Rojas - Obra de arte, Pintura de Cristóbal Rojas (1857–1890) Galería de Arte Nacional, Caracas- Venezuela. - 150 Pinturas Antológicas. Juan Calzadilla. Fundación Museos Nacionales, Galería de Arte Nacional, Caracas, 2012, Public Domain, https://commons.wikimedia.org/w/index.php?curid=2566264

6.5.2. Methods for Monitoring Treatment Efficacy

Successful monitoring techniques are vital to the success of DS-TB treatment, especially considering the patient variability seen in clinical practice. Sputum culture conversion remains the gold standard for treatment efficacy monitoring, such that a negative culture at the two-month time point is taken as a good bacteriological response. This technique provides an early sign of reduced bacterial load and is widely used to predict treatment outcomes. For example, comparative trials with shorter, four-month regimens document sputum culture conversion rates that, although somewhat lower, are statistically similar to the conventional six-month therapy, emphasizing the consistency of this measure in clinical trials and daily practice (Feng et al., 2025). This type of monitoring enables clinicians to detect patients at risk of treatment failure or relapse and hence provide early intervention and regimen modification necessary for successful disease management. Besides microbiologic evaluations, clinical parameters relevant to each patient are also critical for the follow-up of treatment response, particularly in high-risk groups. For pregnant DS-TB women, HIV viral load, anemia status, and the status of EPTB have all been recognized as key predictors of unsuccessful treatment outcomes (Hernandez-Morfin et al., 2025). Monitoring these parameters helps clinicians identify patients who might need extra clinical support or individualized treatment strategies. For instance, a quantifiable HIV RNA viral load is associated with strong correlations with treatment failure, thereby identifying the importance of combined management of the two infections. Therefore, thorough monitoring incorporating bacteriological information and individualized clinical variables is responsible for enhanced treatment outcome and lowered mortality, especially in co-morbidity complicating TB control. Improvements in monitoring methods also highlight the need for real-time safety and compliance evaluations to avoid treatment discontinuation, a situation that can undermine efficacy. Although most often minor, adverse events have been highlighted as frequent causes of therapy termination, particularly among elderly and drug intolerance cohorts with lower drug tolerance (Feng et al., 2025). The regular assessment of patient tolerance by symptom reporting and laboratory indicators allows for prompt detection of toxicities, permitting dose modification or supportive care to maintain treatment compliance. In addition, ongoing patient monitoring through direct observation or electronic adherence technology guarantees the completion of prescribed therapeutic regimens. This comprehensive monitoring system, integrating microbiological, clinical, and pharmacovigilance information, is the basis for effective DS-TB treatment, preventing the occurrence of resistance development and failure of treatment.

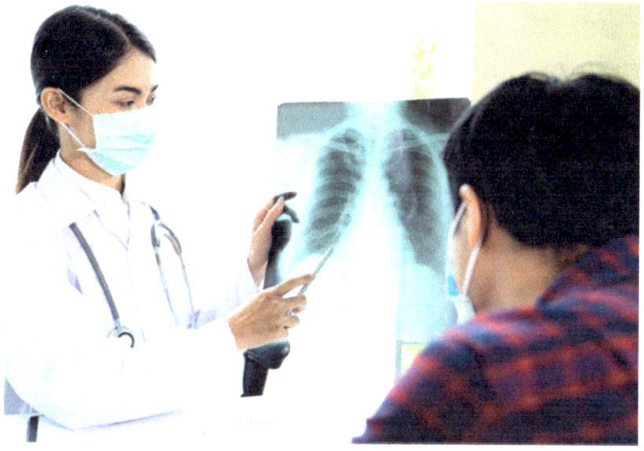

Source: Allen County Department of Health. (n.d.). *Doctor explaining chest X-ray results to a tuberculosis patient.* https://s3.us-east-2.amazonaws.com/assets.allencountyhealth.com/uploads/_960xAUTO_fit_center-center_none/Tuberculosis-lungs-xray-allen-county-department-of-health-indiana.jpg?v=1643832084.

6.5.3. Addressing Treatment Failures

One of the most important challenges in DS-TB management is the occurrence of treatment failure, which severely impairs efforts towards the eradication of the disease. Although regular TB treatment courses have demonstrated efficacy, patient-related factors such as age, nutritional status, and bacterial load can negatively impact results. The evidence indicates that elderly people and underweight individuals are most susceptible to poor treatment outcomes, such as failure, death, or LTFU. These parameters require an adaptive treatment strategy with intensified monitoring and supportive care such as nutritional support. Further, baseline smear grading, as a measure of bacterial burden, has correlated with increased failure rates and highlights the need for early and proper evaluation of severity to guide the intensity of treatment. Therefore, management of these complex risks with patient-centered, individualized strategies constitutes the first-line step in preventing DS-TB treatment failures and enhancing overall success rates (Sugiyono et al., 2025). Concurrently, the solution to treatment failure involves a wider scope focusing on healthcare system determinants of adherence and effectiveness. Drug supply chain disruptions, poor diagnostic infrastructure, and patient education deficits can lead to suboptimal adherence to therapy, creating an environment for treatment failure. Incorporating ongoing monitoring of treatment and quick response systems to developing complications is necessary in timely reaction to early signs of failure. In addition, it is crucial to promote a patient-friendly healthcare environment aligned with social and economic conditions of patients since these determinants influence treatment continuity extensively. Lessons from the management of MDR-TB emphasize the complexities in handling failures of treatment; individualized regimens, extended therapies, and intensified follow-up have become the necessity. Although the treatment for DS-TB is typically shorter and simpler, the same rule of tailoring care and system support applies to averting failure and ensuring success (Sugiyono et al., 2025). In addition, maximizing treatment outcomes for DS-TB includes proactive measures of detecting and correcting risk factors prior to and during treatment. Preemptive nutritional care among underweight patients can enhance immunocompetence and drug tolerance, thus avert failure. Likewise, advanced diagnostics that allow for quick identification of bacterial burden and drug resistance support timely modification of therapy. Integration with patient-focused models of health education, psychological support, and social services confronts obstacles to medication adherence that frequently lead to treatment failure. Use of digital health technologies for real-time monitoring might also assist healthcare professionals in monitoring patient outcomes and managing promptly adverse events. In general, an integrated approach that integrates clinical watchfulness, patient activation, and system-level interventions is essential in minimizing treatment failures in DS-TB as a step towards the achievement of world TB control goals (Sugiyono et al., 2025).

SUMMARY

The complex interaction between MTB genetic mutations and treatment duration highlights the intricacy of DS-TB management. Genomic and transcriptomic analyses within recent studies indicate that some mutations and gene expression patterns may impact increased treatment durations. Such molecular features likely affect bacterial virulence, immune evasion, and persister cell formation, all of which may complicate the efficacy of the standard six-month treatment. Recognizing these biological factors is critical for creating more personalized therapeutic approaches that can shorten treatment regimens and enhance overall patient outcome. Nevertheless, because of the small sample size and the complex nature of such findings, larger-scale and comprehensive studies are needed to conclusively determine the genetic markers linked with treatment difficulty in DS-TB (Ko et al., 2024). The treatment success dynamics among tuberculosis-HIV co-infected patients also underscore the importance of integrated clinical strategies. Evidence from DKI Jakarta illustrates that despite a high rate of successful outcomes for TB-HIV patients, the figure lags behind international targets, and there are still gaps in the care. The setting of treatment and administration of ART are among the factors that significantly contribute to successful treatment. This underscores the need for holistic care models that guarantee sustained monitoring, medication compliance, and support systems specific to vulnerable populations. Closing these gaps is vital to bring treatment success rates closer to the hoped-for 90% level, thus enhancing survival and lowering transmission within DS-TB burdened communities (Budiyani et al., 2024). The management of DS-TB is strongly driven by both microbial and patient-centric clinical practices. The convergence of the genetic data from MTB and the epidemiological data from co-morbid diseases like HIV emphasizes the many-sided aspects of TB treatment effectiveness. A strong conclusion must call for the continued research into the molecular processes of the pathogen in addition to the improved healthcare delivery mechanisms that increase patient compliance and the support. With the alignment of scientific progress and practical interventions, the international community for global health is able to progress toward more impactful treatment strategies, reduced durations of therapy, and eventually, improved tuberculosis control at the population level (Budiyani et al., 2024; Ko et al., 2024).

Successful management of DS-TB depends on high success rates in treatment, which in turn have a direct influence on patient outcomes and wider public health objectives. Recent evidence shows that about three-quarters of patients can successfully complete therapy, highlighting the need to determine factors that are predictors of successful outcomes. Baseline body weight, weight gain on treatment, HIV co-infection status, ADRs, and initial mental health status are important predictors of treatment success. Importantly, patients who gained three or more kilograms of weight during the course of treatment and had no risk of depression at baseline were significantly more likely to be completed effectively. These results indicate that treatment protocols need to extend beyond pharmacologic interventions and include nutritional support and psychological evaluation to maximize treatment effectiveness and patient compliance. Such integrative strategies are necessary in reducing LTFU, treatment failure, and death rates among DS-TB patients (Djochie et al., 2025). One area often given less attention in DS-TB treatment is the danger of acute kidney injury (AKI), which recent evidence shows to be higher than thought. Unlike conventional beliefs that TB medications are the major reason for renal impairment, kidney injury rates are found to be high even in the short-term following TB diagnosis, occurring in almost one-third of patients. This finding warrants systematic renal function assessment from the time of diagnosis, especially in endemic areas with high co-infection rates like HIV. The coexistence of proteinuria or hematuria at admission increases the risk of AKI, which in turn is independently linked with higher mortality within the first month after diagnosis. The early detection of renal impairment enables intervening measures that can potentially limit fatal consequences and enhance the safety and efficacy of TB treatment regimens (Kansiime et al., 2024). Integrating these findings brings into perspective the complexities of managing DS-TB. Combating both physiological and psychosocial risk factors is essential to improving patient outcomes and transmission restraint. Comorbid conditions such as HIV, mental well-being, and nutritional status all play a significant role in determining treatment effectiveness, and close monitoring of renal function can prevent potentially lethal complications. Models of patient-centered care that incorporate integrated comprehensive health assessments and ongoing monitoring are thus essential. Ultimately, these interventions uphold the need for customized treatment regimens for each patient based on their individual clinical profile, promoting greater adherence, fewer adverse effects, and improved global TB control (Djochie et al., 2025; Kansiime et al., 2024).

CLOSER LOOK

PATHOGENESIS AND THE ROLE OF ANTI-TB DRUGS

Tuberculosis (TB) pathogenesis, especially in cases of pulmonary TB, is caused by the complex interplay between Mycobacterium tuberculosis (M. tuberculosis) and the host immune system. Infection often starts as a result of inhalation of airborne droplets that harbor Mtb and their deposition in the lung's alveoli. The bacteria are subsequently phagocytosed by alveolar macrophages, which form the front line of the respiratory protective system. In most patients, the immune system responds by confining the infection, and granulomas form, which are groups of immune cells that try to enclose the bacteria. The granulomas prevent the infection from spreading, but the bacteria might be in a latent state in the granulomas for years and cause latent TB.

On occasion, the immune response is not sufficient to contain the infection, and the bacteria go on to grow and spread beyond the lungs, resulting in EPTB. This happens when the Mtb spreads into the bloodstream or lymphatic system and becomes potentially infective in other organs like the CNS, bones, and kidneys. The clinical presentation of active TB is a consequence of the tissue destruction due to the bacteria and the resulting immune response. This immune destruction, coupled with direct action of the bacteria, results in inflammation, necrosis of tissue, and the hallmark signs of TB such as cough, weight loss, night sweats, and fever.

The management of TB is mainly based on a combination of anti-tuberculosis (anti-TB) medications. These medications are targeted against various phases of the bacterial life cycle to kill the bacteria and avoid resistance effectively. The cornerstone of TB management is isoniazid and rifampicin, which function by inhibiting bacterial cell wall formation and RNA synthesis, respectively. Isoniazid blocks the formation of mycolic acid, an important cell wall component of the bacteria, resulting in bacterial death. Rifampicin, however, blocks the bacterial RNA polymerase and so bacterial transcription and consequently the synthesis of vital proteins.

PZA is yet another significant drug employed in TB treatment that acts by interfering with the bacterial membrane potential and enhancing acidification within the bacterial environment, eventually killing the bacteria in acidic areas of granulomas. Ethambutol acts by inhibiting mycobacterial cell wall synthesis through disruption of the arabinogalactan layer, further destabilizing the bacteria's structural integrity.

The combination of more than one drug is important in preventing drug-resistant strains, including MDR-TB and XDR-TB. These resistant strains arise when the bacteria become mutated in a way that they can survive even in the presence of drugs. The combination of drugs for TB, coupled with drug administration as per the treatment schedule, is important in successful management and the avoidance of drug resistance. The therapeutic function of anti-TB drugs is their capacity to decrease bacterial load, curtail transmission, and eventually heal the disease when used in the right manner for the entire duration of treatment.

REFERENCES

1. Ai, T., Jiang, L., Liu, Q. B., Bai, Y., Yang, Y., Sun, F. J., Jia, Y. T., et al. (2024). Efficacy and safety of first-line anti-tuberculosis drugs combined with linezolid for the treatment of pediatric tuberculous meningitis in real-world practice. *Zhonghua Er Ke Za Zhi = Chinese Journal of Pediatrics, 62*(8), 715–720. https://www.semanticscholar.org/paper/24cd13133cdeffc8a788947f9fd38242259308fd (accessed on 10 May 2025).
2. Ang, M. L. T., Chan, S. M., Cheng, L. T., Cheong, H. Y., Chew, K. L., Chlebicki, P. M., Hsu, L. Y., Kaw, G. J. L., Kee, A. C. L., Ng, M. C. W., Ong, R. T. H., Ong, C. W. M., Quah, J. L., Selvamani, D. B., Sng, L. H., Tan, J. B. X., Tan, C. H., Tay, J. Y., Teo, L. L. S., Thoon, K. C., ... Yang, Q. (2024). Singapore tuberculosis (TB) clinical management guidelines 2024: A modified Delphi adaptation of international guidelines for drug-susceptible TB infection and pulmonary disease. *Annals of the Academy of Medicine, Singapore, 53*(3), 170–186. https://doi.org/10.47102/annals-acadmedsg.2023391 (accessed on 10 May 2025).
3. Arango, D., Cintron, C., Beckhorn, C., Wong, M., Senador, L., Altamirano, E., Lecca, L., et al. (2025). Care for adolescents with drug-susceptible pulmonary tuberculosis in Lima, Peru: A qualitative assessment. *BMJ Open, 15.* https://www.semanticscholar.org/paper/bc9d738daf6ceaebeb1ade1562e1ae7bf1fd6297 (accessed on 10 May 2025).
4. Backues, K. A., & Wiedner, E. (2019). Recommendations for the diagnosis, treatment and management of tuberculosis, *Mycobacterium tuberculosis*, in elephants in human care. *International Zoo Yearbook, 53*, 116–127. https://doi.org/10.1111/izy.12221.
5. Barteka, G., Bwayo, D., Matovu, J. K. B., Wanume, B., Alunyo, J. P., Sseguya, R., Masaba, J. P., et al. (2025). Treatment outcomes and predictors of success for multidrug-resistant tuberculosis (MDR-TB) in Ugandan regional referral hospitals. *Scientific Reports, 15(1)*, 14144. https://www.semanticscholar.org/paper/1988f60527f427f586cdd274fe6766b7f55649ae (accessed on 10 May 2025).
6. Bracchi, M., van Halsema, C., Post, F. A., Awosusi, F., Barbour, A., Bradley, S. M., Coyne, K., et al. (2019). British HIV Association guidelines for the management of tuberculosis in adults living with HIV 2019. *HIV Medicine, 20.* https://doi.org/10.1111/hiv.12748.
7. Budiyani, P. I. R., Djuwita, R., Mahkota, R., & Handayani, D. (2024). Factors associated with successful drug-susceptible tuberculosis treatment among tuberculosis–human immunodeficiency virus patients in DKI Jakarta Province 2020–2022. *Asian Journal of Engineering, Social and Health.* Vol 3 No 4. https://doi.org/10.46799/ajesh.v3i4.287 (accessed on 10 May 2025).
8. Chakaya, J., Khan, M., Ntoumi, F., Aklillu, E., Fatima, R., Mwaba, P., Kapata, N., et al. (2021). Global tuberculosis report 2020–Reflections on the global TB burden, treatment and prevention efforts. *International Journal of Infectious Diseases, 113*, S7–S12. https://doi.org/10.1016/j.ijid.2021.02.107.
9. Chiang, S., Graham, S., Schaaf, H. S., Marais, B., Sant'Anna, C., Sharma, S., Starke, J., et al. (2023). Clinical standards for drug-susceptible TB in children and adolescents. *The International Journal of Tuberculosis and Lung Disease, 27*, 584–598. https://www.semanticscholar.org/paper/3abe7f02f80860c7537fe98c29471462b9d681ca (accessed on 10 May 2025).
10. Chihota, V., Gombe, M. M., Gupta, A., Salazar-Austin, N., Ryckman, T., Hoffmann, C. J., LaCourse,

S., et al. (2024). Tuberculosis preventive treatment in high TB-burden settings: A state-of-the-art review. *Drugs, 85*, 127–147. https://www.semanticscholar.org/paper/5b0d38aa635e4cb3a49dfc08867c000088702713 (accessed on 10 May 2025).

11. Cintron, C., Dauphinais, M., Fiogbe, A. A., Dogo, M. F., Ate, S., Adjonou, C., Agossou, K., et al. (2025). Impact of nutritional support for tuberculosis on intermediate and terminal undernutrition and treatment outcomes (INSTITUT) study: A protocol for a quasi-experimental study to assess the impact of nutritional support on tuberculosis treatment outcomes in Benin and Togo. *BMJ Open, 15.* https://www.semanticscholar.org/paper/bef552f3ae880c838e56b13a39d2c62922a6111a (accessed on 10 May 2025).
12. Cioboată, R., Biciușcă, V., Olteanu, M., & Vasile, C. M. (2023). COVID-19 and tuberculosis: Unveiling the dual threat and shared solutions perspective. *Journal of Clinical Medicine, 12*, 4784. https://doi.org/10.3390/jcm12144784.
13. Cumming, B. M., Addicott, K. W., Maruri, F., Pillay, V., Asmal, R., Moodley, S., Barreto-Durate, B., et al. (2024). Longitudinal mitochondrial bioenergetic signatures of blood monocytes and lymphocytes improve during treatment of drug-susceptible pulmonary tuberculosis patients. *Frontiers in Immunology, 15.* https://www.semanticscholar.org/paper/e1825d0c4e70aa8b3d02cd527c96ab266bac90d7 (accessed on 10 May 2025).
14. DeHart, Ciera, "Health Concerns in Cambodia Compounded by Historical and Rural Setbacks" (2020). Senior Honors Theses. 967. https://digitalcommons.liberty.edu/honors/967 (accessed on 10 May 2025).
15. Dartois, V., & Rubin, E. J. (2022). Anti-tuberculosis treatment strategies and drug development: Challenges and priorities. *Nature Reviews Microbiology, 20*, 685–701. https://doi.org/10.1038/s41579-022-00731-y.
16. Djochie, R. D. A., Anto, B., Opare-Addo, M., & Boakye-Yiadom, J. (2025). Factors influencing treatment success in drug-susceptible tuberculosis patients in Ghana: A prospective cohort study. *PLOS Global Public Health, 5.* https://www.semanticscholar.org/paper/fc7030beac1069cb19b1ca51efd28b21ac3b7777 (accessed on 10 May 2025).
17. Schulthess, B., & Egli, A. (2024). Tuberculosis in Times of War and Peace. *Conexus*, *7*(1), 186-212. https://doi.org/10.24445/conexus.2024.07.011 (accessed on 10 May 2025).
18. Feng, J. Y., Shu, C. C., Lin, S. M., Weng, Y. W., Chen, J. K., Wu, K. S., & Tsai, H. (2025). P-792. Evaluation of the efficacy and safety of a short-course, daily, 4-month regimen including isoniazid, pyrazinamide, rifapentine, and moxifloxacin (2HZPM/2HPM) for the treatment of drug-susceptible pulmonary tuberculosis in Taiwan (ESCAPE-TB): A multicenter study. *Open Forum Infectious Diseases, 12.* https://www.semanticscholar.org/paper/42953681526fc4c630fd1510f61836f6e929c3e1 (accessed on 10 May 2025).
19. Grace, K., Aklilu, A. M., Baluku, J., Yasmin, F., Kanyesigye, M., Muzoora, C., Wilson, F. P., et al. (2024). Incidence of acute kidney injury and associated mortality among individuals with drug-susceptible tuberculosis in Uganda. *Kidney360, 5*, 1446–1454. https://www.semanticscholar.org/paper/a112697246d42505b4cc8c63adf63aaccb8f9c25 (accessed on 10 May 2025).
20. Haworth, C., Banks, J., Capstick, T., Fisher, A. J., Gorsuch, T., Laurenson, I. F., Leitch, A., et al. (2017). British Thoracic Society guidelines for the management of non-tuberculous mycobacterial pulmonary disease (NTM-PD). *Thorax, 72*, ii1–ii64. https://doi.org/10.1136/thoraxjnl-2017-210927.

21. Hernandez-Morfin, N., Cohn, S., Waja, Z., Chaisson, R., Martinson, N., & Salazar-Austin, N. (2025). Assessing TB treatment outcomes in pregnant women living with HIV with drug-susceptible TB. *Public Health Action, 15*, 33–37. https://www.semanticscholar.org/paper/4714d51a2a7f45e4e2a9ef2a572040be097d7bfa (accessed on 10 May 2025).

22. Jadhav, S., Nair, A., Mahajan, P., & Nema, V. (2024). The crosstalk between HIV-TB co-infection and associated resistance in the Indian population. *Venereology*. https://www.semanticscholar.org/paper/ec0ba917b4046b6d47f5697dc3a65b87697fc87b (accessed on 10 May 2025).

23. Jeffry, E. P., & Seikka, C. S. (2025). A comprehensive literature review of diagnosis and management of multi-drug resistant tuberculosis. *The Indonesian Journal of General Medicine*. https://www.semanticscholar.org/paper/63e59789a6b8f7d7ec23747ecff63f951e4e4d7c (accessed on 10 May 2025).

24. Jorge, M. J., Esporlas, C. B., Largoza, M. L. E., & Zamora, R. (2024). Adverse drug events from first-line anti-tuberculosis drugs in a tertiary medical center. *European Medical Journal*. https://www.semanticscholar.org/paper/f2b2760ff576494fdead79d46619a5e1f11657b5 (accessed on 10 May 2025).

25. Kangongwe, M. H., Mwanza, W., Mwamba, M., Mwenya, J., Muzyamba, J., Mzyece, J., Hamukale, A., et al. (2024). Drug resistance profiles of *Mycobacterium tuberculosis* clinical isolates by genotype MTBDRplus line probe assay in Zambia: Findings and implications. *JAC-Antimicrobial Resistance, 6*. https://www.semanticscholar.org/paper/57e57ba8272fac79e3766a7396c819961817f9b3 (accessed on 10 May 2025).

26. Kaur, P., Singh, S., Kaur, K., Mahesh, K., Tigari, B., Sehgal, V., Takkar, A., et al. (2022). The genetics of ethambutol-induced optic neuropathy: A narrative review. *Neuro-Ophthalmology, 46*, 304–313. https://www.semanticscholar.org/paper/dae500c219ca8b323042af4b9534e63a483ff6a2 (accessed on 10 May 2025).

27. Ko, E. M., Min, J., Kim, H., Jeong, J. A., Lee, S. K., & Kim, S. H. (2024). Molecular characteristics of drug-susceptible *Mycobacterium tuberculosis* clinical isolates based on treatment duration. *Osong Public Health and Research Perspectives, 15*, 385–394. https://www.semanticscholar.org/paper/76d9dc65f3f7626d2d11ece12a111fc7dd0090cd (accessed on 10 May 2025).

28. Koroma, J. A., Mahmoud, M., Molleh, B., Sevalie, S., Chan, A., Mishra, S., Lakoh, S., et al. (2025). Effect of the COVID-19 pandemic on drug-resistant tuberculosis treatment outcomes at a national referral hospital in Sierra Leone, 2017 to 2022: A retrospective study. medRxiv 2025.03.17.25324153; doi: https://doi.org/10.1101/2025.03.17.25324153(accessed on 10 May 2025).

29. Murray, C. J. L., Ikuta, K. S., Sharara, F., Swetschinski, L. R., Robles Aguilar, G., Gray, A. P., Han, C., et al. (2022). Global burden of bacterial antimicrobial resistance in 2019: A systematic analysis. *The Lancet, 399*, 629–655. https://doi.org/10.1016/s0140-6736(21)02724-0.

30. Muteeb, G., Rehman, M. T., Shahwan, M., & Aatif, M. (2023). Origin of antibiotics and antibiotic resistance, and their impacts on drug development: A narrative review. *Pharmaceuticals, 16*, 1615–1615. https://doi.org/10.3390/ph16111615.

31. Nahid, P., Mase, S., Migliori, G. B., Sotgiu, G., Bothamley, G., Brożek, J., Cattamanchi, A., et al. (2019). Treatment of drug-resistant tuberculosis: An official ATS/CDC/ERS/IDSA clinical practice guideline. *American Journal of Respiratory and Critical Care Medicine, 200*, e93–e142. https://doi.org/10.1164/rccm.201909-1874ST.

32. Neja, S. A. (2020). Overview on the phenotypic drug resistance in *Mycobacterium tuberculosis*. https://www.semanticscholar.org/paper/c1222960523b9d6cd6078ff33a6fc8c9b5b60fb9 (accessed on 10 May 2025).

33. Olarewaju, S., Adeyemo, S. C., Kayode, A. T., Ayinmodu, J. O., Oladeji, O. O., Odedele, J. T., Victoria, D., et al. (2025). Prevalence, pattern, and correlates of depression among drug-susceptible tuberculosis patient enrollees in Ogbomoso, Oyo State: A cross-sectional study. https://www.semanticscholar.org/paper/1ad7c6093f4358449c540e409ba3e4161dd8490c (accessed on 10 May 2025).

34. Opito, R., Kwenya, K., Ssentongo, S. M., Kizito, M., Alwedo, S., Bakashaba, B., Miya, Y., Bukenya, L., Okwir, E., Onega, L. A., Kazibwe, A., Othieno, E., Kirya, F., & Olupot, P. O. (2024). Treatment success rate and associated factors among drug susceptible tuberculosis individuals in St. Kizito Hospital, Matany, Napak district, Karamoja region. A retrospective study. *PloS one*, *19*(5), e0300916. https://doi.org/10.1371/journal.pone.0300916(accessed on 10 May 2025).

35. Prikhodchenko, O., Arbuzova, Y., Serikbayeva, K., Zhakhina, G., Rakisheva, A., Mussabekova, G., Akhmedullin, R., et al. (2025). Epidemiology, detection, diagnosis and treatment of TB in children in Kazakhstan. *The International Journal of Tuberculosis and Lung Disease, 29*(3), 135–140. https://www.semanticscholar.org/paper/08dac1490d4e7fb86b24e844647673f716c3aa2d (accessed on 10 May 2025).

36. Rashid, F., Iqbal, S., Tahseen, S., & Zhao, Y. (2025). Investigation of bedaquiline heteroresistance among *Mycobacterium tuberculosis* isolates from Pakistan. *Microbiology Spectrum, 13*. https://www.semanticscholar.org/paper/cd2b758b5e1f41e3a3e082a6a639ff27541af551 (accessed on 10 May 2025).

37. Shah, D., Bhide, S., Deshmukh, R., Smith, J. P., Kaiplyawar, S., Puri, V., Yeldandi, V., et al. (2024). Test and treat approach for tuberculosis infection amongst household contacts of drug-susceptible pulmonary tuberculosis, Mumbai, India. *Frontiers in Tuberculosis, 2*. https://www.semanticscholar.org/paper/bc6cb7ab974abb8efe5efed214fed7ffeb338e70 (accessed on 10 May 2025).

38. Shin, J., Jeon, D., Mok, J., Yim, J. J., Kwon, Y. S., Jo, K. W., & Shim, T. S. (2024). Compliance with new drug use and the effect of discrepant drug susceptibility testing on MDR/RR-TB treatment. *The International Journal of Tuberculosis and Lung Disease, 28*(2), 18–24. https://www.semanticscholar.org/paper/b1dbe9ccf7c45ea3f06c7109d2a76ca8d1c329d2 (accessed on 10 May 2025).

39. Sugiyono, R. I., Naysilla, A. M., Susanto, N. H., Handayani, D., Burhan, E., Karuniawati, A., Kusmiati, T., et al. (2025). Treatment outcomes of pulmonary TB in adults in Indonesia. *IJTLD OPEN, 2*, 145–152. https://www.semanticscholar.org/paper/2b14c26129dd8b501b34290ddeae07c4828e4aea (accessed on 10 May 2025).

40. Tasca, B. G., Mganga, A., Leung, C. L., Shilugu, L., Pell, C., Onjare, B., Luvanda, N., et al. (2024). Factors related to the utilization of digital adherence technologies in tuberculosis care: A qualitative study among adults in DS-TB treatment, health care providers, and other key actors in Tanzania. *PLOS Global Public Health, 4*. https://www.semanticscholar.org/paper/38a7b51d80c1c43654bb0f810b37ae9a803ad02a (accessed on 10 May 2025).

41. Torres, T., Brembilla, N., Langley, R., Warren, R. B., Thaci, D., Kolios, A., Prinz, J., et al. (2024). Treatment of psoriasis with biologic and non-biologic targeted therapies in patients with latent tuberculosis infection or at risk for tuberculosis disease progression: Recommendations

from a SPIN-FRT expert consensus. *Journal of the European Academy of Dermatology and Venereology.* https://www.semanticscholar.org/paper/460ecb61ba168d760c3c48b88c68129952e2292c (accessed on 10 May 2025).

42. Uddin, T. M., Chakraborty, A., Khusro, A., Zidan, B. M. R. M., Mitra, S., Emran, T. B., Dhama, K., et al. (2021). Antibiotic resistance in microbes: History, mechanisms, therapeutic strategies and future prospects. *Journal of Infection and Public Health, 14*, 1750–1766. https://doi.org/10.1016/j.jiph.2021.10.020.

43. Walsh, K., Lee, M. H., Chaguza, C., Pamphile, W., Royal, G., Escuyer, V., Pape, J. W., et al. (2024). Molecular epidemiology of isoniazid-resistant *Mycobacterium tuberculosis* in Port-au-Prince, Haiti. *Open Forum Infectious Diseases, 11.* https://www.semanticscholar.org/paper/13e942d6a8bc3acceb1c918128755dbb4cce82d3 (accessed on 10 May 2025).

44. Yamin, D., Usković, V., Wakil, A. M., Goni, M. D., Shamsuddin, S. H., Mustafa, F. H., Alfouzan, W., et al. (2023). Current and future technologies for the detection of antibiotic-resistant bacteria. *Diagnostics, 13*, 3246–3246. https://doi.org/10.3390/diagnostics13203246.

45. Zhang, S. X., Wang, J. C., Yang, J., Lv, S., Duan, L., Lü, Y., Tian, L. G., et al. (2024). Epidemiological features and temporal trends of the co-infection between HIV and tuberculosis, 1990–2021: Findings from the Global Burden of Disease Study 2021. *Infectious Diseases of Poverty, 13.* https://doi.org/10.1186/s40249-024-01230-3.

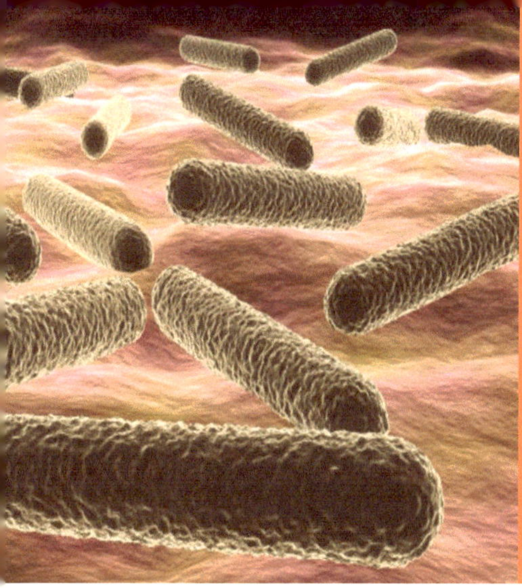

Chapter 7

DRUG-RESISTANT TUBERCULOSIS

Contents

Introduction

The global rise in drug-resistant infectious illness is a major public health issue, of which tuberculosis (TB) occupies a central position due to its long-term morbidity and mortality rates. Despite advances in medical science, TB remains one of the leading causes of infectious agent deaths worldwide. The onset and transmission of drug-resistant tuberculosis (DR-TB), specifically rifampicin-resistant and multidrug-resistant strains, intensified the momentum towards control by diminishing the effectiveness of treatment and increasing the transmission risk. It is a public health crisis that necessitates an understanding of resistance mechanisms and an urgent necessity for development in diagnosis and treatment strategies. The biological complexity of DR-TB is fueled by both internal biological factors in the *Mycobacterium tuberculosis* (MTB) bacterium and systemic challenges like accessibility to healthcare and treatment protocol compliance, necessitating coordinated international interventions and ongoing research (Bimo et al., 2025; Nanavare, 2024). Drug resistance in tuberculosis is mainly a result of individual genetic mutations within MTB bacteria that make them insensitive to first- and second-line anti-TB medications. The distinctive cell envelope of the bacterium also plays a role in its survival against antimicrobial treatment as a barrier that increases drug resistance and affects host-pathogen interactions. These are biological aspects that are important to consider when explaining why standard treatment regimens fail against resistant bacteria. Besides, the development of multi-drug resistant (MDR) and extensively drug-resistant (XDR) TB strains complicates clinical management and calls for new diagnostic instruments capable of identifying speedily and precisely to guide effective treatment interventions. Recent developments include universal drug susceptibility testing (DST) and development of shorter, all-oral regimens to improve patient results and reduce transmission (Bimo et al., 2025).

These scientific results place the urgent demand for innovation in DR-TB treatment and control into context. Adolescents, and particularly girls, form a vulnerable population in the fight against DR-TB, as social stigma and health system limitations particularly affect this group. Though TB has increased notification rates in males, females are confronted with barriers that curb their access to timely diagnosis and proper treatment. This gap highlights the need for age-specific interventions addressing the particular requirements of adolescent girls, who have distinctive psychosocial stress factors and risks during treatment. National TB Programs (NTP) may not have adolescent-specific guidelines, which hinders efficient case handling and increases the risk of recurrence. The World Health Organization's (WHO) overall strategy focuses on expanding diagnostic and treatment service coverage with the addition of new drugs like Delanamid and Bedaquiline to enhance outcomes. These initiatives indicate continued global action for not only controlling DR-TB but also for providing equitable care to heterogeneous populations (Nanavare, 2024).

Definition of Drug-Resistant Tuberculosis (DR-TB)

The worldwide burden of tuberculosis (TB) is made more complex by the rise of strains which do not respond to standard treatment regimens. The reason for this complexity is that some MTB bacteria have become resistant to antibacterial drugs essential in treating the disease. One of the major categories under DR-TB is multi-drug-resistant tuberculosis (MDR-TB), which literally refers to resistance to at least isoniazid and rifampicin, the two most effective first-line anti-TB drugs.

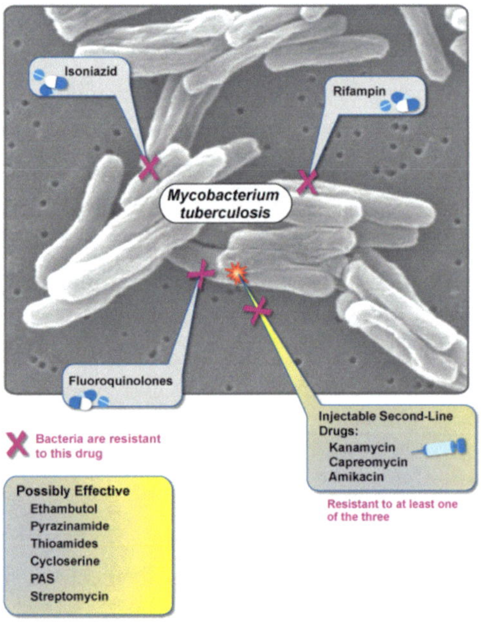

Figure 7.1. Overview of key focus areas in addressing drug-resistant tuberculosis (DR-TB).

Source: By NIAID - Extensively Drug-Resistant Tuberculosis (XDR TB) Diminishing Options for Treatment, CC BY 2.0, https://commons.wikimedia.org/w/index.php?curid=39933280

The occurrence of resistance to these drugs greatly reduces treatment effectiveness, necessitating even longer and more toxic therapeutic regimens. Familiarity with the clinical and microbiological operational definitions of MDR-TB is critical since it dictates both diagnostic algorithms and treatment plans. The diagnosis of MDR-TB relies on drug susceptibility detection in the laboratory, but it is also about identifying clinical resistance patterns that inform prompt intervention and containment actions (Ibrahim et al., 2024) (Figure 7.1).

Apart from MDR-TB, DR-TB covers other categories defined by resistance to a wider range of drugs. Perhaps the most troubling type is extensively drug-resistant (XDR) tuberculosis (XDR-TB), which comprises resistance to isoniazid and rifampicin, in addition to any fluoroquinolone, and one of the three second-line injectable drugs. The World Health Organization (WHO) revised the pre-XDR and XDR-TB definitions in 2021 to more accurately represent the changing resistance patterns observed in practice. This new classification importantly influences treatment planning because XDR-TB is linked to much worse outcomes than both drug-susceptible TB and MDR-TB. As per recent data, treatment success rates for XDR-TB are considerably lower, highlighting the importance of early and proper diagnosis in an effort to apply more effective treatment regimens (Dahl et al., 2024). The definition of DR-TB also finds its way into the field of immunohematological reactions, which can be used as adjunctive prognostic markers. Changes in blood parameters like inflammatory markers, immune cell populations, and global hematological profiles have been observed in patients with MDR-TB. Such biological alterations are indicative of the host-pathogen interactions characteristic of drug-resistant strains and may hold clues to disease severity as well as the patient's probable response to treatment. Incorporation of these immunohematological indices into standard assessment may enable enhanced clinical decision-making, providing a complementary method to conventional microbiological diagnosis. This emphasizes the complexity of classifying DR-TB not only on the basis of microbial susceptibility but also on the basis of changing biomarkers that could enhance prognosis and therapeutic responses (Ibrahim et al., 2024) (Figure 7.2).

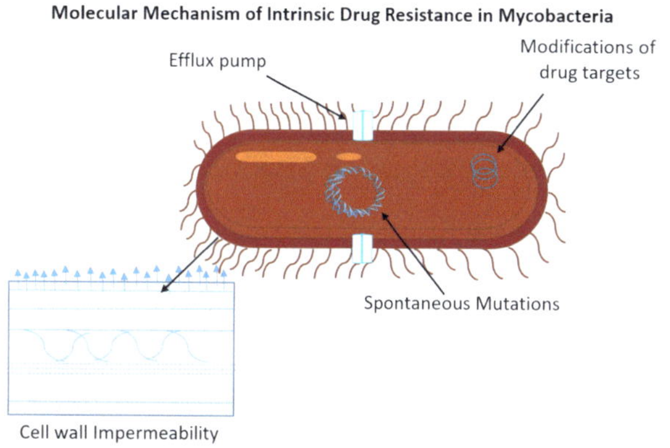

Figure 7.2. Evolution of drug resistance in TB: *Mtb* has been evolving with various strains having different extents of resistance to available anti-TB drugs.

Source: Rabaan AA, Mutair AA, Albayat H, Alotaibi J, Sulaiman T, Aljeldah M, Shammari BRA, Alfaraj AH, Al Fares MA, Alwarthan S, et al. Tools to Alleviate the Drug Resistance in *Mycobacterium tuberculosis*. Molecules. 2022; 27(20):6985. https://doi.org/10.3390/molecules27206985

7.1. Mechanisms of Drug Resistance

The survival of tuberculosis against long-course antibiotic therapy underlines the intricacy of bacterial adaptation and resistance. At the heart of DR-TB is the genetic adaptability of *Mycobacterium tuberculosis* (MTB), which allows it to endure antibiotic pressure through mutations in crucial genes coding for drug targets. Such mutations change the molecular configuration of enzymes and proteins, making first-line drugs such as isoniazid and rifampicin ineffective.

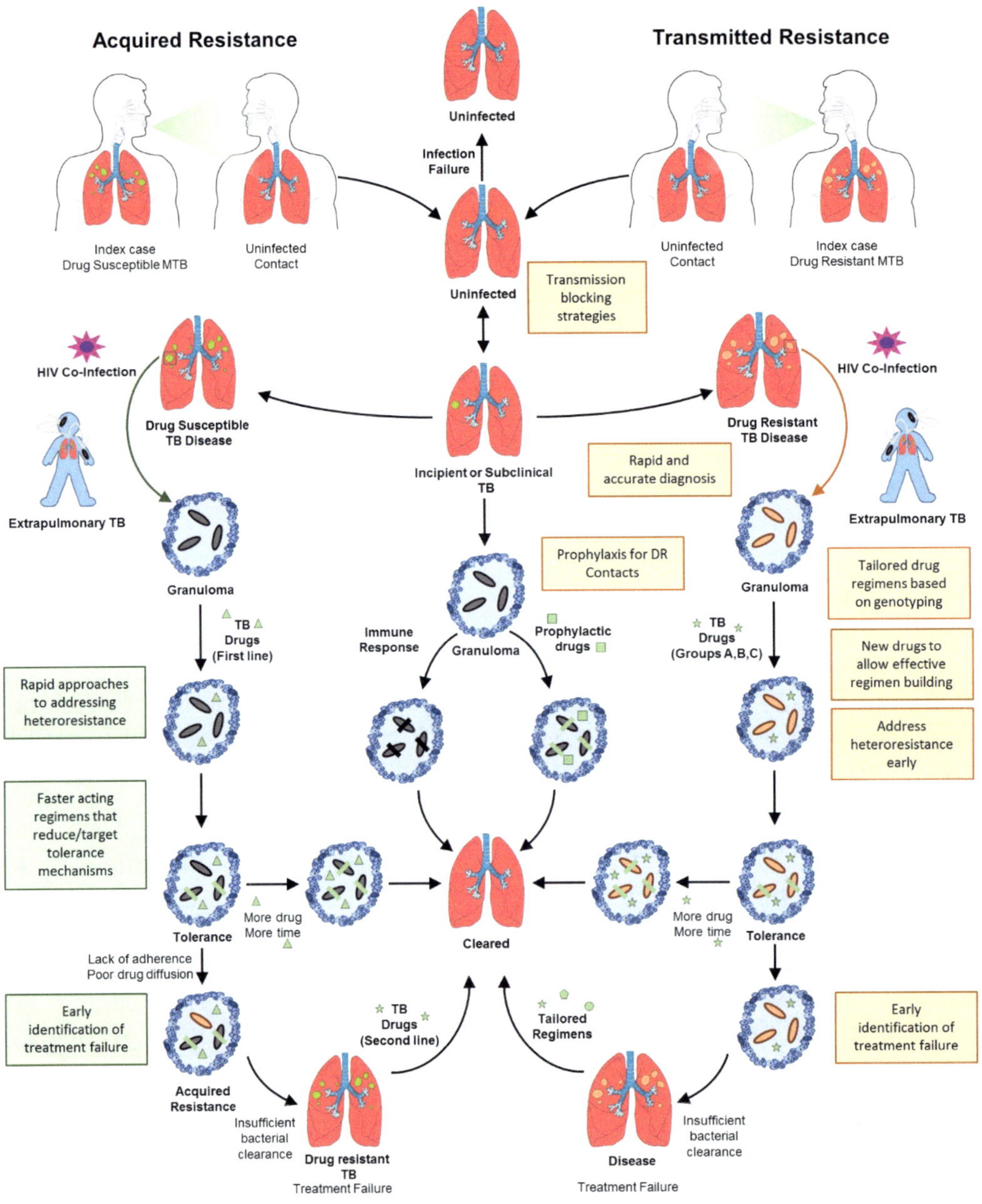

Figure 7.3. Schematic diagram showing the drug resistance mechanisms in *Mycobacterium tuberculosis*.

Source: Liebenberg D, Gordhan BG and Kana BD (2022) Drug resistant tuberculosis: Implications for transmission, diagnosis, and disease management. Front. Cell. Infect. Microbiol. 12:943545. doi: 10.3389/fcimb.2022.943545

Further, the efflux pump overexpression also helps in resistance by actively pumping out the antibiotics from the bacterial cells, lowering the intracellular drug levels to sublethal concentrations. This complex defense mechanism makes the bacterium resistant to eradication, complicating treatment schedules and facilitating the development of multi-drug resistant (MDR) and XDR strains, as evidenced by several epidemiological studies (Arslan et al., 2025). Comprehension of these molecular and genetic processes is essential to devise targeted therapeutics that avoid bacterial defense mechanisms. In addition to genetic mutation, MTB's physiological status at infection determines drug susceptibility. In latent infection or within granulomas, the bacterium enters a resting or slow-growing phase, where decreased metabolic activity reduces the effectiveness of antibiotics acting on active cellular functions. Such phenotypic tolerance also makes treatment more challenging and enhances survival against extended therapy (Figure 7.3).

In addition, the host immune response and pathogen interaction can induce stress responses in the bacterium, triggering genes that increase survival under antibiotic pressure. These adaptive responses, in combination with genetic resistance, create a powerful barrier to current treatment modalities. Diagnostic research, such as the use of molecular tests such as GeneXpert MTB/RIF, has enhanced detection of drug-resistant strains, but the full range of bacterial survival strategies requires further study of genotypic as well as phenotypic resistance mechanisms (Arslan et al., 2025). Current research has started investigating the contribution of the host's gut microbiota to modulating drug resistance in tuberculosis, further enhancing the new dimension to the complicated resistance process. The gut microbiota contributes significantly to modulating the host immunity and metabolic processes that impact the potency of anti-tuberculosis medication. Disturbance in microbial homeostasis, potentially caused by repeated antibiotic treatment, can weaken immune function or enhance bacterial survival, indirectly contributing to the development of drug resistance. Additionally, microbiota-drug interactions may impact the adaptability as well as resistance patterns of the pathogen, implying a microbiome-mediated factor for treatment failure. These new findings present new avenues for adjunct therapy that will restore microbiome health to increase drug efficacy and offset resistance. Incorporating microbiota into the management of TB may therefore be a promising avenue for attacking DR-TB (Figure 7.4).

Gene	Rv number	Cellular function	Description	Final product
glmU	Rv1018c	PG biosynthesis LU biosynthesis	UDP-N-acetylglucosamine pyrophosphorylase	UDP-GlcNAc
murA	Rv1315	PG biosynthesis	UDP-N-acetylglucosamine enolpyruvyl transferase	UDP-MurNAc
murX	Rv2156c	PG biosynthesis	Phospho-N-acetylmuramoyl-pentapeptide-transferase	Lipid I
ponA1/A2	Rv3682	PG biosynthesis Cell wall formation	Lipid II transglycoylase/transpeptidase	Classical (3→4) cross-linked PG
alr	Rv3423c	Alanine metabolism	Alanine racemase	D-alanine
ddl	Rv2981c	Alanine metabolism	d-Alanine–d-alanine ligase	D-alanyl-D-alanine
Ldt	Rv0116c	PG biosynthesis	L,D-transpeptidases	Nonclassical (3→3) cross-linked PG
rmlC	Rv3465	AG biosynthesis LU biosynthesis	dTDP-4-keto-6-deoxyglucose 3,5-epimerase	dTDP-rhamnose
accD6	Rv2247	MA biosynthesis	acyl-CoA carboxylases	methylmalonyl-CoA
pks12	Rv2048c	DIM biosynthesis	Polyketide synthase	Dimycocerosyl phthiocerol
ag85	–	MA biosynthesis	mycolyltransferase	trehalose mycolate

PG, peptidoglycan; AG, arabinogalactan; LU, linker unit; MA, mycolic acid; DIM, Phthiocerol dimycocerosates.

Figure 7.4. Diagrammatic illustration of the intrinsic mechanism of *Mtb* for drug resistance.

Source: Nasiri MJ, Haeili M, Ghazi M, Goudarzi H, Pormohammad A, Imani Fooladi AA and Feizabadi MM (2017) New Insights in to the Intrinsic and Acquired Drug Resistance Mechanisms in Mycobacteria. Front. Microbiol. 8:681. doi: 10.3389/fmicb.2017.00681

7.1.1. Genetic Mutations in Mycobacterium tuberculosis (MTB)

The fight against tuberculosis (TB) has been made more difficult by the ability of the pathogen to become resistant through genetic mutation. This is largely chromosomal mutations and not genes that are horizontally transferred, making MTB a particularly formidable enemy. While most bacteria are resistant through a complex cell envelope and enzymatic activity, drug resistance in *Mtb* arises primarily by genetic mutation causing changes in the drug target or inability to activate prodrugs. The genomic adaptation leads to changes like overexpression or conformational changes in target proteins, enabling the bacterium to survive in the presence of antibiotics. However, the acquisition of advantageous mutations is usually at the expense of bacterial fitness and *in vitro* growth rates. To balance this out, compensatory mutations can occur, counteracting fitness loss and stabilizing resistance in bacterial populations and illustrating a dynamic evolutionary process at the molecular level that makes treatment approaches challenging (Sebastian et al., 2017). Elucidation of the function of particular drug-resistance mutations has been facilitated by whole-genome sequencing (WGS) of spontaneous resistant mutants. Studies highlight mutations in key genes like *mmpL3*, which encodes a protein in cell envelope biosynthesis, as key nodes in resistance networks. Identification of *mmpL3* mutations not only explains the mechanism of resistance but also highlights targets for new drug development. The corresponding phenotypic effects of these mutations are the storage of cell envelope components, like trehalose monomycolate, that can be biochemically detected following challenges with new anti-tubercular (ATT) compounds (Iwuji et al., 2013). These findings illustrate how genetic mutations are not only responsible for drug resistance but also affect bacterial metabolism and cell wall structure, thus impacting both the physiology and pathogenicity of *Mtb* (Hill et al., 2013). Additionally, the assessment of the effectiveness of novel ATT compounds has to account for the genetic diversity and plasticity of *Mtb*. The moving balance between genetic background and resistance mutations implies that new therapies directed towards such features as mmpL3 have to be able to overcome a range of mutational landscapes. Infected animal models with drug-resistant strains carrying these essential mutations have demonstrated that a few next-generation compounds could effectively lower bacterial burden *in vivo*. These therapeutic developments reflect the process by which knowledge of the genetic mutations underlying drug resistance guides drug development and optimization of anti-TB drugs. However, the ongoing mutation-driven evolution of *Mtb* requires that TB control programs remain committed to active surveillance and tailored measures (Hill et al., 2013; Sebastian et al., 2017) (Figure 7.5).

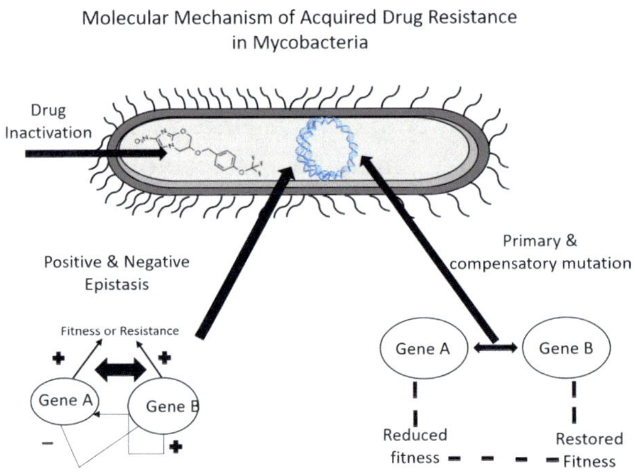

Figure 7.5. The mechanism for acquired drug resistance in *Mtb*.

Source: Rabaan AA, Mutair AA, Albayat H, Alotaibi J, Sulaiman T, Aljeldah M, Shammari BRA, Alfaraj AH, Al Fares MA, Alwarthan S, et al. Tools to Alleviate the Drug Resistance in *Mycobacterium tuberculosis*. Molecules. 2022; 27(20):6985. https://doi.org/10.3390/molecules27206985

7.1.2. Inadequate Treatment Regimens

Optimal DR-TB management is inherently complicated and frequently threatened by the limitations of available regimens. The longer treatment duration and toxicity of MDR-TB regimens contribute to low patient compliance, heightening the prospect of treatment failure and resistance escalation. For instance, in Uganda, which is among the most heavily affected countries by MDR-TB, treatment success in Uganda has remained below national targets because of these problems. Research indicates that close to one-third of MDR-TB patients face unfavorable outcomes, such as death or treatment failure, highlighting the insufficiency of current regimens.

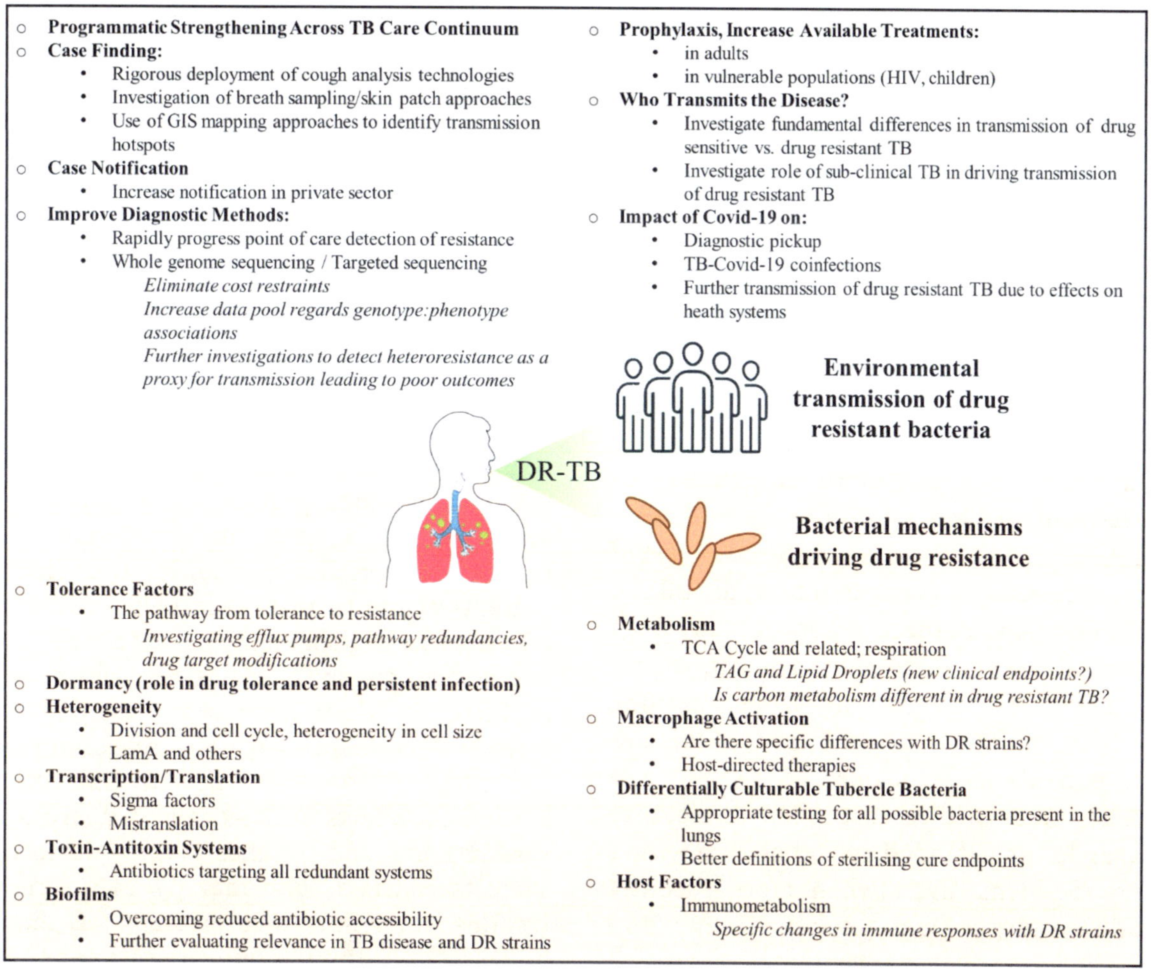

Figure 7.6. Schematic presentation of multi-drug-resistant tuberculosis (MDR-TB) and extensively drug-resistant tuberculosis (XDR-TB).

Source: Liebenberg D, Gordhan BG and Kana BD (2022) Drug resistant tuberculosis: Implications for transmission, diagnosis, and disease management. Front. Cell. Infect. Microbiol. 12:943545. doi: 10.3389/fcimb.2022.943545

Low body weight at the commencement of treatment has been associated with poor prognosis, implying that standardized treatments may not take into consideration individual patient factors adequately. Therefore, the recurrence of poor outcomes emphasizes the need for new and individualized therapeutic approaches to improve efficacy and mitigate the MDR-TB burden (Barteka et al., 2025). The development of resistance against newer antituberculosis drugs also complicates treatment paradigms further and reinforces the issue of suboptimal regimens. Linezolid, as a key element in new multidrug regimens such as BPaLM and BPaL, has shown significant success in enhancing outcomes for MDR-TB. Resistance to linezolid has been increasingly reported, particularly in settings of high burden such as India. This resistance usually results from the addition of linezolid to failing or inadequate current regimens and from treatment discontinuation due to side effects or loss to follow-up (LTFU). These situations worsen the acquisition of additional drug resistance, highlighting the effects of inadmissible drug combinations and regimen formation. Therefore, the inadequacy of treatment regimens not only inhibits near-term results but also creates a vicious cycle of spiraling resistance (Vengurlekar et al., 2023). Additionally, a retrospective cohort study from a Mumbai-based Médecins Sans Frontières clinic shows the clinical difficulties resulting from inadmissible treatment models for DR-TB. In patients with documented resistance to linezolid, most of them had been exposed to the drug for an extended period of time within failing regimens. Even when more recently introduced drugs such as bedaquiline and delamanid are available, treatment success rates were quite variable and reflect that even newer regimens remain subject to constraints due to resistance profiles and patient comorbidities like diabetes. The research also identified that comorbidities and persistent positive cultures had a significant influence on treatment outcomes, supporting the theory that treatment regimens need to be adjusted to the individual clinical and microbiological features of patients. This evidence emphasizes the imperative to fine-tune treatment programs to avoid the failures of traditional protocols in MDR-TB management (Vengurlekar et al., 2023) (Figure 7.6).

7.1.3. Role of Patient Non-Adherence

The development of DR-TB is closely tied to causes outside of microbial genetics, with drug regimen adherence by the patient being a critical component. TB treatment is often long and with multiple drugs, and can be draining for patients both emotionally and physically. Most people, particularly in developing-world contexts, experience social stigma related to TB that dissuades them from pursuing or maintaining care. These stigmatized attitudes worsen isolation feelings and can result in treatment course interruptions that create conditions for resistance development of MTB strains. The social aspect of non-adherence emphasizes the necessity of incorporating stigma reduction and supportive care into programs of TB control because interruption of treatment by patient-related reasons eventually reduces the effectiveness of global containment efforts as well as enhances transmission hazards (Meershoek et al., 2018). In addition, the complicated MDR-TB treatment regimens are also a reason for poor adherence outcomes. Patients are subjected to severe side effects, such as nausea, neurological disturbances, and tiredness, which demotivate them to continue with therapy. In contrast to treating other infectious diseases, TB therapy necessitates long-term commitment over many months, which conflicts with patients' socioeconomic stressors and routine obligations. These problems are augmented by insufficient healthcare infrastructure that precludes regular patient monitoring and follow-up. Taking cues from HIV treatment interventions, where early and prolonged antiretroviral therapy (ART) significantly lowers the viral load and rates of transmission, highlights the need for early intervention and patient-centered adherence support for TB too (Bazin et al., 2013). Inadequate use of full-range adherence interventions allows resistant TB strains to develop and circulate, making public health responses harder. The implications of patient non-compliance reach beyond individual results, threatening the wider public health with serious problems. Discontinuation or abnormal consumption of TB drugs not only fosters the selection of resistant bacilli but also extends infectivity, thus enhancing the resistant case burden in the community. Such situations put diagnostic services to the test and inflate healthcare expenditures owing to more intense treatments. Moreover, non-adherence reinforces cycles of transmission among at-risk populations, with stigma and socio-economic disadvantages further increasing barriers to the completion of treatment. Thus, successful control of TB requires multifaceted approaches aimed at patient education, reduction of stigma, psychosocial support, and accessibility of healthcare to dampen non-adherence and drug resistance. In the absence of addressing such issues, attempts to contain DR-TB risk being undercut at a root level (Meershoek et al., 2018).

7.2. Types of Drug-Resistant Tuberculosis (DR-TB)

The clinical diversity of tuberculosis is largely amplified by the development of multiple drug-resistant types, each with its own set of challenges to control and treatment. Two of these, Rifampicin-resistant tuberculosis (RR-TB) and MDR-TB, are the most common and carry high public health burdens. RR-TB involves resistance to rifampicin, a key agent in first-line treatment, whereas MDR-TB includes resistance to isoniazid as well, another main anti-tuberculosis agent. These patterns largely occur among working-age populations and mirror demographic trends seen in highly incident TB countries. Less frequent but clinically important are Pre-XDR-TB and XDR-TB, which exhibit resistance patterns beyond rifampicin and isoniazid to fluoroquinolones and second-line injectables, radically limiting treatment options and outcomes. The prevalence of these forms is consistent between the genders, with RR-TB and MDR-TB accounting for the majority of cases in men and women (Faye et al., 2024). Beyond the microbiological differences, socioeconomic and environmental conditions have their impact deeply interwoven with the epidemiology of DR-TB forms. Indian studies demonstrate that low socioeconomic status, overcrowding, undernutrition, and indoor air pollution exposure greatly amplify the risk for both drug-sensitive and DR-TB. Smoking, specifically, is a significant lifestyle factor that increases susceptibility to drug resistance, perhaps because it compromises lung function and immune protection. In addition, poor prior treatment and nosocomial exposures are key selective pressures that promote the emergence of resistance outside the initial drug-sensitive setting, greatly contributing to the processes of MDR and XDR-TB generation. It is essential to appreciate these interconnected determinants to customize prevention interventions and maximize resource investment in high-burden settings (Shah et al., 2024). Although the DR-TB classification highlights biological features, the interaction with factors related to the patient reflects the depth of complexity in treating these infections. HIV co-infection, for instance, is associated with increased DR-TB rates but does not serve to meaningfully change the proportional spread of TB types. It does, however, have a profound effect on survival, with HIV-infected individuals showing significantly poorer treatment success. Also, occupational hazards, such as mining and imprisonment, add particularly to higher rates of RR-TB and MDR-TB, which confirm environmental exposure is critical in resistance phenomena. The points of convergence confirm that DR-TB is not pharmacologically controlled alone but involves combined methods tending to clinical, social, and economic factors aimed at enhancing patient outcomes as well as disrupting transmission (Faye et al., 2024) (Figure 7.7).

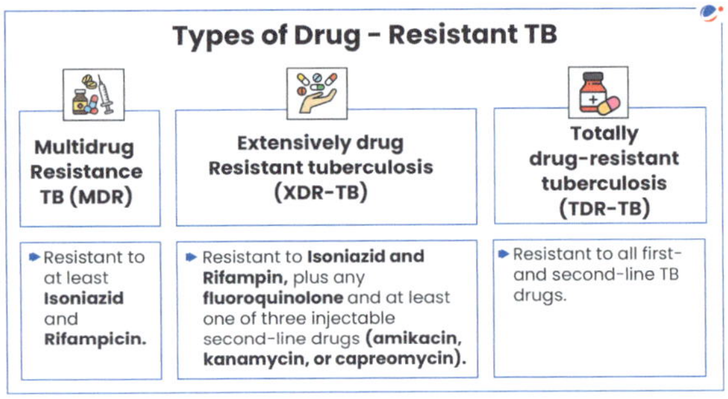

Figure 7.7. Types of drug-resistant tuberculosis (DR-TB).

Source: Cloudfront. (n.d.). *Types of drug-resistant TB: MDR, XDR, and TDR tuberculosis.* https://d2av8kbir6lh9m.cloudfront.net/uploads/ Azurue4jp9V2CslMb0pnDR3r6NptUfGvsPcXBedC.png.

7.2.1. Multi-Drug Resistant Tuberculosis (MDR-TB)

The challenge in treating infectious disease is greatly compounded when resistance to first-line medications occurs, as in the case of MDR-TB. One of the most at-risk groups is those coinfected with HIV, in whom the risk of acquiring tuberculosis and the severity of its comorbidities are greatly exaggerated. Treating MDR-TB in such patients presents a fine balance owing to drug interactions between ART and second-line tuberculosis drugs. The existence of resistance tends to require second-line drugs, which are often more toxic and demand strict adherence to treatment to prevent further resistance. Moreover, the epidemiology of MDR-TB reflects challenges with monitoring the patient, treatment regimen adherence, and adverse effect management, all of which are seen to attribute to the high mortality rates reported, particularly in limited resources and healthcare systems countries (Natália et al., 2022). Economic factors play a crucial role in the availability and efficiency of MDR-TB drug treatment worldwide. In nations such as China, which have a high burden of MDR-TB patients, new drugs like bedaquiline have shown encouraging results in clinical trials. When used as an adjunct to background regimens, bedaquiline reduces culture conversion time drastically and increases quality-adjusted life years (QALYs), which implies better patient outcomes. Utilizing economic models, research has identified that while bedaquiline raises initial treatment expenditures, its cost-effectiveness is underpinned by improved long-term health gains and lower disease burden. The evidence supports including such new drugs within national reimbursement programs to reduce patients' economic burdens and enhance adherence and results in MDR-TB treatment (Zhang et al., 2020).

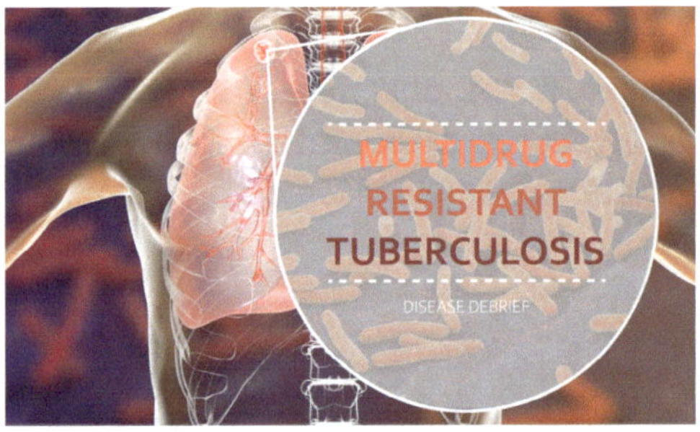

Source: NCCID. (2023). *Multidrug-resistant tuberculosis – Disease debrief.* https://nccid.ca/wp-content/uploads/sites/2/2023/01/Multidrug-Resistant-TB-DD-graphic_Twitter_2.png.

The worldwide struggle against MDR-TB highlights the intersection of clinical complexity and health system capacity. Control of MDR-TB requires success not only in the discovery of new medicines but also in improving healthcare delivery systems to enforce adherence, mitigate side effects, and halt transmission. Tactics such as directly observed therapy (DOT) are essential but have to be modified to meet the varied challenges of coinfected patients, especially HIV, which need well-coordinated treatment regimens. Additionally, ongoing monitoring and research into drug repositioning and new therapeutics are important to counteract resistance strategies. Alongside policy changes to enhance drug supply and access, these comprehensive efforts are necessary to prevent the MDR-TB crisis and curb its global health consequences (Zhang et al., 2020; Natália et al., 2022).

7.2.2. Extensively Drug-Resistant Tuberculosis (XDR-TB)

The emergence and spread of XDR-TB are one of the most frightening dilemmas in contemporary infectious disease management. In contrast to MDR-TB, which is resistant at least to isoniazid and rifampicin, XDR-TB is also resistant to these first-line drugs as well as to any fluoroquinolone and at least one of the three second-line injectable agents. This widespread resistance substantially restricts treatment possibilities, making treatment regimens more complicated and putting patients at greater risk of treatment failure and death. The development of XDR-TB is largely due to incorrect use of antibiotics, either as a result of inappropriate regimens, patient non-adherence to therapy, or excessive and inappropriate use of antimicrobials in human and animal medicine, creating the selection pressure for resistant organisms (Md. Salam et al., 2023).

XDR-TB treatment outcomes.

Study	Study location	XDR-TB patients	HIV status	Treatment success rate
Gandhi *et al.*	KwaZulu Natal, Republic of South Africa	53	positive	2%
Migliori *et al.*	Europe (Estonia, Germany, Italy, and Russian Federation)	64	negative	39%
Keshavjee *et al.*	Tomsk, Russia	29	negative	48%
Chan *et al.*	United States	10	negative	50%
Mitnick *et al.*	Peru	48	negative	60%
Kim *et al.*	South Korea	75	negative	29%

Figure 7.8. Description of extensively drug-resistant tuberculosis (XDR-TB).

Source: Haydel SE. Extensively Drug-Resistant Tuberculosis: A Sign of the Times and an Impetus for Antimicrobial Discovery. Pharmaceuticals. 2010; 3(7):2268-2290. https://doi.org/10.3390/ph3072268

These emphasize the urgent need for strict antimicrobial stewardship and monitoring interventions to counteract the progress of antimicrobial resistance (AMR) in tuberculosis. Treatment of XDR-TB poses daunting challenges requiring creative solutions and individualized treatment regimens. XDR-TB patients need regimens including newer, more costly, and less readily available drugs like bedaquiline and linezolid that have been introduced to reverse resistance in extensive bacterial populations (Nahid et al., 2019). Treatment is frequently extended and burdened with extreme side effects, adding to patient non-compliance and further enabling the development of resistance. The clinical challenge also extends to the need for comprehensive diagnostic facilities capable of rapidly detecting resistance patterns, enabling timely and appropriate intervention. These complexities demand robust healthcare infrastructures capable of integrating drug susceptibility testing (DST), individualized treatment plans, and continuous monitoring to improve outcomes in XDR-TB patients. The public health implications of XDR-TB extend beyond individual cases, threatening broader tuberculosis control efforts on a global scale. Spread of XDR strains defies routine infection control measures in communities and healthcare facilities alike, requiring enhanced contact tracing, isolation procedures, and sensitization campaigns to curb spread (Md. Salam et al., 2023). Further, the financial cost of treating XDR-TB is considerably elevated, with longer hospital stays, more expensive therapeutics, and the use of specialized healthcare services. Global partnership and funding are essential to enable these augmented efforts, as is the priority of research into new therapeutic agents and vaccines. Unless concerted action and commitment are made towards finding solutions to the underlying causes of resistance, such as overuse of antibiotics throughout sectors, the XDR-TB threat will keep on growing and threatening decades of tuberculosis control success (Nahid et al., 2019) (Figure 7.8).

7.2.3. Rifampicin-Resistant Tuberculosis (RR-TB)

The development of RR-TB seriously hampers the global battle against tuberculosis since rifampicin is a backbone drug used in first-line TB treatment. *rpoB* gene mutations, which specifically occur in the region of rifampicin resistance determining region (RRDR), are largely implicated in the resistance to rifampicin. A recent report analyzing 192 rifampicin-resistant isolates highlighted the heterogeneous character of these mutations and their different implications on treatment outcomes. Although most mutations are associated with high-level resistance, some controversial mutations may appear to express as low-level resistance, thereby diminishing the reliability of phenotypic DST. For instance, the Leu430Pro mutation in the *rpoB* gene had a significant potential correlation with rifampicin resistance, even though it was statistically not significant, indicating the complexities in interpreting resistance patterns and clinical prediction. These results highlight the need for advanced diagnostic techniques and individualized treatment approaches to enhance therapeutic outcomes in RR-TB patients (Vadakunnel et al., 2025). Adolescents, especially females, form a vulnerable group in the case of RR-TB, wherein complexities of treatment cross with biological and social issues. Research points out that DR-TB in this age group tends to need specialist care because of increased stigma, possible effects on mental well-being, and distinct clinical presentation from younger children. The RR-TB burden is high globally, with an estimated 4,50,000 new cases each year, highlighting the need for age-appropriate interventions. New treatment protocols with new anti-TB drugs like Delamanid and Bedaquiline have been added according to adult protocols but must be applied with caution to adolescents. Health systems stress the need for holistic approaches that encompass diagnostic coverage, prevention, and access to care tailored to the specific needs of such a population (Nanavare, 2024). Reaching RR-TB demands not just medical breakthroughs but also programmatic strategic interventions aimed at early case detection and successful treatment compliance. The different levels of resistance associated with particular *rpoB* mutations modify the disease course and may require more intensive regimens, particularly in the case of low-level resistance. Optimizing outcomes calls for linking molecular diagnostic tests able to identify these patterns of resistance with treatment protocols that alter dosing and drug combinations based on such identifications. Global approaches emphasize the importance of expanding diagnostic technologies and improving the delivery of care for high-risk populations, such as adolescents and extrapulmonary patients. As a whole, bridging the divide between molecular knowledge and public health efforts is paramount in preventing the morbidity and mortality of RR-TB (Nanavare, 2024; Vadakunnel et al., 2025) (Figure 7.9).

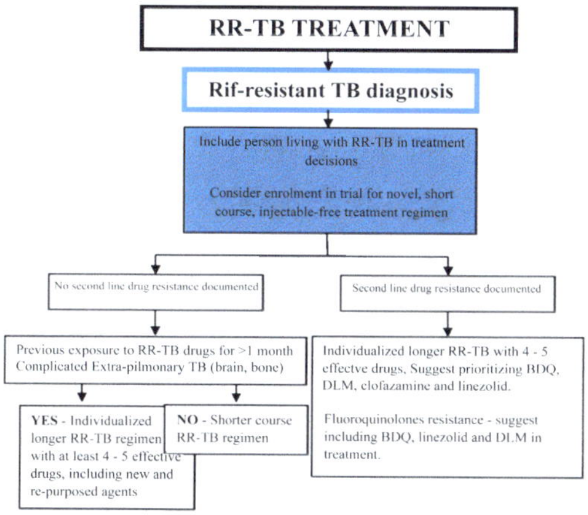

Figure 7.9. Treatment algorithm for rifampicin-resistant TB (RR-TB) and HIV.

Source: ResearchGate. (n.d.). *Treatment algorithm for rifampicin-resistant TB (RR-TB) and HIV.* https://www.researchgate.net/figure/Treatment-algorithm-for-rifampicin-resistant-TB-RR-TB-and-HIV_fig1_323149426.

7.3. Diagnosis of Drug-Resistant Tuberculosis (DR-TB)

Timely and correct diagnosis of DR-TB is essential to preventing the spread of the disease and enhancing outcomes for patients. Even though diagnostic technologies have improved, implementation problems still abound, particularly in resource-constrained settings. For example, a large percentage of patients who are eligible for TB testing still are not being tested for rifampicin resistance, an important marker of MDR-TB, because of logistical challenges as well as knowledge gaps among healthcare providers. Among such factors are limited capabilities for sputum collection and transport issues, which further limit the coverage of diagnosis in remote regions with no access to molecular testing laboratories. Closing the existing gaps is complex, involving increased training of healthcare providers to identify drug resistance testing eligibility criteria and improved sample collection and transport infrastructure to cover patients in remote areas (Oo et al., 2019). Traditional culture-based detection methods for drug resistance, though accurate, are time-consuming and cause a delay in instituting proper therapy. This delay compromises patient prognosis and allows for continued spread of resistant strains. Rapid molecular diagnostic methods are hence integrated into DR-TB diagnosis as a cornerstone. Molecular tests like GeneXpert and line probe assays (LPA) allow for the concomitant detection of MTB and associated drug resistance genetic mutations, enabling early and targeted therapy. These tests have much shorter diagnostic turnaround time than culture approaches, increasing the likelihood of starting appropriate, individualized regimens. Their application, though, relies on strong laboratory infrastructure, trained staff, and quality control systems within National TB Programs (NTPs) to guarantee uniformity and accuracy of DST (Dheda et al., 2019). Due to the dynamic state of drug resistance trends and changing treatment guidelines, regular reassessing diagnostic approaches is necessary. Universal baseline and ongoing DST can avert the progression to multidrug- or extensively DR-TB from isoniazid-resistant by facilitating early therapeutic modifications. In addition, ongoing surveillance via national surveys offers invaluable epidemiological data, guiding public health interventions and resource deployment. The surveys are nevertheless resource-dependent and performed sporadically, which is why sustainable routine DST capacity is very important. Combining rapid molecular diagnostics with regular surveillance activities is the cornerstone of an effective diagnostic strategy, which can reduce the burden of DR-TB globally (Dheda et al., 2019) (Figure 7.10).

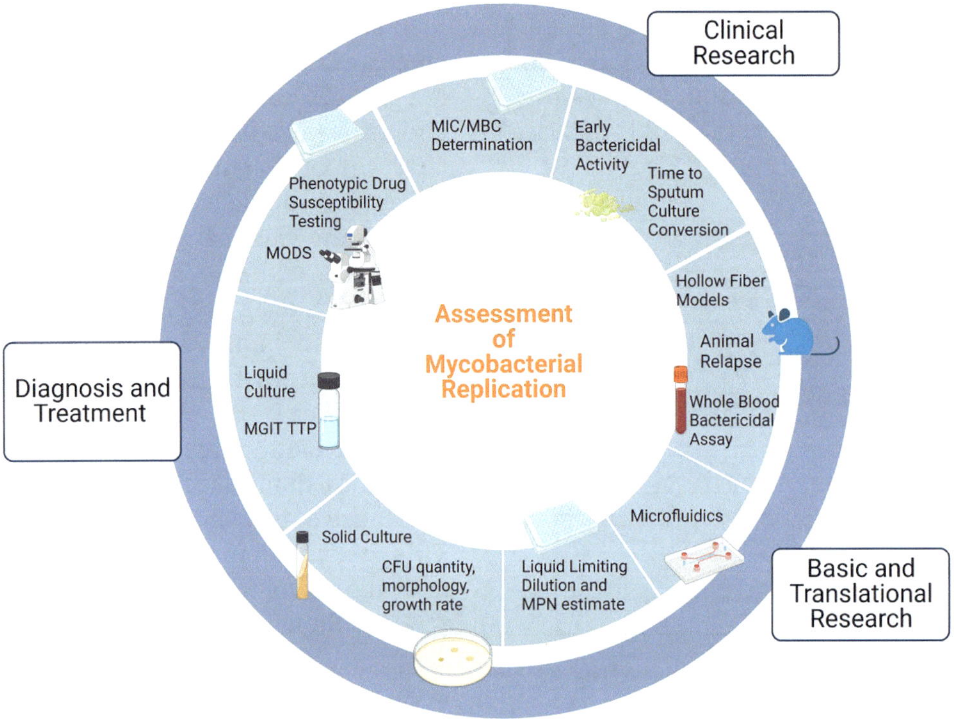

Figure 7.10. Phenotyping methods for determination of drug resistance TB.

Source: Mishra S and Saito K (2022) Clinically encountered growth phenotypes of tuberculosis-causing bacilli and their in vitro study: A review. Front. Cell. Infect. Microbiol. 12:1029111. doi: 10.3389/fcimb.2022.1029111

7.3.1. Traditional Diagnostic Methods

Proper diagnosis is still the basis of successful tuberculosis control, particularly in relation to drug-resistant forms. Sputum smear microscopy has long been a major diagnostic tool because of its low cost and ease of use. It identifies *acid-fast bacilli* (AFB) when examined under a microscope, enabling provisional detection of MTB infection. Nevertheless, conventional smear microscopy is not highly sensitive, especially in patients with low bacterial load or extrapulmonary tuberculosis (EPTB), making drug-resistant types difficult to diagnose. Moreover, culture-related methods, traditionally the reference standard, allow for identification and DST but take weeks to produce results because of the slow growth rate of *Mtb*. Such delay can accelerate spread as well as interfere with timely initiation of responsive treatment. Although these are the limitations, conventional diagnostics have played a significant role in TB control activities globally, providing the groundwork for the establishment of more sophisticated testing modalities (S. K. et al., 2024). Advances in molecular biology have led to nucleic acid-based methods, which provide quicker and more specific diagnoses of tuberculosis and drug resistance. Despite these, even these classical molecular tests, like traditional PCR, have challenges such as technical sophistication and the need for well-equipped laboratories, making them less accessible in most high-burden settings. DST through culture continues to be important for resistance pattern detection but is time-consuming and not always possible in resource-constrained settings. In addition, standard diagnostic methods may yield false positives or negatives, especially in previously *Bacillus Calmette-Guérin* (BCG) vaccinated populations, children, or HIV co-infected individuals, thereby complicating clinical decision-making. These issues highlight the imperative need for optimizing and integrating diagnostic techniques for increased accuracy and efficiency, thereby facilitating early intervention of DR-TB cases (Khutade et al., 2024). The combination of conventional approaches with new diagnostic methods has the potential for enhanced tuberculosis control, particularly for multi-drug resistant (MDR) and XDR bacteria. While culture and smear microscopy form the foundation, their constraint necessitates the integration of molecular diagnostics such as GeneXpert MTB/RIF, which provides rapid rifampicin resistance detection suggestive of MDR-TB. The technique is consistent with international efforts aimed at hastening diagnosis and commencement of treatment. Yet even the most sophisticated conventional tools are handicapped by questions of accessibility, expense, and turnaround time, especially in low-resource environments where TB prevalence is greatest. Ongoing refinement of these traditional techniques, in combination with new technologies, is essential to improving diagnostic delay and inaccuracy. As such, maximizing traditional diagnostic paradigms is an indispensable step toward better control of DR-TB (Khutade et al., 2024).

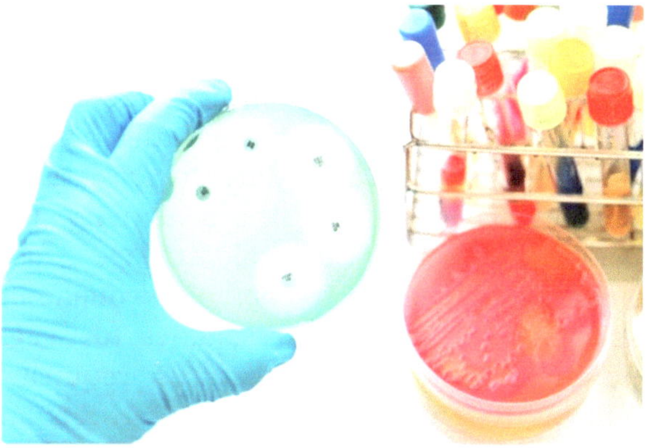

Source: Cloudfront. (2019). *Antibiotic susceptibility testing using disc diffusion method in petri dish*. https://d2jx2rerrg6sh3.cloudfront.net/image-handler/picture/2019/11/shutterstock_392702701.jpg.

7.3.2. Molecular Testing Techniques

Molecular testing technologies have had a significant influence on the diagnosis and management of DR-TB, an affliction that poses a challenge to international health efforts. Conventional tests tend to involve lengthy culture times, where MTB and resistance pattern cannot be identified in time. Molecular assays, on the other hand, allow direct detection of drug resistance-associated genetic mutations from clinical specimens quickly. These assays, including polymerase chain reaction (PCR)-based tests and nucleic acid amplification tests (NAATs), are directed against known genetic markers of resistance and allow for accelerated clinical decision-making. Yet, even with these developments, a large gap exists in the creation of easily accessible, rapid, and reliable point-of-care tests for tuberculosis, which hinders the use of such tools to slow transmission. The natural complexities of the pathogen as well as resource constraints in endemic areas complicate matters further. Hence, ongoing research and forward planning are necessary to enhance molecular diagnostics in tuberculosis control programs (McNerney et al., 2012). MTB strain heterogeneity directly affects the performance and interpretation of results from molecular diagnostic tests. Research conducted in different geographic settings, like Nepal, underscores the genetic diversity of tuberculosis lineages that can carry different resistance mechanisms influencing the sensitivity and specificity of tests. For example, Lineage 2, also referred to as the Beijing genotype, is commonly associated with greater resistance to drugs and unique molecular signatures, requiring specific diagnostic strategies. Molecular testing methods need to consider lineage-specific polymorphisms to preclude false-negative outcomes and achieve optimal targeted resistance detection. In addition, knowledge of the phylogenetic structure of strains circulating in a given population can inform the design of targeted molecular probes and primers that maximize detection efficiency and clinical utility. Therefore, incorporating molecular epidemiology into diagnostic approaches is critical for the adaptation of molecular tests to the changing genetic environment of tuberculosis pathogens (Sandgren et al., 2012). The field application of molecular testing for DR-TB depends not just on the technology but also on the infrastructural and operational platforms for its implementation. Whereas molecular tests provide rapid and accurate results, their usability is dependent on accessibility, affordability, and healthcare worker competence in impacted areas. Most of the molecular assays available today need advanced laboratory facilities, which restricts their application in low-resource settings where tuberculosis burden is highest. Additional logistical issues including shipment of specimens, quality control, and data management affect program sustainability of molecular testing. Overcoming these operational challenges through the creation of portable, user-friendly molecular platforms and extensive training programs can improve early case detection and treatment outcomes. Ultimately, integrating molecular test innovations with practical healthcare delivery models is key to fighting DR-TB globally (McNerney et al., 2012).

7.3.3. Challenges in Early Detection

The complexity of DR-TB diagnosis arises from several interlinked factors that greatly hinder early detection. One major hindrance is the non-specificity of symptoms in the early stages, which tend to mimic drug-sensitive tuberculosis or other respiratory illnesses, leading to many misdiagnoses. Also, the shortage of adequate healthcare facilities in high-burden areas aggravates delays since most of the facilities lack the necessary advanced diagnostic equipment required for early detection of resistant strains. Socioeconomic barriers also discourage patients from accessing healthcare early, as economic constraints and limited awareness regarding the disease lead to treatment disengagement. These problems in aggregate extend the infectious duration, enabling disease transmission prior to when DR-TB is diagnosed and properly treated (Mphothulo et al., 2025). The combined impact of these challenges risks derailing global efforts at containing the spread of drug resistance. There is a pledge of improvement held out by advancements in diagnostic technology, but their adoption into everyday clinical practice is constrained by a number of obstacles. Current phenotypic methods, while reliable, are often time-consuming and require specialized laboratory environments, making them less feasible in low-resource settings. Molecular diagnostic tools such as GeneXpert and next-generation sequencing (NGS) offer rapid detection of resistance mutations, but their high costs and technical requirements restrict widespread accessibility. Also, the genetic heterogeneity of MTB makes it difficult to interpret results from molecular tests with constant updates in assay design for capturing emergent resistance mechanisms. Apart from these impediments, despite constant innovations, slowing down the clinical translation of novel approaches, they extend the time between infection and precise diagnosis, which is necessary to bring to bear effective regimens promptly (Xiong et al., 2024). Until these obstacles are remedied, early detection issues will continue to be a major bottleneck. Beyond infrastructural and technological concerns, patient-oriented factors have a crucial influence on the early detection of DR-TB. Tuberculosis stigma, especially for drug-resistant types, establishes psychological barriers that deter patients from accessing timely diagnosis or follow-up care. Meanwhile, intolerable drug side effects and treatment complexity can demoralize individuals, causing diagnostic processes to be dropped or testing to be left incomplete. Community involvement and family support have also been established as enablers of retention in care but are responsible for attrition from diagnostic care pathways when they are missing. Transportation challenges and food deprivation are also essential factors in determining limited access to diagnostic services, particularly among marginalized groups (Mphothulo et al., 2025). Tackling early detection challenges therefore necessitates a multisectoral response that includes social, psychological, and economic interventions in addition to technological advances for better participation and ensuring timely case finding of DR-TB (Iwuji et al., 2013).

7.4. Treatment Options

Treating DR-TB, especially MDR-TB, is a complicated clinical problem, most notably in vulnerable groups like children. Treatment approaches are discouraged by the unavailability of pediatric-specific information and the absence of formulations that are appropriate for young patients. Most of the second-line drugs that are the mainstay of treating MDR-TB have serious side effects, making long-term adherence and follow-up difficult. Therefore, treatment protocols need to be individually tailored with the aim of balancing efficacy and toxicity. Clinical monitoring must be close, with routine laboratory and radiologic investigations to maximize outcomes and control side effects optimally. Because of the complexities involved, it is highly advisable that pediatric presentations of MDR-TB be treated in multidisciplinary centers to provide complete care from diagnosis to successful completion of treatment (Boss et al., 2022). This individualized strategy is aimed at both pharmacologic and practical issues essential in mitigating morbidity within this population. Treatment paradigms in adults for DR-TB have changed in recent years, with largely a global guideline-driven approach, where there is an increasing focus on shorter, more potent regimens as much as possible. New drug combinations have enhanced treatment efficacy and tolerability, with new drugs specifically active against resistant organisms. Furthermore, management strategies that are integrated and take into account comorbidities like HIV have become essential with their implications for therapeutic choice. Global recommendations now point to the consideration of drug–drug interactions as well as the possibility of regimen adjustment among HIV co-infected patients. These sophisticated guidelines reflect the importance of individualized medicine with consideration of resistance patterns, possible side effects, and individual patient variables to maximize outcomes (Rosa et al., 2020). This progress is a key step in the battle against DR-TB towards becoming both patient-friendly and effective regimens. Prophylactic therapy for contacts of DR-TB is another essential element in curbing transmission. Preventive measures are limited by scarcity of evidence and the high toxicity profile of existing regimens. Risk-benefit assessments are particularly important, most notably in children, where less is known about long-term effects of preventive drugs. More intensive surveillance and early recognition are essential adjuncts to prevention. In addition, research and implementation of newly developed therapeutic agents with better safety profiles are necessary to increase preventive modalities. Specialized referral clinics are essential in treating such cases, to orchestrate the multifaceted interaction between therapy and prevention and avoid complications. This strategy highlights the multidimensional path of combating DR-TB, involving alertness, creativity, and expertise to contain the epidemic effectively (Boss et al., 2022).

7.4.1. Standard Treatment Protocols for Drug-Resistant Tuberculosis (DR-TB)

Successful control of DR-TB requires a strategy that is both accurate and responsive to resistance pattern complexity. Standard treatment regimens frequently break down as a result of wide resistance to first-line anti-TB therapy, which calls for the use of standardized protocols that include second-line and novel pharmaceutical agents. DST largely influences the choice of treatment by detecting resistance markers and informing therapy decisions. This individualized strategy aids in reducing the risk of treatment failure and ongoing resistance emergence. Nevertheless, standardization of these protocols is still important to provide a standardized approach in delivering care in varied healthcare facilities while ensuring efficacy is matched with safety concerns. The latest developments in diagnostic technology are central to enhancing the timing for treatment initiation, hence patient outcomes through tailoring drug combinations based on the resistance pattern. Diagnostic technologies, especially WGS, have greatly improved the accuracy of DR-TB treatment regimens. In contrast to traditional molecular and phenotypic assays, WGS offers whole-genome information on resistance-conferring mutations, allowing for more personalized treatment regimens. Delivery of WGS via affordable and easy-to-use pipelines, like those that combine Oxford Nanopore Technologies (ONT) with sophisticated data analysis tools, has accelerated time-to-diagnosis to about four weeks, an improvement from conventional methods (Elton et al., 2025). Quick turnaround allows for timely implementation of effective therapy, which is crucial in breaking transmission and enhancing prognosis. In addition, concordance of WGS outcomes with phenotypic DST reinforces its dependability, enabling integration into evidence-based treatment guidelines for DR-TB (Elton et al., 2024). Despite such technological progress, there are challenges with standard treatment guidelines for DR-TB, mainly in low-resource settings. Standardized regimens need to meet treatment complexity, drug course duration, toxicity, and patient compliance while being flexible to accommodate varying resistance patterns. The use of optimized diagnostic pipelines that integrate effective DNA extraction techniques with advanced base calling and analytical software enhances accessibility and accuracy and makes the latest treatment guidance more accessible throughout the world (Elton et al., 2024, 2025). Treatment protocols thus increasingly depend on molecular information to fine-tune drug selection and minimize dependence on slower phenotypic techniques. The ongoing development of these protocols, driven by both diagnostic innovation and clinical evidence, continues to be necessary for effective management and control of DR-TB globally (Figure 7.11).

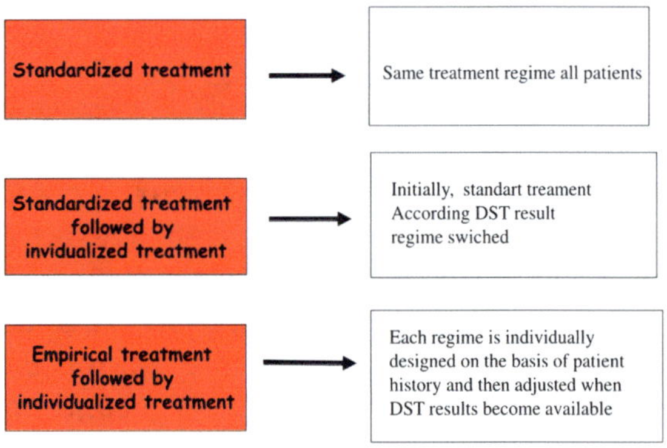

Figure 7.11. Recommended treatment strategies for MDR-TB.

Source: Slideserve. (n.d.). *Recommended treatment strategies for MDR-TB.* https://image.slideserve.com/1404321/recommended-treatment-strategies-for-mdr-tb-l.jpg.

7.4.2. New and Emerging Therapies

Important progress has been made in elucidating the complex interaction between *Mycobacterium tuberculosis* (Mtb) and the host immune system, opening the door for new therapeutic approaches. *Mtb's* capacity to subvert host cellular functions, including autophagy and metabolic pathways, allows it to survive within macrophages, escaping immune elimination. Studies on these bacterial survival strategies have emerged as new targets for therapy to interfere with the pathogen's protective niches. New strategies, such as host-directed therapies (HDTs) that amplify immune function or inhibit bacterial immune evasion strategies, have also been identified as promising adjuvants to conventional antimicrobials. By combining advances in molecular biology and immunology, these therapies hope to not just enhance bacterial clearance but also minimize tissue damage and target drug-resistant strains, holding the promise of more successful TB control in the future (Nasiri & Venketaraman, 2025). Recent clinical practice points to the possibilities of the conjunction of repurposed medications with new immunomodulatory drugs in treating MDR-TB. These conjunctions have indicated encouraging outcomes in those instances when standard treatment was unsuccessful, pointing to the shortcomings of existing regimens. One such case was particularly striking, in which bacteriophage therapy was combined with immunomodulators and repurposed medication, followed by impressive sputum culture conversion and long-term patient recovery. This case demonstrates the therapeutic promise of combining innovative modalities to meet the ongoing challenge of DR-TB. In addition, it highlights the demand for tailored treatment protocols taking into account complex infections that are increasingly aided by technological breakthroughs in clinical decision-making (Pandey, 2024). The convergence of artificial intelligence (AI) and high-performance computational technology is an evolving frontier in treating DR-TB. AI applications hold the promise of optimizing treatment regimens by analyzing vast datasets encompassing microbial genetics, patient response patterns, and drug pharmacodynamics. This technology can facilitate faster identification of effective drug combinations and monitor treatment adherence, thereby improving clinical outcomes and reducing the development of further resistance. Despite its potential, AI's role in TB therapy remains underexplored and requires rigorous validation through clinical trials and multidisciplinary collaboration. Addressing this challenge will require a coordinated global response, employing both biomedicine innovation and technological progress, to overcome the ever-present risk of DR-TB and improve patient prognosis (Pandey, 2024).

7.4.3. Importance of Personalized Medicine

The complexity of DR-TB is a worldwide threat to health, and it calls for innovative strategies beyond the traditional treatment paradigm. Advances in genomic technology, such as the use of next-generation sequencing (NGS), have revolutionized our capacity to investigate the genetic diversity of MTB strains. This enables the more accurate determination of resistance patterns and pathogen heterogeneity, which is essential to personalize effective therapeutic regimens. By taking advantage of these genomic data, personalized medicine can help clinicians choose antibiotics that will most probably be effective against particular bacterial mutations, and this could decrease treatment failure and contain the emergence of resistant bacteria. Personalized interventions are not only benefiting patient outcomes but also maximizing public health program resource utilization, both reducing individual and community burdens of DR-TB (Satam et al., 2023). In addition, personalized medicine holds the promise of tailoring treatment duration and regimen to a patient's individual disease severity, immune system response, and genetic makeup.

Conventional "one-size-fits-all" practice in TB treatment is often not sensitive to the heterogeneity of host-pathogen interactions that condition treatment success. With incorporating clinical biomarkers and host genomics, personalized approaches can predict response to therapy and select individuals at risk of relapse or toxicity. This personalized strategy facilitates the optimization of multidrug regimens for maximal bacterial eradication with minimal toxicity and patient nonadherence, which are key drivers of controlling drug resistance. The challenge is to apply such customized protocols at scale, but constant collaborative work continues to enhance clinical trial designs to facilitate this revolution (Véronique et al., 2022). Beyond enhancing therapeutic accuracy, personalized medicine also enables the discovery and qualification of new diagnostic and predictive markers essential to the management of DR-TB. Discovery of host- and pathogen-specific biomarkers offers reagents for early latent infection detection likely to progress, tracking real-time responses to treatment, and relapse prediction. These biomarkers are the basis for adaptive treatment algorithms that can be constantly updated as new data become available, supporting dynamic TB management. As drug resistance makes treatment challenging, host and microbial genomic data combined allow physicians to predict treatment failure and alter regimens promptly. Inclusion of personalized medicine into TB control programs is a seminal milestone toward overcoming biological uncertainties and speeding up the process of developing successful therapeutic approaches (Véronique et al., 2022; Satam et al., 2023) (Figure 7.12).

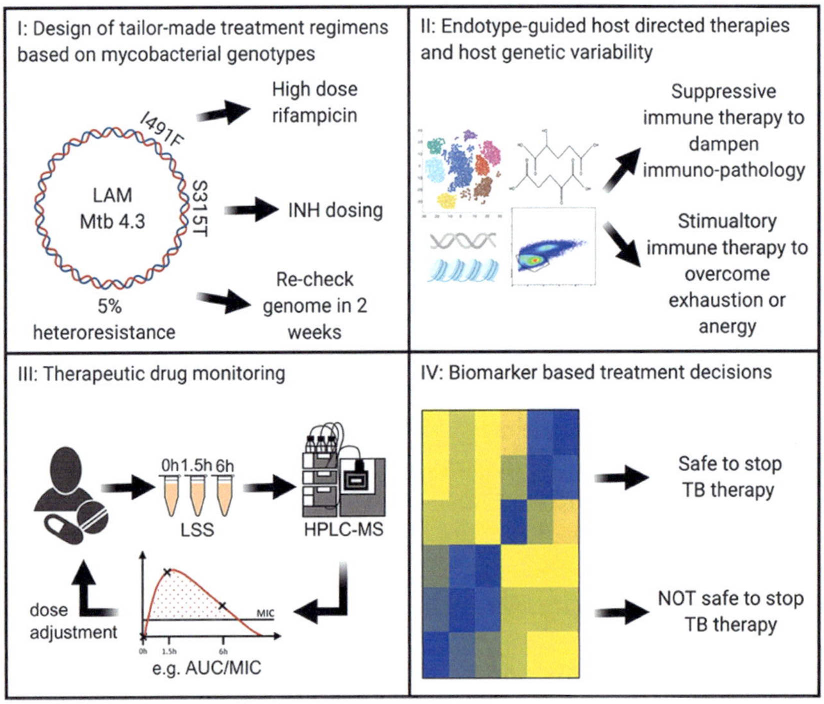

Figure 7.12. Towards precision medicine in tuberculosis (TB).

Source: Lange C, Aarnoutse R, Chesov D, van Crevel R, Gillespie SH, Grobbel H-P, Kalsdorf B, Kontsevaya I, van Laarhoven A, Nishiguchi T, Mandalakas A, Merker M, Niemann S, Köhler N, Heyckendorf J, Reimann M, Ruhwald M, Sanchez-Carballo P, Schwudke D, Waldow F and DiNardo AR (2020) Perspective for Precision Medicine for Tuberculosis. Front. Immunol. 11:566608. doi: 10.3389/fimmu.2020.566608

7.5. Public Health Implications

The problems of DR-TB are more than clinical challenges, such as the implications on public health on a wider scale that require urgent response. DR-TB patients tend to have lengthy and cumbersome treatment processes, which may exaggerate physical, psychosocial, and economic burdens. For example, the patients develop mental illnesses due to loneliness, stigma, and physical decline from their illness, especially on long hospital stays for the isolation process. This is exacerbated within immigrant communities who may further experience language barriers and cultural dislocation, additionally complicating treatment and follow-up care adherence. These factors establish the necessity of holistic support systems that combine psychosocial care with medical treatment to enhance patient outcomes and public health safety. Late diagnosis in certain instances even intensifies risk transmission, extending community exposure and challenging containment measures (Storvig et al., 2024). Globally, appearance and dissemination of DR-TB pose a serious threat to the health security of the world, questioning the sustainability of existing tuberculosis control initiatives. The added economic cost associated with longer treatment regimens, expensive second-line medications, and related healthcare resources makes public health planning more problematic, particularly in low- and middle-income nations (LMICs) with weak healthcare systems. The advances of new drug therapies such as the approval of bedaquiline and pretomanid have opened the way for improved control of multi-drug-resistant infections. The integration of these therapeutic choices into international guidelines marks an important measure toward reducing the public health burden of DR-TB through better cure rates and lowered transmission potential. Yet the likelihood of additional resistance development calls for aggressive drug resistance surveillance and stewardship to help maintain the effectiveness of these new treatments (Shah et al., 2024). In addition, the ongoing transmission of DR-TB requires intensified global collaboration and coordinated public health action to maximize prevention, diagnosis, and treatment activities. Surveillance mechanisms should be enhanced to identify drug resistance patterns early and inform directed interventions to minimize transmission in healthcare facilities as well as in the community. Furthermore, incorporating novel technologies like enhanced diagnostic equipment and nanotechnology-derived treatments can assist in bridging obstacles concerning detection and compliance. Policymakers and health organizations need to make investments a priority in research, healthcare infrastructure, and psychosocial care programs catering to the complex nature of DR-TB. It is only by taking a fully integrated, multi-sectoral approach that it is possible to control the public health threat presented by DR-TB effectively, reducing the impact on infected populations globally (Shah et al., 2024; Storvig et al., 2024).

7.5.1. Impact on Global Health Systems

The development and spread of DR-TB pose serious challenges to health systems worldwide, reflecting weaknesses in infrastructure and allocation of resources. As AMR worsens, it further overloads already-stressed healthcare facilities with diminished diagnostic ability and inadequate laboratory capacity, especially in low-resource environments. DR-TB treatment courses are long, requiring longer hospital stays and increased clinical monitoring, placing additional burdens on healthcare staff and fiscal resources. These are further aggravated by gaps in data hindering effective surveillance and targeted intervention measures, compromising efforts towards controlling transmission as well as managing treatment outcomes (Dartois & Rubin, 2022). Health systems, therefore, have an increasing imperative to invest in better diagnostics, transport specimen networks, and capacity building for their staff to fight both drug-susceptible and resistant types of tuberculosis on a holistic scale. Simultaneously, the COVID-19 pandemic has severely disrupted tuberculosis control programs worldwide, demonstrating the fragility of global health systems amid overlapping infectious disease crises. Redirection of healthcare infrastructure and personnel toward COVID-19 management has led to diminished testing, diagnosis, and treatment continuity for tuberculosis, causing a drastic reduction in case detection and treatment adherence. This system disruption disproportionately impacts DR-TB patients by amplifying delays in treatment and creating situations that promote additional resistance growth. The collateral damage of the pandemic has, in effect, undone decades of progress, underlining the necessity for holistic, person-centered responses that build health systems' resilience to TB as well as to other public health emergencies that occur at the same time. Combating these challenges necessitates joined-up, multisectoral efforts to restore and strengthen tuberculosis services under continuing global health emergencies (Wingfield et al., 2021). Additionally, the economic and social burdens DR-TB places take a further toll on global health systems and pose risks to equity in care provision. Protracted and frequently harmful regimens for MDR-TB impose significant direct and indirect expenses to both health systems and patients, such as protracted medication, inpatient stays, and socioeconomic suffering. Most LMICs are unable to absorb these expenses with limited budgets and lack of international funding, which restricts access to new therapeutics and diagnostics. Further, stigma and fear of tuberculosis can discourage patients from accessing care early enough, leading to community transmission and hindering public health response. It is therefore vital to enhance social protection systems and universal coverage to counteract such effects, provide accessible quality treatment, and avoid catastrophic expenditure among the affected populations. Construction of resilient and fair health systems is central to fighting the dynamic worldwide threat of DR-TB (Wingfield et al., 2021; Dartois & Rubin, 2022) (Figure 7.13).

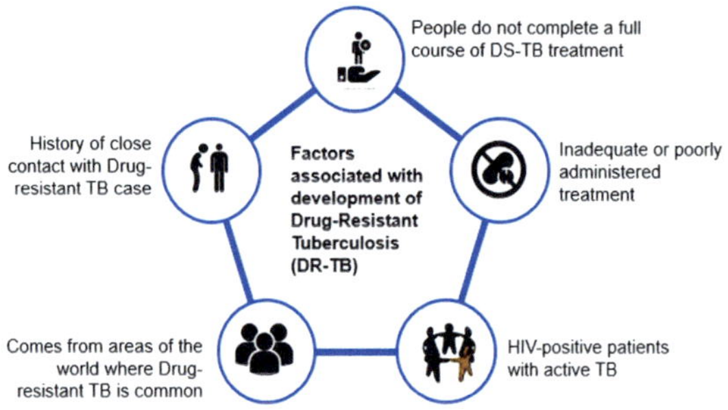

Figure 7.13. High risk for drug-resistant tuberculosis (DR-TB).

Source: National Tuberculosis Elimination Program (NTEP). (n.d.). *Factors associated with development of drug-resistant tuberculosis (DR-TB).* https://ntep.in/node/595/CP-drug-resistant-tuberculosis-dr-tb.

7.5.2. Economic Burden of Drug-Resistant Tuberculosis (DR-TB)

The ongoing burden of DR-TB not only overstretches healthcare systems but also imposes a heavy economic burden on infected communities. DR-TB treatment lasts for long durations, often consisting of costly second-line drugs with major side effects, which cause higher hospitalization and outpatient visits. Direct medical costs are augmented by indirect costs like lost productivity, permanent disability, and early death. In areas with poor healthcare infrastructure, the economic burden can be crippling for individuals and for public health budgets, finally hindering economic growth. The economic cost is compounded by the requirement of sophisticated diagnostic equipment and prolonged treatment monitoring to contain resistance effectively. Such needs highlight the need to invest in prevention and early detection measures to lessen economic burdens from drug-resistant infections, as evident in the bigger picture of AMR's drain on global health resources (Christopher et al., 2022). In addition to the direct costs of treating DR-TB infections, long-term complications add to the economic burden. Post-tuberculosis lung disease (PTLD), the prevalent sequela among survivors of TB particularly those infected with drug-resistant strains, causes chronic respiratory disease that necessitates recurrent medical treatment and rehabilitation. These ongoing health disabilities reduce patients quality of life and productivity, creating sustained economic burdens on families and healthcare systems. Lack of uniform management and preventive measures for PTLD results in most individuals who are affected experiencing repeated episodes of health crises, leading to frequent healthcare attendance and further treatment costs. Chronic morbidity perpetuates the vicious cycle of economic burden associated with DR-TB, where treatment costs and lost income accumulate, heavily contributing to the social burden (Allwood et al., 2021). The economic implications of DR-TB also extend to the social level, compromising economic stability and growth, especially in areas where TB is highly prevalent. Public health systems are forced to invest a lot of resources in controlling MDR-TB cases, redirecting those funds from other vital health services. The diversion can increase healthcare inequalities and hinder other disease access to care. In addition, the social economic cost goes beyond healthcare spending to encompass the effects on workforce activity and community productivity, particularly in economically at-risk populations. Policymakers should take these complex costs into account when crafting interventions, highlighting multimodal approaches that integrate antimicrobial stewardship, optimal treatment, and rehabilitation care. Enhancing surveillance and laboratory infrastructure to monitor resistance patterns is still essential in diminishing the clinical as well as economic impact of drug-resistant pathogens (Allwood et al., 2021; Christopher et al., 2022).

7.5.3. Strategies for Prevention and Control

Addressing the increasing threat of DR-TB requires a multifaceted approach that combines early detection with targeted therapeutic interventions. Surveillance systems play a critical role in monitoring resistance patterns and informing clinical decisions. For example, comprehensive DST, as demonstrated in Guangzhou City, revealed important resistance profiles indicating the urgent need for personalized treatment regimens to prevent treatment failures and further resistance development (Alibrahim et al., 2024). Application of routine screening programs to risk groups like previous treatment for TB or co-morbid conditions like diabetes would enhance early diagnosis of drug-resistant cases. Early detection by such proactive measures enables the timely administration of suitable drug regimens, thereby controlling transmission and resistance amplification. Provision of access to quality diagnostic equipment and establishment of molecular testing technologies are also essential in order to optimize diagnostic precision, delay reduction, and treatment outcome improvement in infected communities. Along with the diagnostic advancements, public health interventions need to focus on the consistency and completion of anti-TB medication regimens to avoid resistance development. DR-TB most commonly results from irregular or incomplete administration of anti-TB medications, leading to the emergence of resistant mycobacterial strains. DOT and patient support programs have been found effective in improving compliance and decreasing relapse rates. Education campaigns addressed to vulnerable populations, such as expatriates or younger people classified as being of higher risk in the Gulf Cooperation Council countries, can educate patients with information on the value of adherence and diminishing stigma (Li et al., 2024). In addition, targeting social determinants such as poverty, nutrition, and healthcare facility accessibility creates a setting that is supportive of treatment success and overall disease control. Intersectoral partnerships among healthcare professionals, policymakers, and populations are critical to coordinating resources and maintaining long-term intervention efforts. Prevention of new infections should also be focused on through environmental controls and infection control policies, particularly within healthcare facilities where transmission risk is high. Dissemination of airborne infection control measures, ventilation improvement, and utilization of personal protective equipment for healthcare personnel minimize nosocomial transmission of resistant strains. Community-based approaches involve contact tracing and screening of close contacts to break chains of transmission. Combining these prevention measures with strong surveillance data enhances the ability to rapidly respond to developing trends in resistance. In addition, research and development of new therapeutics and vaccines will ensure long-term solutions to address DR-TB. As emphasized by regional research, ongoing surveillance, public health promotion, and clinical creativity need to coexist to be able to successfully manage this dynamic public health problem (Alibrahim et al., 2024; Li et al., 2024).

SUMMARY

The current challenge of DR-TB underscores the need for upgrading therapeutic regimens with effective bacterial clearance, as well as reducing adverse effects for enhanced patient compliance and outcomes. Recent pharmacokinetic research on bedaquiline and delamanid shows encouraging plasma drug concentrations that correlate with intended therapeutic concentrations, revealing an exposure–response relationship essential for maximizing culture conversion rates in pre-extensively DR-TB patients. This data further supports the importance of personalized medication strategies, especially with regard to factors like BMI that affect drug exposure. These findings set the stage for more targeted dosing regimens that might decrease treatment time and toxicity and thereby improve the overall effectiveness of multidrug regimens intended to target resistant strains (Anuj et al., 2024). Such observations represent a crucial step in the fine-tuning of treatment regimens for limiting the worldwide burden of DR-TB. Further, the investigation of new pharmacological compounds with enhanced safety profiles remains of highest priority for the control of DR-TB. The therapeutic efficacy of contezolid as an effective substitute for linezolid among patients with severe adverse effects represents advancements in safer long-term regimens. Since linezolid-associated toxicities like suppression of bone marrow and peripheral neuropathy negatively affect patient quality of life and therapy success, having alternatives like contezolid, which is as potent but less toxic, is a critical development. These case reports also highlight the need for ongoing clinical trials and real-world studies to support widespread use of such agents without sacrificing efficacy for tolerability (Xiong et al., 2024). In the end, including safer drugs into routine treatment protocols will overcome critical gaps in therapy completeness and compliance levels. DR-TB treatment needs an interdisciplinary treatment with optimization of drug dosing, monitoring pharmacokinetic parameters, and incorporation of safer alternatives into therapy. The evolving context of tuberculosis treatment means that integration of pharmacokinetic data with new drug candidates can significantly enhance treatment effectiveness and diminish side effects. Such an interdisciplinary strategy is vital for avoiding the limiting constraints brought about by resistance and toxicity, which are major deterrents to international tuberculosis control. Continued investment in research and development, along with optimal use of customized treatment regimens, will likely reduce the public health burden of DR-TB and bring us closer to its eventual eradication. Intimate interaction among clinicians, researchers, and policymakers will be essential to achieving these gains in the real world and maximizing patient outcomes worldwide.

The complete picture of DR-TB requires an awareness of the essential diagnostic and therapeutic difficulties that continue to challenge the world. A decade of technological advancements in diagnostic tools has enhanced the diagnosis of TB as well as its drug-resistant variants immensely. Automated liquid culture platforms, integrated with molecular LPAs, are now established as the gold standard for first-line DST, offering increased accuracy and reliability in detecting resistance patterns. Second-line DST, on the other hand, remains complex and costly with some of the drugs available without effective tests. These developments, although crucial, again show that the world still needs quick, reliable, and affordable point-of-care tests that are multi-purpose across a wide variety of healthcare providers globally, particularly in resource-constrained settings where TB burden is highest (O'Grady et al., 2011). These developments are key to successful clinical management and drug-resistant strain containment. With technological progress, epidemiological data show particular demographic and clinical determinants of TB and MDR-TB prevalence and detection.

Recent research using large datasets shows that some populations, such as males, adults, and those with previous TB treatment, share a greater probability of TB infection and rifampicin resistance. On the other hand, older individuals have significantly lower RR-TB risk among all ages. The threat to children is of special concern, as children reflect odds of resistance to rifampicin that are similar to adults. Notably, there are regional differences, as are found in Mumbai, where female patients with definite TB are at higher risk of MDR-TB than male patients. These observations highlight the nuances of TB epidemiology and the need for specific diagnostic and therapeutic approaches (Nair et al., 2016). In conclusion, the management of DR-TB calls for an interdisciplinary strategy that marries innovative diagnostic methods with a sensitive assessment of risk factors within and between populations. Although molecular and culture-based diagnostics are today's gold standard, the hope still lies in an assailable point-of-care test that simultaneously identifies both TB and drug resistance with rapidity and affordability. In parallel, identification of demographic and clinical predictors facilitates priority setting for high-risk groups to undertake strengthened surveillance and interventions. These concerted efforts are critical to stem the worldwide epidemic of DR-TB and progress toward holistic disease control and ultimately eradication. Ongoing research and directed policy interventions will be critical in overcoming current challenges and maximizing results for populations affected globally (O'Grady et al., 2011; Nair et al., 2016).

CLOSER LOOK

RIFAMPICIN-RESISTANT TUBERCULOSIS (RR-TB)

RR-TB is a type of tuberculosis (TB) due to rifampicin-resistant MTB strains, which is one of the key first-line anti-TB drugs. Resistance to rifampicin usually is a sign of more extensive drug resistance and may complicate the treatment process of TB. It results from mutations in the rpoB gene of the bacteria that codes for the bacterial RNA polymerase. These mutations prevent rifampicin from binding to its target, rendering the drug ineffective. RR-TB can be diagnosed through molecular tests, such as the GeneXpert MTB/RIF assay, which can rapidly detect resistance to rifampicin.

The clinical consequences of RR-TB are serious. Rifampicin is a cornerstone of TB treatment regimen, and resistance to this drug results in the failure of the conventional TB therapy. Consequently, patients who have RR-TB are at increased risk for treatment failure, prolonged disease, and transmission. RR-TB is most common in persons with incomplete or inappropriate treatment of TB but may also develop in previously untreated persons, especially in high transmission settings with inadequate infection control practices.

The management of RR-TB requires the administration of second-line drugs, which are less effective and induce more side effects than the first-line drugs. The most common second-line drugs include fluoroquinolones, aminoglycosides, and injectables, together with newer drugs such as bedaquiline and delamanid. These agents are administered in combination for long durations, usually 18–24 months. Because of the treatment complexity and the potential for additional resistance, RR-TB is managed with specialized care, close observation, and compliance with a more intensive and longer treatment course. The development of RR-TB underscores the urgent need for early detection, correct treatment regimens, and measures to avert the acquisition of drug resistance.

REFERENCES

1. Agnes Meershoek, Alice Zwerling, Amrita Daftary, Brian Citro, Caoimhe Smyth, Dean Lewis, Deirdre Ni Cheallaigh, Elaine Byrne, Ellen M. H Mitchell, Gill Craig, Ieva Leimane, James Malar, Jens Levy, Julia van der Land, Kate Macintyre, Lisa G. Johnston, Nadine Ferris France, Nora Engel, Olive Mumba, Rajita Bhavaraju, Ronan R. Conroy, Sarah van de Berg, Stephen H-F Macdonald, Timur Abdullaev, and Tushar Nair. (2018). *TB Stigma–Measurement Guidance.* The United States Agency for International Development (USAID), !nancially supports this publication through Challenge TB under the terms of Agreement No. AID-OAA-A-14-00029. This publication was made possible by the generous support of the American people through USAID. https://core.ac.uk/download/287580942.pdf (accessed on 10 May 2025).

2. Adamu, I. A., Samson, E., Kwoegbu, I. M., Emmanuel-Funsho, A. A., Amarachi, B. J., & Musa, M. A. (2024). Immuno-haematological indices in multi-drug resistant tuberculosis: Implications for prognosis. *Sokoto Journal of Medical Laboratory Science.* SJMLS Volume 9, Number 2 June, 2024. https://www.semanticscholar.org/paper/93fe49c2975df624503fadd509dd9852f1b6a8d4 (accessed on 10 May 2025).

3. O'Grady, Justina,b; Maeurer, Markusc; Mwaba, Peterb,d; Kapata, Nathanb,d; Bates, Matthewa,b; Hoelscher, Michaele; Zumla, Alimuddina,b. New and improved diagnostics for detection of drug-resistant pulmonary tuberculosis. Current Opinion in Pulmonary Medicine 17(3):p 134-141, May 2011. | DOI: 10.1097/MCP.0b013e3283452346 (accessed on 10 May 2025).

4. Alibrahim, A., Alqahtani, H., Thirunavukkarasu, A., & Qazi, I. (2024). Prevalence, patterns, and determinants of drug-resistant tuberculosis in Gulf Cooperation Council countries: An updated systematic review. *PeerJ, 12.* https://www.semanticscholar.org/paper/8a415f77c9b6da1c6c985452cd6cc84aff3e46f7 (accessed on 10 May 2025).

5. Allwood, B., Byrne, A., Meghji, J., Rachow, A., van der Zalm, M. M., & Schoch, O. D. (2021). Post-tuberculosis lung disease: Clinical review of an under-recognised global challenge. *Respiration, 100,* 751–763. https://doi.org/10.1159/000512531.

6. Almeida, N. R., Lima, C. A., Freitas, N. L. D., & Brandão, F. (2022). Pharmacological treatment of multidrug-resistant tuberculosis (MDR-TB) in patients co-infected with HIV and its incidence in Federal District–Brazil. *Research, Society and Development.* https://www.semanticscholar.org/paper/6fa742773d7cb80337e6e27384ca648ce7de36b3 (accessed on 10 May 2025).

7. Iwuji, C. C., Orne-Gliemann, J., Tanser, F., Boyer, S., Lessells, R. J., Lert, F., Imrie, J., Bärnighausen, T., Rekacewicz, C., Bazin, B., Newell, M. L., Dabis, F., & ANRS 12249 TasP Study Group (2013). Evaluation of the impact of immediate versus WHO recommendations-guided antiretroviral therapy initiation on HIV incidence: the ANRS 12249 TasP (Treatment as Prevention) trial in Hlabisa sub-district, KwaZulu-Natal, South Africa: study protocol for a cluster randomised controlled trial. *Trials, 14,* 230. https://doi.org/10.1186/1745-6215-14-230

8. Nair SA, Raizada N, Sachdeva KS, Denkinger C, Schumacher S, Dewan P, et al. (2016) Factors Associated with Tuberculosis and Rifampicin-Resistant Tuberculosis amongst Symptomatic Patients in India: A Retrospective Analysis. PLoS ONE 11(2): e0150054. https://doi.org/10.1371/journal.pone.0150054 (accessed on 10 May 2025).

9. Arslan, M., Arshad, R., Hameed, F., Iqbal, S., Ahmad, I., Mubeen, A., Ud, I., et al. (2025). A comprehensive review of drug-resistant tuberculosis: Mechanisms, epidemiology, and diagnostic approaches. *Insights–Journal of Health and Rehabilitation.* Volume 3 Issue 2: Drug

Resistance in Tuberculosis. https://www.semanticscholar.org/paper/9d2329a1bbe06e6745067642392b7d196518aaff (accessed on 10 May 2025).

10. Barteka, G., Bwayo, D., Matovu, J. K. B., Wanume, B., Alunyo, J. P., Sseguya, R., Masaba, J. P., et al. (2025). Treatment outcomes and predictors of success for multidrug-resistant tuberculosis (MDR-TB) in Ugandan regional referral hospitals. *Scientific Reports, 15*(1), 14144. https://www.semanticscholar.org/paper/1988f60527f427f586cdd274fe6766b7f55649ae (accessed on 10 May 2025).

11. Bhatnagar, A. K., Hemanthkumar, A., Vijayalakshmi, M. M., Vohra, V., Padmapriyadarsini, C., Ramesh, P. M., Taneja, G., et al. (2024). Effect of bedaquiline and delamanid pharmacokinetics on sputum culture conversion and adverse events in drug-resistant tuberculosis. *Therapeutic Drug Monitoring, 46*, 363–369. https://www.semanticscholar.org/paper/beea92ba4f6b49a3fbcda19420db6cc7786cef78 (accessed on 10 May 2025).

12. Bimo, K., Nugroho, C., & Sasanti, R. R. (2025). A comprehensive literature review of *Mycobacterium tuberculosis* drug resistance. *The International Journal of Medical Science and Health Research*. https://www.semanticscholar.org/paper/a83f57ce2b78a3c6f9a8d6cc5bdb134e4a164c70 (accessed on 10 May 2025).

13. Sebastian M. Gygli, Sonia Borrell, Andrej Trauner, Sebastien Gagneux, Antimicrobial resistance in Mycobacterium tuberculosis: mechanistic and evolutionary perspectives, FEMS Microbiology Reviews, Volume 41, Issue 3, May 2017, Pages 354–373, https://doi.org/10.1093/femsre/fux011 (accessed on 10 May 2025).

14. https://doi.org/10.1080/17512433.2023.2148653. Bossù, G., Autore, G., Bernardi, L., Buonsenso, D., Migliori, G. B., & Esposito, S. (2023). Treatment options for children with multi-drug resistant tuberculosis. *Expert review of clinical pharmacology, 16*(1), 5–15. https://doi.org/10.1080/17512433.2023.2148653

15. Buckley, R. M., d'Arminio Monforte, A., Bracchi, M., Dedes, N., Horban, A., Katlama, C., Латышева, И. Б., et al. (2020). 2019 update of the European AIDS Clinical Society guidelines for treatment of people living with HIV version 10.0. *HIV Medicine, 21*, 617–624. https://doi.org/10.1111/hiv.12878.

16. Dahl, V. N., Butova, T., Rosenthal, A., Grinev, A., Gabrielian, A., Vashakidze, S., Shubladze, N., et al. (2024). Drug-resistant tuberculosis, Georgia, Kazakhstan, Kyrgyzstan, Moldova, and Ukraine, 2017–2022. *Emerging Infectious Diseases, 30*, 831–833. https://www.semanticscholar.org/paper/c150e919c615a2f4ad47e9cb75b503e920808eb3 (accessed on 10 May 2025).

17. Dartois, V., & Rubin, E. J. (2022). Anti-tuberculosis treatment strategies and drug development: Challenges and priorities. *Nature Reviews Microbiology, 20*, 685–701. https://doi.org/10.1038/s41579-022-00731-y.

18. Datiko, D. G., Habte, D., Jerene, D., & Suarez, P. (2019). Knowledge, attitudes, and practices related to TB among the general population of Ethiopia: Findings from a national cross-sectional survey. *PLoS ONE, 14*, e0224196. https://doi.org/10.1371/journal.pone.0224196.

19. Dheda, K., & Sharma, S. K. (2019). What is new in the WHO consolidated guidelines on drug-resistant tuberculosis treatment? *The Indian Journal of Medical Research, 149*, 309. https://doi.org/10.4103/ijmr.ijmr_579_19.

20. Elton, L., Aydin, A., Stoker, N., Rofael, S., Wildner, L. M., Abdul, J. B. P. A. A., Tembo, J. M., et al. (2024). A pragmatic pipeline for drug resistance identification in *Mycobacterium*

tuberculosis using whole genome sequencing. https://www.semanticscholar.org/paper/f0e8b6ecdba312059c12a0edbd5ff9fefe85ed56 (accessed on 10 May 2025).

21. Elton, L., Aydin, A., Stoker, N., Rofael, S., Wildner, L., Abdul, J., Tembo, J. M., et al. (2025). A pragmatic pipeline for drug resistance and lineage identification in *Mycobacterium tuberculosis* using whole genome sequencing. *PLOS Global Public Health, 5*. https://www.semanticscholar.org/paper/04e7ded51f169aba5206dd610c87e04f501e2648 (accessed on 10 May 2025).

22. Faye, L. M., Hosu, M. C., & Apalata, T. (2024). Drug-resistant tuberculosis in rural Eastern Cape, South Africa: A study of patients' characteristics in selected healthcare facilities. *International Journal of Environmental Research and Public Health, 21*. https://www.semanticscholar.org/paper/266bebd4302258aed5406dd43ff0c819f46e7fc5 (accessed on 10 May 2025).

23. McNerney, R., Maeurer, M., Abubakar, I., Marais, B., McHugh, T. D., Ford, N., Weyer, K., Lawn, S., Grobusch, M. P., Memish, Z., Squire, S. B., Pantaleo, G., Chakaya, J., Casenghi, M., Migliori, G. B., Mwaba, P., Zijenah, L., Hoelscher, M., Cox, H., Swaminathan, S., … Zumla, A. (2012). Tuberculosis diagnostics and biomarkers: needs, challenges, recent advances, and opportunities. *The Journal of infectious diseases*, *205 Suppl 2*, S147–S158. https://doi.org/10.1093/infdis/jir860 (accessed on 10 May 2025).

24. Hill, A., Koul, A., Grzegorzewicz, A. E., Mendoza-Losana, A., Tyagi, A. K., Dye, C., Varela, C., et al. (2013). Tetrahydropyrazolo[1,5-a]pyrimidine-3-carboxamide and N-benzyl-6′,7′-dihydrospiro[piperidine-4,4′-thieno[3,2-c]pyran] analogues with bactericidal efficacy against *Mycobacterium tuberculosis* targeting MmpL3. https://core.ac.uk/download/18328074.pdf (accessed on 10 May 2025).

25. Jeffry, E. P., & Seikka, C. S. (2025). A comprehensive literature review of diagnosis and management of multi drug resistant tuberculosis. *The Indonesian Journal of General Medicine*. https://www.semanticscholar.org/paper/63e59789a6b8f7d7ec23747ecff63f951e4e4d7c (accessed on 10 May 2025).

26. Dachuan Jin, Shunqin Jin (2025) Gut Microbiota and Comprehensive Analysis of Drug Resistance Mechanisms in Tuberculosis. Journal of Medicine and Healthcare. SRC/JMHC-379. DOI: doi.org/10.47363/JMHC/2025(7)298(accessed on 10 May 2025).

27. Karmakar, M., Ragonnet, R., Ascher, D., Trauer, J., & Denholm, J. (2022). Estimating tuberculosis drug resistance amplification rates in high-burden settings. *BMC Infectious Diseases, 22*. https://www.semanticscholar.org/paper/ee5e925ba5d2f3887c4c72db185b49a1151369d6 (accessed on 10 May 2025).

28. Li, X., & Liu, J. (2024). Analysis of the results of tuberculosis drug resistance surveillance in Yuexiu District, Guangzhou City, 2013–2022. *Immunity, Inflammation and Disease, 12*(11), e70060. https://www.semanticscholar.org/paper/e9704451424b4207d437ce58bfaa45d3acb7e684 (accessed on 10 May 2025).

29. Mphothulo, N., Hlangu, S., Furin, J., Moshabela, M., & Loveday, M. (2025). Navigating DR-TB treatment care: A qualitative exploration of barriers and facilitators to retention in care among people with history of early disengagement from drug-resistant tuberculosis treatment in Johannesburg, South Africa. *BMC Health Services Research, 25*. https://www.semanticscholar.org/paper/024dedb6e895068ccf089cb463878bd158928f64 (accessed on 10 May 2025).

30. Murray, C. J. L., Ikuta, K. S., Sharara, F., Swetschinski, L. R., Robles Aguilar, G., Gray, A. P., Han, C., et al. (2022). Global burden of bacterial antimicrobial resistance in 2019: A systematic

analysis. *The Lancet, 399*, 629–655. https://doi.org/10.1016/s0140-6736(21)02724-0.

31. Mustafa, G., & Almarshad, F. (2024). Burden and patterns of multidrug-resistant tuberculosis in pediatric and adolescent patients at a tertiary care hospital in Pakistan. *Cures, 16*. https://www.semanticscholar.org/paper/e83c83bdc7418ba8cd9211ef1bf90219440f1032 (accessed on 10 May 2025).

32. Nahid, P., Mase, S., Migliori, G. B., Sotgiu, G., Bothamley, G., Brożek, J., Cattamanchi, A., et al. (2019). Treatment of drug-resistant tuberculosis: An official ATS/CDC/ERS/IDSA clinical practice guideline. *American Journal of Respiratory and Critical Care Medicine, 200*, e93–e142. https://doi.org/10.1164/rccm.201909-1874ST.

33. Nanavare, R. T. (2024). Piloting the complex ground of drug-resistant extrapulmonary tuberculosis in adolescent females: Unraveling challenges and shaping future strategies. *Journal of Medical Science and Clinical Research*. https://www.semanticscholar.org/paper/33308143284d22e505ae1e024360709e0dea3287 (accessed on 10 May 2025).

34. Nasiri, M. J., & Venketaraman, V. (2025). Advances in Host-Pathogen Interactions in Tuberculosis: Emerging Strategies for Therapeutic Intervention. *International journal of molecular sciences, 26*(4), 1621. https://doi.org/10.3390/ijms26041621(accessed on 10 May 2025).

35. Oo, T., Kyaw, K. W. Y., Soe, K., Saw, S., Satyanarayana, S., & Aung, S. T. (2019). Magnitude and reasons for pre-diagnosis attrition among presumptive multi-drug resistant tuberculosis patients in Bago Region, Myanmar: A mixed methods study. *Scientific Reports, 9*. https://doi.org/10.1038/s41598-019-43562-3.

36. Pandey, A. (2024). Emerging therapeutic approaches to drug-resistant tuberculosis: A case report and review of novel treatments. Case Report Frontiers in Medical Case Reports, ISSN: 2582-8142 DOI: http://dx.doi.org/10.47746/FMCR.2024.5503 (accessed on 10 May 2025).

37. S. K., Parivakkam Mani, A., Geethalakshmi, S., & Yadav, S. (2024). Advancements in artificial intelligence for the diagnosis of multidrug resistance and extensively drug-resistant tuberculosis: A comprehensive review. *Cures, 16*. https://www.semanticscholar.org/paper/516896b524b0a53c07897f47d460d84b86137bc5 (accessed on 10 May 2025).

38. Salam, M. A., Al-Amin, M. Y., Salam, M. T., Pawar, J. S., Akhter, N., Rabaan, A. A., & Alqumber, M. A. A. (2023). Antimicrobial resistance: A growing serious threat for global public health. *Healthcare, 11*, 1946. https://doi.org/10.3390/healthcare11131946.

39. Sandgren, A., Hirsh, A. E., Malik, A. N., de Jong, B. C., Maharjan, B., Shrestha, B., Malla, B., et al. (2012). First insights into the phylogenetic diversity of *Mycobacterium tuberculosis* in Nepal. https://core.ac.uk/download/18261343.pdf (accessed on 10 May 2025).

40. Satam, H., Joshi, K., Mangrolia, U., Waghoo, S., Zaidi, G., Rawool, S., Thakare, R. P., et al. (2023). Next-generation sequencing technology: Current trends and advancements. *Biology, 12*, 997. https://doi.org/10.3390/biology12070997.

41. Shah AM, Shah SV. Recent advances in drug therapy for tuberculosis. Natl J Physiol Pharm Pharmacol. 2024; 14(5): 805-814. doi:10.5455/njppp.2024.14.04164202416042024

42. Shah, V., Yogesh, M., Kothari, D. R., Gandhi, R., & Nagda, J. (2024). Audit of risk factors of drug-sensitive, drug-resistant tuberculosis disease: A case-control study of patients registered under NTEP, Gujarat. *Journal of Family Medicine and Primary Care, 13*, 3614–3620. https://

www.semanticscholar.org/paper/930713795d2cdf731cef4e9b1ed798b4c002f453 (accessed on 10 May 2025).

43. Shangase, P. Z., Shaw, B. S., & Shaw, I. (2025). Characteristics and smoking behaviors among patients with drug-resistant tuberculosis (DR-TB) in South Africa. *BMC Public Health, 25.* https://www.semanticscholar.org/paper/9d9efb5d650eb45dba4f62630217b5f7903f7ea9 (accessed on 10 May 2025).

44. Shuaib, Y. A., Khalil, E. A. G., Wieler, L. H., Schaible, U. E., Bakheit, M. A., Mohamed-Noor, S. E., Abdalla, M. A., et al. (2020). *Mycobacterium tuberculosis* Complex Lineage 3 as causative agent of pulmonary tuberculosis, Eastern Sudan. *Emerging Infectious Diseases, 26*, 427–436. https://doi.org/10.3201/eid2603.191145.

45. Storvig, E., Harstad, I., Ehrnström, B., & Iversen, V. C. (2024). Beyond the diagnosis of drug-resistant tuberculosis in Norway: Patients' experiences before, during and after treatment. *BMC Public Health, 24.* https://www.semanticscholar.org/paper/c2ab3fa69d01d8fb09c26d9eb450be17246a2ed2 (accessed on 10 May 2025).

46. Vadakunnel, M. J., Nehru, V. J., Brammacharry, U., Ramachandra, V., Palavesam, S., Muthukumar, A., Mani, B. R., et al. (2025). Impact of *rpoB* gene mutations and rifampicin-resistance levels on treatment outcomes in rifampicin-resistant tuberculosis. *BMC Infectious Diseases, 25.* https://www.semanticscholar.org/paper/7415657ef147332de48dc33c2a1d09919df36405 (accessed on 10 May 2025).

47. Valença, M. S., Scaini, J. L., Abileira, F. S., Gonçalves, C. V., von Groll, A., & Silva, P. E. A. (2015). Prevalence of tuberculosis in prisons: Risk factors and molecular epidemiology. *The International Journal of Tuberculosis and Lung Disease, 19*, 1182–1187. https://doi.org/10.5588/ijtld.15.0126.

48. Vengurlekar, D., Walker, C., Mahajan, R., Dalal, A., Chavan, V., Galindo, M. A., Iyer, A., et al. (2023). Linezolid resistance in patients with drug-resistant TB. *The International Journal of Tuberculosis and Lung Disease, 27*, 567–569. https://www.semanticscholar.org/paper/38848dc206bf7b23c3c0d33b7cd6df803d81da8c (accessed on 10 May 2025).

49. Khutade K J, Wagh S, Shah H, An array of various microbiological diagnostic modalities for pulmonary tuberculosis: A review. Indian J Microbiol Res 2024;11(3):147-155 (accessed on 10 May 2025).

50. Wingfield, T., Karmadwala, F., MacPherson, P., Millington, K., Walker, N. F., Cuevas, L. E., & Squire, S. B. (2021). Challenges and opportunities to end tuberculosis in the COVID-19 era. *The Lancet Respiratory Medicine, 9*, 556–558. https://doi.org/10.1016/S2213-2600(21)00161-2.

51. Xiong, X. S., Zhang, X. D., Yan, J. W., Huang, T. T., Liu, Z. Z., Li, Z. K., Wang, L., et al. (2024). Identification of *Mycobacterium tuberculosis* resistance to common antibiotics: An overview of current methods and techniques. *Infection and Drug Resistance, 17*, 1491–1506. https://www.semanticscholar.org/paper/7c1fa3a299f20d26180765ad4dbcc4560330b6de (accessed on 10 May 2025).

52. Xiong, Y. J., Xiao, Y., Xie, L., Gao, L., Han, Y., Huang, P. F., Liu, S., et al. (2024). Contezolid for the treatment of drug-resistant tuberculosis in China: A clinical case series. *Infection and Drug Resistance, 17*, 3491–3499. https://www.semanticscholar.org/paper/f2b9aaf0df3ae4f093e708429225f23a98c029f7 (accessed on 10 May 2025).

53. Zhang, F., Liu, Y., Liu, Z., Guo, Z., Yang, J., & Zhao, K. (2020). PP400: Cost-effectiveness analysis of adding bedaquiline to drug regimens for multidrug-resistant tuberculosis treatment in China. *International Journal of Technology Assessment in Health Care, 36*, 33–34. https://www.semanticscholar.org/paper/2184604803df0eebe9d0494d36b8fd54f8ec4a94 (accessed on 10 May 2025).

54. Zhang, H., Sun, R., Wu, Z., Liu, Y., Chen, M., Huang, J., Lv, Y., Zhao, F., Zhang, Y., Li, M., Jiang, H., Zhan, Y., Xu, J., Xu, Y., Yuan, J., Zhao, Y., Shen, X., & Yang, C. (2024). Spatial pattern of isoniazid-resistant tuberculosis and its associated factors among a population with migrants in China: a retrospective population-based study. *Frontiers in public health*, *12*, 1372146. https://doi.org/10.3389/fpubh.2024.1372146.

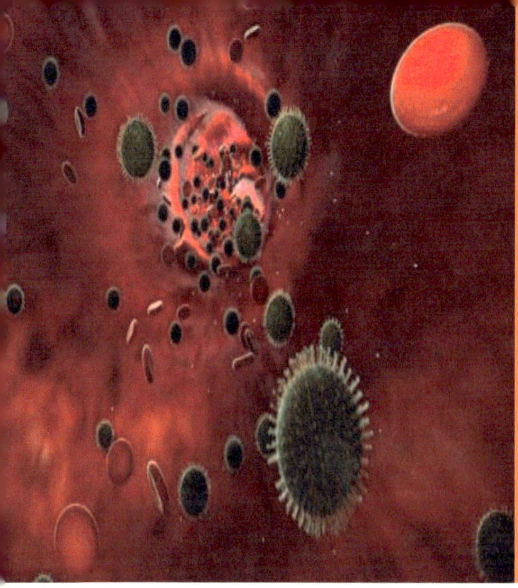

Chapter 8

TB-HIV CO-INFECTION

Contents

Introduction

The international health environment is often assaulted by diseases that overlap and exacerbate one another's effects, making prevention and treatment more difficult. This phenomenon is well illustrated in the relationship between tuberculosis (TB) and human immunodeficiency virus (HIV), two communicable diseases with a large impact on vulnerable populations around the globe. TB continues to be among the primary causes of mortality in HIV-infected individuals, as HIV-induced immunosuppression makes it easier for latent tuberculosis infections (LTBIs) to reactivate and progress. The interaction between these pathogens adds an aggregate burden on healthcare systems, especially in areas where both diseases are endemic. Knowledge of the epidemiological, immunological, and clinical determinants of TB-HIV co-infection is central to the development of comprehensive therapeutic interventions and patient outcomes. The complexity of TB-HIV co-infection is highlighted by the influence that it has on disease progression and control. HIV weakens the immune system, compromising the body's capacity to suppress *Mycobacterium tuberculosis* (MTB) and hence making active TB disease more likely. Conversely, the presence of active TB can accelerate the decline in immune function associated with HIV. This bi-directional relationship complicates diagnosis and treatment, requiring healthcare providers to adopt multifaceted approaches that address both infections simultaneously. Advancements in diagnostic tools and biomarkers, such as the investigation of microRNAs (miRNAs), portend better early detection and customized treatment of co-infected patients, thus improving treatment outcomes and mortality rates (Tribolet et al., 2020). Such developments are a harbinger of precision medicine in the management of infectious disease. TB-HIV co-infection management requires the intervention of multiple disciplines based on evidence-based clinical guidelines. Existing treatment protocols have to reconcile antiretroviral therapy (ART) and anti-tubercular (ATT) medications, managing drug interactions and adherence issues. Emerging consensus recommendations prepared by global experts provide a platform for standardizing treatment protocols, maximizing drug combinations, and taking into account comorbidities and contexts of patients (Wollenberg et al., 2022). The recommendations highlight the need for delivery of integrated care, patient-centered interventions, and ongoing monitoring to prevent complications. As co-infection is an unresolved major public health concern, constant research and refinement of guidelines are essential to ensuring that practice continues to advance in tandem with increasing knowledge of the complex relationships between TB and HIV.

Definition of Human Immunodeficiency Virus (HIV)

The nature of infectious diseases is heightened when two or more pathogens interact in a host, especially when immune function is impaired. One of these, the human immunodeficiency virus (HIV), is particularly noteworthy for its ability to methodically compromise the immune system, making patients increasingly vulnerable to opportunistic pathogens, such as tuberculosis (TB). HIV is a retrovirus that primarily infects $CD4^+$ T lymphocytes, which are key participants in coordinating immune defense. By infecting and killing these cells, HIV increasingly weakens the host immune surveillance and response, resulting in acquired immunodeficiency syndrome (AIDS) in case of no treatment.

Gradual loss lowers the body's capacity to suppress latent infections like MTB, hence enabling latent to active TB progression. A grasp of the definition and biological effects of HIV is crucial in appreciating the dynamics of co-infection of TB and HIV and challenges in treatment and diagnosis. At the molecular level, HIV has an RNA genome contained in a lipid envelope that is derived from the host cell membrane. The virus enters host cells by attaching to the CD4 receptor and co-receptors like CCR5 or CXCR4, facilitating fusion and subsequent reverse transcription of its RNA into DNA.

This viral DNA is incorporated into the genome of the host, creating a chronic infection that defies immune surveillance and antiviral treatments. HIV's life cycle compromises immune cell function and facilitates chronic immune activation, which worsens tissue damage and undermines antimicrobial defense mechanisms. Such a mechanism accounts for the fact that TB, a disease that relies strongly on cell-mediated immunity for control, is so severe and hard to contain among HIV-infected patients. Such interactions also highlight the need for targeted therapies that take into account the complexities of both pathogens among co-infected patients (Chauhan et al., 2024) (Figure 8.1).

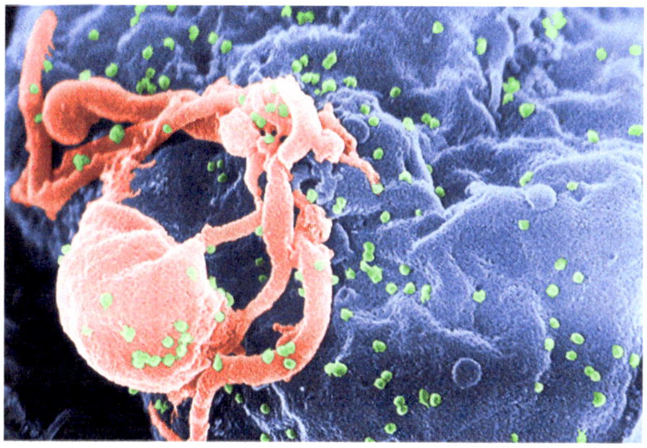

Figure 8.1. HIV structure.

Source: By Photo Credit: C. GoldsmithContent Providers: CDC/ C. Goldsmith, P. Feorino, E. L. Palmer, W. R. McManus - This media comes from the Centers for Disease Control and Prevention's Public Health Image Library (PHIL), with identification number #10000.Note: Not all PHIL images are public domain; be sure to check copyright status and credit authors and content providers.العربية | Deutsch | English | македонски | slovenščina | +/−, Public Domain, https://commons.wikimedia.org/w/index.php?curid=3909584

The clinical presentation of HIV infection is also made complicated by the presence of other infections like TB or syphilis. HIV-induced immunosuppression changes the presentation and course of these diseases, necessitating complex diagnostic and therapeutic strategies. For example, HIV can alter the immune response to TB and thus influence disease progression and treatment outcomes. Co-infections also require close drug interaction consideration and immune reconstitution inflammatory syndrome (IRIS) that has the potential to exacerbate symptoms paradoxically at treatment initiation. This nuance is brought out by clinical scenarios when HIV-positive patients have several concomitant infections, calling for combined therapy approaches to enhance prognosis (Melin & Dharmasanti, 2024). Hence, the definition of HIV in the context of TB co-infection transcends the field of virology to involve an all-encompassing clinical problem necessitating a thorough understanding and handling.

Importance of Studying TB-HIV Co-Infection

The dynamics between tuberculosis (TB) and HIV infection pose a strong challenge to the health systems of the world, particularly in the areas that are plagued by high prevalence levels. Knowledge of the dynamics of TB-HIV co-infection is important since co-infected patients tend to have more adverse disease progression and complications than TB-only patients. Research has shown that the success of TB treatment is lower in co-infected individuals, with both loss to follow-up (LTFU) and mortality rates significantly greater, highlighting the complexities of clinical management in this population (Omara et al., 2025). Without specific studies, these overlapping epidemics can continue to hamper public health measures. Accumulating more in-depth understanding of outcomes of treatment and obstacles can make it possible to create more integrated care models that enhance prognosis, mitigate transmission, and ultimately enhance patient survival and quality of life. Apart from treatment outcomes, understanding predictors of mortality among TB-HIV co-infected patients is crucial to the development of effective intervention approaches. Various factors, such as nutritional status, opportunistic infection, and treatment regimen adherence, strongly affect survival rates. For instance, studies have shown that low body mass index (BMI), extrapulmonary tuberculosis (EPTB) manifestations, and poor adherence to anti-tuberculosis therapy are strongly associated with higher mortality among co-infected individuals (Kegne et al., 2024). Recognizing these predictors allows healthcare providers to identify high-risk patients early and tailor interventions that address these specific factors. Therefore, systematically studying TB-HIV co-infection is essential for improving patient management protocols and resource allocation in healthcare systems, particularly in low-income settings where the burden is disproportionately severe. In addition to clinical implications, studying TB-HIV co-infection holds vital public health significance for controlling the spread of both diseases. Co-infection synergistically exacerbates transmission dynamics, accelerating the proliferation of TB among immunocompromised populations and complicating efforts to contain HIV. The intertwined nature of these diseases demands integrated surveillance and diagnostic frameworks to promptly detect cases and monitor treatment efficacy effectively. Moreover, understanding the epidemiological links and treatment challenges through focused research can inform policy-making and guide investment in targeted prevention programs. Ultimately, prioritizing studies on TB-HIV co-infection is crucial to devising comprehensive public health strategies that not only improve individual patient outcomes but also contribute to the broader goal of disease elimination globally (Kegne et al., 2024; Omara et al., 2025) (Figure 8.2).

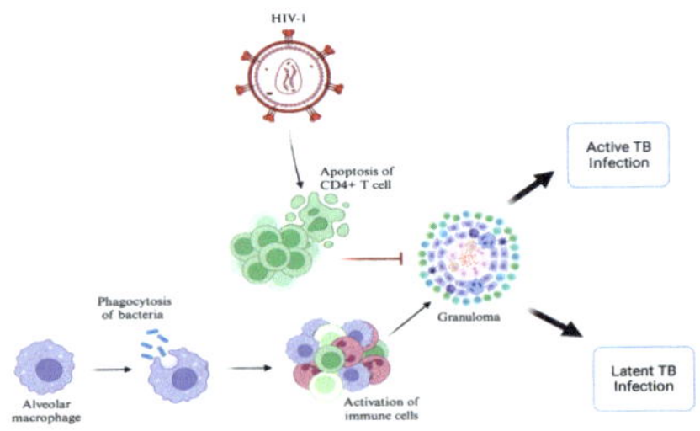

Figure 8.2. Impact of HIV-induced immunosuppression on host CD4⁺ T cell response to TB infection. In immunocompetent individuals infected with *Mtb*, CD4⁺ T lymphocytes along with other immune cells work synergistically to combat infection.

Source: Navasardyan I, Miwalian R, Petrosyan A, Yeganyan S, Venketaraman V. HIV–TB Coinfection: Current Therapeutic Approaches and Drug Interactions. Viruses. 2024; 16(3):321. https://doi.org/10.3390/v16030321

8.1. Epidemiology of TB-HIV Co-Infection

The interaction between tuberculosis (TB) and human immunodeficiency virus (HIV) is a vital public health concern, especially because of their synergistic effects on mortality. Research indicates that HIV-infected individuals, particularly those who have developed acquired immunodeficiency syndrome (AIDS), have a higher vulnerability to opportunistic infections such as TB. For example, a detailed meta-analysis with more than 23,000 participants from Vietnam, China, Japan, Ethiopia, and South Africa revealed that co-infection with TB nearly doubles the risk of death among HIV-positive patients on antiretroviral therapy (aHR = 1.89) (Anindita et al., 2024). This illustrates the synergistic interaction between the two conditions, whereby the immune suppression offered by HIV promotes the reactivation and rapid development of latent TB, enhancing negative health outcomes. TB is thus the most prominent cause of mortality among individuals with HIV (PLHIV), highlighting the need for integrated disease control and targeted interventions among such populations. Similarly, pediatric HIV populations have a distinct epidemiological pattern for TB co-infection that mirrors both the biological susceptibility and transmission patterns. A retrospective case study comparing pediatric HIV cases reported a high TB co-infection rate of 16%, where the patients were predominantly under four years old (Bashir et al., 2023). The dominance of mother-to-child transmission identifies key challenges in preventing HIV vertical transmission and the control of TB where the disease is endemic. Clinical manifestations among these children are often a combination of fever, cough, and weight loss, a presentation which coincides with that of TB, making it difficult to diagnose on time. The co-infection burden in children further increases morbidity, highlighting the importance of stricter screening processes and early prophylactic therapy to address the increased risk of TB in HIV-infected children. Geographical and demographic influences have a major impact on the epidemiology of co-infection for TB-HIV, affecting both outcomes and prevalence. Gender disparities have been noted with evidence indicating that female HIV patients on antiretroviral therapy (ART) were at lower risk of mortality than males (aHR = 0.70) (Anindita et al., 2024). These variations could be attributed to biological, social, and healthcare access determinants influencing disease advancement and treatment compliance. In addition, regional differences in co-infection rates highlight the role endemic TB environments play in exposing HIV groups to increased vulnerability. For instance, high TB prevalence nations report more cases of co-infections, making it challenging to control the disease. Recognizing these epidemiological details is essential in developing policy responses that integrate gender-neutral frameworks and site-specific interventions to effectively stem the double epidemic.

8.1.1. Global Prevalence Rates

The complex relationship between HIV and TB has resulted in a co-infection pattern that is disproportionately high in areas of high HIV prevalence, with sub-Saharan Africa being particularly high on the list. re frameworks addressing both infections simultaneously (Yirsaw et al., 2025) (Figure 8.3).

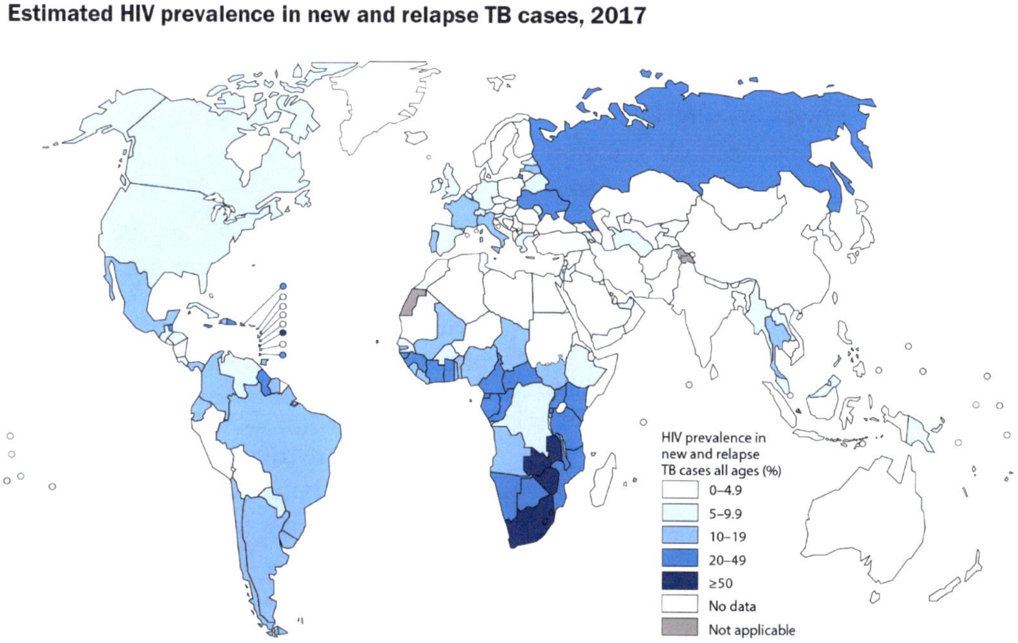

Figure 8.3. Estimated HIV prevalence in new and relapse TB cases, 2017.

Source: Archivos de Bronconeumología. (2020). *Estimated HIV prevalence in new and relapse TB cases, 2017.* https://www.archbronconeumol.org/en-tuberculosis-hiv-co-infection-progress-challenges-after-articulo-S1579212920301518.

Co-existence of the infectious diseases brings together individual susceptibility, hence enhancing the disease burden. For example, in Ethiopia, the pooled pulmonary tuberculosis prevalence is 15% among HIV/AIDS adults, a high rate that observes the synergistic epidemic in the region. This higher prevalence is determined by immunosuppression variables like low CD4 levels and high HIV clinical stages that weaken the host defenses and allow for TB activation and progression. Smoking and decreased physical mobility also increase vulnerability. These results emphasize the way compromised immune systems in HIV-positive patients provide a setting for infection and advancement of TB, placing a premium on holistic, integrated ca

At the global level, the epidemiology of TB-HIV co-infection is characterized by heterogeneity of incidence and mortality rates, which mirror differential healthcare capacity and epidemic severity in different countries. The Global Burden of Disease Study data highlight that in 2021, the age-standardized incidence rate (ASIR) of HIV-infected drug-susceptible tuberculosis (HIV-DS-TB) was around 11.59 per 1,00,000 population globally. Also on the rise are cases of more drug-resistant TB types—HIV-MDR-TB and HIV-XDR-TB—albeit lower in absolute numbers, exhibit alarming increasing trends. The estimated annual percentage change (EAPC) reveals increasing incidence rates for these resistant types, inferring widening problems in disease control. These worldwide trends note long-standing public health issues, especially in regions where treatment and diagnostic capacities are low, and act as important predictors for directing intervention resources to stem both HIV and TB incidence concurrently (Zhang et al., 2024). Developing a global understanding of TB-HIV co-infection also involves noting the continued changes in mortality and disease incidence over time. Though the case number is the major concern, morbidity and mortality due to co-infection reflect the entire burden on public health systems. The age-standardized mortality rate (ASMR) for HIV-DS-TB in 2021 continued high at 2.22 per 1,00,000 population across the world, the drug-resistant types demonstrating smaller but rising death rates. These death trends mirror incidence trends, the latter demonstrating the growing complexity of resistance presented by resistant TB strains among HIV-infected populations. Since co-infection results in added disability-adjusted life years (DALYs), the need for more diagnostic accuracy, robust healthcare infrastructure, and greater access to combined care is heightened. Global health policy must thus become responsive to these changing prevalence and death profiles to contain this lethal co-epidemic more effectively (Zhang et al., 2024) (Figure 8.4).

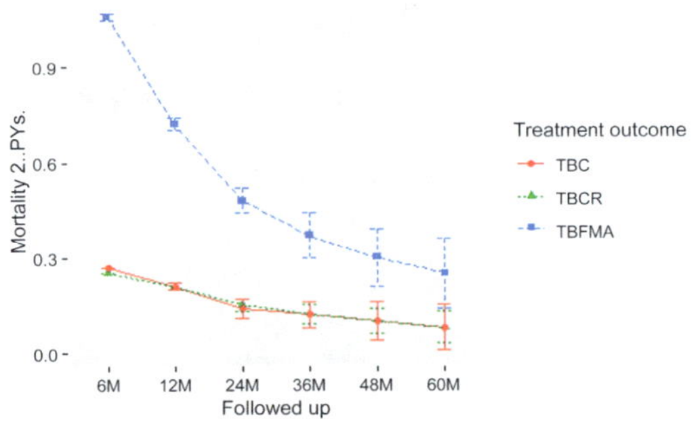

Figure 8.4. Annual prevalence of TB/HIV co-infection stratified by sex.

Source: Zheng, Z., Nehl, E.J., Zhou, C. *et al.* Insufficient tuberculosis treatment leads to earlier and higher mortality in individuals co-infected with HIV in southern China: a cohort study. *BMC Infect Dis* **20**, 873 (2020). https://doi.org/10.1186/s12879-020-05527-0

8.1.2. High-Risk Populations

Populations with socio-economic vulnerabilities tend to carry the bulk of infectious disease burdens, such as TB and HIV. In areas like South Africa's Northern Cape Province, there is a mix of demographic factors and living conditions that raises the risk of disease. As an illustration, gender was an independent predictor of tuberculosis in this high-incidence environment, with approximately a threefold raised risk compared to women. In addition, other factors like rural birthplace with residence in more urban townships increase exposure and susceptibility. These patterns represent rapid socio-economic change where mobility, poverty, and community structure shape transmission patterns. Even though lifestyle issues like smoking and alcohol use have long been associated with TB, their contribution was not present in this population, so other systemic and environmental factors could be more pertinent. It is crucial to understand these subtle risk profiles in the formulation of public health interventions attuned to localized epidemiology (Oshiomah et al., 2023). Some stigmatized groups, such as injecting drug users, men having sex with men, and sex workers, have enhanced risks as a result of intersecting social and medical vulnerabilities. Syndemic states—where interacting co-occurring epidemics reinforce each other, exacerbate the risk of HIV acquisition and co-infection with tuberculosis. These groups often have in place barriers like stigma, discrimination, poverty, and limited access to health care, which compromise treatment adherence and health outcomes. The presence of comorbid infections and related social determinants not only increases susceptibility but also makes clinical management challenging. This difficulty calls for an integrated approach that brings together medical, psychological, and social services to tackle the multifaceted nature of risk. By targeting interventions at these groups, public health action can efficiently break chains of transmission and enhance prognosis (Moneke et al., 2022). Identification of high-risk groups within TB-HIV co-infection settings highlights the paramount significance of targeted prevention and treatment approaches. Epidemiological data supports the deployment of tailored harm reduction interventions, in combination with culturally sensitive screening and care. Policies must be directed at the unique vulnerabilities engendered by socio-behavioral and biophysical circumstances particular to these populations. For example, combining community outreach efforts with specialized healthcare staff can improve treatment program engagement and retention. Policymaker, healthcare provider, and community organization intersectoral collaboration is essential to making interventions sustainable and effective. In addition, reducing stigma and discrimination by means of education and advocacy has the potential to enhance access and compliance among such vulnerable populations. Such strategic guidelines have the potential not only to diminish disease prevalence but also to mitigate the larger social inequalities responsible for the syndemic of TB-HIV (Moneke et al., 2022; Oshiomah et al., 2023).

8.1.3. Geographic Distribution of Co-Infection

Recognition of the geographical distributions of TB-HIV co-infection is important for the establishment of focused public health interventions. Disproportionate co-infection burden is centrally located in areas of co-endemicity for the two diseases, frequently compounded by socioeconomic and healthcare inequalities. Sub-Saharan Africa, for instance, is still the focus of TB-HIV co-infection cases, indicating overlapping epidemics fueled by high levels of HIV prevalence and continued TB transmission. Geographic patterns vary also due to demographic density, healthcare facilities, and access to diagnostic and treatment facilities. Capturing these patterns with exactitude through sophisticated modeling is crucial, as it allows policymakers to predict trends more accurately and target resources where they are most urgently required, thereby making intervention strategies more precise (Abade et al., 2024). These geographically stratified models illuminate the complex interplay between the dynamics of disease and social determinants of health, reinforcing the necessity of customized regional strategies in the fight against co-infection. Ethiopia provides a striking case study of how geographically conditioned context influences the extent of TB-HIV co-infection, with mortality rates mirroring localized issues within the healthcare system. Epidemiological analysis demonstrates that some Ethiopian areas have significantly greater mortality rates among those with co-infection, depending on widespread comorbidities and stages of disease progression. Conditions like advanced immunosuppression, extrapulmonary tuberculosis (EPTB), and functional impairment disproportionately hit patients in regions with poor access to ART and prophylaxis. These geographic inequalities not only influence patient outcomes but point toward the urgent need for region-specific data informing public health policies. In addition, systematic reviews in Ethiopia demonstrate the potential of aggregation of regional mortality data to pinpoint hotspots where intensified screening, early treatment initiation, and full care should be provided to stem the disproportionate burden borne by the affected population (Moges et al., 2024). The uneven geographic distribution of TB-HIV co-infection calls for the confluence of biases-free epidemiological surveillance with cutting-edge predictive analytics. Current developments in machine learning and deep learning have been found especially efficient in capturing inherent non-linear co-infection relationships within co-infection data from all regions. Through the integration of temporal case information with geospatial attributes, the predictive models are able to refine patterns of disease transmission and pick out emerging high-risk areas. Precision of this kind is crucial in low-resource environments where blanket interventions can be unproductive or unaffordable. Using methods such as Bidirectional LSTM and CNN-LSTM networks makes it possible to perform high-fidelity predicting that take into consideration seasonal trends as well as complex disease dynamics in particular communities. Therefore, using these technologies enables more adaptive and evidence-informed distribution of health resources to communities facing the highest burden of co-infection (Abade et al., 2024) (Figure 8.5).

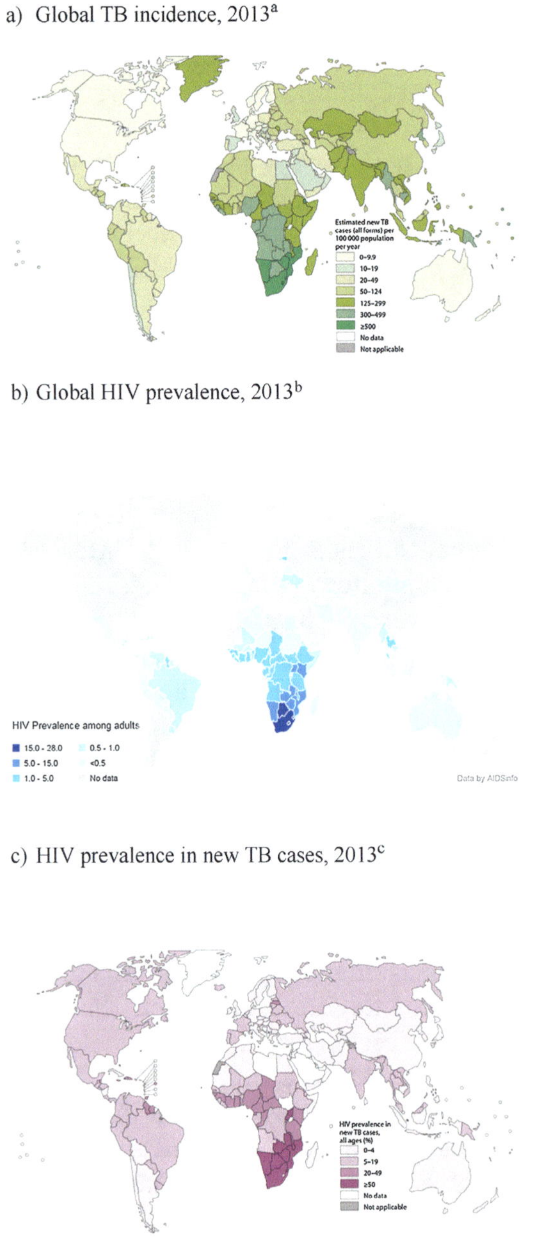

Figure 8.5. Global disease burden associated with TB and HIV.

Source: ScienceDirect. (2014). *Global TB incidence and HIV prevalence, 2013.*

8.2. Pathophysiology of TB-HIV Co-Infection

The interaction between *Mycobacterium tuberculosis* (MTB) and HIV-1 tightly dysregulates immune homeostasis, resulting in accelerated disease advancement among co-infected subjects. In the case of spinal tuberculosis, diagnostic examinations have produced markedly higher MTBC DNA levels in HIV-infected patients, reflecting higher bacterial loads at the site of disease. Elevated bacterial load accelerates local inflammation and tissue damage, thereby worsening neurological and physical impairment. Sensitive diagnostic technologies like Xpert MTB/RIF Ultra and droplet digital PCR have shown greater sensitivity in identifying *Mtb*, particularly in paucibacillary samples characteristic of co-infection situations. These results highlight not just the diagnostic difficulties but also complex pathophysiology where HIV-1 infection compromises immune control over *Mtb* to facilitate greater bacterial replication and dissemination in spinal tissues. Identification of these interactions is vital to maximize therapeutic interventions and reduce TB-HIV co-infection morbidity (Waters et al., 2023).

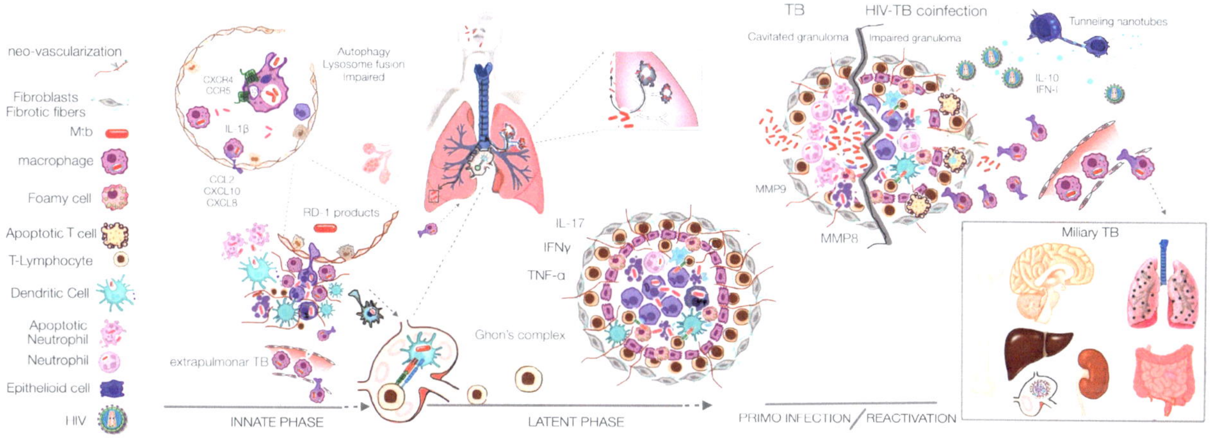

Figure 8.6. Pathogenesis of *Mtb* infection: implications in HIV co-infection. Inhaled aerosols containing up to three bacilli reach the alveoli in the lower part of the lung.

Source: Azevedo-Pereira JM, Pires D, Calado M, Mandal M, Santos-Costa Q, Anes E. HIV/Mtb Co-Infection: From the Amplification of Disease Pathogenesis to an "Emerging Syndemic". Microorganisms. 2023; 11(4):853. https://doi.org/10.3390/microorganisms11040853

A key component of pathophysiology of TB-HIV co-infection is defective immune regulation by immune checkpoint molecules and cytokines. Studies have shown that co-infected patients have a heightened level of PD1 expression on $CD8^+$ T cells in conjunction with heightened IL-10 secretion. This immunosuppressive environment is a consequence of dysfunctional antigen presentation fueled by impaired transporter associated with antigen processing (TAP) function in dendritic cells (DCs) and macrophages. These impairments lower efficient T cell activation, enabling MTB immune evasion, and supporting chronic infection. The disruption of host immune defense mechanisms therefore enables *Mtb* to take over the host system, which is further exacerbated by HIV-induced immunosuppression. These molecular observations of PD1, IL-10, and TAP pathways identify essential immune evasion mechanisms that drive TB reactivation and disease progress among HIV-infected individuals, presenting complex challenges in the design of innovative immunotherapeutic interventions (Sunder et al., 2020). The combined pathophysiologic impacts of TB and HIV extend from localized infection to generalized immune dysregulation, significantly raising inflammatory mechanisms. High plasma biomarkers that correlate with increased mycobacterial burden suggest that co-infection maintains an enhanced inflammatory condition, which paradoxically does not clear infection efficiently. HIV-1-induced CD4⁺ T cell depletion impairs granuloma formation, destabilizing the hosts primary defense against *Mtb* containment. Destabilization permits mycobacterial dissemination and chronic infection, leading to greater morbidity. Moreover, the interaction between *Mtb* and HIV worsens tissue damage by recruiting inflammatory cells and the release of cytokines, further making clinical outcomes more difficult. These interactions at both systemic and local levels help present the conceptual framework that is critical in creating a combined diagnostic and therapeutic strategy to control TB-HIV co-infection effectively (Waters et al., 2023) (Figure 8.6).

8.2.1. Interaction Between TB and HIV

The dynamic interaction between HIV and TB greatly hampers disease control and enhances morbidity and mortality globally. HIV infection severely compromises the immune system, specifically $CD4^+$ T cells that are critical in the maintenance of *Mycobacterium tuberculosis* (Mtb) containment. This immunosuppression tremendously raises the risk of developing active disease from latent tuberculosis infection (LTBI) by over 20-fold. Despite ART, which plays a central role in the recovery of immune competence and lowering TB incidence, risk among HIV-infected persons continues to be significantly increased compared with the general population. This continued susceptibility points to an incomplete immune reconstitution by ART, implying that other immunological disturbances provoked by HIV remain to sustain TB reactivation. Knowing these cellular and molecular mechanisms of the increased TB susceptibility in co-infected individuals is crucial to guide the development of better therapeutic and preventive methods (Kaushal et al., 2023). DCs become central to the pathogenesis of HIV-TB co-infection because they act as a bridge between innate and adaptive immunity. Both HIV and some retroviruses hijack DC function to facilitate evading immune recognition and viral spread. In co-infection, HIV uses DCs to infect $CD4^+$ T cells more effectively, further compromising immune system integrity. DC impairment also impairs antigen-presenting activity, inhibiting the induction of effective immune responses required to contain *Mtb* infection. In addition, the neurologic sequelae seen with HIV infections, creating conditions like HIV-associated neurocognitive disorders (HAND), can worsen the overall health complications of the patient. These complex interactions reflect that the immune dysregulation in the case of HIV/TB co-infection is not merely due to straightforward depletion of the immune cells but includes complex neuro-immunological mechanisms (Mulherkar et al., 2022) (Figure 8.7).

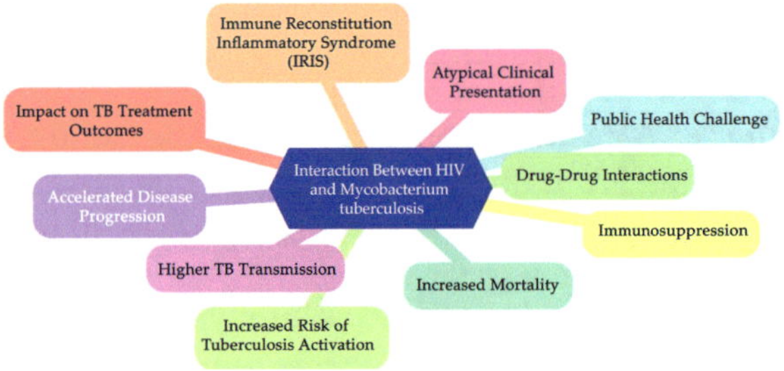

Figure 8.7. The interaction between HIV and *Mycobacterium tuberculosis.*

Source: Patel A, Pundkar A, Agarwal A, et al. (September 06, 2024) A Comprehensive Review of HIV-Associated Tuberculosis: Clinical Challenges and Advances in Management. Cureus 16(9): e68784. doi:10.7759/cureus.68784

The chronic immune activation in TB-HIV co-infection presents enormous challenges for disease and treatment control. Even with successful ART suppressing viral replication, immune system dysfunctions persist, creating a setting that is conducive to reactivation of *Mtb* and disease progression. This chronic immune activation fosters systemic inflammation that can cause host tissue damage and damage protective immunity, making the course of both infections more complex. Treatment of these immunological disturbances involves holistic therapeutic approaches, which blend anti-TB therapy with interventions aimed at HIV-driven immune dysregulation. Existing treatments emphasize viral suppression and bacterial clearance, but future treatments need to include modulation of chronic immune activation for improved patient outcomes. These observations highlight the importance of a multi-faceted strategy with molecular, immunological, and pharmacological foundations in TB-HIV co-infected groups (Kaushal et al., 2023).

8.2.2. Immune System Implications

The delicate balance of the human immune system is severely compromised in the co-infection of TB and HIV, and this gives rise to aggravated difficulties in controlling the pathogens. The adaptive immune response, especially the function of $CD8^+$ T cells, is very important in fighting off the two infections. Yet, in co-infected patients, the cells are prone to experience hierarchical differentiation characterized by a progressive process of exhaustion, which compromises their cytotoxicity functions. Of particular interest are memory stem T cells (TSCM), which constitute a reservoir of highly resistant and potent immune cells with the ability to maintain long-term immunological memory. Changes in TSCM frequency and functionality of $CD8^+$ TSCM cells during co-infection suggest that immune exhaustion impairs the ability to launch strong responses against both HIV and MTB. Targeting the repair or improvement of these cells may provide new therapeutic options to enhance disease outcomes in co-infected patients (Xiao et al., 2024). Apart from adaptive immunity, innate immune factors such as natural killer (NK) cells are important for the early defense against TB and HIV. The phenotypic profile of NK cells is drastically altered in TB/HIV co-infection with an increased size of the $CD56^-$ NK cell subset, which has functional deficits. This defective NK cell phenotype is linked with decreased ability to eliminate mycobacterial infection, hence disease progression. Interestingly, successful TB treatment results in partial recovery and re-tuning of NK cell subsets, underscoring the dynamic interaction between therapeutic treatment and immune recuperation.

Furthermore, phenotypic characteristics like NKp46 expression on $CD56^{+dim}$ NK cells are associated with reduced lung cavitation, suggesting that certain NK cell phenotypes both control pathogens and disease severity (Maseko et al., 2023). The combined disruption of adaptive and innate immune responses in TB and HIV co-infection creates a precarious immune environment that challenges effective pathogen clearance and heightens disease severity. Exhausted $CD8^+$ T cells and impaired NK cell subsets illustrate how both arms of immunity are compromised, allowing for unchecked MTB proliferation under the influence of HIV-induced immunosuppression. These immunological changes play a central role in co-infection pathogenesis and highlight the utility of immune-directed therapeutic approaches. Augmenting $CD8^+$ TSCM cell function and rectifying NK cell dysfunctions may reconstitute immune competence, decrease bacterial burden, and enhance clinical presentation in co-infected patients. Therefore, the immune system consequences of HIV and TB co-infection represent a multifaceted interplay of cellular depletion and functional compromise in several compartments of the immune system, necessitating an integrated strategy for treatment (Maseko et al., 2023; Xiao et al., 2024) (Figure 8.8).

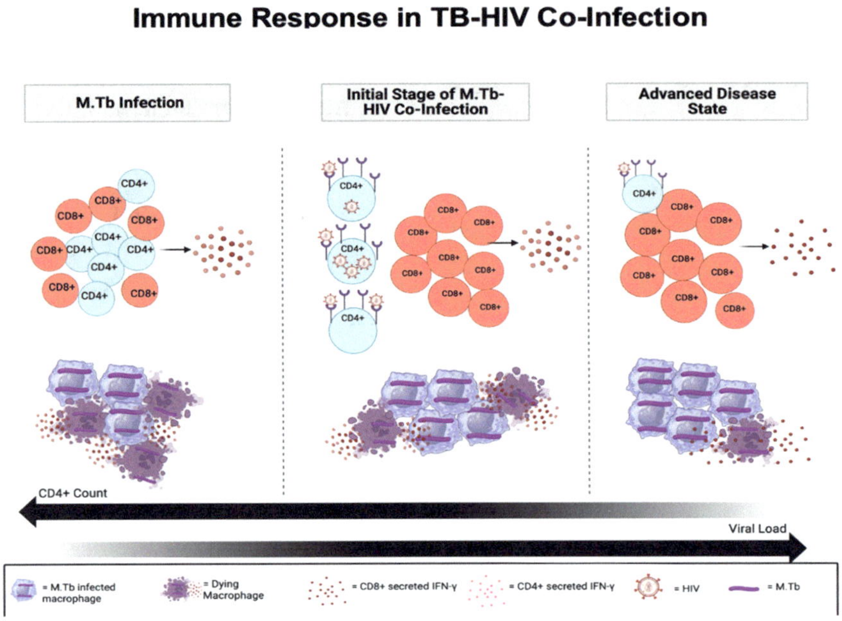

Figure 8.8. Immune response in TB and HIV co-infection.

Source: Hosseinian K, Gerami A, Bral M, Venketaraman V. *Mycobacterium tuberculosis*–Human Immunodeficiency Virus Infection and the Role of T Cells in Protection. Vaccines. 2024; 12(7):730. https://doi.org/10.3390/vaccines12070730

8.2.3. Progression of Disease in Co-Infected Individuals

The dynamic interaction between HIV and TB infections plays a critical role in determining the course of disease in patients with co-infection. Immunosuppression induced by HIV accelerates the natural course of TB by compromising cellular immune mechanisms responsible for containing MTB. Not only does this immunologic impairment allow LTBIs to reactivation, but it also makes the patients susceptible to primary progressive TB. As a result, patients with co-infection tend to develop more virulent clinical manifestations and worse outcomes. Experiments have emphasized that lower CD4 cell counts—a characteristic of HIV progression—positively correlate with susceptibility to TB co-infection and accelerated disease progression. In addition, TB causes HIV viral replication to occur, further accelerating immune degradation and AIDS progression. These cross-talk pathological processes set up a vicious cycle of waning immunity and rising pathogen burden in co-infected individuals, reflecting the interdependence of disease advancement in this group (Clarence, 2020; Bayabil et al., 2021). Clinical markers like body weight, hemoglobin concentration, and WHO clinical staging are essential prognostic indicators of TB-HIV co-infection progression and severity. Weight and hemoglobin declines, which are characteristic of late HIV disease, are associated with lower CD4 cell counts and compromised susceptibility to opportunistic infections such as TB. Interestingly, patients in more advanced AIDS clinical stages are characterized by a pronounced susceptibility to TB, with frequent aggressive progression and unfavorable response to treatment. Adherence to ART and TB treatment has a strong moderating effect on disease progression. Adherence is protective against immunosuppression and the acquisition of opportunistic infections and thus improves the clinical course. In addition, greater healthcare visit frequency works to enhance patient outcomes by allowing for closer surveillance and prompt treatment of co-infection complications. Such clinical parameters, in combination with immunological indicators, explain how biological and behavioral variables come together to influence disease progression in individuals who are co-infected (Bayabil et al., 2021). Social determinants and systemic inequities also exacerbate TB-HIV co-infection progression by determining disease susceptibility and treatment availability. Structural determinants like poverty, poor healthcare infrastructure, and stigma hinder early diagnosis and uniform treatment compliance, thus compounding prognoses. Syndemic theory highlights that concurring epidemics do not only co-exist but also synergistically interact in adverse social environments to exacerbate health inequalities. For instance, institutionalized racism and socio-economic exclusion both compromise immune system function and exposure risk, resulting in increased disease burdens and more rapid progression among stigmatized populations. The interactive nature of biological, social, and environmental factors requires concerted public health interventions that tackle both medical and social aspects of co-infection. By acknowledging these multifactorial determinants, interventions can be more suitably designed to minimize disease progression and maximize survival rates among co-infected individuals (Clarence, 2020; Bayabil et al., 2021).

8.3. Clinical Manifestations

The co-infection TB-HIV is complex not only in its epidemiological load, but also in the subtlety and heterogeneity of its clinical presentation. Patients with TB-HIV co-infection tend to present overlapping symptoms between both conditions, making it difficult to diagnose and treat in the early stages. Common presenting clinical features are chronic cough, fever, chronic diarrhea, and excessive weight loss, all of which signal immune system compromise with added effects of co-infection. Laboratory reports usually show low hemoglobin levels with normal leukocyte and platelet counts, indicating the hematological effects co-infection has on the host. These manifestations underscore the immunosuppressive synergy between TB and HIV, as the body struggles with impaired CD4 cell counts and the systemic effects of two opportunistic infections acting in tandem (Ketaren et al., 2025). The clinical spectrum of TB-HIV co-infected patients extends to both pulmonary and extrapulmonary presentations, which further complicates clinical management. For example, mesenteric tuberculosis, as uncommon as it is, illustrates the extrapulmonary disease in co-infected patients and is characterized by manifestations of abdominal pain, distension, and systemic symptoms such as fever and anorexia. Such atypical manifestations require a high degree of suspicion in HIV-infected patients with nonspecific gastrointestinal complaints. Physical examination may also yield signs such as ascites and diminished breath sounds, indicative of advanced disease states involving multiple organ systems. Optimal clinical assessment therefore necessitates careful diagnostic work incorporating radiologic imaging, tissue biopsies, and laboratory tests in an attempt to apprehend the multimodal nature of TB-HIV co-infection (Maulidiyah et al., 2024). The clinical variation in presentations calls for a holistic, multidisciplinary strategy in diagnosis and management. As much as pulmonary and EPTB occur with a high degree of frequency together in HIV-infected patients, clinical suspicion is important to recognize combinations of symptoms that would otherwise be inappropriately attributed to one disease process. Early detection of symptoms such as chronic cough with extrapulmonary signs such as abdominal rigidity or lymphadenopathy can avoid diagnostic delay. Treatment regimens that integrate anti-TB treatment with antiretroviral therapy, together with supportive care such as prevention of opportunistic infections, are all dependent on proper clinical evaluation to achieve maximum benefit for patients. Finally, proper knowledge of clinical presentations in TB-HIV co-infection is critical for minimizing morbidity and mortality of this dual epidemic (Maulidiyah et al., 2024; Ketaren et al., 2025).

8.3.1. Symptoms of TB in HIV-Positive Patients

The clinical presentation of TB among HIV-positive persons tends to deviate from classic symptoms in immunocompetent persons, making it challenging to diagnose and treat on time. Though pulmonary TB continues to be the leading form, co-infection with HIV enhances the risk of extrapulmonary types, which are often uncharacteristic and subtle. For instance, the symptoms of uncontrolled fever, dramatic weight loss, nocturnal sweats, and generalized weakness are general but nonspecific and coexist with other opportunistic diseases prevalent in HIV-positive patients. In addition, cough—the classic sign of pulmonary TB—is occasionally absent or diminished in advanced immunocompromised patients, making diagnosis difficult.

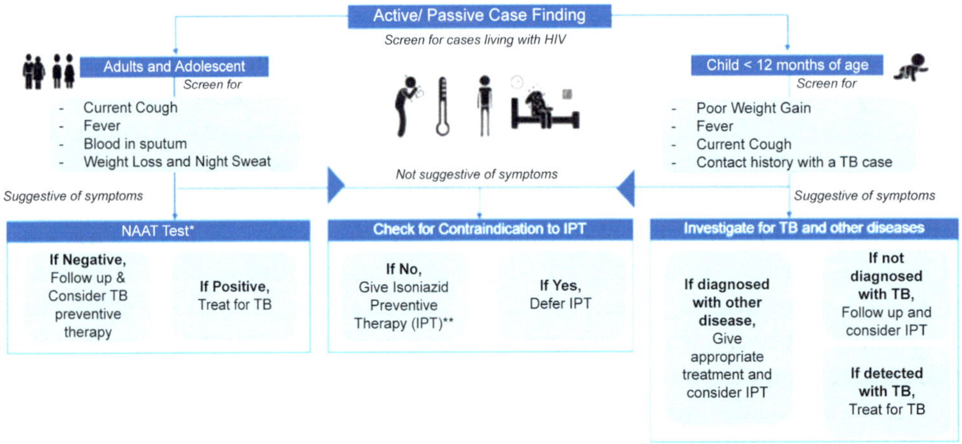

Figure 8.9. Screening steps for TB-HIV patients.

Source: National Tuberculosis Elimination Program (NTEP). (n.d.). *Screening and management algorithm for TB in people living with HIV.* https://ntep.in/node/580/CP-hiv-tb-patients.

These differences highlight the importance of increased clinical suspicion and thorough diagnostic methods when assessing HIV-infected patients for TB to reduce morbidity and mortality from late diagnosis. Interaction between HIV-mediated immunocompromise and TB infection plays an important role in symptom manifestation and disease course. HIV-infected patients tend to present with a more disseminated type of TB, affecting several organ systems outside the lungs, including lymph nodes (LNs), the central nervous system (CNS), and the abdomen. These extrapulmonary manifestations manifest with varied symptoms, such as lymphadenopathy, neurological impairment, and abdominal discomfort or ascites, not typically seen in classical pulmonary TB. Moreover, co-infection causes accelerated disease progression and more serious constitutional symptoms, complicating clinical evaluation. This requires dependency on sophisticated laboratory equipment and extensive clinical evaluation to effectively recognize and treat these unusual presentations, especially in resource-poor settings where both infections are endemic (Benjamin, 2023). Laboratory diagnostic techniques such as urine lateral flow–lipoarabinomannan (LF-LAM) testing have been suggested to enhance detection of TB among HIV-positive patients because of their unusual symptom presentation. Recent evidence, however, identifies pitfalls such as false positives resulting from infections with nontuberculous mycobacteria (NTM) or other opportunistic infections such as nocardiosis and cryptococcosis. These conditions simulate TB manifestations and make it difficult for clinical decision-making, highlighting the absolute necessity of prudent interpretation of test results in the overall clinical context. Notably, false positives can cause unnecessary treatment and worsen patient morbidity when confirmatory diagnosis through culture or molecular techniques is not available. Thus, while symptom awareness is most important, it has to be combined with meticulous diagnostic evaluation to prevent mismanagement in HIV-TB co-infected patients (Sharma & Kumar, 2025) (Figure 8.9).

8.3.2. Symptoms of HIV in TB Patients

The interaction of HIV and TB significantly impacts the clinical presentation seen in the co-infected individuals. During early HIV infection, patients may have nonspecific flu-like illness, which may make it difficult to identify coexisting TB. As HIV advances and the immune function becomes more impaired, the risk for opportunistic infection such as TB increases dramatically. More pronounced symptoms such as chronic cough, weight loss, night sweats, and prolonged fever commonly occur in patients with these symptoms being the classic signs of tuberculosis. In HIV, however, the symptoms might occur atypically or with increased intensity as a result of dysregulation of the immune system. TB in HIV-positive patients thus can occur in extrapulmonary locations, further complicating the symptomatology and necessitating cautious clinical assessment for diagnosis and treatment (Hoque et al., 2024). Immunosuppression due to HIV changes the pathophysiology of tuberculosis, leading to an increased, more complex symptomatic spectrum. In co-infected individuals, TB often appears in atypical locations like the spine, LNs, and disseminated organs, where the symptoms may be inconspicuous or masquerade as other diseases. Spinal tuberculosis is a case in point, which can result in localized pain, neurological impairment, and physical disability if it goes undiagnosed. HIV-induced immunodeficiency promotes increased bacterial loads in infected tissues, increasing local inflammation and systemic manifestations. More advanced diagnostic methods, including molecular tests for detecting *Mycobacterium tuberculosis* complex (MTBC) DNA, have played a central role in detecting TB in HIV-infected persons, verifying the increased bacterial burden and its association with symptom intensity (Waters et al., 2023). This assessment calls for implementing sensitive and prompt diagnostic means to tackle the complex clinical presentations among co-infected individuals. HIV-TB co-infected patients' systemic symptoms are a reflection of the additive immune impairment due to viral and bacterial pathogens. The decline of the immune system in HIV allows for ongoing MTB replication, tending to result in aggressive disease evolution. Subtle common symptoms such as unexplained weight loss, fatigue, and lymphadenopathy can be accentuated while pulmonary presentations of cough and hemoptysis may vary with immune reconstitution inflammatory syndrome (IRIS) when antiretroviral therapy (ART) starts. Laboratory indicators of immune activation and inflammation have also been associated with bacterial load at the sites of disease, which reflects the systemic nature of co-infection. Improved awareness of the overlapping and distinctive clinical features of TB in the context of HIV is essential for early recognition, timely diagnostic testing, and effective management (Waters et al., 2023; Hoque et al., 2024).

8.3.3. Diagnostic Challenges

The difficulty in diagnosing TB among HIV co-infected patients is mainly a function of the atypical presentations and overlapping symptomology of the two illnesses. Patients with weakened immune systems may not present with typical tuberculosis symptoms, like chronic cough or specific radiographic findings, making it difficult to identify the infection on time. Also, EPTB presentations, such as uncommon forms like mesenteric TB, further complicate the diagnostic picture because of their nonspecific symptoms and vague clinical features. This complexity of the case requires a holistic and multidisciplinary effort for proper diagnosis, incorporating tissue biopsies, radiographic imaging, and laboratory tests to separate dual infections appropriately. The need for combinational diagnostic approaches is reinforced by the risk of delayed treatment initiation and poor outcomes in the absence of timely and accurate disease classification (Maulidiyah et al., 2024). The insidious presentation of co-infection scenarios emphasizes the imperative to refine and modify existing diagnostic protocols for better patient prognosis. Metabolic changes among TB-HIV co-infected patients add extra layers of diagnostic complexity beyond clinical and microbiological evaluations. The interconnected metabolic perturbations, especially in fatty acid and protein metabolism, have been discovered through targeted metabolomics studies, revealing distinctive urinary biomarkers that may improve disease detection. Altered amino acid profiles and increased medium-chain acylcarnitine's indicate a physiological environment that mimics diabetes and cachexia, making clinical interpretation of symptoms and biomarker readouts challenging. These metabolic alterations not only impact diagnostic accuracy but also determine disease progression and response to treatment, being essential factors for consideration in diagnostic assessment. Elucidating these biochemical signatures via sophisticated methods like liquid chromatography mass spectrometry could enable more accurate differentiation between TB, HIV, and co-infection statuses, hence resolving crucial diagnostic challenges in clinics (Pretorius et al., 2024). Incorporating metabolic profiling into diagnostic frameworks promises to refine identifying co-infected patients with complex presentations. Despite advances in diagnostic technology, the integration of TB and HIV care remains hindered by systemic and logistical challenges that impact diagnosis quality and timeliness. Where co-infection rates are high in resource-poor environments, access to thorough diagnostic modalities such as sophisticated imaging, biopsy facilities, and metabolomics remains limited, leading to underdiagnosis or misdiagnosis. Additionally, interacting treatment regimens require careful planning to ensure lack of drug interactions and resistance, rendering timely and precise diagnosis crucial. The partnership model between TB and HIV/ AIDS control programs becomes necessary to overcome such limitations, ensuring coordinated testing, treatment monitoring, and follow-up. This was reflected in clinical examples of effective EPTB and HIV co-infection management through combined diagnostic and treatment approaches (Maulidiyah et al., 2024). Resolution of these operational barriers will be imperative to enhancing detection levels and maximizing health outcomes among co-infected individuals worldwide.

8.4. Treatment Strategies

Optimal management of TB-HIV co-infection requires an integrated strategy attacking the two infections jointly to maximize patient outcomes and curtail transmission. Mathematical modeling identifies the potential benefit of dual vaccine and treatment approaches in controlling disease transmission. By examining different compartments of a population, such as susceptible, infected, and recovered individuals—studies show how elevating vaccination coverage rates coupled with prompt treatment can effectively lower the rates of TB, HIV, and their co-infection. This substantiates the fact that interventions in public health need to focus on preventive and curative measures of equal importance, scaling up vaccine campaigns aimed at high-risk groups while granting access to regimens of treatment. These models emphasize the significance of multifaceted approaches integrating vaccination and treatment interventions as complementary tools to reduce the burden of these interlinked epidemics (Toaha et al., 2024). Treatment protocols for TB–HIV co-infection need to be well coordinated because of the challenges posed by drug–drug interactions between the anti-tuberculosis drugs and ART. Such interactions affect drug metabolism and may diminish efficacy or enhance toxicity, making clinical decision-making challenging. Individualized therapeutic approaches that take these interactions into account are essential to maximize the efficacy of treatment and minimize adverse effects. Adjustments of doses and second-choice drugs might be required to balance antagonistic outcomes while ensuring effective suppression of pathogens. Therefore, clinicians need to handle patients on combination therapy cautiously and use evidence-based protocols to direct treatment. This is a prudent strategy that prevents the delicate balance of treating two infections at once from undermining overall patient well-being (Navasardyan et al., 2024). In addition, treatment regimens should include ongoing monitoring and patient education to maximize adherence and mitigate problems with adverse effects and regimen complexity. Combining anti-HIV and anti-TB treatments requires multidisciplinary coordination to mitigate side effects and strengthen compliance. By individualizing regimens and providing supportive care, health systems can optimize long-term outcomes.

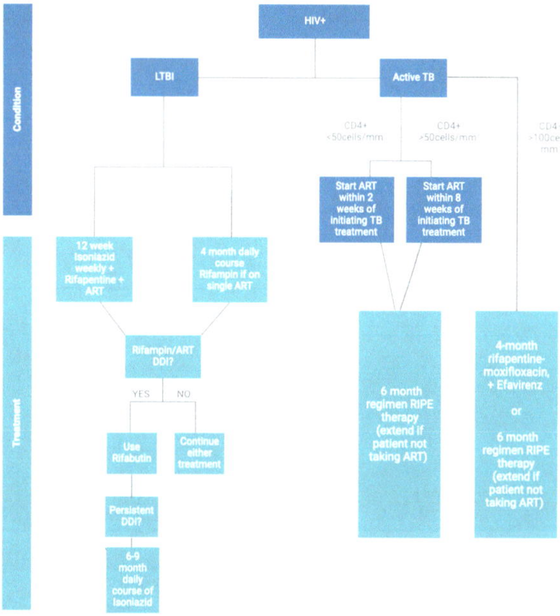

Figure 8.10. Treatment regimen for individuals co-infected with HIV and LTBI or Active TB. HIV-positive individuals with untreated LTBI can be treated with a 12-week once-weekly regimen of isoniazid and rifapentine in combination with ART or four-month daily course of rifampin if on ART monotherapy.

Source: Navasardyan I, Miwalian R, Petrosyan A, Yeganyan S, Venketaraman V. HIV–TB Coinfection: Current Therapeutic Approaches and Drug Interactions. Viruses. 2024; 16(3):321. https://doi.org/10.3390/v16030321

The dynamic pattern of co-infection necessitates flexible protocols responding to new resistance patterns and clinical outcomes, highlighting the necessity for continuous research and development of new therapeutic strategies. Finally, through the integration of vaccination, maximized pharmacotherapy, and patient-centered interventions, an overall framework becomes crucial for effective control of TB-HIV co-infection (Navasardyan et al., 2024; Toaha et al., 2024) (Figure 8.10).

8.4.1. Antiretroviral Therapy (ART) for HIV

Treating HIV and tuberculosis co-infections requires a thorough understanding of the underlying biological processes and treatment interventions. ART has become a backbone in the repression of HIV replication, hence enhancing immune function and limiting opportunistic infections like TB. In the absence of an irreversible cure or vaccine for HIV, ART substantially reduces viral loads, increases patient lifespan, and lowers disease transmission risks. Mathematical modeling of HIV-TB co-infection, as illustrated in fractional-order models, emphasizes how treatment regimens affect disease courses and epidemiology.

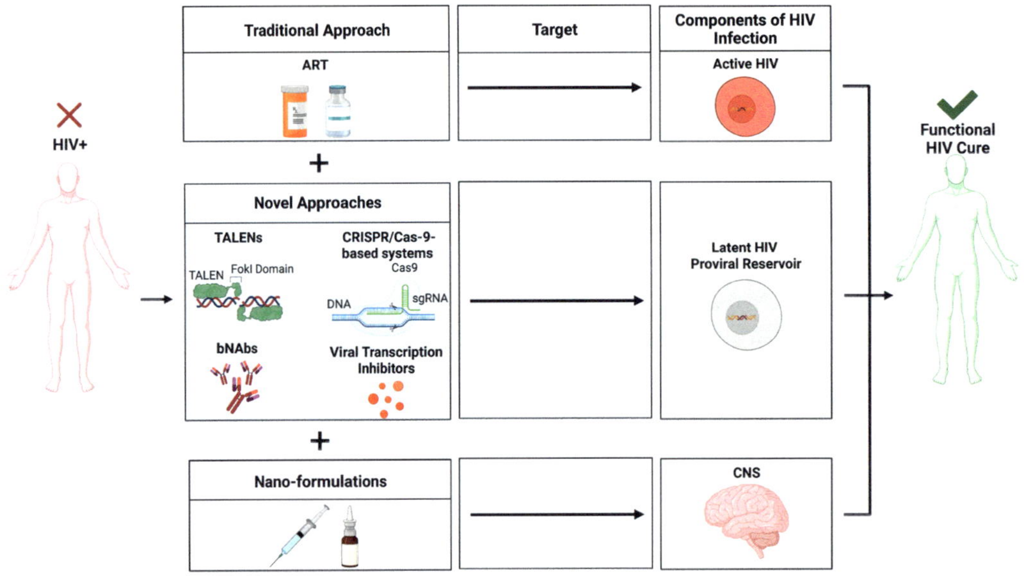

Figure 8.11. Antiretroviral therapy (ART) for HIV.

Source: Rudd H, Toborek M. Pitfalls of Antiretroviral Therapy: Current Status and Long-Term CNS Toxicity. Biomolecules. 2022; 12(7):894. https://doi.org/10.3390/biom12070894

Such models factor in ART's role in conjunction with TB treatment, investigating stability thresholds in terms of reproduction numbers and evaluating long-term dynamics. Such analytical perspectives provide useful insights into the optimization of co-management approaches, such that implementing ART is informed by sound scientific principles to manage the complex interaction between the two pathogens (Raza et al., 2025). The balancing of the initiation and delivery of ART in co-infected patients with HIV and TB needs cautious clinical judgment owing to possible drug interactions and IRIS-related complications. IRIS is a paradoxical presentation of increasing symptoms after initiating ART, typically due to the enhanced immune recovery that reveals previously latent TB or other opportunistic diseases. IRIS complicates both adherence to and outcome of treatment, especially in resource-constrained settings with a high prevalence of multi-drug-resistant strains of TB (DR-TB). Co-infected individuals also have to contend with additive toxicities of antiretroviral and antituberculosis medications that can amplify side effects and diminish therapeutic benefits. The complex interface of ART efficacy and treating latent TB emphasizes the need for combined care pathways, where the early diagnosis of HIV and the early initiation of ART reduce the progression of TB to an active state and enhance the general prognosis (Jadhav et al., 2024) (Figure 8.11).

Execution of ART as a component of an integrated co-infection control policy is imperative in the management of the HIV-TB burden at the global level, particularly in areas with high prevalence. From the epidemiological evidence, it appears that about one-third of HIV-infected persons also carry MTB infection, in the form of either latent or active TB. Successful ART inhibits viral replication, enhancing host immune responses and decreasing the risk of reactivation of TB. Yet, there are ongoing challenges posed by DR-TB strains and diagnostic and monitoring gaps that complicate treatment outcomes. In such a context, ART programs must be accompanied by strict TB screening, adherence assistance, and co-treatment guidelines individualized to patient risk profiles. Strategic ART integration into TB-HIV treatment not only improves survival for the individual patient but also reduces risks to public health by breaking chains of transmission and preventing the emergence of resistance (Jadhav et al., 2024).

8.4.2. Treatment Regimens for TB

The complexities of treating tuberculosis (TB) among patients co-infected with HIV require a balanced consideration of therapeutic regimes and their complexities. Comorbidities, resistance to drugs, and adherence by the patient are major factors in determining outcomes. Mental illness, for instance, makes TB therapy in co-infected patients challenging by significantly lowering sputum conversion and cavity closure rates, which are important indicators of the success of therapy. Patients with concurrent mental health conditions show almost half the treatment success rate of those without it, along with a significantly high mortality rate. These observations highlight the importance of creating tailored treatment protocols targeting both TB and comorbid mental health issues to enhance the overall healthcare effectiveness and survival of the TB/HIV co-infected patients (Kazemian et al., 2024). Pharmacological progress has brought about bedaquiline as a potential addition to extensive DR-TB and multi-drug-resistant treatment regimens, especially for those battling additional HIV infection. When bedaquiline has been added to ART, it has shown significant success, increasing treatment efficacy up to 70.6%, and significantly enhancing the outcomes of those with intact immunity. The interaction between bedaquiline and ART minimizes mortality and poor treatment outcomes and underscores the critical role of modern TB treatment in co-infected patient populations. Cautious choice of regimens of ART is important as their combination with selected non-nucleoside reverse transcriptase inhibitors and protease inhibitors raises levels of adverse events, requiring close monitoring (Borisova et al., 2024). The addition of new pharmacotherapies to TB treatment regimens is part of larger attempts to individualize treatment for the complicated pathophysiological interaction of HIV co-infection. Treatment regimens including bedaquiline have been relatively safe and well-tolerated, with side effects in a minority of patients. These improvements in treatment come with a decreased rate of relapse after several years following the end of chemotherapy, with sustained therapeutic benefits. However, the complex balancing of drug interactions, immune status, and resistance patterns continues to be critical to maximally optimize treatment regimens. Ongoing research and patient-centered care models are vital to successfully manage the multidimensional treatment issues confronting TB/HIV-infected patients (Borisova et al., 2024) (Figure 8.12).

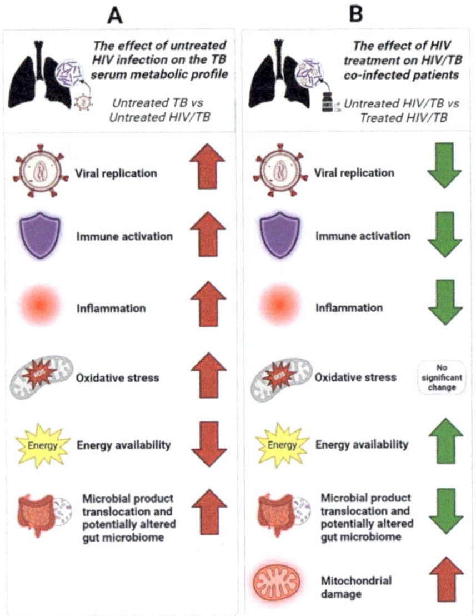

Figure 8.12. The potential effects of HIV infection and its treatment on patients with TB, as elucidated by this metabolomics investigation. A Shown are the implications of the metabolites found to be significantly different between the untreated TB and untreated HIV/TB co-infected groups, representing the effect of HIV infection on an individual who already has TB. B The implications of the metabolites were found to be significantly different between the untreated and ART-treated HIV/TB co-infected groups, representing the effect of ART on HIV/TB co-infection. Although ART improved the effects of HIV infection to some extent, implying that some metabolites returned to a value closer to, but not equal to, those of healthy controls, many metabolites were unaffected by ART.

Source: Herbert, C., Luies, L., Loots, D.T. *et al.* The metabolic consequences of HIV/TB co-infection. *BMC Infect Dis* **23**, 536 (2023). https://doi.org/10.1186/s12879-023-08505-4

8.4.3. Considerations for Co-Treatment

Successful management of TB and HIV co-infection needs to have a subtle understanding of how the diseases interact in the host and influence treatment outcome. The sequence and timing of ART with tuberculosis treatment are essential to maximize improvement while reducing side effects. One such concern is the possibility of drug-drug interactions, reducing efficacy or enhancing toxicity of medications. For example, rifampicin, a drug of choice in the treatment of TB, may induce hepatic enzymes that enhance the metabolism of many antiretroviral drugs, perhaps requiring dose adjustments. In addition, IRIS that occurs upon starting ART in individuals with active TB presents challenges in co-treatment strategies. Personalizing treatment regimens through consideration of these interactions and patient-specific characteristics has the potential to enhance survival and minimize complications among co-infected individuals, based on the value placed on emphasizing the early diagnosis and treatment of TB and effective ART initiation (Bolaji et al., 2024). Socioeconomic and demographic considerations are crucial to the success of co-treatment strategies for TB-HIV patients. Findings suggest that survival and death are significantly determined by social factors such as education, employment status, and access to health services. Low-educated or unemployed patients experience significant obstacles to compliance and timely treatment, accelerating disease progression. In addition, the immunological state, shown by CD4 levels and the presence of comorbidities such as diabetes or renal disease, has a significant influence on tolerance and response to combined treatments. These factors compel health workers to embrace an integrated patient-centered model that targets not just biological determinants but also social circumstances that affect treatment continuity and adherence (Rocha et al., 2021). This comprehensive model is imperative for minimizing the total burden of TB-HIV co-infection, given that co-infection alone multiplies the threats of each disease alone. The treatment regimen optimization in TB-HIV co-infection also requires consideration of reinfection risks, especially for tuberculosis reinfection following treatment. Research on the dynamics of co-infection emphasizes that TB reinfection susceptibility can lead to complex patterns of disease progression, including the occurrences of backward bifurcation, which makes eradication difficult when the basic reproduction number is less than unity. Thorough co-treatment guidelines should thus stress extended follow-up and potentially extended prophylactic treatment to decrease reinfection rates among HIV-positive subjects, who are particularly susceptible. Prior treatment of latent TB, particularly among co-infected patients, can greatly lower subsequent transmission and disease burden. This strategy emphasizes the need to incorporate epidemiological modeling findings into clinical practice to guide intervention efforts targeting active as well as latent infections (Bolaji et al., 2024) (Figure 8.13).

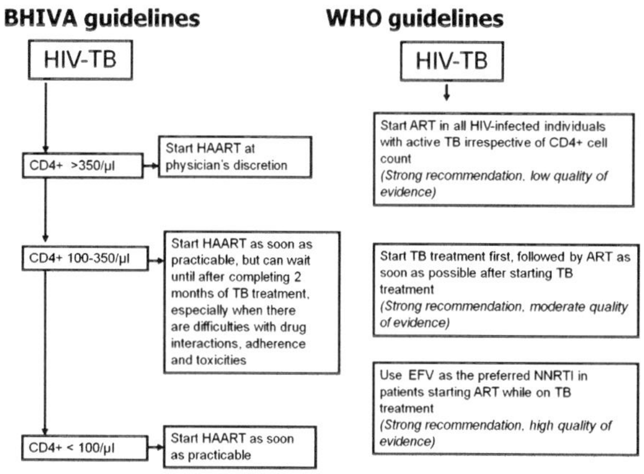

Figure 8.13. Guidelines on timing of antiretroviral treatment in patients with HIV-TB co-infection ART.

Source: ResearchGate. (n.d.). *Guidelines on timing of antiretroviral treatment in patients with HIV-TB co-infection: BHIVA vs. WHO.* https://www.researchgate.net/figure/Guidelines-on-timing-of-antiretroviral-treatment-in-patients-with-HIV-TB-co-infection_fig6_236614590.

SUMMARY

The complex relationship between HIV and tuberculosis greatly complicates clinical management, making a strategic measure to the management of co-infection imperative. Higher treatment failure and mortality rates among TB-HIV co-infected patients stress the need for individualized interventions. Mental illness among co-infected patients further reduces the efficacy of treatment, as reflected in significantly poorer sputum conversion rates and higher lethality. This unique patient subgroup requires tailored care programs to meet the complex challenges of concurrent mental illness disorders, drug resistance, and immunosuppression. The merging of mental health services in TB-HIV treatment programs, therefore, stands out as a critical key to increased therapy success and mortality prevention among this at-risk group (Kazemian et al., 2024). The epidemiologic trends seen since the last decade indicate rates of stagnation of notifications for TB and continued high rates of HIV co-infection, pointing to enduring public health problems. Despite general familiarity with HIV status and the availability of TB care, there are still major barriers in the cascade of care from contact screening to adherence and completion of treatment. Resistance to rifampicin adds to challenges in management, leading to enhanced morbidity and case fatality. These results highlight the need for robust national approaches emphasizing enhanced diagnostic capacity, ongoing patient monitoring, and increased support for adherence to suppress the long-term burden of TB-HIV co-infection. Consolidation of these elements will be pivotal to reversing recent trends and achieving significant reductions in disease incidence and mortality (Commiesie et al., 2024). The overlap of TB and HIV epidemics is a powerful combination posing an extremely challenging situation for which integrated, multisectoral interventions are needed to enhance patient outcomes. Management success will depend on the management of co-infections using combined care models incorporating mental health care, adherence strategies, and resistance handling. Policymakers and health workers need to utilize epidemiological information to optimize national policies, increase resource utilization, and roll out strategic interventions where the disease burden is largest. Ongoing research and monitoring are crucial to the development of these strategies in the context of changes in drug resistance and demographics. In the end, the success of initiatives to prevent TB-HIV co-infection will rely on sustained dedication to balanced, patient-focused care based on evidence-driven practices (Commiesie et al., 2024; Kazemian et al., 2024).

The co-infection dynamics of TB and HIV exhibit complex challenges in disease management, especially among populations with limited general access to ART. Mathematical modeling shows that susceptibility to TB reinfection plays a key role in disease perpetuation, leading to events like backward bifurcation even when the TB basic reproduction number is less than one. This demonstrates the challenge of eliminating TB from HIV-impacted populations without dealing with latent infections and risks of reinfection. In addition, the model shows that targeted intervention approaches aimed at people with latent TB , either singly infected or co-infected with HIV , can greatly decrease both TB and HIV incidence. Hence, the emphasis on treatment interventions in the latent stage of TB infection can represent an important control strategy in high-burden contexts, highlighting the need for early identification and continued management of TB among HIV-affected populations to prevent larger epidemic effects (Bolaji et al., 2024). A more detailed review of real-world data from Kyrgyzstan highlights the added vulnerabilities experienced by persons with TB-HIV co-infection. A large percentage of these patients are also members of several overlapping key population groups that are marked by increased exposure, reduced access to healthcare, and greater risk of TB. Outcomes of treatment are significantly worse among those who are members of three or more of these groups, and treatment failure greatly increases in line with other risk factors such as comorbidities, migration, and drug use. In the face of large ART and prophylactic treatment rates, complexity in social determinants perpetuates high levels of treatment failure and unfavorable clinical outcomes. This finding highlights the need for population-based, integrated intervention models that treat not only biomedical but also socio-economic and behavioral aspects to enhance the prognosis of TB-HIV co-infected individuals (Goncharova et al., 2023). Synthesizing theoretical modeling with empirical data highlights essential considerations for advancing TB-HIV co-infection management. Identifying critical parameters influencing transmission and disease progression informs strategic prioritization of limited healthcare resources, such as focusing on latent TB treatment and interrupting reinfection cycles. Simultaneously, the uneven burden imposed by marginalized subgroups requires policy interventions to minimize barriers to care by offering broad-based, equitable health services that respond to the intersecting risks of co-infected persons. In combination, these findings call for an integrated approach merging mathematical epidemiology and operational research results to maximize clinical and public health benefits in TB-HIV co-infection. This strategy is crucial to breaking through the endemic problem of co-epidemics across heterogeneous populations and ensuring health equity across impacted areas (Goncharova et al., 2023; Bolaji et al., 2024).

CLOSER LOOK

THE ROLE OF CD4⁺ T CELLS IN TB PATHOGENESIS

CD4$^+$ T cells are crucial in the pathogenesis of TB because they are central elements in the immune response to M. tuberculosis infection. CD4$^+$ T cells are mainly responsible for the adaptive immune response, coordinating both the containment and clearance of bacteria. After infection, Mtb is phagocytosed by macrophages, but bacteria can survive and replicate inside these cells. CD4$^+$ T cells can recognize Mtb antigens, presented by the infected macrophages, through major histocompatibility complex class II molecules. This action leads to the activation of CD4$^+$ T cells, which in turn secrete cytokines, including interferon-gamma (IFN-γ).

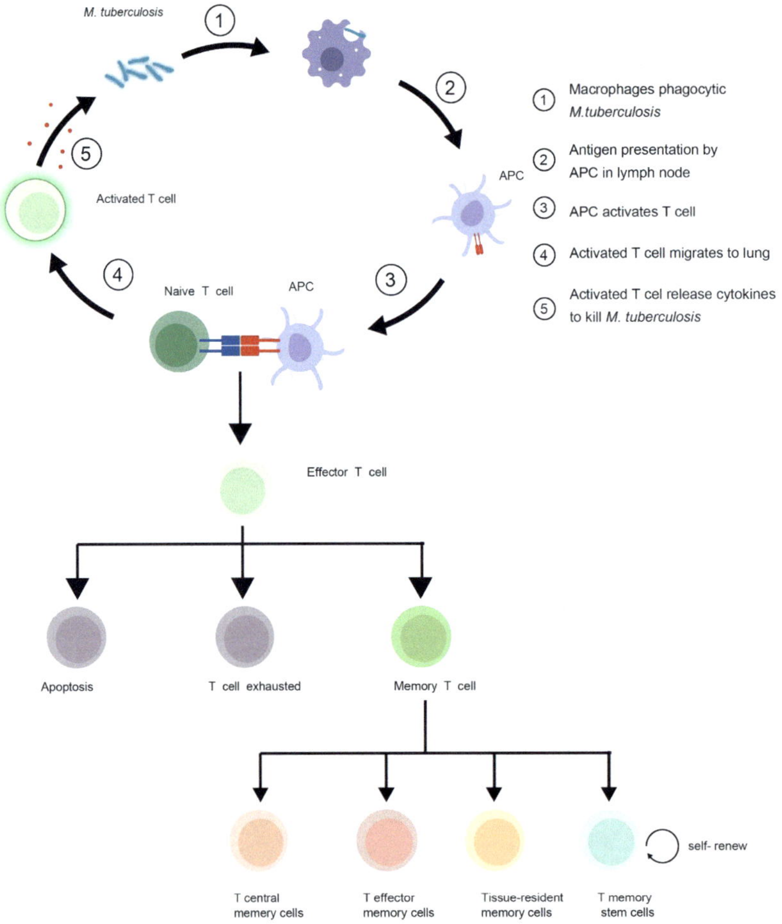

Source: Liu X, Li H, Li S, Yuan J and Pang Y (2023) Maintenance and recall of memory T cell populations against tuberculosis: Implications for vaccine design. Front. Immunol. 14:1100741. doi: 10.3389/fimmu.2023.1100741

One of the major functions of CD4$^+$ T cells in TB disease is macrophage activation through secretion of IFN-γ. The activation increases the killing ability of the macrophage, encouraging granuloma formation—collections of immune cells intended to contain the bacteria. Granulomas are a characteristic feature of TB, serving as a physical barrier limiting infection spread. The $CD4^+$ T cells in the granulomas play a role in regulating macrophage function so that the immune response is potent enough to suppress the infection without inducing too much tissue destruction.

But when $CD4^+$ T cell responses are compromised, for example, in HIV/AIDS or other immunocompromised states, the immune response cannot hold Mtb in check. This results in the progression of the infection, usually to active TB disease. The granulomas are also not formed fully in such a scenario, permitting the bacteria to spread beyond the lung and infect other organs.

In total, $CD4^+$ T cells play a central role in the containment and clearance of TB infection. Their role in activating macrophages and inducing granuloma formation is key to aborting disease progression, indicating their role in TB pathogenesis.

REFERENCES

1. Abade, A., Porto, L. F., Scholze, A. R., Kuntath, D., Barros, N. D. S., Berra, T. Z., Ramos, A. C. V., Arcêncio, R. A., & Alves, J. D. (2024). A comparative analysis of classical and machine learning methods for forecasting TB/HIV co-infection. *Scientific reports*, *14*(1), 18991. https://doi.org/10.1038/s41598-024-69580-4 (accessed on 10 May 2025).
2. Anindita, F. S., Indriani, F., Murti, B., & Veibiani, N. A. (2024). Factors affecting mortality in people living with HIV with antiretroviral therapy: A meta-analysis. *Journal of Epidemiology and Public Health*. Journal of Epidemiology and Public Health (2024), 09(04): 480-494 Meta-analysis Masters Program in Public Health, Universitas Sebelas Maret. https://www.semanticscholar.org/paper/0fca11bb38ec104324831ff81741795abf2d12ec (accessed on 10 May 2025).
3. Antony, B., Tiewsoh, J. B. A., & Boloor, R. (2020). HIV-TB co-infection with clinical presentation, diagnosis, treatment, outcome and its relation to CD4 count: A cross-sectional study in a tertiary care hospital in coastal Karnataka. *Journal of Family Medicine and Primary Care, 9*, 1160–1160. https://doi.org/10.4103/jfmpc.jfmpc_950_19.
4. Bashir, N., Haider, N., Farooq, A., & Hussain, M. (2023). Epidemiology and clinical spectrum of pediatric patients with human immunodeficiency virus (HIV) infection: A 15 years' experience. *Pakistan Journal of Medical Sciences, 39*, 820–824. https://www.semanticscholar.org/paper/1763b4ed478cc867f998a7ed3ef56cdbacbd8335 (accessed on 10 May 2025).
5. Bayabil, S., & Tegegne, A. S. (2021). Joint modeling in detecting predictors of CD4 cell count and status of tuberculosis among people living with HIV/AIDS under HAART at Felege Hiwot Teaching and Specialized Hospital, North-West Ethiopia. *HIV/AIDS – Research and Palliative Care, 13*, 527–537. https://doi.org/10.2147/hiv.s307069 (accessed on 10 May 2025).
6. Kazemian, S. V., Shakeri, M., Nazar, E., Nasehi, M., Sharafi, S., & Dadgarmoghaddam, M. (2024). Prevalence, treatment outcomes and determinants of TB/HIV coinfection: A 4-year retrospective review of national tuberculosis registry in a country in a MENA region. *Heliyon*, *10*(5), e26615. https://doi.org/10.1016/j.heliyon.2024.e26615
7. (accessed on 10 May 2025).
8. Benjamin, M. (2023). Influential factors in TB/HIV co-infection among HIV-positive patients at Jinja Regional Referral Hospital, Uganda. International Digital Organization for Scientific Research ISSN: 2579-0730 IDOSR JOURNAL OF BIOLOGY, CHEMISTRY AND PHARMACY 8(3)94-105, 2023. https://doi.org/10.59298/IDOSR/JBCP/23/11.1118 (accessed on 10 May 2025).
9. Bolaji, B., Onoja, T., Agbata, C., Omede, B. I., & Odionyenma, U. B. (2024). Dynamical analysis of HIV-TB co-infection transmission model in the presence of treatment for TB. *Bulletin of Biomathematics*, *2*(1), 21–56. https://doi.org/10.59292/bulletinbiomath.2024002 (accessed on 10 May 2025).
10. Borisova, S. B., & Borodina, N. Y. (2024). Effectiveness and safety of the regimens containing bedaquiline in patients with TB and HIV-infection. *Tuberculosis and Lung Diseases*. 2024, Tuberculosis and Lung Diseases, № 5, p. 40-49. https://www.semanticscholar.org/paper/a11b239f92d3f68a1431bea6455d2904a11c01aa (accessed on 10 May 2025).
11. Chauhan, S., Nusbaum, R. J., Huante, M., Holloway, A., Endsley, M., Gelman, B. B., Lisinicchia, J. G., et al. (2024). Therapeutic modulation of arginase with nor-NOHA alters immune responses in experimental mouse models of pulmonary tuberculosis including in the setting

of human immunodeficiency virus (HIV) co-infection. *Tropical Medicine and Infectious Disease, 9.* https://www.semanticscholar.org/paper/15dc38073a9fdedf79b903bbb86e846ef6428ea3 (accessed on 10 May 2025).

12. Clark, Kendall B.; Cortez, Mayleen; Hernandez, Cristian; Thomas, Beth E.; and Lewis, Allison L. (2019) “Combating Tuberculosis: Using Time-Dependent Sensitivity Analysis to Develop Strategies for Treatment and Prevention,” Spora: A Journal of Biomathematics: Vol. 5, 14–23. DOI: http://doi.org/10.30707/SPORA5.1Clark (accessed on 10 May 2025).

13. Commiesie, E., Stijnberg, D., van den Boogaard, J., Gopie, F., Vreden, S., & de Vries, G. (2024). Key drivers of the TB epidemic in Suriname and priority actions to reduce incidence and mortality. *IJTLD Open, 1*, 34–40. https://www.semanticscholar.org/paper/fe8926ef2e665047aa88e88006ad62c8e381805b (accessed on 10 May 2025).

14. Devarbhavi, H., Asrani, S. K., Arab, J. P., Nartey, Y. A., Pose, E., & Kamath, P. S. (2023). Global burden of liver disease: 2023 update. *Journal of Hepatology, 79*, 516–537. https://doi.org/10.1016/j.jhep.2023.03.017.

15. Goncharova, O., Abrahamyan, A., Nair, D., Beglaryan, M., Bekbolotov, A., Zhdanova, E., Kadyrov, A., et al. (2023). Triple priority: TB/HIV co-infection and treatment outcomes among key populations in the Kyrgyz Republic: A national cohort study (2018–2022). *Tropical Medicine and Infectious Disease, 8.* https://www.semanticscholar.org/paper/c8d925943db1272448ab4b16e5c145aab03e187a (accessed on 10 May 2025).

16. Gravlee C. C. (2020). Systemic racism, chronic health inequities, and COVID-19: A syndemic in the making?. *American journal of human biology : the official journal of the Human Biology Council, 32*(5), e23482. https://doi.org/10.1002/ajhb.23482Hoque, K. A., Khan, M. M. R., Das, M., & Roy, B. L. (2024). Knowledge about HIV-AIDS and co-infection rate among HIV-AIDS patients: A study among different community clinics of Chattogram District, Bangladesh. *International Journal of Science and Healthcare Research*. olume: 9 | Issue: 4 | Pages: 403-417. DOI: https://doi.org/10.52403/ijshr.20240446. https://www.semanticscholar.org/paper/a9aa4920f34a4473570e5a07bc9d3b1db86c3001 (accessed on 10 May 2025).

17. Jadhav S, Nair A, Mahajan P, Nema V. The Crosstalk Between HIV-TB Co-Infection and Associated Resistance in the Indian Population. Venereology. 2024; 3(4):183-198. https://doi.org/10.3390/venereology3040015(accessed on 10 May 2025).

18. Kaushal, D., Singh, D., & Mehra, S. (2023). Immune responses in lung granulomas during Mtb/HIV co-infection: Implications for pathogenesis and therapy. *Pathogens, 12*. https://www.semanticscholar.org/paper/0dfe14e05677cb57a9cc40e3486178481d224239 (accessed on 10 May 2025).

19. Kegne, T., Anteneh, Z. A., Bayeh, T., Shiferaw, B. M., & Tamiru, D. (2024). Survival rate and predictors of mortality among TB-HIV co-infected patients during tuberculosis treatment at public health facilities in Bahir Dar City, Northwest Ethiopia. *Infection and Drug Resistance, 17*, 1385–1395. https://www.semanticscholar.org/paper/382712d34521a197d15b3303f6524376dbe97363 (accessed on 10 May 2025).

20. Ketaren, T. N. B., Wahyunitisari, M., Rusli, M., & Widodo, A. D. W. (2025). Clinical profile of TB-HIV coinfected patients at RSUD Dr. Soetomo Surabaya in 2022. *International Journal of Scientific Advances*. https://www.semanticscholar.org/paper/c3e881ee9e172fdeb9ef95a68898b55ed1d37ba3 (accessed on 10 May 2025).

21. Maseko, T. G., Rambaran, S., Ngubane, S., Lewis, L., Ngcapu, S., Hassan-Moosa, R., Archary, D., et al. (2023). NK cell phenotypic profile during active TB in people living with HIV—Evolution during TB treatment and implications for bacterial clearance and disease severity. *Scientific Reports, 13.* https://www.semanticscholar.org/paper/1cd605e4b756015d956b78c8e202b8668bc30b05 (accessed on 10 May 2025).

22. Maulidiyah, N., Wicaksono, R., Retnowulan, A., Santoso, B., Subianto, A., Mashudi, L., & Kurniawan, F. (2024). Successful resolution of mesenteric tuberculosis and HIV co-infection following 6 months of anti-tuberculosis therapy: a case report. *Deka in Medicine, 1*(1), e738. https://doi.org/10.69863/dim.v1i1.2(accessed on 10 May 2025).

23. Melin, U. N., & Adhi Dharmasanti, P. (2024). Secondary Syphilis with Multiple Co-Infections of Human Immunodeficiency Virus (HIV), Tuberculosis (TB), and Oral Candidiasis in a 19-Year-Old Men Who Have Sex with Men (MSM): A Case Report. *Berkala Ilmu Kesehatan Kulit Dan Kelamin, 36*(3), 225–231. https://doi.org/10.20473/bikk.V36.3.2024.225-231

24. (accessed on 10 May 2025).

25. Moges, S., & Lajore, B. A. (2024). Mortality and associated factors among patients with TB-HIV co-infection in Ethiopia: A systematic review and meta-analysis. *BMC Infectious Diseases, 24.* https://www.semanticscholar.org/paper/0a67ae6e17345a05f24fcc0fb905f18446a31605 (accessed on 10 May 2025).

26. Moneke, K. C., Mosaku, L., & Ogunboye, I. (2022). Unraveling hidden trends: A syndemic approach to HIV epidemiology and co-infections in high-risk populations. *World Journal of Advanced Research and Reviews, 2022, 16(03), 1203-1216*

27. *Article DOI: 10.30574/wjarr.2022.16.3.1388*(accessed on 10 May 2025).

28. Mulherkar, T., Gómez, D. J., Sandel, G., & Jain, P. (2022). Co-infection and cancer: Host–pathogen interaction between dendritic cells and HIV-1, HTLV-1, and other oncogenic viruses. *Viruses, 14.* https://www.semanticscholar.org/paper/785a900ff35ee54c833edbdd01ba5cf21452c4d0 (accessed on 10 May 2025).

29. Murray, C. J. L., Ikuta, K. S., Sharara, F., Swetschinski, L. R., Robles Aguilar, G., Gray, A. P., Han, C., et al. (2022). Global burden of bacterial antimicrobial resistance in 2019: A systematic analysis. *The Lancet, 399*, 629–655. https://doi.org/10.1016/S0140-6736(21)02724-0.

30. Navasardyan, I., Miwalian, R., Petrosyan, A., Yeganyan, S., & Venketaraman, V. (2024). HIV–TB co-infection: Current therapeutic approaches and drug interactions. *Viruses, 16.* https://www.semanticscholar.org/paper/e39fae19bf35aa8cdee7f17a4c99e855c2815b1e (accessed on 10 May 2025).

31. Omara, G., Bwayo, D., Mukunya, D., Nantale, R., Okia, D., Matovu, J. K., Wanume, B., et al. (2025). Tuberculosis treatment success rate and its predictors among TB-HIV co-infected patients in East and North Eastern Uganda. *Scientific Reports, 15.* https://www.semanticscholar.org/paper/15aca373bc60dc191055ae0c040a460ed59cd91f (accessed on 10 May 2025).

32. Oyageshio OP, Myrick JW, Saayman J, van der Westhuizen L, Al-Hindi DR, Reynolds AW, et al. (2024) Strong effect of demographic changes on Tuberculosis susceptibility in South Africa. PLOS Glob Public Health 4(7): e0002643. https://doi.org/10.1371/journal.pgph.0002643 (accessed on 10 May 2025).

33. Pretorius, C., & Luies, L. (2024). Characterising the urinary acylcarnitine and amino acid

profiles of HIV/TB co-infection, using LC–MS metabolomics. *Metabolomics, 20.* https://www.semanticscholar.org/paper/4740daeac61df325193c24778b5fb450508ef9a3 (accessed on 10 May 2025).

34. Putri, N. K., Arfijanto, M. V., & Setiabudi, R. J. (2025). The intersection of HIV and tuberculosis: A comprehensive literature review on co-infection challenges and management. *Magna Scientia Advanced Research and Reviews, 2025, 13(01), 042-049*

35. *Article DOI: 10.30574/msarr.2025.13.1.0235* (accessed on 10 May 2025).

36. Ravimohan, S., Kornfeld, H., Weissman, D., & Bisson, G. P. (2018). Tuberculosis and lung damage: From epidemiology to pathophysiology. *European Respiratory Review, 27,* 170077. https://doi.org/10.1183/16000617.0077-2017.

37. Raza, N., Irum, S., Niazai, S., Ullah, M. A., Alshahrani, M. Y., & Omame, A. (2025). A mathematical framework of HIV and TB co-infection dynamics. *Scientific Reports, 15.* https://www.semanticscholar.org/paper/1fcb412bb06b97b42a82d230d82a1bca685fe1d9 (accessed on 10 May 2025).

38. Rocha, A. C., Chenini de Carvalho Reis, N. F., & Gonçalves, M. J. (2021). Factors associated with mortality or survival of patients with tuberculosis: An integrative review. *Revita Eletrônica Acervo Saúde.* REAS Vol.13(12) DOI: https://doi.org/10.25248/REAS.e9352.2021 (accessed on 10 May 2025).

39. Seibert, A. M., Matheu, M. M., Buckel, W., Moores Todd, T., Vines, C. M. D., Bledsoe, J., Balls, A., et al. (2025). 388. Co-Testing: Increasing HIV testing in patients undergoing sexually transmitted infection evaluation in a large integrated healthcare network. *Open Forum Infectious Diseases, 12.* https://www.semanticscholar.org/paper/4ab6ae21e6793b69dd39cc9dc76f968426b15af2 (accessed on 10 May 2025).

40. Shivang Sharma, Deepak Kumar, P-795. Unravelling the Enigma: Evaluating False Positive and Invalid Results in Urinary TB LAM Test among HIV Patients with Opportunistic Infections, Open Forum Infectious Diseases, Volume 12, Issue Supplement_1, February 2025, ofae631.987, https://doi.org/10.1093/ofid/ofae631.987 (accessed on 10 May 2025).

41. Ramaseri Sunder, S., Suryadevara, N. C., Pydi, S. S., Neela, V. S. K., & Valluri, V. L. (2020). Defective Antigen Presentation Leads to Upregulation of PD1 and IL-10 in HIV-TB Co-Infection. *Journal of interferon & cytokine research : the official journal of the International Society for Interferon and Cytokine Research, 40*(6), 310–319. https://doi.org/10.1089/jir.2019.0243 (accessed on 10 May 2025).

42. Toaha, S., Sukmawati, Kasbawati, Firman, & Wan Muhamad, W. Z. A. (2024). Stability Analysis of the Transmission Model of TB-HIV Co-Dynamics with Vaccination and Treatment. *Journal of Advanced Research in Applied Sciences and Engineering Technology, 54*(2), 143–156. https://doi.org/10.37934/araset.54.2.143156 (accessed on 10 May 2025).

43. Tribolet, L., Kerr, E., Cowled, C., Bean, A. G. D., Stewart, C. R., Dearnley, M., & Farr, R. J. (2020). MicroRNA biomarkers for infectious diseases: From basic research to biosensing. *Frontiers in Microbiology, 11.* https://doi.org/10.3389/fmicb.2020.01197.

44. Waters, R., Held, M., Dunn, R., Laubscher, M., Adikary, N., & Coussens, A. (2023). Improving the diagnosis of spinal tuberculosis and our understanding of its pathophysiology and interaction with HIV-1 co-infection. *Orthopaedic Proceedings.* https://doi.org/10.1302/1358-992X.2023.15.036(accessed on 10 May 2025).

45. Wollenberg, A., Kinberger, M., Arents, B. W. M., Aszodi, N., Avila Valle, G., Barbarot, S., Bieber, T., et al. (2022). European guideline (EuroGuiDerm) on atopic eczema: Part I–Systemic therapy. *Journal of the European Academy of Dermatology and Venereology, 36*, 1409–1431. https://doi.org/10.1111/jdv.18345.

46. Xiao, J., Wang, F., Yan, H., Wang, B., Su, B., Lu, X., & Zhang, T. (2024). Memory stem CD8+ T cells in HIV/Mtb mono- and co-infection: Characteristics, implications, and clinical significance. *Frontiers in Cellular and Infection Microbiology, 14*. https://www.semanticscholar.org/paper/241575b14aa192675d797eda29642c9b3e94ab5f (accessed on 10 May 2025).

47. Yirsaw, A. N., Mengistie, B. A., Getachew, E., Mekonnen, G. B., Shibabaw, A. A., Chereka, A. A., Kitil, G. W., Wondie, W. T., & Lakew, G. (2025). Prevalence of pulmonary tuberculosis and associated factors among adults living with HIV/AIDS in Ethiopia, systematic review and meta-analysis. *BMC infectious diseases, 25*(1), 49. https://doi.org/10.1186/s12879-024-10419-8(accessed on 10 May 2025).

48. Zhang, SX., Wang, JC., Yang, J. *et al.* Epidemiological features and temporal trends of the co-infection between HIV and tuberculosis, 1990–2021: findings from the Global Burden of Disease Study 2021. *Infect Dis Poverty* **13**, 59 (2024). https://doi.org/10.1186/s40249-024-01230-3(accessed on 10 May 2025).

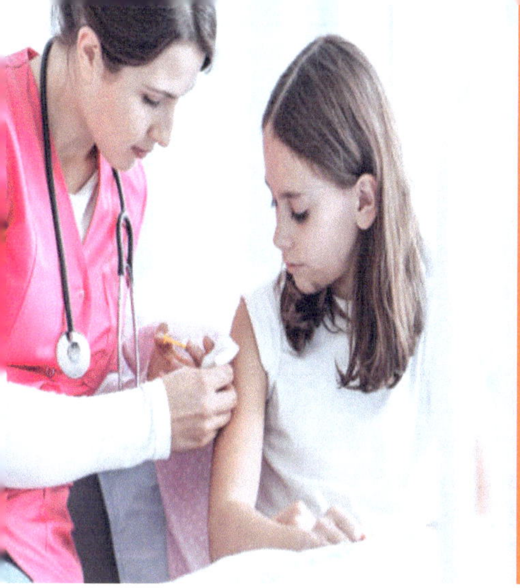

Chapter 9

PEDIATRIC TUBERCULOSIS

Contents

Introduction

Tuberculosis is still a major health concern worldwide, especially among vulnerable populations including children. *Mycobacterium tuberculosis* (MTB) causes the disease, and it presents specific diagnostic as well as therapeutic challenges in the case of children because of variation in immune response and disease presentation compared to adults. Children present with non-specific symptoms, which do not allow timely and correct diagnosis, thus delaying treatment. Additionally, pediatric tuberculosis is more likely to be more severe when left undiagnosed or untreated, leading to greater morbidity and mortality. Such complexity highlights the need for specialized strategies in tuberculosis management in children in a bid to enhance early detection as well as guarantee effective intervention measures. The difficulty in the diagnosis of tuberculosis in children is increased by challenges in accessing appropriate clinical specimens. Pediatric patients can sometimes not voluntarily expectorate sputum, decreasing access to bacteriological validation. Induced sputum collection is then a useful alternative, providing a minimally invasive but effective method of diagnostic sampling. The process has been established as safe and standardized, averting more invasive methods such as fiberoptic bronchoscopy (Farrugia et al., 2013). Application of such strategies is important not only for proper diagnosis but also for early initiation of treatment, which is important in avoiding the spread and progression of tuberculosis in children. Treatment of pediatric tuberculosis involves more than clinical management and should incorporate funding, research, and public health strategies. Investments from different sources, such as investments made by foundations located in the United States, have played an important role in health-related activities used to fight tuberculosis, especially in areas of high disease burden like Africa (Mutima, 2004). These investments fund programs that facilitate better access to diagnosis, treatment, and preventive services among children. As such, combining these resources with clinical and public health approaches can augment efforts to control pediatric tuberculosis and diminish its worldwide impact, and emphasis on sustained support and interdisciplinarity is warranted.

Definition of Pediatric Tuberculosis (TB)

Assessment of the nuances of tuberculosis in children involves not only an assessment for the infectious nature of the disease but also an understanding of its distinct clinical presentation in the child. Unlike in adults, children tend to develop a more disseminated tuberculosis after primary infection because of their immature immune system. Pediatric tuberculosis exists mainly as a pulmonary disease but can also involve extrapulmonary sites, including lymph nodes (LNs), the central nervous system (CNS), and bones. This is important in defining pediatric tuberculosis precisely since the pathology and course can be quite different from that of adult tuberculosis. The diagnostic difficulties are increased because children have a generally lower bacterial load, so microbiological confirmation is challenging. Furthermore, in children, symptoms can be nonspecific, such as failure to thrive, persistent cough, or fever. Identification of these factors forms the basis of the overall definition of pediatric tuberculosis as a systemic infectious disease with unique clinical features and diagnostic implications. The epidemiology of pediatric tuberculosis further defines it by emphasizing the susceptibility and transmission patterns unique to children. Children usually get infected from close contacts, usually active pulmonary tuberculosis (PTB) adult cases, highlighting the contagious nature of the diseases in families and communities. Pediatric tuberculosis has a huge burden, particularly in high-prevalence areas, where millions of children can become infected or at risk each year. Notably, pediatric tuberculosis is a closer indicator of recent transmission than adult tuberculosis, serving as an indicator of community transmission ongoing. The World Health Organization (WHO) and other governmental public health agencies have focused more attention on pediatric cases to better understand and contain tuberculosis transmission. This influence structures the definition of pediatric tuberculosis to include not only the clinical illness but also epidemiological importance and the need for early detection and intervention among at-risk groups (Gudeta et al., 2023). Progress in clarifying the immunological and environmental interactions that contribute to tuberculosis in children also broadens its definition further beyond mere infection. Investigations of immune responses in children indicate that disease development and progression are influenced by genetic predispositions as well as environmental conditions, including nutritional status and the presence of concomitant infections. For instance, investigations into the interrelation between tuberculosis and other immune-mediated conditions illustrate complex interactions that may have implications for diagnosis and treatment in the pediatric patient. While particular investigations of co-infections and immune phenomena such as celiac disease autoimmunity in children note varying immunogenetics without immediate tuberculosis connections, these observations emphasize immune system complexity in the involvement of pediatric tuberculosis (Gudeta et al., 2023). Pediatric tuberculosis can thus be most accurately described as a multifaceted condition with microbiological, immunological, and environmental influences that requires an integrated public health and clinical response to its prevention and management.

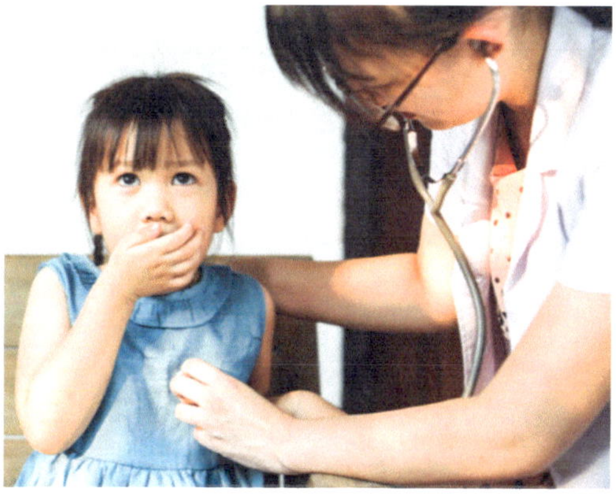

Source: Murdoch Children's Research Institute. (n.d.). *Doctor examining a child with suspected tuberculosis symptoms.* https://www.mcri.edu.au/images/impact/az/Tuberculosis/A_Z_TB_resized_1.jpg.

9.1. Epidemiology of Pediatric Tuberculosis (TB)

Proper disease pattern analysis in children needs extensive epidemiological information to inform prevention and treatment. Pediatric tuberculosis (TB) is unique from adult TB in the manner it presents and spreads and needs particular concern because of its high morbidity and mortality globally. Emerging epidemiological research identifies the complexity of pediatric TB with demonstrating differing incidence and presentation dependent on geographic, ethnic, and socio-economic determinants. For instance, trends in Southwest China over more than two decades pointed to a heterogeneous pediatric TB population dominated by mixed presentations of TB involving multiple body sites. These observations reinforce the need for longitudinal studies to reflect trends in disease and the proper adjustment of public health interventions accordingly (Wang et al., 2024). This is a method that provides detailed insight that is essential in tackling the specific vulnerabilities of children's populations in TB epidemic countries. Exploring the geographic prevalence and ethnic susceptibilities found in pediatric TB contributes another layer of investigation to epidemiological studies. Much of the cases of pediatric TB in China have been found to originate from ethnic minority groups, especially Tibetans, and this mirrors larger social determinants of health and access to healthcare. The increasing trend among these populations indicates the necessity of culturally responsive, targeted health policies to limit spread and enhance outcomes. Knowledge of these demographic trends helps to apportion resources and create community-specific health programs that are potentially more efficient in suppressing transmission and enabling earlier diagnosis. Therefore, this epidemiological knowledge not only shapes clinical practice but also influences public health priorities and resource allocation in heterogeneous pediatric populations (Wang et al., 2024). While tuberculosis mainly affects the lungs, childhood cases often present with extrapulmonary forms, adding to diagnostic difficulty and affecting epidemiological evaluation. The frequency of disseminated TB, lymphadenitis, pleural TB, and meningitis in children is the indicator of the severity and complexity of disease presentations beyond pulmonary infection and which could also make surveillance complicated. Younger children are also more likely to be affected by severe extrapulmonary disease like TB meningitis, making age a vital determinant in the epidemiology of child TB. This clinical range requires strong epidemiological models that take into account various presentations of disease and their demographic counterparts. This complete collection of data permits improved clinical identification and eventually more efficient treatment protocols, highlighting the dynamic relationship of clinical and epidemiological dimensions in the war against pediatric TB (Wang et al., 2024).

9.1.1. Global Incidence Rates

The incidence dynamics of pediatric tuberculosis show an alarming increasing pattern in the last decades, particularly regarding multi-drug resistant tuberculosis (MDR-TB) among young children and adolescents. Latest examinations highlight that the global burden of MDR-TB in people aged less than 20 has significantly amplified since 1990, with an estimated annual percentage increase of around 4.15%. This rise is uneven and disproportionately impacts areas of lower sociodemographic indices such as Southern sub-Saharan Africa, Eastern Europe, and South Asia. The children of less than the age of five years are the hardest hit by the burden, with increased mortality and disability-adjusted life years (DALYs) for this group in comparison to their older counterparts. These trends indicate a pressing requirement for focused health intervention and collaborative research initiatives that counteract the socio-economic inequities influencing MDR-TB incidence rates among pediatric populations globally (Zhong et al., 2025). Knowledge of the socio-economic and environmental drivers of tuberculosis spread makes a significant contribution to the understanding of its global patterns of incidence. Ecological-level drivers like climate and air quality have presented themselves as pivotal determinants shaping TB incidence as well as mortality rates. Systematic reviews demonstrate a positive association between elevated humidity, rainfall, and the presence of airborne pollutants such as sulfur dioxide and fine particulate matter with high TB incidence. Additionally, socio-economic factors such as poverty, urbanization, and immigrant population percentages also relate to increased tuberculosis risk, connoting underlying social and environmental vulnerabilities. On the contrary, indicators like gross domestic product, wealth indices, and effective treatment success rates are inversely correlated with incidence, enumerating the protective effects of economic development and access to healthcare (Liyew et al., 2024).

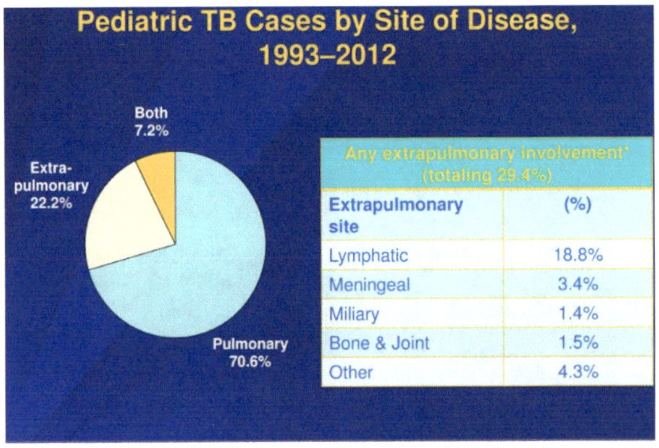

Figure 9.1. Epidemiology of pediatric tuberculosis in the United States, 1993–2012.

Source: Slideserve. (n.d.). *Pediatric TB cases by site of disease, 1993–2012.* https://image1.slideserve.com/2681165/pediatric-tb-cases-by-site-of-disease-1993-2012-l.jpg.

The complex dynamics between demographic, climatic, and socio-economic determinants create a scenario for pediatric tuberculosis globally, further obscuring eradication. High-density, poor-air-quality, and insufficient social infrastructure sites provide fertile terrain for TB dissemination among vulnerable child cohorts. Disparities in access to care and treatment also worsen the predicament faced by children of multi-drug resistant exposure. This multi-dimensional setting requires concerted public health intervention that goes beyond conventional biomedical care, including management of the environment, economic improvement, and stringent social welfare schemes. Mitigating these worldwide incidence determinants involves combined efforts in various industries to stifle the increased tide of pediatric tuberculosis and protect future generations (Liyew et al., 2024; Zhong et al., 2025) (Figure 9.1).

9.1.2. High-Risk Populations

Within the urban environments where rapid population growth tends to overwhelm public health infrastructure, children are at special risk factors which predispose them to greater tuberculosis risk.

The complexities of urban living, including habitation in unauthorized colonies and contact with increased air pollution, augment pediatric populations' vulnerability to drug-resistant tuberculosis (DR-TB). Malnutrition, often intermixed with poverty in such environments, further weakens immune guard, making children more susceptible to infection and disease progression. Empirical evidence from a New Delhi tertiary care center shows that almost half of pediatric patients with DR-TB are from such vulnerable living conditions, highlighting the way social determinants intersect with biology to exacerbate disease burden among kids. This complex risk profile suggests that treating pediatric tuberculosis in high-density urban settings calls for more than medicine; it needs holistic approaches that address root socioeconomic inequalities and environmental risks (Viswanathan, 2025). The interaction between long-term health issues and tuberculosis complications heightens concerns among pediatric populations under heightened risk. Children with comorbidities like HIV, diabetes mellitus (DM), or other serious diseases present complex therapeutic problems, rendering traditional tuberculosis therapy unpredictable in terms of both effectiveness and safety. Therapeutic drug monitoring (TDM) becomes an essential breakthrough here, allowing health practitioners to individualize anti-tuberculosis regimens according to serum drug levels measured. In children, where pharmacokinetics vary substantially from adults, individually tailored dosing based on TDM can reduce ADRs and increase the rate of successful treatment. This is particularly critical in children with slow onset of treatment response or those at risk for serious complications and emphasizes the need to incorporate pharmacological monitoring as part of pediatric tuberculosis treatment protocols to maximize outcomes for these high-risk subgroups (Ivanova et al., 2025). Socioeconomic and demographic factors further add to the difficulties experienced by vulnerable children in the battle against pediatric tuberculosis. Male children are slightly more affected, but gender by itself does not capture the extent of risk enhancers. The most affected age group consists of school children at around eight years old, a developmental period characterized by growing social contact and environmental exposure. MDR-TB represents a substantial majority of pediatric patients within these facilities, highlighting the need for focused public health interventions that account for both prevalence of drug-resistant strains and the social environments driving their spread. Achievements in treatment outcomes show that with proper strategies, even populations at high risk can gain positive outcomes, but continued efforts towards early diagnosis, nutritional status, and reduction of environmental risks remain crucial to tuberculosis control among children (Viswanathan, 2025) (Figure 9.2).

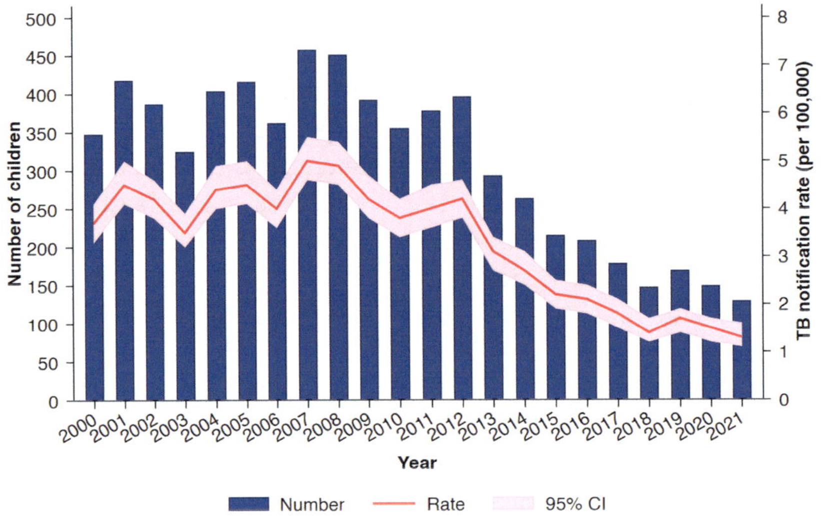

Figure 9.2. The overall number and rate of TB notifications in children aged less than 15 years, England, 2000 to 2021.

Source: UK Government. (2022). *TB in children: incidence, epidemiology, and microbiology in England, 2000–2021.* https://www.gov.uk/government/publications/tuberculosis-in-england-2022-report-data-up-to-end-of-2021/tb-in-children-incidence-epidemiology-and-microbiology-in-england-2021.

9.1.3. Geographic Distribution

The epidemiology of childhood TB exhibits differing geographic patterns that are important to recognize to grasp the dissemination of the disease and for developing specific public health interventions. In some regions, like the Rambipuji District of Indonesia, spatial analysis has identified TB case clusters within vulnerable subgroups, namely stunted children. Using geographic information system (GIS) technology, the researchers found intense case clustering in Rambigundam village, revealing spatial correlations of disease occurrence. Yet the larger geographic pattern among numerous villages evidenced dispersed case distributions, such that infection does not occur within contained pockets but has diffusion patterns within broader areas. This geographic nuance highlights the necessity of thorough monitoring and specific control strategies to contain both localized epidemics as well as the general dissemination of pediatric TB in endemic areas (Utami et al., 2024).

Epidemiological research from Southwest China also demonstrates the dynamic geographic pattern of pediatric tuberculosis, extending to several provinces such as Sichuan, Tibet, Qinghai, and Yunnan. During a 20-year period, hospitalization data signaled dynamic case flows, emphasizing the utility of temporal and spatial analysis for TB epidemiology. Most conspicuous is the increasing incidence in ethnic minorities, particularly in Tibetan children, which reveals the way sociocultural and environmental determinants interact with geography to modulate TB burden. These observations emphasize that control measures for TB should take into consideration affected population heterogeneity and variability in the distribution of disease presentations within different geographic and demographic strata for effective control (Wang et al., 2024). It is also possible to attribute geographic differences in pediatric tuberculosis to environmental and socioeconomic determinants that affect disease transmission and outcomes. Areas with higher malnutrition and stunted growth rates among children usually overlap with higher rates of TB prevalence, just as in the spatial concentration of cases. The environmental factors, including population density and healthcare resource availability, additionally influence disease distribution, with scattered patterns reflecting extensive but sometimes cryptic transmission networks. Understanding geographic distribution, therefore, necessitates integrating spatial epidemiology with local health risk factors to identify hotspots and optimize resource allocation. Such an approach supports comprehensive public health policies aimed at reducing pediatric TB incidence by addressing geographic disparities and enhancing localized interventions (Utami et al., 2024; Wang et al., 2024) (Figure 9.3).

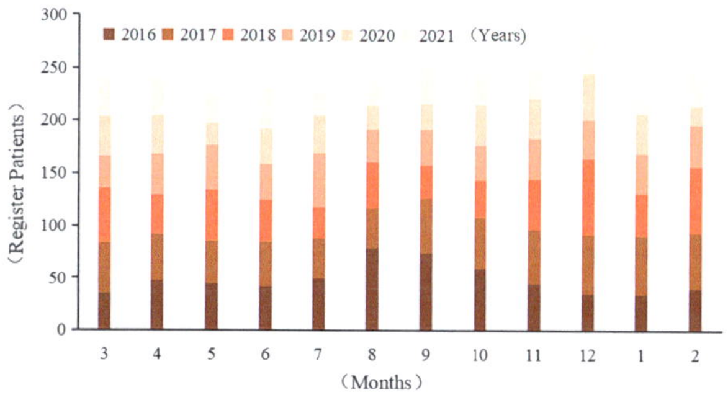

Figure 9.3. Worldwide geographic distribution of TB incidence.

Source: Wang Q, Zhu J, Zhang L and Xie L (2023) Regional and epidemiological characteristics of tuberculosis and treatment outcomes in West China. Front. Public Health. 11:1254579. doi: 10.3389/fpubh.2023.1254579.

9.2. Pathophysiology of Tuberculosis (TB) in Children

The interaction of the immune systems with *Mycobacterium tuberculosis* (MTB) is a significant factor in the pathophysiology of TB in children when cellular immunity is not yet fully developed. When inhaled, the bacteria settle within the alveoli, and an initial innate immune response is initiated. Macrophages capture the bacilli but might not always kill them, resulting in the establishment of latent infection. In children, especially in children below the age of five, the immature immune response will lead to a more pronounced clinical presentation because the bacilli are not properly contained. The process incorporates the process of granuloma formation, which is the body's effort to wall off the infection. The efficacy of the granulomas is inconsistent in children, and the direct influence on disease progression is notable. Genetic and immunologic determinants, such as HLA phenotypes, can affect susceptibility and immune response to TB infection, as they do in vaccine response to other childhood illnesses (Anania et al., 2017). Once infected, the course of these diseases in children is generally more rapid and widespread than in adults because of anatomic and immunologic differences in the lung. The spread of MTB beyond the primary site via lymphatic and hematogenous routes can lead to disseminated disease, including miliary TB and TB meningitis, which are more prevalent in pediatric cases. This systemic dissemination indicates a failure of the immune containment mechanisms. Additionally, the pediatric lungs smaller size and less mature architecture facilitate more widespread pulmonary involvement. Imaging modalities like computed tomography (CT), while more frequently mentioned elsewhere in the pediatric respiratory disorders like cystic fibrosis, highlight the need for early identification of pathological changes to avoid serious outcomes, implying potential similarities in pediatric TB management (Aghahosseini et al., 2018). Knowledge of these mechanisms highlights the necessity for early diagnosis and individualized treatment in children. Host factors underlying the pathophysiology of pediatric TB include complex interactions between genetic predisposition, immune maturation, and environmental factors. Protective immunity development is regulated by various factors, including antigen presentation and resultant antibody formation, modulated by genetic heterogeneity of the human leukocyte antigen (HLA) system, as seen in other pediatric immunologic disorders (Anania et al., 2017). Such heterogeneity has the potential to result in variable vaccine efficacy and susceptibility to infection. Additionally, children in resource-rich environments frequently have repeat exposure, which influences immune priming and manifestation of disease. These multi-determination factors require a more sophisticated understanding of TB pathophysiology to guide enhanced diagnostic and therapeutic interventions specifically tailored for the child population to provide improved disease control and prevention (Figure 9.4).

Age	Number of population	Number of patients	The reported incidence (1/10,0000)	Standardized incidence (1/10,0000)
0-4	301,797	0	0.00	0.00
5-14	788,629	12	1.52	26.40
15-24	815,761	312	38.25	608.12
25-34	884,362	315	35.62	702.05
35-44	791,547	320	40.43	619.34
45-54	1,298,072	762	58.70	702.67
55-64	759,667	576	75.82	537.58
65-74	590,094	468	79.31	385.44
75-	316,267	134	42.37	94.91
Summation	6,549,196	2,899	44.29	36.77

Figure 9.4. Pathogenesis of tuberculosis in children.

Source: Wang Q, Zhu J, Zhang L and Xie L (2023) Regional and epidemiological characteristics of tuberculosis and treatment outcomes in West China. Front. Public Health. 11:1254579. doi: 10.3389/fpubh.2023.1254579

9.2.1. Transmission Mechanisms

The transmission of tuberculosis among child populations is inextricably linked to social and environmental conditions that allow for the first exposure to MTB. Young children are especially at risk as a result of close and extended contact with infected adults, frequently in families or group living situations. These settings increase the probability of transmission through the air when an infected person exhales or coughs respiratory droplets carrying the bacterium. In addition, the natural course of TB disease in children is significantly varied by age, and infants and young children are more likely to become progressively ill after initial infection, highlighting that not just exposure but host susceptibility is also involved in transmission. These aspects underscore why pediatric TB transmission dynamics are complex, determined not just by bacilli presence but also by socioeconomic and immunological factors that affect disease evolution following infection (Seddon et al., 2014). Environmental factors are key drivers in perpetuating the transmission cycle of child tuberculosis. Crowding within housing and poor ventilation greatly amplify the density of infectious droplet nuclei, increasing transmission risk in contexts with limited resources in which children tend to spend time near adult cases of TB. Moreover, variables such as poor nutrition and the presence of comorbid diseases compromise children's immune protection, allowing for acquisition of infection and development of active disease. Epidemiologic data from historical as well as recent studies show that advances in living standards, sanitation, and nutrition have lowered TB transmission rates and related mortality considerably. These observations imply that control of transmission among children implies multi-factor interventions that address both pathogen exposure and host susceptibility (Clay & Troesken, 2006).

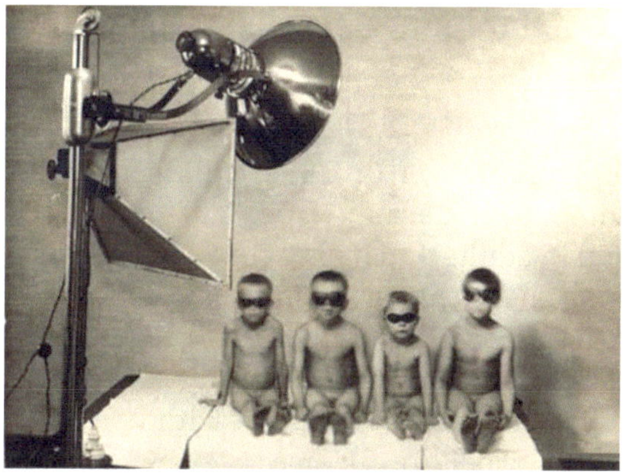

Source: By Unknown author - http://www.pohjois-savonmuisti.fi/verkko_nayttelyt/pohjoissavonlehtikuvia/01/index-13.htm, Public Domain, https://commons.wikimedia.org/w/index.php?curid=7564674

Transmission dynamics among pediatric tuberculosis also call for a focus on community-level factors that affect the spread of the disease. Limited healthcare access and late diagnosis of adult TB cases in most high-burden areas extend infectious periods, heightening the likelihood that children with close contact are exposed. Transmission is also made more complicated by the absence of symptoms in latent tuberculosis infection (LTBI) in children, which usually goes unnoticed but preserves the latent reservoir for the reactivation of future disease. These threaten to emphasize the need for targeted contact investigation and preventive treatment of children exposed to infected adults. Identifying and interrupting early transmission routes has the potential to curb the burden of childhood TB, highlighting that effective control involves an integrated strategy that cuts across the biological, social, and health system determinants (Seddon et al., 2014).

9.2.2. Immune Response in Pediatric Patients

The immune system of children patients has certain distinct features that determine the course and treating tuberculosis infection. In children, especially less than three years old, the immune response to MTB is strikingly different from adults, which makes diagnosis and containment challenging. One of the distinguishing observations in children with LTBI is a major impairment of the phagocytic function of leukocytes by about 30%, which impairs the primary intracellular killing of the pathogen. Furthermore, concomitant ailments like obesity, connective tissue dysplasia, and allergic disorders are commonly associated with LTBI, suggesting an abnormal immuno-metabolic status that could impede immune protection. The retention of a positive Diaskin test despite prolonged treatment indicates the role of resident memory T-cells, which are integral to immune vigilance but could also indicate sustained immune activation against persistent reservoirs of pathogen (Salova et al., 2025). New research has also identified the molecular mechanisms of immune responses in pediatric tuberculosis through the investigation of autophagy-related mechanisms. Autophagy, a cellular process needed for the degradation of intracellular pathogens, seems to be directly involved in differentiation between latent and active tuberculosis disease in children. Gene expression profiling has shown the presence of distinct autophagy-related molecular clusters, each with corresponding immune patterns. One cluster demonstrated reduced adaptive cellular immunity accompanied by heightened inflammatory activity, reflecting a potential deviation from protective immunity to immune pathology. This heterogeneity of immune responses indicates that there is a complicated interaction between autophagy and immune regulation, such that abnormalities or changes in autophagy may disrupt the clearance of bacteria and lead to disease progression among children (Yu et al., 2024).

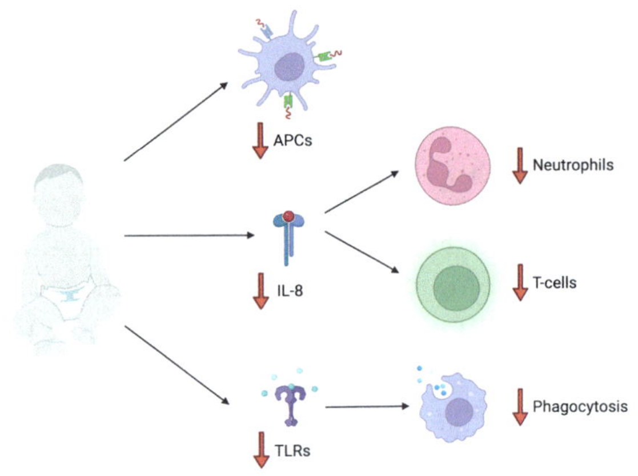

Figure 9.5. Infants are more susceptible to acquiring TB due to an immature immune system, including reduced antigen-presenting cells (APCs), reduced IL-8 chemokine production leading to impaired chemotaxis of neutrophils and T-cells, reduced toll-like receptors (TLRs), and, therefore, decreased phagocytosis for fighting infection.

Source: Rangchaikul P, Ahn P, Nguyen M, Zhong V, Venketaraman V. Review of Pediatric Tuberculosis in the Aftermath of COVID-19. *Clinics and Practice*. 2022; 12(5):738-754. https://doi.org/10.3390/clinpract12050077

The complexity of immune mechanisms in pediatric tuberculosis makes it necessary to have personalized and targeted therapies for effective disease management. The immuno-metabolic profile of children with LTBI without known exposure highlights the importance of individualized vaccination strategies and long-term multidisciplinary follow-up to deal not only with the infection but also with concomitant health conditions. Molecular diagnostics advances, such as gene expression-based biomarkers, provide promising directions to better differentiate latent versus active disease. Such precision in disease state detection may lead to earlier intervention and improved treatment outcomes. Additionally, the knowledge of autophagy function in immune modulation opens up possibilities of new therapeutic targets to augment intracellular bacterial killing, thereby improving the control of pediatric tuberculosis and minimizing the risk of disease progression (Yu et al., 2024; Salova et al., 2025) (Figure 9.5).

9.2.3. Differences from Adult Tuberculosis (TB)

The presentation of TB in children tends to deviate considerably from the presentation found in adults and makes timely diagnosis and management challenging. In contrast to adults, who have pulmonary disease with manifestations of chronic cough and hemoptysis, children's tuberculosis tends to present with non-specific features of failure to thrive, fever, and loss of weight. Additionally, children are at risk for developing extrapulmonary manifestations of the disease, including lymphadenitis or meningitis, illustrating variations in disease and immune response. These differences, in turn, affect clinical suspicion, as well as prompt increased caution on the part of physicians to prevent delayed and missed diagnoses. The more subtle nature of symptomatology in children leads to underreporting and underdiagnosis, thereby compromising public health strategies to control transmission of tuberculosis in children (Seddon et al., 2014). Apart from symptomatology, diagnostic difficulties prominently characterize pediatric tuberculosis from that seen in adults. The paucibacillary presentation of TB in children renders microbiological diagnosis by sputum smears or cultures challenging, in contrast to adults in whom sputum is more easily accessible and has higher bacterial concentrations. Young children are also not able to bring up sputum on command, requiring invasive methods like gastric aspiration or induced sputum, which cannot always be performed in resource-poor environments. These diagnostic challenges result in increased dependence on clinical and radiological criteria, which may be subjective and highly variable across practitioners. Combined with delays in diagnosis, these contributory factors yield a unique epidemiological picture among children requiring adjusted strategies to detection and control (Leining, 2019; Seddon et al., 2014). The epidemiology and transmission dynamics of tuberculosis among children also serve to demonstrate significant divergence from the case of adult TB. Children mostly learn infection from close contact with infected adults, representing a sentinel for recent transmission within the community. Nonetheless, their poor TB transmission capacity due to paucibacillary disease is in contrast to adults, who are mostly the key source of infection in the community through aerosolized bacilli. Geographic and socioeconomic conditions also have a heightened impact since children residing in remote or under-resourced communities are more likely to encounter significant obstacles to healthcare access, worsening disease burden and transmission (Leining, 2019). Detection of such distinctive patterns of transmission justifies the need for child-centered public health interventions that focus on early case detection and treatment among high-risk groups.

9.3. Clinical Manifestations

The clinical presentation of tuberculosis among children is usually problematic in terms of diagnosis because of its varied clinical presentations. In contrast to adults, tuberculosis in children is generally characterized by non-specific symptoms that may resemble other prevalent pediatric infections, making early detection more complicated. Clinical manifestations tend to rely on the location and severity of infection. Pulmonary infection continues to be the most common and tends to manifest as chronic cough, fever, loss of weight, and night sweats. Yet, the manifestation of extrapulmonary tuberculosis (EPTB) is varied and can involve lymph nodes (LNs), the central nervous system (CNS), bones, or abdominal organs. The insidious and overlapping nature of presentation with other conditions in childhood requires a high level of suspicion by clinicians. Prompt recognition is crucial since it prevents morbidity of a severe kind, especially in cases of tuberculous meningitis (TBM) where neurologic complications occur rapidly. Neurological presentation in childhood tuberculosis is one of the most serious manifestations, with TBM having complicated clinical pictures and possibly disastrous results. They usually begin with protracted fever, irritability, lethargy, and headache, followed by neurological dysfunction in the form of cranial nerve palsies, seizures, or altered consciousness as the illness advances. Complications such as hydrocephalus and cerebral infarctions are frequent and significantly contribute to morbidity and mortality if not treated early. Proper management relies on early detection of these clinical manifestations and prompt institution of anti-tubercular (ATT) treatment with the addition of adjunct therapies such as corticosteroids. Case reports highlight that even with timely intervention, patients might need extra therapeutics to avoid sequelae, highlighting the urgent need for increased vigilance in clinical practice (Ajassa et al., 2018). Although most pediatric tuberculosis has respiratory symptoms or neurological involvement, there are other rarer presentations complicating the clinical picture. For example, gastrointestinal tuberculosis can masquerade as inflammatory bowel diseases (IBDs) and present from abdominal pain and diarrhea to malnutrition, so differentiation becomes difficult. Such a presentation may result in strictures, fistulas, or ulcerations that are endoscopically visible and histologically demonstrable, showing granulomatous inflammation quite similar to that in Crohn's disease. Pediatric patients can be asymptomatic or present with subtle symptoms that necessitate extensive investigation, such as imaging and biopsy. Treatment is a combination of ATT medications and supportive treatments with the aim of mucosal healing and systemic symptom resolution. Clinical overlap with other chronic conditions necessitates careful diagnostic evaluation to provide proper therapy (Vale Rodrigues et al., 2019).

9.3.1. Common Symptoms in Children

Children with infectious diseases usually exhibit a cluster of nonspecific signs, which can make timely and precise diagnosis difficult. In tuberculosis in children, these signs often involve fever, chronic cough, and respiratory distress, which indicate underlying pulmonary pathology. Fever, an acute systemic reaction, is usually persistent despite initial antibiotic therapy, which calls for further investigation. Cough in pediatric tuberculosis can be of prolonged and refractory nature to conventional therapies, in contrast to that of common viral or bacterial infections.

The morbidity of respiratory distress can be variable but can elicit urgent clinical intervention with impaired airway function. These early symptoms are vital indicators that help medical professionals distinguish between tuberculosis and other respiratory conditions, particularly in regions of high prevalence where tuberculosis in children is a major issue (Loembe et al., 2025). Identifying the symptoms early allows for quick diagnostic procedures and intervention, hence enhancing outcomes. Apart from respiratory manifestations, failure to thrive and weight loss are characteristic signs in pediatric tuberculosis that herald a systemic infection on a child's general well-being. Chronic cough and prolonged fever could be associated with significant weight loss, indicative both of the metabolic consumption of the infection and also loss of appetite. Such a presentation highlights the chronicity of the disease and its interference with growth and development. Also, pain in the abdomen can present in scenarios where tuberculosis is extrapulmonary, adding to the symptomatology. Other laboratory indicators such as high inflammatory indexes including C-reactive protein and erythrocyte sedimentation rate (ESR) tend to reflect disease severity, offering more assistance in diagnosis. These symptoms are a call for complete clinical evaluation for tuberculosis in children presenting with chronic systemic symptoms, highlighting the necessity of a heightened index of suspicion in endemic regions (Sevliya et al., 2025). The diagnostic dilemma in pediatric tuberculosis is the overlap of its presentation with more frequently encountered childhood conditions, which calls for cautious clinical observation and directed investigations. Unilateral pleural effusion detected on imaging may itself prove to be a useful marker of tuberculous involvement, commonly manifesting in the company of clinical evidence such as fever and respiratory distress. Pleural ultrasounds and chest radiographs are radiological methods that aid in establishing the accumulation of fluid in the pleural space, which, along with clinical evidence, is suggestive of tuberculosis in most instances. The occurrence of staphylococcal infections as frequent differential diagnoses requires empiric and later adjusted antimicrobial therapy to deal with bacterial co-infections, but refractory symptoms in the face of such treatment bolster the suspicion for tuberculosis (Loembe et al., 2025). Proper identification of the symptom constellation and correlation with diagnostic imaging ultimately leads to the initiation of proper antitubercular regimens, enhancing pediatric patient prognoses (Figure 9.6).

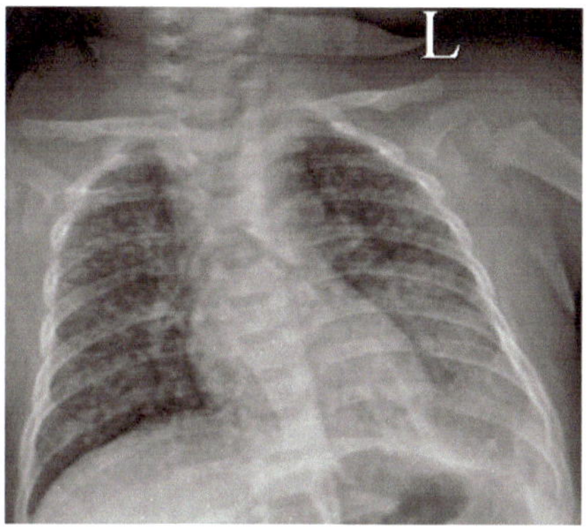

Figure 9.6. Tuberculosis symptoms.

Source: Nguyen PTK, Thai TTB, Huynh J, Marais BJ. An Infant with Xpert® Confirmed TB Meningitis in Central Viet Nam. *Journal of Clinical Medicine*. 2018; 7(11):397. https://doi.org/10.3390/jcm7110397

9.3.2. Asymptomatic Cases and Their Risks

The difficulty of diagnosing tuberculosis in children is exacerbated by the prevalence of asymptomatic cases, which makes early diagnosis and intervention difficult. Unlike adult patients, pediatric patients with LTBI may not present with open symptoms, thus routine screening is critical, particularly in healthcare facilities. Medical students and health trainees are a population at risk, as evidenced by research showing a quantifiable prevalence of LTBI even in young adults in medical training. This silent infection reservoir underscores the importance of meticulous screening practices like tuberculin skin test (TST) and interferon-gamma release assays (IGRAs) in identifying latent infections before they develop into active disease, especially because untreated LTBI becomes infectious. Thus, detecting asymptomatic cases is a central component of tuberculosis control, highlighting awareness gaps and the importance of preventive care among high-risk populations (Verso et al., 2019). Socioeconomic and geographic factors also impact the likelihood of occult pediatric tuberculosis, particularly in remote or underserved areas.

Children who reside far from health facilities tend to have barriers to early diagnosis and treatment because of restricted access and hence experience increased rates of TST-positive status even among asymptomatic individuals. Spatial inequality in access accounts for the continuation of latent infections, which are undetectable but cause a severe public health problem by maintaining transmission in the community. Without aggressive outreach and targeted intervention, especially to distant communities, asymptomatic cases will be missed for prolonged durations. This delays the public health burden to enable progression to active disease and household and community transmission, underscoring the pivotal position of accessibility to healthcare in pediatric tuberculosis management (Leining, 2019).

Given these challenges, the dangers of asymptomatic tuberculosis in children require a multi-pronged strategy that merges early identification, vaccination, and education. The presence of LTBI in children's populations not only means that there is an underlying risk for disease activation but also raises awareness of the possibility that these children may act as reservoirs for continued cycles of transmission. Preventive strategies must therefore address both medical and social determinants, including prompt screening of high-risk groups and comprehensive community health initiatives. Particularly in healthcare training environments, where latent infections show a measurable prevalence, enhanced surveillance and vaccination efforts can mitigate future cases. Detection and control of asymptomatic disease in children is critical to the interruption of tuberculosis transmission and better long-term public health (Verso et al., 2019) (Figure 9.7).

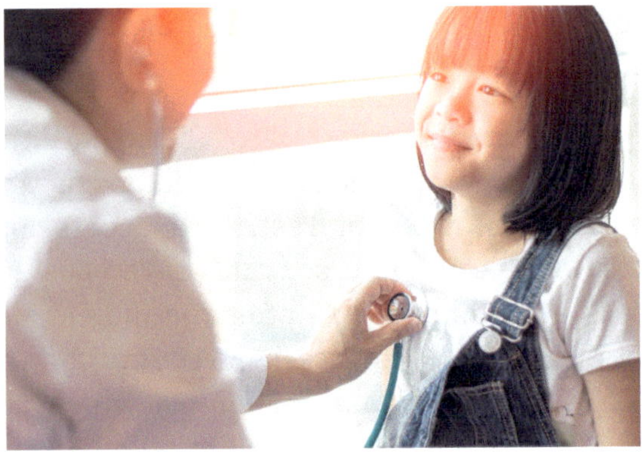

Figure 9.7. Diagnosing latent tuberculosis infection (LTBI) in children.

Source: T-SPOT Asia. (2021). *Pediatrician examining a young girl during a health check-up.* https://tspot.asia/wp-content/uploads/2021/07/professional-general-medical-pediatrician-doctor-in-white-uniform-gown-listen-lung-and-heart-sound-of-asia-child-patient-with-stethoscope-physician-check-up-asian-kid-female-after-consult-in-hospital-scaled.jpeg.

9.3.3. Complications Associated with Pediatric Tuberculosis (TB)

Tuberculosis usually presents a complicated clinical course in affected children depending on their age, immune status, and underlying conditions. Most at risk are those below the age of 18 months, whose immature immune system makes them victims of increased morbidity and mortality. Complications in these children are often superimposed in those with HIV/AIDS, where immunodeficiency worsens the progression of disease and predisposes to opportunistic infections. Research has shown that low baseline hemoglobin levels in children are strongly associated with higher mortality risk during treatment, making early detection and intervention particularly critical. Collectively, these factors underscore the clinical difficulty in managing children with tuberculosis, especially in decentralized or resource-constrained healthcare settings where expert care is not readily available. Therefore, the integration of thorough diagnostic and therapeutic plans is essential in reducing outcomes for vulnerable child populations hit by tuberculosis (Janssen et al., 2010). Inpatient management is very vital in treating complicated or severe pediatric tuberculosis, weighing clinical demands and public health needs. The indications for inpatient treatment go beyond clinical severity to host-related parameters like malnutrition, immune suppression, or infancy under 12 months. Additionally, logistic hurdles and social determinants influence admission and isolation decisions. Precautionary respiratory isolation is still a critical step for children waiting for confirmatory diagnosis, irrespective of age, to preclude nosocomial transmission and protect public health. Effective hospitalization protocols also include discharge and return to the community criteria, focusing on continued treatment compliance and microbiological clearance to limit relapse or dissemination. These maneuvers are critical to preventing complications and promoting recovery in the patient, as well as addressing larger epidemiologic issues (Vecchio et al., 2015). Complications of pediatric tuberculosis are more than simple respiratory findings and frequently involve systemic and extrapulmonary complications that complicate management. CNS involvement, such as TBM, is a serious complication with risk for long-term neurological impairment if not diagnosed early. Also, spreading to lymphatic, skeletal, and abdominal locations threatens clinical control via diagnostic difficulty and long therapy demands. Patients with comorbidities like malnutrition or HIV are most at risk of life-threatening disease courses and complications from treatment, warranting multidisciplinary management strategies. The dynamics of host immune response, severity of disease, and therapeutic outcomes decide the potential for unfavorable consequences, requiring individually directed interventions and constant surveillance. Identification and management of these complex complications are essential processes toward lowering mortality and enhancing the quality of life in tubercular children (Janssen et al., 2010; Vecchio et al., 2015) (Figure 9.8).

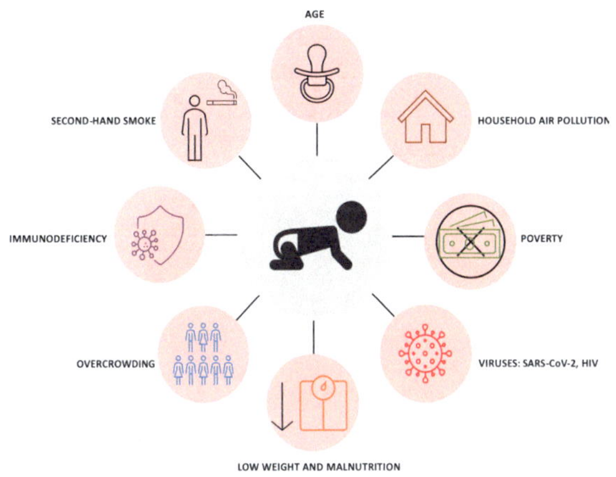

Figure 9.8. The likelihood of acquiring childhood TB is impacted by age, where infants and children below five years have the greatest risk, household air pollution, poverty, SARS-CoV-2 and HIV infection, low weight and malnutrition, overcrowding, immunodeficiency, and second-hand smoke exposure.

Source: MDPI. (2021). *Risk factors contributing to tuberculosis in children.* https://www.mdpi.com/2039-7283/12/5/77.

9.4. Diagnosis of Pediatric Tuberculosis (TB)

Early detection of childhood tuberculosis is frequently hampered by the insidious and non-specific nature of childhood symptoms, making clinical diagnosis more difficult. In addition, the paucibacillary nature of the disease, with a low bacterial load, restricts the utility of conventional diagnostic tests based on smear microscopy that need a high number of bacteria to yield detectable results. With these limitations in mind, more complex methods, such as molecular diagnostic methods, have been put in place to enhance sensitivity and specificity. Polymerase chain reaction (PCR) and nucleic acid amplification tests (NAATs) have transformed the diagnosis of TB by being able to identify tiny amounts of bacterial genetic material, thereby bypassing some of the hurdles posed by low numbers of bacteria. The World Health Organization (WHO) advises cartridge-based nucleic acid amplification testing (CBNAAT) to be the main diagnostic tool in childhood TB because it can give accurate results within a short time, leading to early treatment initiation and minimizing mortality. The innovations highlight the value of using molecular techniques to increase the accuracy of pediatric tuberculosis diagnosis (Srinidhi et al., 2025). As a supplement to molecular testing, the application of noninvasive sample sources has also been noted as a viable option for use in children. Young children have difficulty coughing up sputum, hindering collection of the classic samples that are used to identify MTB. New programs have looked into the diagnostic value of stool specimens, which are less painful and less difficult to collect than respiratory samples. A pilot project in Ukraine showed the effectiveness of stool examination in the diagnosis of TB in children, with bacteriologic confirmation established in the majority of instances in which stool was the only positive source sample. Identification of drug resistance indicators like rifampicin resistance by stool examination is another example of the advantage of this method, justifying specific treatment regimens. This noninvasive approach has the potential for widespread application and is a patient-friendly option that may enhance early diagnosis and control of childhood TB (Diuzheva et al., 2024). Technology notwithstanding, the diagnosis of tuberculosis among children is complex and still calls for an integration of the clinical, radiologic, and lab findings. The characteristic immunological and pathological presentation of TB in children requires an integrative approach that accounts for host response markers in addition to direct pathogen identification. Biomarkers such as lipoarabinomannan, a mycobacterial cell wall-specific glycolipid, have been useful urinary indicators, especially in immunocompromised groups such as children with HIV. Culturing techniques, while less rapid and more costly, offer valuable confirmatory information by amplifying bacterial loads in samples to dilute for direct detection. Diagnostic excellence therefore relies on a synergy of methods that are appropriate to resource status and patient capacity, ultimately demanding clinical judgment to negotiate such nuances. Ongoing research and innovation, in addition to pragmatic adoption of new diagnostic methods, are needed to enhance pediatric tuberculosis care outcomes (Srinidhi et al., 2025) (Figure 9.9).

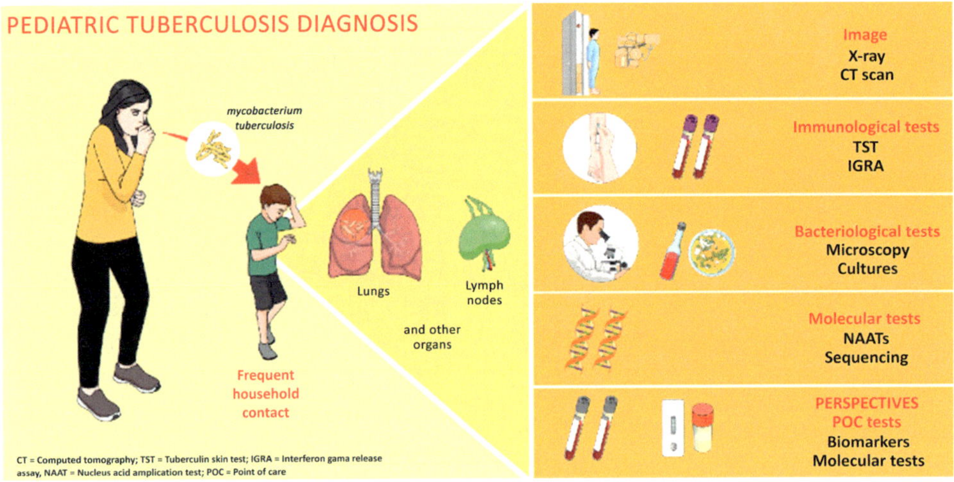

Figure 9.9. Pediatric tuberculosis diagnosis.

Source: Springer Nature. (2023). *Pediatric tuberculosis diagnosis: Transmission and diagnostic approaches.* https://media.springernature.com/lw685/springer-static/image/chp%3A10.1007%2F978-3-031-15955-8_11/MediaObjects/497831_1_En_11_Figc_HTML.png?as=webp.

9.4.1. Diagnostic Tests and Procedures

Diagnosis of TB in children is particularly challenging because pediatric TB is frequently paucibacillary and it is challenging to obtain suitable clinical specimens. In contrast to adults, children most commonly have EPTB, which calls for varied diagnostic strategies other than the usual sputum examination. Radiographic imaging, such as chest X-rays, continues to be a useful initial measure for detecting pulmonary involvement, but its specificity may be compromised, particularly in discriminating TB from other respiratory pathogens. Cytopathological assessment of LN aspirates and other extrapulmonary sites becomes particularly important in resource-constrained environments. In addition, molecular tests like CBNAAT have transformed detecting TB by enabling prompt and specific detection of MTB, with added drug resistance profiling. Yet, only a small percentage of the cases are microbiologically confirmed through such techniques, making it important to have complementary diagnostic tests that can successfully record the diverse pediatric TB presentations (Ramanthan et al., 2025). New diagnostic technologies aim to surmount the invasiveness and sensitivity constraints inherent in existing pediatric TB testing. Breath analysis, for instance, is an exciting area that has the potential to provide a quick and non-invasive option to detect volatile organic compounds in association with MTB infection. This could prove especially useful for children, who have difficulty producing sputum and need less invasive approaches to diagnosis. However, this strategy is still in its infancy stages of development, with research continuing towards standardizing the collection of breath and ascertaining biomarker sensitivity and specificity. Application of breath tests to the diagnostic program would go a long way in improving early detection, particularly in HIV co-infected children and extrapulmonary and DR-TB, where standard approaches have lower efficacy (Lotte et al., 2025). However, overall clinical integration requires additional strong validation to provide consistent, replicable results. Despite advances in diagnostic methods, practical application in most endemic areas is confronted with serious barriers such as poor laboratory facilities and unavailability of high-level molecular assays.

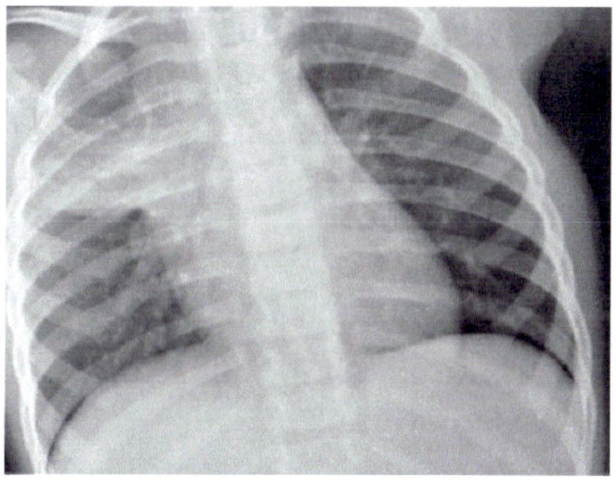

Figure 9.10. Primary tuberculosis in a small child. Antero-posterior chest X-ray demonstrates homogeneous consolidation with air bronchogram in the right middle lung zone.

Source: ResearchGate. (n.d.). *Primary tuberculosis in a small child: Antero-posterior chest X-ray.* https://www.researchgate.net/figure/Primary-tuberculosis-in-a-small-child-Antero-posterior-chest-X-ray-demonstrates_fig1_262386090.

The dominance of EPTB disease among children in rural and underdeveloped communities complicates diagnosis due to the impossibility of using standard sputum microscopy. Thus, the health systems need to place emphasis on scaling up diagnostic modalities like CBNAAT in conjunction with cytopathology and imaging-based testing to raise detection rates. Moreover, treatment of malnutrition and other co-morbid conditions that predispose individuals to TB infection is needed to enhance diagnostic yield and treatment outcomes. Enhancing diagnostic competency through training, funding, and including innovative technologies would eliminate existing gaps and eventually alleviate the burden of pediatric TB by allowing for timely and correct diagnosis of the disease (Ramanthan et al., 2025) (Figure 9.10).

9.4.2. Challenges in Diagnosing Pediatric Tuberculosis (TB)

Diagnosis of tuberculosis in children poses a special combination of challenges that are often responsible for delayed and inaccurate detection of the disease. In contrast to adults, children with TB tend to develop a paucibacillary form of the disease, i.e., possess a smaller number of bacteria, which severely diminishes the diagnostic power of standard testing procedures. Furthermore, pediatric patients are often characterized by nonspecific and overlapping clinical features with other frequent conditions in childhood, further confusing clinicians. Radiological features can be subtle or unusual, particularly in younger children, making imaging-dependent diagnosis challenging. Such diagnostic difficulty is compounded in resource-poor environments where access to sophisticated laboratory facilities or specialized expertise can be limited, thereby hindering early identification and intervention. Overcoming these obstacles demands technical innovations as well as clinician skill and confidence reinforcement among frontline health care providers to accurately and authoritatively read complex presentations (Brittany et al., 2024). Innovative strategies introduced in recent programmatic attempts improve detection of pediatric tuberculosis despite these challenges, as shown in demonstration of pragmatic solutions in overcoming the limitations of diagnosis. For example, nations such as Ukraine have tested stool sample testing as a noninvasive substitute for the conventional sputum samples that are notoriously hard to get from young children. Stool testing allows bacteriological confirmation of MTB, including drug-resistant strains, which is crucial in tailoring effective treatment regimens. The pilot test proved that stool samples indicated tuberculosis in a few instances when no other positive samples existed, highlighting the value of this method as a diagnostic tool. Innovations like these enhance patient comfort and diagnostic yield while facilitating the timely onset of safer and more effective treatment. The successful incorporation of stool testing into regular pediatric TB services showcases how new diagnostic technologies can fill current gaps, especially in high-burden, low-resource settings (Diuzheva et al., 2024). Despite such promising technologies, considerable systemic and operational challenges remain, limiting implementation and scale-up of enhanced diagnostic approaches for pediatric tuberculosis. Implementing evidence and policy guidelines into standard practice tends to be faced with obstacles concerned with healthcare infrastructure, training of the workforce, and budgetary allocation. Most clinicians might not yet have the confidence or expertise in diagnosing TB in children because of its diverse presentation and paucity of diagnostic equipment. Thus, enhancing the capacity of the healthcare providers by way of thorough guidelines, education, and support is needed to facilitate clinical decision-making. In addition, political will and long-term funding to extend access to new diagnostics and roll out prevention, detection, and treatment services at the community level are still essential. To address these complex challenges in an integral manner will be necessary to decrease the pediatric tuberculosis burden worldwide by enhancing diagnosis and ensuring children are treated in a timely and proper manner (Brittany et al., 2024) (Figure 9.11).

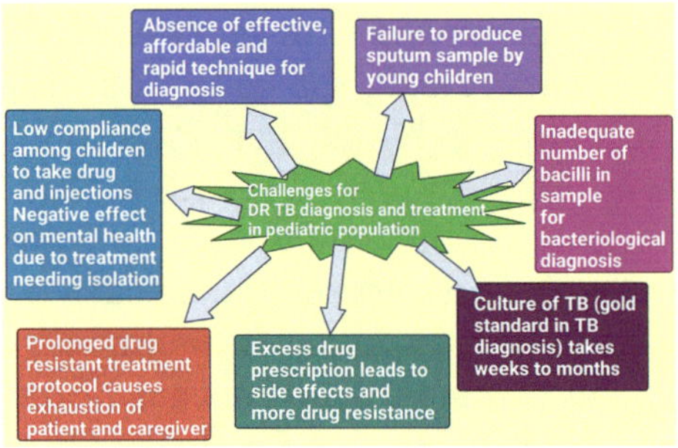

Figure 9.11. Depicting the various challenges for diagnosing and treating drug-resistant tuberculosis (DR-TB) among the pediatric population.

Source: ResearchGate. (n.d.). *Challenges for diagnosing and treating drug-resistant tuberculosis in pediatric populations.* https://www.researchgate.net/figure/Depicting-the-various-challenges-for-diagnosing-and-treating-Drug-Resistant-Tuberculosis_fig2_368636983.

9.4.3. Importance of Early Detection

The complexities involved in the diagnosis of disease in children usually provide tall orders because presentation is usually not typical and symptoms cross-match with those of other diseases. In the case of TB, earlier detection is critical to differentiate it from other diseases, like malignancies, which have similar presentation symptoms like lymphadenopathy. Delayed or incorrect diagnosis could result in further advancement of the disease, and hence morbidity, as well as causing transmission risk. Diagnostic precision is dependent to a great extent on confirmatory methods, and pathological biopsy still stands as the gold standard for confirming TB infection among symptomatic children of cervical lymphadenopathy. Additionally, selection of diagnostic method can affect detection sensitivity; for instance, fine needle aspiration can provide less representative samples than surgical LN biopsies, which increase rates of detection. Thus, accurate and prompt diagnostic testing is essential to begin proper therapy and achieve optimal pediatric patient outcomes in the management of TB (Lawrence et al., 2024). In treating pediatric tuberculosis, delays between collection of specimens and confirmation of results play a critical role in clinical decision-making and initiation of treatment. Delays in testing can hinder timely therapeutic action, leading to increased severity of the disease and transmission risk among vulnerable populations. Diagnostic workflow innovations, like in-site point-of-care testing, also have much lower turnaround times than off-site laboratory assays. Moving from off-site high-sensitivity troponin testing to in-site assays in pediatric care, for instance, had a median decrease of more than 50% in verification times for results, and this showcases the advantages of being in close proximity and immediate in terms of testing capabilities. While targeted at cardiac injury markers, these results highlight the wider significance of quick diagnostics that, if extended to detecting TB in children, would enable the starting of treatment earlier and prevent adverse outcomes. This approach emphasizes the need to enhance diagnostic infrastructure to streamline the detection process in cases of pediatric tuberculosis (Luo et al., 2024). Early diagnosis of pediatric tuberculosis assumes central importance not just in clinical prediction but also in disease spread control in communities. Children are especially at risk for accelerated disease progression and serious extrapulmonary complications, making early detection and treatment a necessity. Early diagnosis allows healthcare practitioners to provide correct antimicrobial treatment, thus preventing risks of complications such as disseminated infection and drug resistance. In addition, from a public health standpoint, early case detection supports the breaking of chains of transmission, particularly in high-burden environments where children are often sentinel markers of active community spread. As such, investment in diagnostic sensitivity and access through improved sampling methods and rapid on-site diagnosis, becomes a critical strategy in modern pediatric tuberculosis control, supporting both clinical and epidemiological mandates (Lawrence et al., 2024; Luo et al., 2024).

9.5. Treatment Options

Effective control of child TB requires thorough treatment planning aimed at the individualized physiological and immunological nature of children. As opposed to TB in adults, child TB often involves vigilant adjustment of doses as well as attention to the process of absorption and metabolism of drugs. Routine treatment regimens often include an intensive phase of a combination of multiple antitubercular agents for two months, followed by a continuation phase of four to six months on fewer drugs for pathogen eradication and prevention of relapse. Adherence to therapy in pediatric TB is also a concern, which may be especially difficult given the longer duration and potential side effects of the drugs. Moreover, concomitant conditions like malnutrition or hemoglobinopathies can complicate therapy and require interdisciplinary interaction to maximize treatment outcomes in the pediatric population (Abu-Sharar et al., 2024). Compliance with treatment procedures in pediatric tuberculosis is paramount, as it can result in drug resistance and failure of treatment if therapy is partial or non-uniform. Improving adherence is usually achieved by educating caregivers, employing child-friendly formulations, and frequent follow-up visits that monitor both clinical response and possible ADRs. For MDR-TB, treatment becomes complicated as a result of the side effects and duration of second-line drugs, requiring careful monitoring for drug interactions and side effects. New therapeutic methods are being investigated to minimize treatment time without reducing efficacy, such as innovations in pharmacogenomics and individualized medicine. These advances also seek to counter the problems created by resistant organisms and optimize therapy success rates among pediatric patients, pointing to the need for personalized treatment protocols (Gupta et al., 2024). Surgical treatments, although less frequent, can be indicated in some cases of pediatric TB for which drug therapy would not be adequate, e.g., in severe pulmonary destruction or in complications such as tuberculous lymphadenitis or spinal involvement. Moreover, adjunctive treatments, namely nutritional support and treatment of comorbid illnesses such as anemia or immune dysfunction, are integral parts of global care. Routine monitoring by clinical assessments and imaging tests guarantees early detection of treatment response and prompt identification of possible complications. Multidisciplinary care teams, including pediatricians, infectious disease experts, nutritionists, and social workers, improve treatment compliance and prognosis. Ongoing studies on new drug formulation and diagnostic approaches are critical to enhancing cure rates and survival status for children suffering from tuberculosis (Abu-Sharar et al., 2024; Gupta et al., 2024).

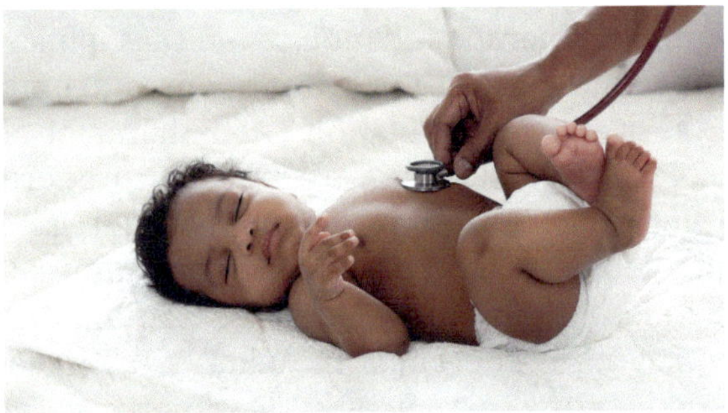

Source: Boston University School of Public Health. (2023). *Physician examining infant for pediatric tuberculosis.* https://www.bu.edu/sph/files/2023/04/PTB-scaled.jpg.

9.5.1. Standard Treatment Regimens

Improvements in treating pediatric tuberculosis have greatly changed the treatment paradigm, particularly for drug-susceptible tuberculosis (DS-TB). In the past, the default strategy involved at least six months of combination treatment, which was frequently difficult because of extended treatment duration and lack of adherence. New treatment regimens have been recently developed that cut down on treatment duration to around four months without affecting effectiveness. These technologies not only simplify therapy but also enhance tolerability, playing a role in improved outcomes among children and adolescents. The use of new and repurposed drugs like bedaquiline, delamanid, and linezolid, along with maximized dosages of approved agents like rifampicin and rifapentine, has transformed treatment regimens. In addition, the existence of child-friendly preparations guarantees the right dosing and administration, which are paramount in the pediatric setting (Garcia-Prats et al., 2022). These advances highlight the dynamic evolution in TB management and the promise of enhanced pediatric patient care. Central nervous system tuberculosis (CNS-TB) poses special therapeutic challenges among pediatric patients with its severe clinical presentation and high morbidity and mortality. Treatment recommendations classically support an extended course with prolonged therapy of nine or even 12 months using a multidrug regimen of isoniazid, rifampin, pyrazinamide (PZA), and ethambutol. Adjunctive corticosteroid treatment is also routine to prevent inflammatory outcomes in the initial phases of treatment. However, new data from some recent clinical trials indicate that more intense and sometimes truncated regimens of treatment can produce superior clinical outcomes, possibly reducing neurological complications. Even with these encouraging advances, achieving an ideal balance between treatment duration and regimen intensity continues to be a focus of investigation. Early and correct diagnosis coupled with early institution of therapy is still central to optimizing the prognosis of children with CNS-TB (Ahmed, 2018). Treatment for DR-TB has witnessed profound shifts, reducing the paradigms from the traditionally long and toxic regimens. In the past, treatment involved 18 to 24 months of therapy that usually involved injectable drugs that come with dreadful side effects and create huge challenges to drug adherence, particularly in children. Existing treatments focus on shorter, all-oral durations that are more tolerable and have proved to have more favorable safety profiles. The treatments utilize the new anti-TB medications bedaquiline and delamanid, in addition to repurposed drugs clofazimine and linezolid, to enable successful treatment with less harm. The availability of pediatric formulations has significantly boosted individualized dosing plans and compliance. Together, these developments mark a paradigm shift towards enhanced and child-focused pediatric DR-TB care (Garcia-Prats et al., 2022) (Figure 9.12).

Drug	Daily dose and range (mg/kg body weight)	Daily maximum (mg)
Isoniazid	10 (10-15) mg	300mg
*Rifampicin	15 (10-20)	600
Pyrazinamide	35(30-40)	2000

Figure 9.12. Treatment of tuberculosis in children—special considerations.

Source: SlideShare. (n.d.). *Daily pediatric dosing of first-line anti-TB drugs by body weight.* https://image.slidesharecdn.com/treatmentofchildhoodtb-160729150013/95/treatment-of-childhood-tb-12-638.jpg?cb=1496942837.

9.5.2. Considerations for Drug Resistance

A fine-grained assessment of clinical presentation is of great importance when identifying DR-TB in children early on. Radiological findings are central to this diagnostic work since certain features seen on chest X-rays can indicate resistance even before a microbiological diagnosis can be made. Specifically, cavitary and consolidation areas have been statistically correlated with DR-TB cases. These characteristic radiographic features aid in discriminating between drug-sensitive and drug-resistant types so that clinicians can initiate suitable therapy more quickly. Early detection, which is critically important in children, is especially so since disease advancement and transmission risk would be heightened if there were postponement in effective treatment. This radiological information not only supplements microbiological testing but also provides a useful tool in resource-constrained environments where lab results may not be immediately available (Gupta et al., 2025). Finally, combining imaging findings with clinical suspicion is crucial to enhancing outcomes in pediatric DR-TB. Advances in diagnostic technology have significantly enhanced the detection and treatment of drug resistance in pediatric tuberculosis. Among numerous available approaches, NAATs like GeneXpert and CBNAAT have become front-line reagents because of their speed of reporting and sensitivity. These molecular assays detect MTB effectively and concurrently screen rifampicin resistance, a defining marker for multidrug resistance, much faster than conventional techniques. In contrast to Ziehl-Neelsen staining, which tends not to pick up low bacterial burdens encountered in children, CBNAAT is more sensitive, especially for paucibacillary presentation. Additionally, upon receiving positive results, follow-up tests such as the line probe assay (LPA) or culture-based testing may yield supplementary resistance profiling. Hence, the mass use of these molecular diagnostic technologies in high-burden nations also emphasizes their utility both in early diagnosis and timely treatment initiation, curbing drug resistance development (Shah et al., 2024). In addition to diagnostics, treatment protocols for pediatric tuberculosis have to carefully deal with the issues of drug resistance. Development of resistance requires changes in the therapeutic regimen, such as the administration of second-line ATT agents, which is usually accompanied by greater toxicity and longer duration of treatment. Early detection of resistance patterns through integrated clinical, radiological, and molecular evaluation is hence important to prevent treatment failure and minimize the risk of enhanced resistance multiplication. Also, socioeconomic and healthcare infrastructure conditions affect access to drugs and diagnostics, impacting treatment compliance and outcome. Pediatric-specific issues, including dosing and formulation, make treatment challenging but are still of highest priority to maximize efficacy with minimal side effects. A multi-disciplinary strategy with watchful monitoring and patient education is needed to cater to the complexities of drug resistance in pediatric tuberculosis and ensure positive outcomes (Shah et al., 2024; Gupta et al., 2025).

9.5.3. Role of Directly Observed Therapy (DOT)

Good management of pediatric tuberculosis depends not only on proper diagnosis and drug regimens but also on the provision of regular treatment adherence. Of relevance in this regard is the use of directly observed therapy (DOT) as a key method of strengthening adherence and warding off the onset of drug resistance. By making it mandatory for healthcare providers or trained monitors to follow each dose given to the child, DOT covers challenges associated with pediatric TB treatment, including low compliance and risk of incomplete treatment. Research that has explored adherence levels with self-administered treatment has also noted the challenge of many patients sustaining strict drug schedules, thus demonstrating the necessity for such interventions as DOT that ensure a formal and answerable structure of treatment administration (Nackers et al., 2012). Not only does this approach enhance individual health outcomes, but also supports public health by preventing transmission threats from untreated or incompletely treated cases of TB. In addition to its express benefit for adherence, DOT has been linked to cost-effectiveness and enhanced long-term health outcomes in treating chronic infectious illnesses, which can be extended to pediatric tuberculosis therapy. Similar experiences among other infectious illnesses, like applying DOT in ART among HIV-infected pregnant women, show how directly observed drug administration can notably decrease vertical transmission yet is economically reasonable (McCabe et al., 2010). While pediatric TB is distinct in pathology and demographics, the basic tenet of ensuring stringent adherence through observation applies. The augmentation of adherence through DOT reduces complications of unfinished treatment, consequently lowering both morbidity and prospective healthcare costs. Therefore, DOT not only fits with clinical necessities but also plays a beneficial role in resource allocation in pediatric TB control programs, making it an indicator for its larger function in maximizing therapy outcome. However, operationalizing DOT in pediatric tuberculosis care does invoke challenges, including resource intensiveness, potential stigmatization, and caregiver burden, which must be navigated carefully. To maximize efficacy, DOT programs must balance rigorous supervision with sensitivity to the social and economic contexts of affected families. Other models like community-based DOT or employment of digital technologies for observation are being considered in view of these challenges to maintain the essential advantages of adherence monitoring with decreased intrusiveness (Nackers et al., 2012). Adapting the DOT method according to the specific requirements of pediatric populations, along with education and psychosocial support for caregivers, can increase acceptance and rate of completion. Accordingly, the DOT role is more than passive observation, acting as an integrative force in integrated pediatric TB care that promotes adherence, transmission reduction, and holistic treatment (Figure 9.13).

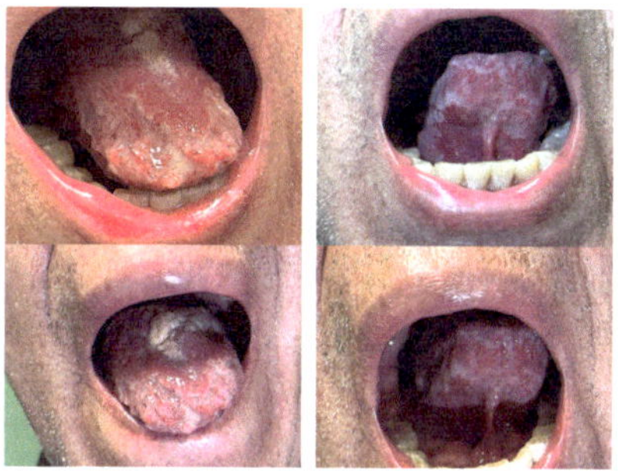

Figure 9.13. Way to better recovery in tuberculosis.

Source: Sevilla-Fuentes S, Mendoza-Vargas LÁ, Araiza-Rodríguez JF, Berthaúd-González B, Falfán-Valencia R, Bautista-Becerril B. Tongue Tuberculosis as a Complication of Pott's Disease in a Patient on Systemic Steroid Therapy without Pulmonary Tuberculosis. *Medicina*. 2024; 60(8):1282. https://doi.org/10.3390/medicina60081282

SUMMARY

Despite international measures against tuberculosis, pediatric tuberculosis is still a serious public health problem, especially among countries with high disease burdens. Recent estimates show that success rates in treatment are usually below critical national and global benchmarks, giving clues to operational gaps of existing control programs. Patient age, nature of disease presentation such as EPTB, and heterogeneity of care practices are among the noteworthy reasons for variable results. Targeted interventions that take these determinants into consideration are critical to prognosis improvement and transmission reduction among children. Institutional studies' lessons highlight the need to adapt TB control measures to the unique needs of pediatric populations to maximize effectiveness and overall survival rates (Nurfeta et al., 2024). These lessons point to the imperative of creating targeted policies and resource allocation to fill these treatment gaps. Additionally, new solutions in public health policy have proven to enhance pediatric TB results on a mass scale. As an example, instituting pre-entry screening policies for immigrants in certain nations has resulted in significant reductions in native-immigrant disparities among TB patients. The increased early detection and timely initiation of treatment that is linked to these measures has greatly boosted treatment success rates among vulnerable groups, including children. These improvements illustrate how systemic changes and international cooperation can robustly impact pediatric TB management beyond clinical care alone. Strengthening healthcare collaboration frameworks and patient support programs, alongside screening, is imperative for sustaining progress and ensuring equitable health outcomes for all children affected by TB (Yu et al., 2024). Tackling pediatric tuberculosis necessitates a multifaceted approach encompassing clinical, policy, and social dimensions. Despite suboptimal treatment success in many settings, strategic efforts guided by epidemiological information and adapted to pediatric conditions can result in significant gains. Strengthening early diagnosis, maximizing compliance with treatment guidelines, and tackling socioeconomic determinants of TB are pivotal to checking morbidity and mortality. In addition, inclusion of novel public health policy measures, including global screening and collaboration of health systems, provides a promising avenue to achieving equity in TB care. Sustained research, investment, and cooperation are needed to meet global goals and ultimately eliminate pediatric tuberculosis as a public health problem.

Knowledge of pediatric tuberculosis involves the awareness of the specific vulnerabilities and diagnostic difficulties of children. It is significant that children make up approximately 10% of all TB cases worldwide, with the disease having a high pediatric burden. Epidemiological data show that prevalence of pediatric TB can be significantly increased in geographically remote or underserved areas, where access to health facilities is limited. This limited access leads to delayed diagnosis and treatment, hence augmenting transmission risks in communities. Research has highlighted the importance of health outreach by healthcare providers within such distant locations to enhance early detection and therapeutic services in children. These results highlight the need for targeted public health interventions addressing geographical and structural barriers to treatment to effectively decrease pediatric TB incidence and mortality (Nair et al., 2016). The demographic trend of TB infection and drug resistance in children mirrors, but uniquely represents, the larger TB population trends. Whereas adult age and male gender are often linked with increased TB positivity rates, children's cases indicate similar risks of drug-resistant types such as rifampicin resistance. Significantly, contrary to old age with relatively lower risk of resistance, children are still at risk of MDR-TB. This defies any belief that resistance is largely an adult disease and necessitates pediatric-relation diagnostic surveillance and DST. Furthermore, history of treatment continues to be an important predictor of resistance, but geographic location or gender may differentially impact resistance prevalence. These findings underscore the complexity of controlling pediatric TB and the imperative for subtle, context-appropriate strategies (Leining, 2019). Bringing these key findings together shows that control of pediatric tuberculosis requires comprehensive efforts targeting both biological and social determinants. Early and proper diagnosis is hindered by poor access to healthcare, especially in rural or remote communities, necessitating creative outreach and screening programs. Furthermore, identifying pediatric vulnerability to both drug-sensitive and DR-TB strains calls for regular drug resistance monitoring in this population to inform effective treatment regimens. Effective management of pediatric TB also includes identifying demographic risk factors and treatment histories to target high-risk populations. Such a multidimensional perspective is crucial for developing public health policy and resource allocation to decrease the burden of pediatric TB and eventually implement the larger End TB strategy objectives by 2035 (Nair et al., 2016; Leining, 2019).

CLOSER LOOK

IMPACT OF HIV ON THE PROGRESSION OF TB IN CHILDREN

The concurrent presence of HIV and tuberculosis (TB) in children drastically changes the course and clinical outcomes of TB. HIV, a virus that invades and destroys the immune system, specifically CD4$^+$ T cells, profoundly impacts the capacity of the immune system to contain Mycobacterium tuberculosis (M. tuberculosis), the causative pathogen of TB. In children, this co-infection tends to cause more serious manifestations of TB, higher risk of dissemination, and poorer treatment outcomes than in HIV-negative children.

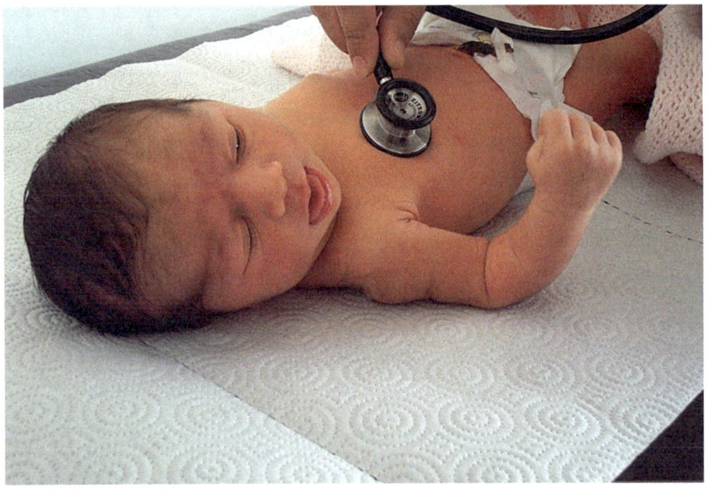

Source: By Nevit Dilmen - Own work, CC BY-SA 3.0, https://commons.wikimedia.org/w/index.php?curid=1428959

Children infected with HIV are also more likely to become infected with TB because of their weakened immune system. The MTB germs can more readily spread within children who have HIV because the immune mechanisms that would usually keep the infection contained, like activating CD4$^+$ T cells and the development of granulomas, are impaired. Therefore, HIV-infected children are more likely to develop active TB from latent TB, which can affect the lungs, LNs, or other extrapulmonary regions such as the brain or kidneys. The lack of effective immune containment allows for more rapid dissemination of infection.

One of the notable impacts of HIV on TB disease in children is a higher risk of disseminated TB, where bacteria spread throughout the body. This type of TB is more prevalent and more dangerous in children infected with HIV, resulting in complications like TB meningitis or miliary TB. Also, the diagnosis of TB among children with HIV tends to be delayed, as the symptoms are less specific or masked by other opportunistic infections that are typical among HIV-infected children.

Another effect is the disrupted response to TB therapy. HIV-infected children are at higher risk of treatment failure, relapse, or drug resistance because of their compromised immunity and the risk of drug interactions between anti-TB agents and ART. This can make it difficult to treat both diseases since both take long, often complex regimens. ART has been found to enhance immune status, but initiation of ART prematurely in children with active TB results in a condition known as immune reconstitution inflammatory syndrome (IRIS), where the reviving immune system generates an enhanced inflammatory response against the TB infection, which exacerbates symptoms.

The overall prognosis for children with both HIV and TB is poorer than for those with TB alone, and they have a higher mortality rate. Timely diagnosis, early initiation of ART, and appropriate TB treatment are essential to improve the outcomes for these children. Efforts to control TB in high-HIV burden settings require integrated care strategies to manage both infections concurrently, emphasizing the need for routine screening for TB in HIV-positive children and vice versa.

REFERENCES

1. Abu-Sharar, A. J., Zayadeen, N. F., & Almanasrah, A. S. (2024). Understanding pediatric hemoglobinopathies: Epidemiology, genetics, and management strategies. *Scholars Academic Journal of Pharmacy; ISSN 2347-9531 (Print) | ISSN 2320-4206 (Online)*(accessed on 10 May 2025).
2. Aghahosseini, F., Bakhshayeshkaram, M., Hassanzad, M., Jamaati, H., et al. (2018). CT-measured pulmonary artery diameter as an independent predictor of pulmonary hypertension in cystic fibrosis. https://core.ac.uk/download/161841179.pdf (accessed on 10 May 2025).
3. Ahmed, A. (2018). Treatment of central nervous system tuberculosis. *Journal of Pediatric Infectious Diseases, 13*, 141–152. https://www.semanticscholar.org/paper/0b85635299765e45f65e73d5d719ff64dc2da8f8 (accessed on 10 May 2025).
4. Caraffa, E., Russo, G., Vita, S., Lichtner, M., Massetti, A. P., Mastroianni, C. M., Vullo, V., Ciardi, M. R., & Ajassa, C. (2018). Intracranial tuberculous mass lesions treated with thalidomide in an immunocompetent child from a low tuberculosis endemic country: A case report. *Medicine, 97*(29), e11186. https://doi.org/10.1097/MD.0000000000011186 (accessed on 10 May 2025).
5. Anania, C., Olivero, F., Spagnolo, A., Chiesa, C., & Pacifico, L. (2017). Immune response to vaccines in children with celiac disease. *World journal of gastroenterology, 23*(18), 3205–3213. https://doi.org/10.3748/wjg.v23.i18.3205 (accessed on 10 May 2025).
6. Reither, K., Katsoulis, L., Beattie, T., Gardiner, N., Lenz, N., Said, K., Mfinanga, E., Pohl, C., Fielding, K. L., Jeffery, H., Kagina, B. M., Hughes, E. J., Scriba, T. J., Hanekom, W. A., Hoff, S. T., Bang, P., Kromann, I., Daubenberger, C., Andersen, P., & Churchyard, G. J. (2014). Safety and immunogenicity of H1/IC31®, an adjuvanted TB subunit vaccine, in HIV-infected adults with CD4+ lymphocyte counts greater than 350 cells/mm3: a phase II, multi-centre, double-blind, randomized, placebo-controlled trial. *PloS one, 9*(12), e114602. https://doi.org/10.1371/journal.pone.0114602 (accessed on 10 May 2025).
7. Nair SA, Raizada N, Sachdeva KS, Denkinger C, Schumacher S, Dewan P, et al. (2016) Factors Associated with Tuberculosis and Rifampicin-Resistant Tuberculosis amongst Symptomatic Patients in India: A Retrospective Analysis. PLoS ONE 11(2): e0150054. https://doi.org/10.1371/journal.pone.0150054 (accessed on 10 May 2025).
8. Vecchio, A. L., Bocchino, M., Lancella, L., Gabiano, C., Garazzino, S., Scotto, R., Raffaldi, I., Assante, L. R., Villani, A., Esposito, S., & Guarino, A. (2015). Indications to Hospital Admission and Isolation of Children With Possible or Defined Tuberculosis: Systematic Review and Proposed Recommendations for Pediatric Patients Living in Developed Countries. [Corrected]. *Medicine, 94*(50), e2045. https://doi.org/10.1097/MD.0000000000002045 (accessed on 10 May 2025).
9. Vale Rodrigues, R., Sladek, M., Katsanos, K., van der Woude, C. J., Wei, J., Vavricka, S. R., Teich, N., Ellul, P., Savarino, E., Chaparro, M., Beaton, D., Oliveira, A. M., Fragaki, M., Shitrit, A. B., Ramos, L., Karmiris, K., & ECCO CONFER investigators (2020). Diagnosis and Outcome of Oesophageal Crohn's Disease. *Journal of Crohn's & colitis, 14*(5), 624–629. https://doi.org/10.1093/ecco-jcc/jjz201 (accessed on 10 May 2025).

10. Janssen, N., Ndirangu, J., Newell, M. L., & Bland, R. M. (2010). Successful paediatric HIV treatment in rural primary care in Africa. *Archives of disease in childhood, 95*(6), 414–421. https://doi.org/10.1136/adc.2009.169367 (accessed on 10 May 2025).

11. Verso, M. G., Serra, N., Ciccarello, A., Romanin, B., & Di Carlo, P. (2019). Latent Tuberculosis Infection among Healthcare Students and Postgraduates in a Mediterranean Italian Area: What Correlation with Work Exposure?. *International journal of environmental research and public health, 17*(1), 137. https://doi.org/10.3390/ijerph17010137 (accessed on 10 May 2025).

12. Clay, Karen B. and Troesken, Werner, Deprivation and Disease in Early Twentieth-Century America (March 2006). NBER Working Paper No. w12111, Available at SSRN: https://ssrn.com/abstract=893766 (accessed on 10 May 2025).

13. Concha-Mora, L. A., Guzman-Guajardo, A., Treviño-Valdez, P. D., Mares-Gil, J., & Tamez-Rivera, O. (2025). P-1433. Characterization and georeferencing of tuberculosis cases in pediatric patients at a reference hospital in México in 13 years. *Open Forum Infectious Diseases, 12*. https://www.semanticscholar.org/paper/af4adb92e45d367dbeec4282b2f017cd7cea6176 (accessed on 10 May 2025).

14. de Koning, L., Seiden-Long, I., Anker, K., Myers, K., & Stang, A. (2024). Whole Blood Cardiac Troponin "Triaging" to Improve Early Detection of Myocardial Injury at a Pediatric Hospital. *The journal of applied laboratory medicine, 9*(3), 540–548. https://doi.org/10.1093/jalm/jfad133(accessed on 10 May 2025).

15. Demir, S. Ö., Bozbeyoğlu, S. G., & Çeliker, K. (2025). The role of clinical and laboratory findings in the diagnosis of tuberculosis in pediatric patients: A 4-year single-center evaluation. *Marmara Medical Journal*. https://doi.org/10.5472/pp.2025.0154.

16. Öcal Demir S, Bozbeyoğlu SG, Çeliker K. The role of clinical and laboratory findings in the diagnosis of tuberculosis in pediatric patients: A 4-year single-center evaluation. Marmara Med J. January 2025;38(1):55-61. doi:10.5472/marumj.1627948 (accessed on 10 May 2025).

17. Diuzheva, O., Skoklyuk, L., Zherebko, N., Barbova, A., Germanovych, M., Klinkenberg, E., Bogdanov, O., et al. (2024). Paving the way to innovative, child-friendly pediatric diagnostic methods for tuberculosis: Introduction of stool-based testing in Ukraine. *Tropical Medicine and Infectious Disease, 9*. https://www.semanticscholar.org/paper/0bef74aeca641f48c69d95091680847a96428725 (accessed on 10 May 2025).

18. Farrugia, B. (2013). Tuberculosis in Malta: A case for sputum induction. https://core.ac.uk/download/46602348.pdf (accessed on 10 May 2025).

19. McCabe, C. J., Goldie, S. J., & Fisman, D. N. (2010). The cost-effectiveness of directly observed highly-active antiretroviral therapy in the third trimester in HIV-infected pregnant women. *PloS one, 5*(4), e10154. https://doi.org/10.1371/journal.pone.0010154

20. Garcia-Prats, A., Starke, J., Waning, B., Kaiser, B., & Seddon, J. (2022). New drugs and regimens for tuberculosis disease treatment in children and adolescents. *Journal of the Pediatric Infectious Diseases Society, 11*(Supplement_3), S101–S109. https://www.semanticscholar.org/paper/4cc8f34cd415f9bd9808e4d3ebca99711bcc57c4 (accessed on 10 May 2025).

21. Gudeta, A. N. (2023). *Aspects of immunogenetics, infections, and nutrition on the risk of celiac disease autoimmunity in an Ethiopian pediatric birth cohort*. [Doctoral Thesis (compilation), Department of Clinical Sciences, Malmö]. Lund University, Faculty of Medicine.(accessed on 10 May 2025).

22. Gupta, S., & Sharma, R. (2024). Pediatric obstructive sleep apnea: Diagnostic challenges and management strategies. *Cureus, 16*(5). https://doi.org/10.7759/cureus.23389.
23. Gupta, S., Khanna, H., Gupta, V., Barman, N. K., Parihar, A., & Kant, S. (2025). Chest X-ray features of drug-resistant tuberculosis in the pediatric population: A prospective study in a high-endemic area. *Pediatric Pulmonology, 60*(3), e71039. https://doi.org/10.1002/ppul.24567.
24. Ivanova, D. A., Litvinova, N. V., Yurovskaya, E. I., Kubrakova, E. P., & Mitrofanova, Y. Y. (2025). Therapeutic drug monitoring in the treatment of tuberculosis patients. *Tuberculosis and Socially Significant Diseases*. https://www.semanticscholar.org/paper/9524b526c05f2fe50b2d30a9cefd35e2bfab932e (accessed on 10 May 2025).
25. Leining, Lauren M., "Geospatial Analysis Of Pediatric Tuberculosis In Bohol, Philippines: Disease Clusters And Access To Care" (2019). *Dissertations & Theses (Open Access)*. 67. https://digitalcommons.library.tmc.edu/uthsph_dissertsopen/67 (accessed on 10 May 2025).
26. Liyew, A. M., Clements, A., Akalu, T., Gilmour, B., & Alene, K. A. (2024). Ecological-level factors associated with tuberculosis incidence and mortality: A systematic review and meta-analysis. *PLOS Global Public Health, 4*. https://www.semanticscholar.org/paper/0268cb04d15668ad2e72f6b072605a0b34328808 (accessed on 10 May 2025).
27. https://www.semanticscholar.org/paper/7fc99f9b409b05eaa8d710ea19fcef57a2d488ce FC, Loembe, Mekame AE, Mintsa, EL, Midili TL, Minto'O, RS, and Nzame, Y. 2025. "Epidemiological, Etiological, Clinical, and Therapeutic Aspects of Pleural Effusion in Children at the Pediatric Department of Libreville University Hospital". *Asian Journal of Pediatric Research* 15 (2):13-18. https://doi.org/10.9734/ajpr/2025/v15i2423. (accessed on 10 May 2025).
28. Luo, Y., Yang, X., Zhou, J., Pu, S., & Wang, Y. (2024). Case report: Reiterating the importance of tissue biopsy in the diagnosis of tuberculosis: Lessons from a case of pediatric pulmonary tuberculosis complicated by Hodgkin's lymphoma. *Frontiers in Pediatrics, 12*. https://doi.org/10.3389/fped.2024.950716.
29. Moore, B. K., Graham, S. M., Nandakumar, S., Doyle, J., & Maloney, S. A. (2024). Pediatric tuberculosis: A review of evidence-based best practices for clinicians and health care providers. *Pathogens, 13*. https://www.semanticscholar.org/paper/51c93f0e21331cebcc90ecaaa4103e40dc4cfa2c (accessed on 10 May 2025).
30. Mutima, N. (2004). Funding for health in Africa: Mapping the U.S. foundation landscape, 2000–2002. https://core.ac.uk/download/75779536.pdf (accessed on 10 May 2025).
31. Nijman, L. W., Cristescu, S. M., & Jansen, R. S. (2025). Broadening the diagnostic landscape of *Mycobacterium tuberculosis* infection: Analyzing exhaled breath. *Journal of Breath Research*. https://www.semanticscholar.org/paper/849e40cb74f482f00fddfb1cee535ce43b3a8e4f (accessed on 10 May 2025).
32. Nurfeta, R., Ababiya, T., Woldeamanuele, N., Ababiya, R., Deregasso, B., Tema, L., Hailu, S., et al. (2024). Tuberculosis treatment outcomes and associated factors at Zewditu Memorial Hospital, Ethiopia. *International Journal of Infectious Diseases and Therapy*. https://doi.org/10.1016/j.ijidt.2024.05.008.
33. Nackers, F., Huerga, H., Espié, E., Aloo, A. O., Bastard, M., Etard, J. F., Sitienei, J., Varaine, F., Chakaya, J., & Bonnet, M. (2012). Adherence to self-administered tuberculosis treatment in a high HIV-prevalence setting: a cross-sectional survey in Homa Bay, Kenya. *PloS one, 7*(3), e32140. https://doi.org/10.1371/journal.pone.0032140 (accessed on 10 May 2025).

34. Ramanthan, R., & Jayapritha, M. (2025). Clinico-epidemiological profile and diagnostic procedures in suspected pediatric tuberculosis in a tertiary care centre in Tamil Nadu. *International Journal of Contemporary Pediatrics*. https://doi.org/10.1007/s13224-025-01614-7.

35. Ricci, V., & Maina, G. (2025). Clinical and public health challenge of handling synthetic cathinone and cannabinoid abuse in pediatric care: A narrative review. *Pediatric Reports, 17*(2). https://doi.org/10.3390/pediatrreps17030054.

36. Salova A.L., Chelnokova O.G., Mozzhukhina L.I. Latent tuberculosis infection in the pediatric population without contact: a prospective controlled study. *Patient-Oriented Medicine and Pharmacy*. 2025;3(1):59-63. (In Russ.) https://doi.org/10.37489/2949-1924-0082. EDN: JRIQBA(accessed on 10 May 2025).

37. Seddon, J. A., & Shingadia, D. (2014). Epidemiology and disease burden of tuberculosis in children: A global perspective. *The Lancet Infectious Diseases*. https://doi.org/10.1016/S1473-3099(14)70103-4.

38. Shah, P., Pol, S., Prabhakaran, E., Karmalkar, B., Gaikwad, V., Dharamshale, S., & Karyakarte, R. (2024). Utility of GeneXpert in diagnosis of pediatric tuberculosis and detection of rifampicin resistance. *Perspectives in Medical Research*. https://www.semanticscholar.org/paper/ba7503561e3541d6d62fef4295b5d03180bbe1ed (accessed on 10 May 2025).

39. Srinidhi, R., Sowmiya, G., Elanthamizh, P., Tamilselvan, J., & Nanthini, R. (2025). Diagnosis of tuberculosis: Part 1–Demonstration of causative organism. *Pediatric Surgery in Tropics*. https://doi.org/10.9735/jpst.2025.1446.

40. Todorov, S., Petrov, P., Kirovakov, Z., & Penchev, P. (2024). Epidemiological study of traumatic brain and spinal injuries in a pediatric population: A one-year analysis of prevalence, causes, and trends. *Cures, 16*(3), e57224. https://doi.org/10.7759/cureus.57224.

41. Utami, W. S., Amrina, A. P. Y., Armiyanti, Y., & Maududie, A. (2024). Spatial analysis of tuberculosis cases among stunted toddlers in Rambipuji District, Jember Regency. *Jurnal Kedokteran dan Kesehatan Indonesia*. https://doi.org/10.20473/jkki.v33i4.467-475.

42. Viswanathan V. Analysis of Sociodemographic Risk Factors in Pediatric Drug-Resistant Tuberculosis: A Single-Center Study. SVOA Paediatrics 2025, 4:1, 05-12. doi: 10.58624SVOA PD.2025.04.002(accessed on 10 May 2025).

43. Wang, D. M., Wang, C., An, Q., Yang, Q., & Liao, Y. (2024). Clinical characteristic, common sites, and geographical distribution of pediatric tuberculosis patients in Southwest China. *Frontiers in pediatrics, 12*, 1327648. https://doi.org/10.3389/fped.2024.1327648 (accessed on 10 May 2025).

44. Willis, M., Van de Wetering, J., Brown, H., Barnowska, E. J., Stuetzle, S. C. W., Nadiruzzaman, M., & Fastenau, A. (2025). Barriers and facilitators to pediatric tuberculosis management in India: A systematic review. *BMC Infectious Diseases, 25*. https://www.semanticscholar.org/paper/623735af20299046ab26040f3790ffbe731c8a7d (accessed on 10 May 2025).

45. Yildirim, I. (2017). Impact of vaccines on diagnosis and outcomes of infectious diseases: All-cause pneumonia in PCV13-era, impact of BCG vaccination on tuberculin skin test, and cost-effectiveness of screening for latent tuberculosis infection. *Boston University School of Public Health*. https://hdl.handle.net/2144/27137; (accessed on 10 May 2025).

46. Yu, S., Jeong, D., Kang, H. Y., Kang, Y. A., Lee, G. I., & Choi, H. (2024). A quasi-experimental study on the effect of pre-entry tuberculosis screening for immigrants on treatment outcomes in South Korea: A difference-in-differences analysis. *Journal of Epidemiology and Global Health, 14*(2), 154–161. https://doi.org/10.1016/j.jegh.2024.04.015.
47. Yu, Y., Hua, J., & Chen, L. (2024). Autophagy-related molecular clusters identified as indicators for distinguishing active and latent TB infection in pediatric patients. *BMC Pediatrics, 24*, 73. https://doi.org/10.1186/s12887-024-03235-7.
48. Zhong, Y. y., Xie, H., Cai, F., Liu, M., Gan, H., Tang, Z., & Bai, Y. (2025). Global burden of multidrug-resistant tuberculosis in children and adolescents. *Pediatric Research*. https://doi.org/10.1038/s41390-025-01899-w.

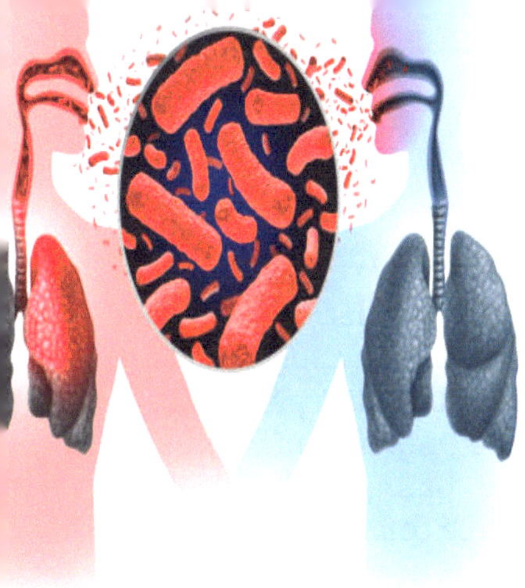

Chapter 10

TUBERCULOSIS IN SPECIAL POPULATIONS

Contents

Introduction

Tuberculosis (TB) continues to be among the most significant infectious diseases globally, imposing a disproportionate disease burden on special and vulnerable populations. Caused primarily by *Mycobacterium tuberculosis* (MTB), the disease continues to exist despite the existence of vaccines and antimicrobial drugs, in part due to complexities of drug resistance and host immunity. The development of antimicrobial resistance (AMR) has mounted challenges, making disease control more difficult and raising mortality rates, particularly in resource-constrained healthcare settings. Estimating the global burden of AMR on tuberculosis and its interaction with different population groups highlights the need for focused interventions and specific healthcare strategies. Identification of these dynamics is critical in policy formulation that addresses not only clinical treatment but also socio-economic and biological considerations of disease spread and outcome in special populations (Dartois & Rubin, 2022). Vaccination programs have long remained a foundation for preventing tuberculosis, but populations' heterogeneity in vaccine efficacy complicates control efforts. The *Mycobacterium bovis*-derived *Bacillus Calmette-Guérin* (BCG) vaccine is the sole licensed tuberculosis vaccine and is extensively used across the globe, especially in newborns. Although it has been used for many years and has been shown to confer protection against life-threatening, disseminated tuberculosis in children, its protective efficacy against adult pulmonary tuberculosis (PTB) varies extensively. New developments in the study of BCG's mechanisms uncover noteworthy nonspecific immune advantages in addition to tuberculosis-specific prevention, including possible protection against other infectious diseases as well as some cancers caused by infection. These attributes are of particular relevance in special populations, who might develop longer-term vaccine responses differently in view of pre-existing medical conditions or immune system status (Locht et al., 2020). In the study of tuberculosis in special populations, it is important to appreciate the intersectionality of biological, social, and healthcare determinants that especially affect disease susceptibility and course. Patients with weakened immune systems, such as those with HIV/AIDS, undernourished children, and chronic disease patients, show heightened infection and poor outcome susceptibility. Socioeconomic determinants like poverty, crowding, and lack of access to quality healthcare also increase risks among marginalized groups. Moreover, the challenges presented by AMR also require new treatment strategies and increased vigilance. By combining epidemiological information with knowledge of vaccine effectiveness and resistance patterns, the medical community will be able to better respond to tuberculosis's effects on these groups, ultimately decreasing morbidity and mortality and promoting equitable healthcare delivery (Locht et al., 2020; Dartois & Rubin, 2022).

Importance of Studying Tuberculosis (TB) in Special Populations

Knowledge about the subtleties of TB in special populations is essential for enhancing not only the individual but also public health outcomes. Vulnerable populations like the immunocompromised, jail populations and residents of low-resource communities typically experience multiplicatively increased risks as a consequence of restricted access to care and greater rates of comorbidities. These groups are disproportionately impacted by DR-TB, a burgeoning issue that destabilizes the efficacy of standard treatments and drives higher mortality. An in-depth examination of TB among these groups identifies resistance and disease progression patterns that vary substantially from the broader population, guiding interventions designed specifically for the group. Additionally, the burden of AMR worldwide establishes the necessity to pay special attention to populations in which strains of TB are found to be more resistant since they are reservoirs for transmission and development of more virulent strains (Dartois & Rubin, 2022). Therefore, giving precedence to research in special populations is imperative in controlling TB worldwide. Healthcare systems in low- and middle-income nations (LMICs) carry the burden of TB's consequences most significantly among their most susceptible residents. While there have been some improvements in health, inequalities in care quality and access continue to exist for marginalized group patients with TB. The problems reach far beyond the availability of care to involve gaps in timely diagnosis, effective care provision, and dignified patient treatment. These structural quality problems fall heavily on special groups, leading to delayed or insufficient TB treatment and worse overall health status (Margaret et al., 2018). TB management in such settings requires an integrated strategy that improves both clinical outcomes and patient satisfaction while promoting equitable delivery of health services. By specific research and policy interventions targeting such vulnerable populations, health systems are better positioned to contribute to the universal health coverage targets and enhance TB-associated morbidity and mortality rates more efficiently than with homogenized approaches themselves (Margaret et al., 2018). In addition, research on TB in special populations is invaluable in generating knowledge on sociocultural and economic determinants influencing disease dynamics as well as treatment compliance. Migrants, indigenous populations, and individuals living with stigmatized health conditions usually experience barriers to care, including mistrust of healthcare systems, discrimination, and lack of economic resources. These elements contribute to therapy discontinuity and enhanced risk of transmission in tight-knit communities. Knowledge of these special determinants makes it possible to create culturally and contextually tailored interventions that take into account both medical and social determinants of health. Such specific strategies are important to prevent the emergence of multi-drug resistant tuberculosis (MDR-TB) strains that disproportionately affect vulnerable populations, causing huge health and economic burden globally (Dartois & Rubin, 2022; Margaret et al., 2018). Thus, incorporating social context into TB research for special populations is crucial for securing sustainable disease control and ultimate eradication (Figure 10.1).

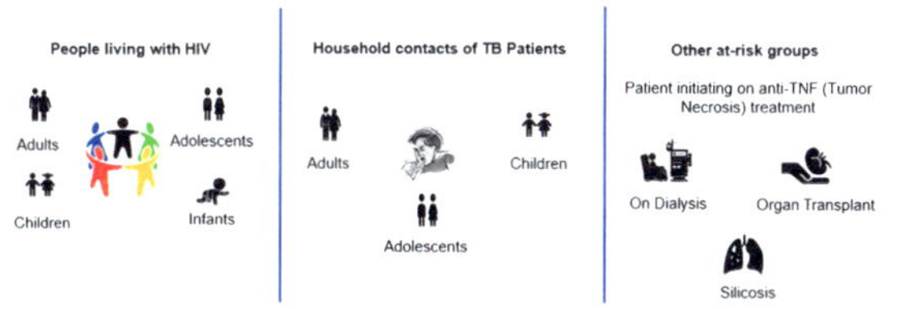

Figure 10.1. Key and vulnerable population for TB Infection.

Source: National Tuberculosis Elimination Program (NTEP). (n.d.). *High-risk groups for tuberculosis preventive treatment (TPT).* https://www.ntep.in/node/6674/tpt-tb-infection-and-epidemiology.

10.1. Tuberculosis (TB) in Children

Children are a particularly susceptible population in the global battle against TB because of their developing immune systems and difficulties in diagnosing the disease at an early phase. In contrast to adults, child TB frequently has nonspecific manifestations, making clinical suspicion problematic and laboratory verification challenging. The subtlety of clinical presentation adds to the difficulty in timely intervention, which is essential to avoid disease progression and long-term complications. In addition, the AMR burden amplifies the threat, especially in resource-constrained environments where diagnostic and treatment choices might be limited. The wider public health implications are substantial, as children tend to become infected with TB from close family contacts, highlighting the need for coordinated family-centered disease control strategies (Dartois & Rubin, 2022). Pediatric TB, thus, needs to be addressed through targeted strategies that consider both biological vulnerability and socio-environmental determinants. Treatment of TB in children is also compounded by other challenges arising from drug resistance and the effect of concomitant diseases, including malnutrition or HIV infection. The emergence of multi-drug resistant tuberculosis (MDR-TB) strains creates a significant impediment to effective treatment, considering the paucity of pediatric formulations of second-line anti-TB drugs and the increased risk of adverse drug reactions (ADRs) among younger patients. Additionally, the contamination of the environment and food chains with antibiotic residues is a factor causing AMR that makes treatment regimens complicated in adults as well as in pediatric patients (Christy et al., 2018). Such dynamics call for strict antibiotic stewardship and the creation of child-friendly diagnostic equipment and medicine. Improving TB control among children also requires enhanced healthcare infrastructure and increased surveillance, essential to obtaining accurate epidemiologic information and informing evidence-based interventions among this special population. Prevention is key to decreasing the prevalence of pediatric tuberculosis, especially through vaccination and early detection of latent infection among high-risk groups. *Bacillus Calmette-Guérin* (BCG) vaccination is still a mainstay of prevention but is geographically variable in its efficacy and only modest in preventing pulmonary TB, the most transmissible form. Thus, an international health priority is the development of more effective vaccines and prophylaxis regimens that are appropriate for children.

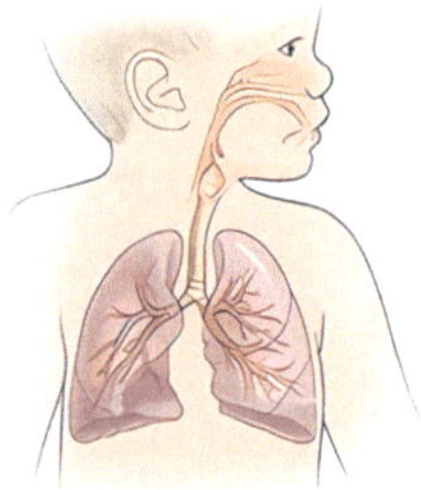

Figure 10.2. Tuberculosis (TB) in children.

Source: BREATH Clinic. (2022). *Illustration showing the respiratory tract and lungs in a child.* https://external-content.duckduckgo.com/iu/?u=https%3A%2F%2Fwww.breathclinic.in%2Fwp-content%2Fuploads%2F2022%2F07%2Fsymptoms-of-TB-in-a-child-1024x585.png&f=1&nofb=1&ipt=c4372928a54bddccaa3ee204ea0ab270ae0929536b28dc24e9648325ecab972b.

Also important are programs of household screening and contact tracing to catch disease transmission in infancy, particularly where children are exposed to adults who have active TB. Integrating these measures into more effective health policies, underpinned by solid data on the disease burden and AMR trends, is essential. This focused action will reduce TB morbidity and mortality among children, allowing for special population needs to be addressed with accuracy and vigilance (Dartois & Rubin, 2022; Christy et al., 2018) (Figure 10.2).

10.1.1. Symptoms and Diagnosis in Pediatric Populations

Pediatric populations pose a special clinical problem in diagnosing tuberculosis because the frequently non-specific and subtle presentation is unlike that of adults. TB can present in children with such manifestations as prolonged fever, weight loss, and chronic cough, but these can overlap with diseases common in pediatrics so as to hinder timely diagnosis. Additionally, young children are unlikely to cough up sputum, the preferred specimen for microbiological confirmation, and thus conventional diagnostic strategies are less efficacious.

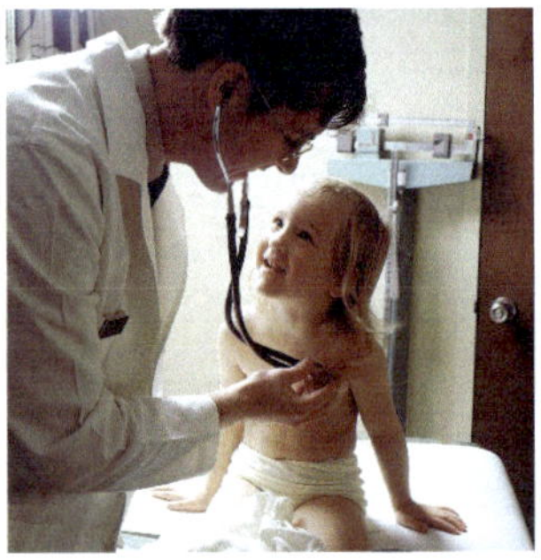

Figure 10.3. The symptoms of tuberculosis in children.

Source: By Unknown author - http://www.defenseimagery.mil; VIRIN: DA-ST-85-12888, Public Domain, https://commons.wikimedia.org/w/index.php?curid=9783736

This limitation emphasizes the role of clinical suspicion in conjunction with an extensive history of exposure and radiologic evaluation in the pediatric population. Children's variable immune response also makes symptom presentation and disease course even more challenging, highlighting the necessity for differential diagnostic criteria that take these physiological variations into account to enhance early detection and intervention results (Bruyn et al., 2016) (Figure 10.3). The pediatric diagnosis of tuberculosis is also hampered by the unavailability of quick, accurate point-of-care tests, an issue that is still of significant concern in resource-poor settings where the majority of cases of pediatric TB take place. The available diagnostic tools, such as tuberculin skin tests (TSTs) and interferon-gamma release assays (IGRAs), are flawed with respect to sensitivity, specificity, and interpretation in children. Furthermore, culture-based testing, although a gold standard, necessitates extended incubation times and is prone to false negatives in the form of paucibacillary disease in pediatrics. Improved detection through advances in molecular tests has occurred, but most of these methods remain laboratory-based, costly, and less accessible. Successful diagnosis therefore not only relies on technological advancement but on higher funding and infrastructural support aimed at pediatric TB diagnosis (McNerney et al., 2012). Emerging research on biomarkers has the potential to improve tuberculosis diagnosis in children through greater accuracy and velocity. With the complex host-pathogen interactions and heterogenous immune patterns in children, identifying host or pathogen-derived biomarkers may offer non-invasive, quick, and more sensitive diagnostic options compared to existing tests. Identification of such biomarkers should be properly validated against end-point clinical events like treatment failure or relapse. In addition, these biomarker-based strategies could require special pediatric and other special population adjustment to accommodate distinctive disease patterns. Prioritization of this research is crucial not only for enhancing diagnosis but also for monitoring response to treatment, which is a major challenge in children because of the heterogeneity of immune responses and subclinical infections (Bruyn et al., 2016) (Figure 10.4).

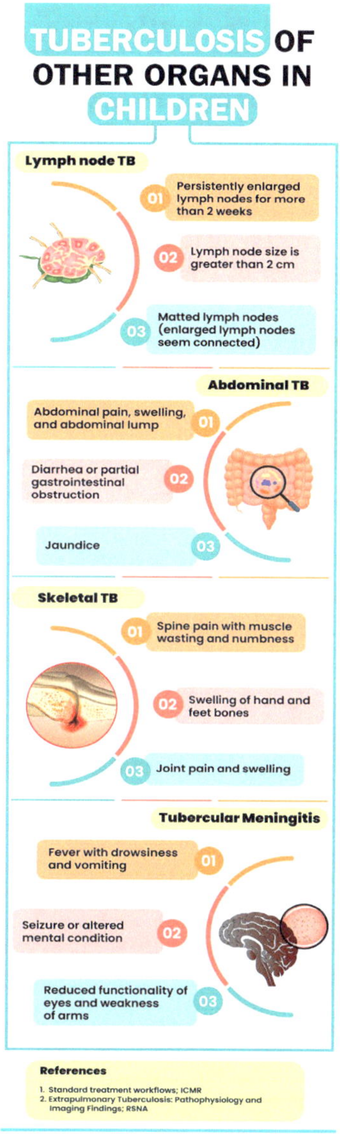

Figure 10.4. Tuberculosis of other organs in children.

Source: MomJunction. (n.d.). *Tuberculosis of other organs in children.* https://external-content.duckduckgo.com/iu/?u=https%3A%2F%2Fcdn2.momjunction.com%2Fwp-content%2Fuploads%2F2022%2F02%2FInfographic-Manifestations-Of-Tuberculosis-In-Organs-Other-Than-The-Lungs.jpg&f=1&nofb=1&ipt=90f1a98eb171b61f5dadfbb36bde0530b871511b41f51e9d417191a19287f837.

10.1.2. Treatment Challenges and Considerations

TB treatment in special populations is made difficult by a number of interrelated factors affecting the treatment response and safety of patients. TB has a greater risk of progression in immunocompromised patients, especially HIV-coinfected individuals, and presenting with atypical manifestations that complicate early diagnosis. Antiretroviral and anti-TB regimens frequently have pharmacokinetic interactions necessitating careful adjustment to avoid suboptimal drug concentrations or toxicity. Additionally, similar side effects such as hepatotoxicity and neuropathy bring challenges in sustaining compliance and treatment discontinuation. These complexities are further compounded in vulnerable populations such as children and pregnant women, where changes in physiology influence drug metabolism and dosing guidelines are less established. Therefore, individualized treatment strategy is crucial, including not only clinical care but also social support systems to deal with adherence barriers, access barriers, and comorbidities (Patel et al., 2024). Development of multi-drug resistant (MDR) and extensively drug-resistant (XDR) tuberculosis strains adds the complexity in populations where pharmacodynamics is changed or there is a higher susceptibility to drug toxicity. More recent agents, including bedaquiline, have transformed MDR-TB treatment but for whom evidence regarding its safety and efficacy in special populations is still meager. Adolescents, pregnant women, and the elderly are populations for which trial data are lacking, leaving these populations with gaps in guidelines and clinical confidence. These groups may need careful monitoring for side effects and dose adjustment because of changed drug absorption or organ function. Therefore, treatment has to weigh the risks of progression to drug resistance against likely toxicities, with continuous research necessary to maximize regimens addressed to these vulnerable groups (Zhang et al., 2023) (Figure 10.5).

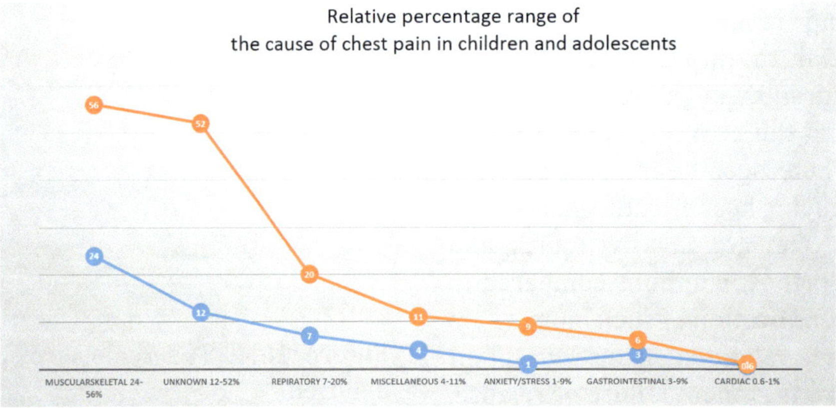

Figure 10.5. Treatment for TB in children.

Source: By Barbara (WVS) - Own work, CC BY-SA 4.0, https://commons.wikimedia.org/w/index.php?curid=45805198

Apart from pharmacological aspects, socioeconomic and health system determinants also have an important impact on treatment outcomes in special groups suffering from TB. Lack of access to healthcare, stigma, and comorbidities like malnutrition and drug addiction may interfere with continuity of care and compliance with long duration regimens. This is most striking among older patients who tend to have several chronic conditions and among pregnant patients where fear of fetal harm may slow the start or completion of treatment. Conjoined models of care that align TB therapy with HIV, maternal-child, and geriatric care allow for more comprehensive treatment and better outcomes. In addition, education of the patient and community are critical to counter misinformation and empower those affected. To meet these multi-faceted challenges, a multidisciplinary strategy uniting biomedical, social, and public health interventions is needed to mitigate morbidity and mortality in special populations (Zhang et al., 2023; Patel et al., 2024) (Figure 10.6).

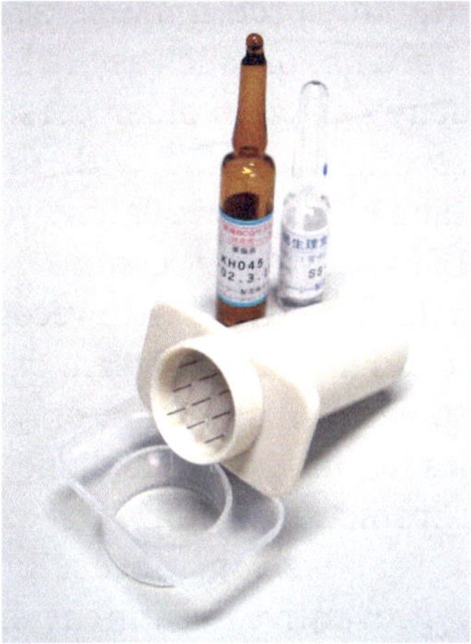

Figure 10.6. The main way to prevent TB in children is to take the BCG (*Bacillus Calmette-Guérin*) vaccine.

Source: By Y tambe - Y tambe's file, CC BY-SA 3.0, https://commons.wikimedia.org/w/index.php?curid=1066227

10.1.3. Long-Term Effects of Tuberculosis (TB) in Children

The course of TB in children commonly goes beyond acute infection, giving rise to a range of long-term health problems that must be closely evaluated. Pediatric TB may disrupt normal lung growth, producing chronic pulmonary complications including bronchiectasis and restrictive lung disease. The sequelae can produce ongoing respiratory symptoms, decreased exercise tolerance, and long-term functional impairment that affects the quality of a child's life. Moreover, TB in extrapulmonary sites, such as the CNS, will result in neurological impairment with permanent cognitive and motor dysfunction. These consequences tend to complicate the child's developmental milestones and school education, which is why there is a need for regular follow-ups and individualized rehabilitation programs. The residual physiological and psychosocial impacts highlight TB as not just an infectious illness but also a condition with immense implications on child health pathways (Devos et al., 2017). In addition, long-term care of child TB involves countering complications from the interaction between the infection and treatment protocols. Antituberculosis drugs, although lifesaving, are toxic and can have adverse effects like ototoxicity, hepatotoxicity, and delayed growth rates, and may worsen long-term morbidity in vulnerable children. The additional challenge of DR-TB strains complicates the treatment, with prolonged and more toxic regimens being the rule. Therapeutic drug monitoring (TDM) advances, such as new sampling methods such as dried blood spots, potentially improve treatment accuracy and lower toxicity levels, yet remain underutilized in children (Hofman et al., 2015). These pharmacological complexities require multidisciplinary interventions to prevent long-term effects of disease and therapy on developing children. Apart from physical wellbeing, the psychosocial impacts of TB in children can appear as delayed stigma, social exclusion, and emotional distress impacting long-term mental health. Children with TB often face interruptions in education as a result of prolonged treatment duration and hospital stays, delaying cognitive and social development. The chronic nature and stigma of TB may contribute to perceptions of marginalization and fear, added to the hardship placed on families with complex care requirements. These psychosocial sequelae justify inclusion of psychological care in TB treatment programs. Identifying the complex and long-term implications of pediatric TB underscores the need for integrated care models that assess and treat both the biological and social aspects of the disease among vulnerable populations (Devos et al., 2017).

10.2. Tuberculosis (TB) in the Elderly

The geriatric population poses special challenges in the diagnosis and treatment of TB because of physiological changes associated with aging and the occurrence of comorbidities. Immune senescence weakens the capacity to develop an effective immune response, which usually results in atypical clinical presentations and delayed diagnosis. In contrast to younger patients, older individuals may present with less severe symptoms like fever or productive cough, making clinical suspicion more difficult to establish. The superimposition of TB symptoms on other prevalent geriatric conditions, such as COPD or pneumonia, also makes timely detection more difficult. In addition, diagnostic tests might be less sensitive in this population; for example, immunologic tests may give false-negative results because of immune suppression. All of these cumulatively put this subgroup at a greater risk for disease worsening and worse outcomes in elderly patients with TB, stressing the requirement for increased surveillance and specific diagnostic approaches in this at-risk population subgroup (Niederman, 2003; Patel et al., 2024). The management of tuberculosis in elderly populations is further confounded by polypharmacy and the likelihood of drug interaction complications. Most geriatric patients receive several medications for chronic illnesses like cardiovascular disease, diabetes, or renal disease and are thus at risk of dangerous interactions with usual anti-TB medications. Hepatotoxicity is especially concerning because aging-related reduction in liver function may potentiate drug toxicity due to drugs such as isoniazid and rifampin. Impaired monitoring and dose adjustment must be done carefully to balance efficacy against safety. Moreover, compliance with complex regimens may be difficult because of cognitive impairment, social isolation, or physical disability, requiring extensive support systems. These factors highlight the need to incorporate geriatric principles into TB treatment regimens to maximize therapeutic outcomes in older patients (Niederman, 2003; Patel et al., 2024). Preventive measures for tuberculosis among the elderly need to take into consideration the enhanced vulnerability and frequently impaired immune status of this population. Vaccination, such as the BCG vaccine, is less frequently given in older persons, and its effectiveness might decline with time. Hence, it is important to diagnose latent tuberculosis infection (LTBI) through screening in elderly persons, particularly those with recognized risk factors like residence in long-term care facilities or prior exposure. Also, commonly occurring comorbidities in this group like diabetes mellitus (DM) and chronic respiratory disease increase the risk of reactivation, necessitating close monitoring. Preventive treatment should also include education and control of co-morbidities to decrease vulnerability. Since public health perspectives, targeted TB control among the older people are integral parts in decreasing disease burden within special groups (Niederman, 2003; Patel et al., 2024) (Figure 10.7).

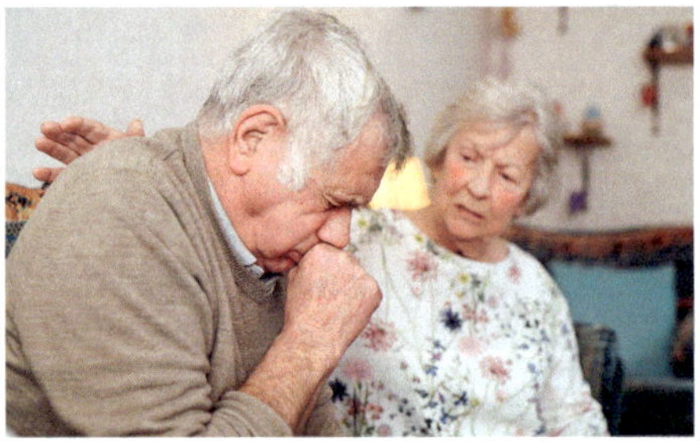

Figure 10.7. Tuberculosis in the elderly.

Source: Getty Images. (2019). *Senior coughing.* https://www.mcknights.com/wp-content/uploads/sites/5/2019/08/seniorCoughing_GettyImages-1132722167_2000x1125.jpg.

10.2.1. Increased Susceptibility and Risk Factors

Recognition of the complex relationship between genetic susceptibility and environmental determinants is necessary in dealing with the increased susceptibility of specific groups to TB. Various research studies have implicated certain genetic markers, including mutations in the vitamin D receptor (VDR) gene, as key determinants of susceptibility to pulmonary TB. For example, polymorphisms such as the FokI CC and ApaI TT genotypes have been associated with higher risk of disease, identifying a genetic factor that disrupts immunity to *Mycobacterium tuberculosis* (MTB). Coupled with these genetic determinants, sociodemographic factors such as reduced educational attainment and smoking behavior enhance this vulnerability, generating a multifactorial risk picture that defies traditional TB control efforts. Combining genetic information from screening results with behavioral evaluations could help enhance the detection of at-risk individuals in TB-endemic multiethnic groups and allow for more targeted and efficient preventive interventions (Ismail et al., 2025). Besides the structural effect of *VDR* gene polymorphisms, new structural findings indicate other structural loci that additionally control TB susceptibility. This supports the concept of a polygenic contribution to the risk of disease. One example of such involves polymorphisms within the *ASAP1* gene, where certain alleles such as rs4733781 and rs10956514 have been found to be linked with an increased susceptibility to TB among indigenous populations. Such genetic factors may influence immune system regulation and response to pathogens, although the precise biological mechanisms have yet to be fully understood. Identifying these gene risk factors underlines the need for using a precision medicine strategy for TB management, an individualized approach to screening and treatment based on the genetic profile of individuals to maximize outcomes, especially for those at-risk groups with unique genetic compositions (Ismail et al., 2025). In addition to genetic disparities, many lifestyle and environmental factors significantly contribute to an increased susceptibility to TB, particularly in special populations with socioeconomic disadvantages. Poor nutrition, crowded living conditions, and restricted access to health services severely undermine immune competence and predispose to bacterial spread, providing an ideal environment for TB epidemics. Coupled with hereditary vulnerabilities, these environmental hazards amplify disease burden and hinder treatment efficacy and compliance. Therefore, effective TB control involves an interdisciplinary approach that not only addresses hereditary predispositions but also targets modifiable social determinants.

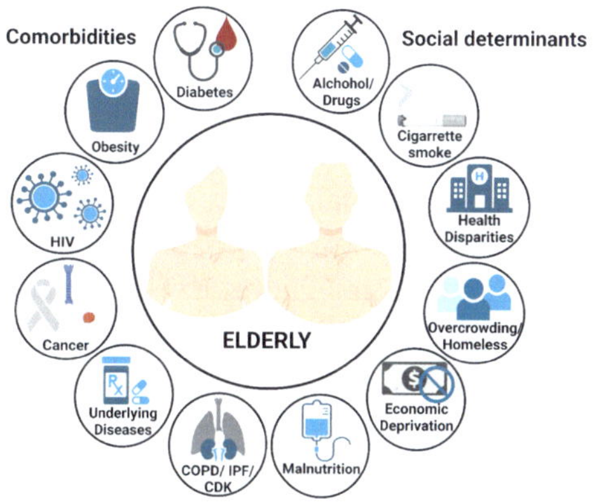

Figure 10.8. Risk factors of TB disease and mortality in the elderly. Aging by itself is a major risk factor for developing and succumbing to TB, partially due to the waning immunity that characterizes the elderly population. Additional risk factors, including comorbidities and socioeconomic determinants, are key drivers to increase even more the susceptibility of the elderly to respiratory infections.

Source: Olmo-Fontánez AM, Turner J. Tuberculosis in an Aging World. *Pathogens*. 2022; 11(10):1101. https://doi.org/10.3390/pathogens11101101

Spending on education, smoking cessation initiatives, and better living conditions remains key to TB incidence reduction and building resilience among vulnerable populations (Ismail et al., 2025) (Figure 10.8).

10.2.2. Comorbidities Affecting Tuberculosis (TB) Treatment

The success of TB treatment is highly dependent on a multitude of factors other than the bacterial infection itself. Sociodemographic and clinical patient characteristics are significant determinants of TB therapy outcomes, particularly when comorbidities are involved. In the COVID-19 pandemic, for example, there were disruptions in healthcare provision, with a significant decline in critical follow-up processes like control smear microscopy and chest X-rays. Patients who had other health issues like HIV infection, mental illness, and drug abuse had significantly worse access to essential treatment steps. Such comorbidities not only add to the complexity of disease pathology but also disrupt the continuity and quality of care and frequently require special treatment protocols and more medical consultations. Therefore, the occurrence of comorbidities can greatly interfere with usual TB treatment, emphasizing the importance of individualized follow-up and integrated care to ensure better adherence and success of the treatment (Antunes et al., 2024) (Figure 10.9).

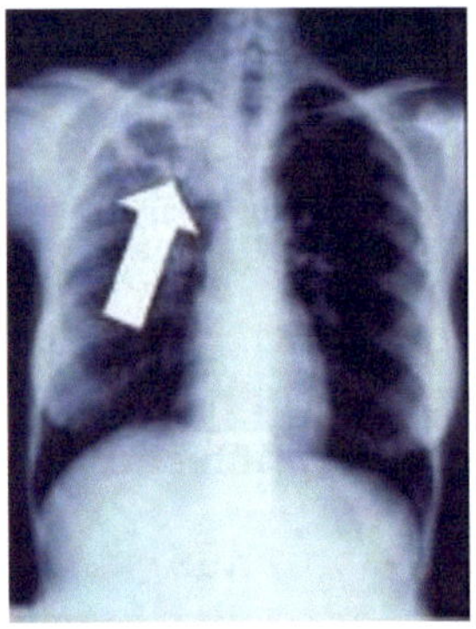

Figure 10.9. Chest X-rays are particularly useful in older patients.

Source: Public Domain, https://commons.wikimedia.org/w/index.php?curid=486608

The interaction between TB and concomitant health conditions goes well beyond communicable diseases and includes a wide range of disabling diseases that undermine immune function or make clinical management challenging. For instance, patients with chronic neurological, psychiatric, or cardiovascular disease can present enhanced susceptibility to TB owing to compromised physiological resilience and the complexity of managing polypharmacy. Also, special populations with severe comorbidities usually present with reduced treatment compliance and more risk of drug interactions with negative consequences, resulting in less desirable outcomes. These multifaceted challenges are reflective of similar challenges in other chronic inflammatory diseases where severe comorbidities strongly affect the effectiveness of treatment as well as patient quality of life. These complexities are addressed by holistic care plans that include both the infectious disease process of TB and the general context of the health status of the patient (Potestio et al., 2024). Proper control of TB among comorbid patients necessitates not just clinical observation but also systemic modifications in the delivery of healthcare. The lower rate of essential diagnostic and monitoring interventions observed for comorbid patients highlights the obstacles that preclude optimal TB treatment. Retreatment and special treatment regimen cases typically illustrate the challenges in ensuring uniform care in the presence of overlapping medical concerns. Intervention through a multidisciplinary framework that involves integrating mental health services, addiction treatment, and individualized medical regimens can potentially overcome gaps in care. Furthermore, increased resource investment in post-pandemic recovery initiatives is imperative to restore timely diagnostics and routine follow-up. Collectively, these interventions are imperative in reducing the negative effect of comorbidities on TB cure and promoting public health objectives in vulnerable populations (Antunes et al., 2024) (Figure 10.10).

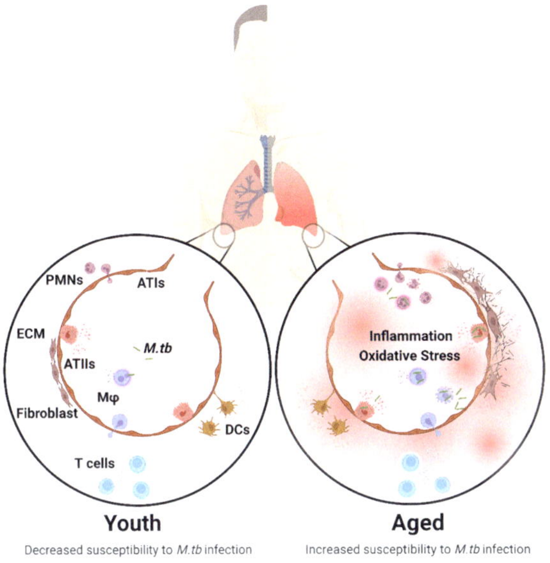

Figure 10.10. Structural and cellular changes in the aging lung. Age-associated changes in the composition and function of pulmonary cells are characterized by increased inflammation and oxidative stress driving impaired lung homeostasis, leading to increased susceptibility to MTB infection.

Source: Olmo-Fontánez AM, Turner J. Tuberculosis in an Aging World. *Pathogens*. 2022; 11(10):1101. https://doi.org/10.3390/pathogens11101101

10.2.3. Strategies for Prevention and Management

Successful prevention and management of TB in vulnerable groups requires a composite, patient-centered response designed according to their singular weaknesses and treatment needs. Co-infection of TB and HIV substantially increases active TB disease development because the HIV-depressed immunity diminishes both macrophage functions and gamma-interferon mechanisms of antimycobacterial immune responses, pointing to timely identification and concerted application of TB medication along with ART. Diagnostic accuracy is essential since overlapping symptoms may mask timely diagnosis, and interactions between TB drugs and antiretrovirals need to be monitored to avoid adverse effects. Comprehensive screening protocols should be adopted by health systems and ensure support for adherence, especially among socioeconomically disadvantaged populations where impediments to access persist. In addition to pharmacologic measures, education and community outreach are crucial in building awareness and eliminating stigma and thereby ensuring early diagnosis and treatment completion. Such combined measures enhance clinical outcomes and mitigate risks of transmission among at-risk subpopulations (Patel et al., 2024). Beyond the complexities of co-infection, TB control among other special groups like pregnant women, children, and older persons entails more sophisticated considerations affecting prevention and treatment measures. In pregnant females, harmonization of successful TB treatment without compromising fetal safety requires personalized regimens and careful follow-up, frequently complicated by physiological alterations with implications for drug metabolism. Age-specific dosing and pediatric formulations are necessary in pediatric patients to guarantee both efficacy and safety, with complementary strategies targeting nutrition and immunization to enhance immunity. In elderly groups, other challenges related to comorbidities and possible polypharmacy pose higher susceptibility to side effects and treatment non-adherence. Individualized clinical evaluation is required to dictate the selection and course of therapy, with multidisciplinary treatment teams ensuring proper management. Preventive interventions among these populations should also target contact tracing and LTBI screening for preemption of disease progression, as the need for specialized protocols that cater to diverse patient populations is critical (Patel et al., 2024). The occurrence of simultaneous health emergencies, like COVID-19, adds to the complexity of TB management protocols, especially in hospitalized patients at risk of thrombosis and other complications. Even though essentially a respiratory infection like TB, COVID-19 offers unique challenges requiring combined prevention protocols taking into account both infections' inflammatory and immune processes. Risk assessment for venous thromboembolism and implementing prophylactic anticoagulation have become increasingly relevant, especially where co-infection is suspected or confirmed. Optimizing treatment regimens demands coordination between antiviral, anti-inflammatory, and anticoagulant therapies, carefully balancing risks of bleeding and thrombotic events to improve prognostic outcomes. Clinical guidelines continue to evolve, advocating for personalized management strategies in special populations to address these intersecting risks effectively. By integrating newer evidence-based thromboprophylaxis guidelines, TB prevention and control programs can evolve to meet the new challenges presented by concurrent infectious diseases.

10.3. Tuberculosis (TB) in Immunocompromised Individuals

Immunocompromised hosts pose a big challenge in infectious disease management with their compromised immune response. Such a state of vulnerability is particularly important in TB where immune suppression can result in a swift conversion from latent to active disease. Several conditions like solid organ transplant, hematopoietic stem cell transplant, cancer, and congenital immunodeficiency account for this vulnerability. The simultaneous occurrence of such immunodeficiencies typically goes along with distorted clinical presentations and a higher risk for severe outcomes from TB. Vaccinations play an important role in preventing infectious diseases in these populations, but their efficacy and safety must be carefully tested. For instance, research evaluating responses to COVID-19 vaccines in comparable immunocompromised populations identifies a sophisticated interaction between vaccine reactogenicity and immune status, highlighting the subtle clinical factors in disease prevention strategies in such groups (Miyaji et al., 2025). The overlap of tuberculosis and immunocompromised conditions is further complicated by the impact of dynamic pathogens. Strains of other causative pathogens, like SARS-CoV-2, have shown varied effects on special groups, including those having compromised immune systems. Studies on such dynamics show that certain viral strains lead to more severe clinical presentations, whereas others result in mild to moderate disease processes accompanied by increased transmissibility. Such a variance makes it imperative to constantly observe and tailor healthcare interventions accordingly, which is similarly relevant in TB care. Immunocompromised patients may need individualized therapeutic and prophylactic regimens due to their heightened susceptibility to opportunistic infections and the risk of unusual disease patterns (Livieratos et al., 2024). These findings underscore the need to modify TB control strategies to the particular requirements of immunocompromised individuals. Treating tuberculosis in immunocompromised populations calls for an integrated strategy that encompasses careful clinical monitoring, proper vaccination practices, and personalized treatment protocols. Ensuring safety of the vaccine and surveillance of adverse events are critical elements of care since immunosuppression can potentially change the anticipated immune response as well as the profile of risk of the intervention. Vaccine-associated complications, although still uncommon in immunocompromised patients, demand careful assessment and further investigation to determine well-defined causative associations. In addition, heterogeneity in this group requires stratification according to underlying conditions to provide effective optimization of outcomes. By integrating concurrent evidence from other related infectious disease literature and those on tuberculosis directly, healthcare professionals can reinforce prevention and treatment efforts, ultimately lowering TB morbidity and mortality among immunocompromised patients (Livieratos et al., 2024; Miyaji et al., 2025) (Figure 10.11).

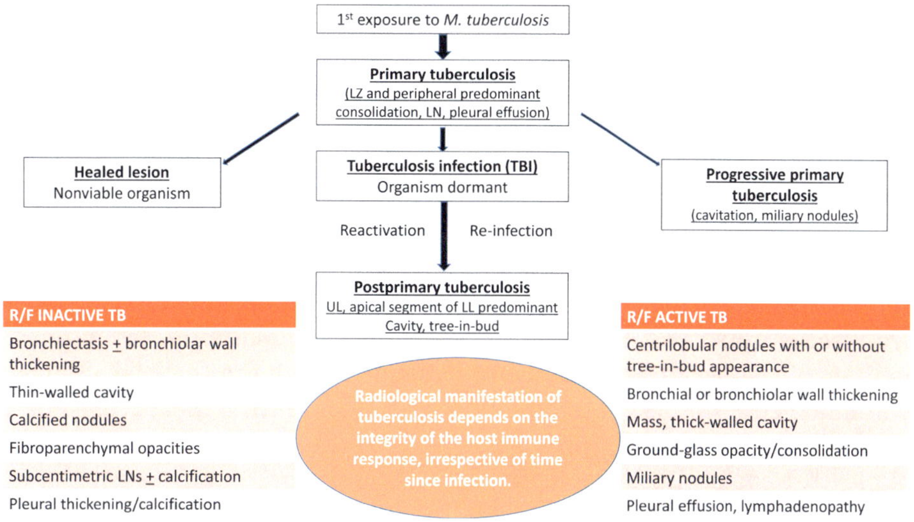

Figure 10.11. Natural history and common radiological features of tuberculosis.

Source: Thieme Connect. (2023). *Tuberculosis in the elderly: Diagnostic challenges and management strategies.* https://www.thieme-connect.com/products/ejournals/pdf/10.1055/s-0044-1787792.pdf.

10.3.1. Definition of Immunocompromised Populations

Persons with compromised immune systems are a special subgroup of the population whose risk of developing infectious illness, including tuberculosis, is significantly higher. This susceptibility stems from a wide range of medical and nonmedical conditions and treatments that compromise the immune response and make the body less able to defend against organisms. For instance, patients who are being treated with cytotoxic cancer treatments, patients who are on biological agents for autoimmune illnesses, and transplant recipients tend to suffer from reduced immune function. Moreover, inherited immunodeficiencies as well as acquired immune disorders add to this defective state. The heterogeneity is the reason behind the complexity of defining immunocompromised populations, since the extent and nature of immune compromise are highly variable, making it difficult to implement standardized clinical practice and research to tackle diseases such as tuberculosis (Cheng et al., 2023). It is important to address these differences to customize prevention and treatment in special populations with tuberculosis. In practice and clinical research, a lack of a global standard definition of immunocompromised individuals provides considerable obstacles to infection control with conditions like pneumonia and tuberculosis. Current community-acquired pneumonia guidelines, for example, often systematically omit immunocompromised hosts, leaving the provision of evidence-based care in these at-risk populations to chance. Such omissions stem from challenges in using standardized empirical treatment owing to varying risk profiles and microbial pathogens within immunocompromised hosts. Efforts have been made to establish consensus-based frameworks using multidisciplinary panels and methods such as the Delphi survey to outline the features of immunocompromised patients. Consensus efforts aim at defining the population, identifying probable pathogens, and outlining principles for diagnostic and therapeutic interventions, which are critical in extrapolating such frameworks to tuberculosis management in similar populations (Cheng et al., 2020). Such strategies highlight the importance of definitional clarity for this population in optimizing clinical outcomes. Appreciating the interaction between immune dysfunction and risk for infectious diseases, especially tuberculosis, that take advantage of compromised host defenses is a prerequisite for comprehending the definition of immunocompromised populations. Immunocompromised status does not refer to one clinical condition but rather to a spectrum of mild to severe immune compromise depending on the cause and its severity. Immunosuppressive drugs, for example, corticosteroids or biologics, add to this spectrum by modifying immune cell function and pathogen perception. Additionally, HIV/AIDS is an example of complex conditions that illustrate acquired immunodeficiency states with significantly increased risk of tuberculosis. Identification and classification of these groups according to their immune deficits allow healthcare professionals to recognize those at increased risk for tuberculosis reactivation or development early on. Therefore, this personalized recognition is crucial for planning effective screening, prophylaxis, and treatment programs in these special populations (Cheng et al., 2023).

10.3.2. Tuberculosis (TB) Risk in HIV/AIDS Patients

The interaction between infectious diseases and immunosuppression has challenged clinical management for years, especially in areas with both HIV/AIDS and TB. HIV's weakened immune system greatly enhances vulnerability to opportunistic disease, with TB being prominent because of its high mortality and morbidity in this population. Research in Hebei Province, China, indicates that HIV/AIDS patients have a significantly higher risk of developing TB, with infection rates varying according to the mode of HIV transmission. Of particular interest, those with same-sex transmission pathways showed almost fivefold higher risk than those infected via blood-borne routes. This correlation highlights the influence of behavioral and immunological factors in disease susceptibility. At the same time, diminished CD4⁺ T lymphocyte levels, a signature of HIV infection, were strongly correlated with TB incidence, with patients who had counts of less than 350 cells/μL having triple the risk (Figure 10.12). These results underscore the multi-factorial etiology of TB risk in HIV patients, to emphasize again the requirement for focused clinical surveillance and intervention measures (Pio, 2024).

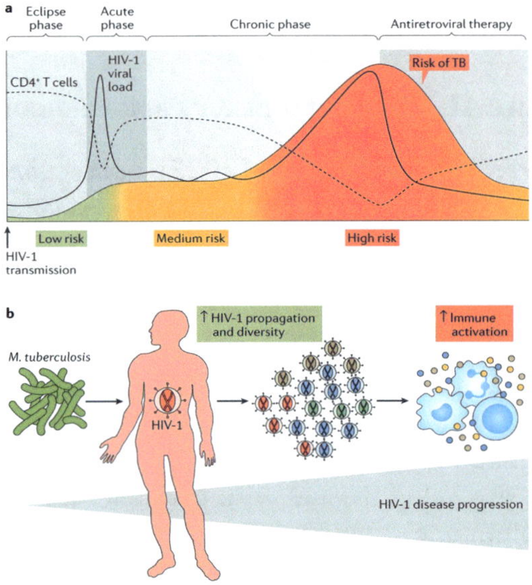

Figure 10.12. Pathogenesis of HIV-1 and *Mycobacterium tuberculosis* co-infection.

Source: Springer Nature. (2018). *Immune response and pathogenesis in tuberculosis infection.* https://media.springernature.com/full/springer-static/image/art%3A10.1038%2Fnrmicro.2017.128/MediaObjects/41579_2018_Article_BFnrmicro2017128_Fig1_HTML.jpg.

The prevalence of PTB in HIV-infected individuals further depicts the complex host immunity-pathogen exposure dynamic, necessitating coordinated healthcare strategies. Cross-sectional analysis of patients visiting ART clinics revealed close to one-fifth of the cohort was exposed to TB co-infection, highlighting its significant contribution. Demographic factors such as increasing age and male sex appeared as independent predictors of the occurrence of pulmonary TB, perhaps indicative of behavioral and biological vulnerabilities in these groups. In addition, alcohol consumption behavior and smoking were identified as modifiable factors that increase the risk of TB, implying avenues for prevention other than pharmacotherapy. The research reaffirmed the pivotal significance of adherence to ART and TB prophylaxis in strengthening immune capacities and reducing disease progression. These findings promote intensive patient education and focused support structures as a means to combat the singular susceptibilities among HIV-positive individuals (Pio, 2024). Mitigation of increased risk of TB among HIV/AIDS patients requires an integrated public health intervention that acknowledges heterogeneity among infected populations. Targeting TB screening and preventive treatment to those with low CD4$^+$ levels and defined risk factors, including men who have sex with men, would enhance early diagnosis and treatment responses. In addition, strengthening healthcare infrastructure to accommodate ongoing monitoring and drug compliance with ART regimens would decrease the immunosuppressive environment conducive to TB reactivation. Prevention measures should also include behavioral risk reduction strategies, such as smoking cessation and moderation of alcohol intake, which enhance susceptibility. These types of extensive interventions need to involve clinical providers, policymakers, and community-based organizations to close gaps in educational activities and the delivery of care. The evidence points out that contexts-sensitive, population-focused responses are needed to effectively combat the double burden of TB and HIV/AIDS (Pio, 2024) (Figure 10.13).

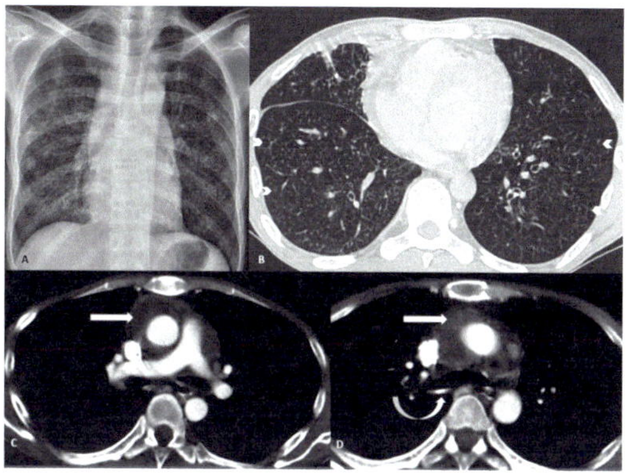

Figure 10.13. Tuberculosis in people living with human immunodeficiency virus (PLHIV). (A) Posteroanterior (PA) radiograph of a 43-year-old with dysphagia and a CD4 count of 80 cells/μL shows bilateral multiple miliary nodules. (B) Computed tomography (CT) axial image of the thorax (lung window) shows multiple miliary nodules in both lower lobes (white arrowheads). (C) The axial image (mediastinal window) shows multiple confluent necrotic nodes (white arrows). (D) Oral contrast opacifies the right main bronchus (white curved arrow), indicating esophagobronchial fistulous communication.

Source: Thieme Connect. (2023). Tuberculosis in the elderly: Diagnostic challenges and management strategies. https://www.thieme-connect.com/products/ejournals/pdf/10.1055/s-0044-1787792.pdf.

10.3.3. Management of Tuberculosis (TB) in Transplant Recipients

The complexities of the management of TB among transplant recipients are highlighted by the complex relationship between immunosuppressive treatment and the potential for opportunistic infection. Such individuals, commonly subjected to lifelong immunosuppression to avoid graft rejection, are at greater risk for reactivation of latent TB as well as for new TB infection. Successful management involves weighing anti-tubercular (ATT) therapy against immunosuppressive protocols, with possible dose adjustments needed to avoid drug interactions and toxicity. Moreover, TDM comes to play as a key tool to maximize pharmacotherapy, especially considering drug metabolism altered in this patient group. Evidence has highlighted the use of TDM in treating pulmonary infections with dried blood spot techniques, which can be applied to the anti-TB drugs to secure efficacy while minimizing side effects in transplant recipients (Hofman et al., 2015). The method can help in individualized treatment, considering both infection control and graft maintenance. Clinically, post-transplant infections such as TB have resulted in high morbidity and mortality. Studies among populations that have undergone kidney transplants bring out the fact that infections such as TB have accounted for a high percentage of post-transplant mortality, with the importance of monitoring and early management strategies (Kumar et al., 2023). Screening for LTBI prior to transplant using a standardized diagnostic test is important to identify the candidates who need prophylaxis. When TB is diagnosed, ATT regimen must be closely incorporated into the treatment schedule of the patient with regular monitoring for drug-drug interactions, particularly with calcineurin inhibitors and mTOR inhibitors being extensively used as immunosuppressants. Monitoring of liver function, renal function, and also possible hematologic adverse effects is also of utmost importance to avoid complications that threaten both graft survival and patient survival. Effective management relies not just on pharmacological therapy but also on a multidisciplinary strategy that includes transplant clinicians, infectious disease experts, and pharmacists. Due to the possibility of changed drug absorption and drug metabolism in such patients, continuous monitoring by newer TDM techniques can markedly maximize therapy efficacy. Technological progress in methods of sampling, including dried blood spots, promises to enable frequent monitoring even beyond the hospital environment, enhance compliance and detection of subtherapeutic drug levels at an early stage (Hofman et al., 2015). In addition, identification and prevention of possible ADRs through close clinical observation can minimize the risk of graft rejection and death associated with TB and other infections. Therefore, careful management strategies that address the specific vulnerabilities of transplant recipients are crucial to enhance prognosis in this vulnerable group (Kumar et al., 2023).

10.4. Tuberculosis (TB) in Refugees and Immigrants

Refugees and immigrants' difficulties in obtaining regular health care are major determinants of their susceptibility to infectious infections such as TB. Most of them come from high TB prevalence countries and usually suffer from the interruption of health care while in transit. During resettlement, clinical screenings are important interventions in detecting latent tuberculosis infection (LTBI) and other infectious diseases. Research has indicated that Iraqi and Afghan SIVH have a high prevalence of LTBI, among adults of Afghan origin, who are found to be twice as likely as Iraqis to present with LTBI. This group also has high vulnerability to hepatitis B and intestinal parasites, which underscores the multiple health hazards of displacement and resettlement. These conclusions highlight the necessity of targeted screening measures at entry to prevent active TB formation and transmission among these high-risk populations (Kumar et al., 2020). Conducting extensive domestic medical examination soon after arrival in the United States is of prime importance in addressing tuberculosis, as well as other infectious diseases, among immigrants and refugees. Evidence has shown that coverage of

TB screening in these tests achieves more than 90%, an effective strategy in the early detection of latent or active disease. The screenings allow timely treatment and acceptance into the healthcare system, thus minimizing the risk of community transmission. Disparities continue to occur in participation and follow-up care due to language, culture, and system barriers encountered among refugee populations. Whereas infection screening rates are high, ancillary health checks like mental health status are under-assessed, pointing to a gap in comprehensive care that indirectly could affect TB control through psychosocial determinants of health (Kumar et al., 2020). The greater burden of LTBI among refugees and some immigrant subgroups necessitates increased attention to culturally sound interventions and ongoing monitoring. Evidence demonstrates significant disparity in LTBI prevalence across populations, with Afghan refugees showing significantly higher levels than Iraqi refugees, mirroring heterogeneity in pre-migration exposures and epidemiologic contexts. Such differences require public health responses that are adapted to include rigorous risk assessments and education regarding TB prophylaxis adherence to guarantee successful therapy. Furthermore, combining TB screening with co-infection evaluation and examinations for conditions like hepatitis B will enhance overall health outcomes and maximize resource use. It is essential that healthcare workers remain aware of the diverse nature of refugee and immigrant health profiles to enhance efforts against tuberculosis among these special groups (Kumar et al., 2020) (Figure 10.14).

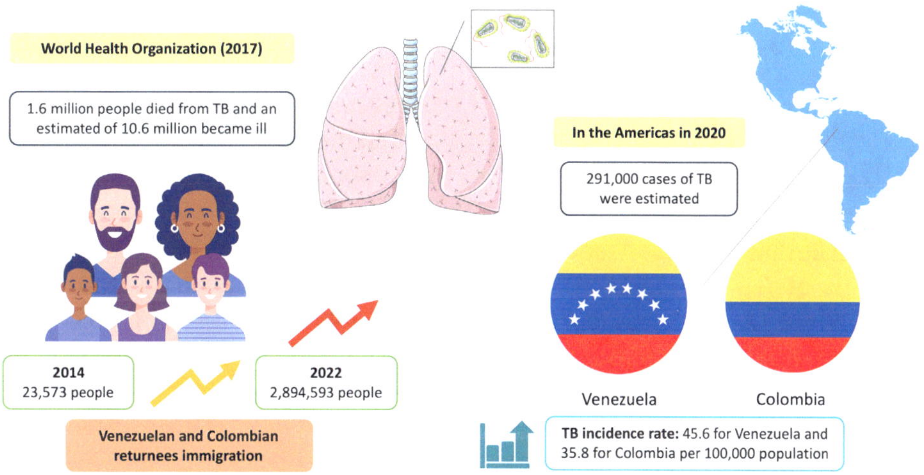

Figure 10.14. Migration flows and the tuberculosis burden: A focus on Colombia and Venezuela.

Source: The Lancet. (2023). *Tuberculosis in older adults: Challenges and opportunities.* https://www.thelancet.com/journals/lanam/article/PIIS2667-193X%2823%2900174-6/fulltext.

10.4.1. Prevalence of Tuberculosis (TB) in Refugee Populations

The refugee populations' health concerns are also complex, usually driven by their specific migration histories and way of life before resettlement. TB, specifically LTBI, is particularly common among these groups because of exposure in high-burden settings and factors like crowding and poor access to healthcare in refugee camps. Recent SIVH analyses from Iraq and Afghanistan showed that about 14% of adults had LTBI, with Afghan refugees having a higher rate than their Iraqi counterparts. This highlights the urgent necessity for targeted screening and prevention according to refugees' unique epidemiological profiles. Detection and control of LTBI in these groups are important to avoid progression to active disease and lower community transmission during settlement (Kumar et al., 2020). Post-arrival domestic medical examination screening coverage is central in managing tuberculosis among refugees. Data collected between 2014 and 2016 reveal that over 90% of refugees underwent TB screening as part of routine health assessments shortly after arriving in the United States. Such high screening rates provide a valuable opportunity to detect LTBI or active TB early, facilitating timely intervention and treatment.

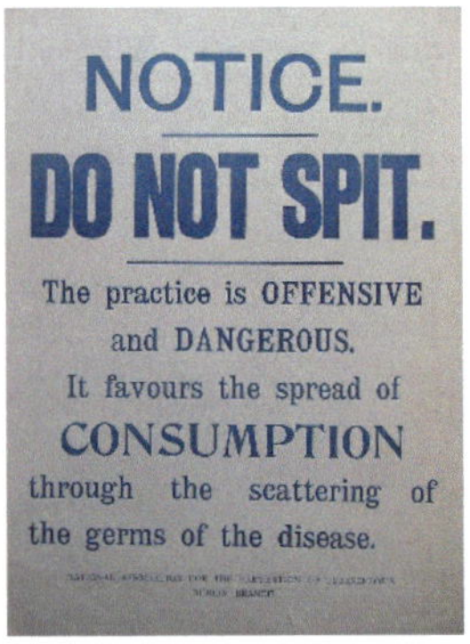

Source: By Unknown authorNational Association for the Prevention of Tuberculosis, Dublin Branch1905 - Google Arts & Culture — notice-do-not-spit-national-association-for-the-prevention-of-tuberculosis-dublin-branch/SAFcCWlmnTtKnw, Public Domain, https://commons.wikimedia.org/w/index.php?curid=92571769

Despite this, efforts are still needed to achieve standardized screening practices in varying states and healthcare settings that can affect the uniformity and quality of TB diagnosis. Refining these screening programs can improve public health outcomes among refugees as well as contribute to TB control among special populations efforts (Kumar et al., 2020). Even with progress in screening activity, inequalities in TB prevalence continue to exist across different refugee subgroups based on country of origin, socio-economic status, and migration routes. Afghan refugees, for example, show increased rates of LTBI compared to Iraqi refugees, consistent with underlying variations in TB exposure before resettlement. Such variation highlights the need for culturally and epidemiologically guided healthcare strategies that acknowledge disparate risk profiles within refugee groups. Public health strategies need to then incorporate in-depth TB surveillance and preventive practices that account for these subtleties as well as co-occurring health problems prevalent among refugees. Such practice encourages a fairer and more effective TB response among such high-risk groups (Kumar et al., 2020).

10.4.2. Barriers to Healthcare Access

Disparities in healthcare access pose significant obstacles to the control and management of tuberculosis in special populations, tending to widen health inequities. Children and youth with special healthcare needs (CYSHCN) in the United States experience particular difficulties in accessing timely and proper treatment, which may increase infectiousness and compound outcomes. For example, even with a general high report of having access to healthcare, patients with long-term health conditions often face barriers like the unavailability of appointments, restricted specialist services, and exorbitant costs. These may hamper diagnosis and treatment initiation, pivotal processes in tuberculosis management. Furthermore, financial issues and weak health insurance cover exacerbate these challenges, making diagnostic and therapeutic care challenging to access. Overcoming these barriers calls for overall improvement in health system funding and targeted augmentation of specialist numbers suited to the priorities of vulnerable child populations (Bogle et al., 2025). In most low-resource environments, particularly rural parts of sub-Saharan Africa, healthcare accessibility barriers even further complicate tuberculosis control among vulnerable populations. These remote communities frequently struggle with under-resourced health systems, acute shortages of skilled healthcare providers, and difficult transportation arrangements that hinder frequent clinic visits or drug adherence. Structural weaknesses like poor infrastructure and few healthcare facilities also limit the potential for early diagnosis and ongoing treatment, thereby enhancing disease transmission and treatment failure risks. Educational and cultural barriers also sustain myths about tuberculosis, thereby deterring people from availing themselves of timely medical treatment. The interplay between these issues sustains a perpetual cycle of poor healthcare access for special populations living in rural settings, emphasizing the imperative of concerted policy actions and resource planning to enhance healthcare provision in these marginalized communities (Anand et al., 2024). Economic and systemic limitations represent a second major hindrance that restricts access to healthcare for tuberculosis control among special populations. Unaffordable out-of-pocket expenditures, incomplete insurance coverage, and the indirect costs of transportation and lost time from work disproportionately burden marginalized populations, such as individuals with disabilities or chronic illnesses. Such financial barriers can discourage patients from finishing TB diagnostic tests or following long regimens of treatment, resulting in increased drug resistance and poor clinical outcomes. In addition, health care service fragmentation frequently results in patients with extensive needs, such as HIV co-infected or children with developmental disorders, having to visit multiple providers, raising the chances of delayed or missed care. To improve tuberculosis outcomes, health systems need to adopt policies that minimize economic barriers and integrate services to offer coordinated, patient-centered care for these special populations (Anand et al., 2024; Bogle et al., 2025).

10.4.3. Public Health Implications and Screening Strategies

Control of TB in special populations has to recognize broader public health consequences with high disease burden and transmission risk. Active TB in vulnerable populations like prisoners, migrants, and people with compromised immunity usually worsens health disparities and undermines disease control in the population. Diagnostic and treatment delays in such groups enable MTB transmission, which leads to cycles of infection that go beyond patient outcomes. Adding to these complexities are underlying systemic disparities in availability of quality healthcare and social determinants of health that complicate early detection and optimal management. In addition, neglect to cure TB fully in such vulnerable populations can lead to augmented morbidity and mortality, along with tremendous socioeconomic expense. Therefore, public health interventions need to include specially focused interventions that not only detect cases early but also tackle root-level structural determinants of disease patterns in these groups. Screening interventions specially focused on special populations are essential in preventing tuberculosis transmission and providing timely treatment. Since TB symptoms are nonspecific and frequently overlap with other illnesses, especially in immunosuppressed persons like HIV-infected individuals, systematic screening with both symptom-based evaluation and diagnostic testing is indicated. For the incarcerated population, routine screening at intake and follow-up screening at regular intervals are necessary to break the chains of transmission in crowded settings where transmission is encouraged by overcrowding and poor ventilation. Migrant and homeless community-based screening programs must involve culturally appropriate strategies to overcome stigma and trust barriers. Progress in molecular testing and radiographic screening enables earlier diagnosis with enhanced outcomes and secondary transmission reduction.

Such strategies integrated into extended health systems capacity building, along with quality assurance measures, guarantee effective and equitable screening (Stovner et al., 2018). The success of tuberculosis control in special populations depends equally on the health system's ability to sustain screening efforts and address quality of care. Weaknesses in diagnostic accuracy, delayed treatment initiation, and poor patient follow-up compromise public health objectives and erode trust in health services, especially among vulnerable groups. Installation of high-quality health systems that emphasize competence, respectful care, and reliable availability of resources is critical to the optimization of screening program performance. Ensuring decision-making backed by data through solid mechanisms of monitoring enables modulation of screening procedures to current epidemiological trends. In addition, incorporating TB screening into core health infrastructure and community outreach and education can increase patient demand for treatment and adherence to cure, and thus magnify the effect of public health programs. These system enhancements decrease health inequities and build resilience against TB recurrence in special populations (Stovner et al., 2018).

10.5. Cultural and Societal Factors

The influence of social norms and cultural beliefs has a profound impact on TB outcomes in special populations. In most communities, TB stigma can discourage patients from presenting early for diagnosis and treatment, leading to increased transmission and poor prognosis. Cultural models of illness often inform health behaviors, such that traditional or misinformation-based remedies for TB delay formal healthcare system utilization. In addition, linguistic, literacy, and health communication differences may be sources of obstacles hindering successful prevention and intervention efforts. Such cultural differences call for community-focused public health initiatives that value and address local traditions and incorporate them while enhancing evidence-based TB treatment. Acknowledgment of such various cultural models is key in crafting interventions that are accessible and acceptable to affected populations and thereby enhancing adherence and outcomes. Social determinants like poverty, housing insecurity, and health care access significantly play a part in the risk vulnerability of particular groups to tuberculosis. Vulnerable populations like older adults and marginalized urban dwellers tend to encounter systemic disparities that compound their vulnerability. These social determinants do not only expand exposure to MTB but also complicate steady treatment compliance, promoting drug resistance and unfavorable clinical outcomes. In elderly people, for example, the co-existence of chronic illness and functional impairment complicates TB control, highlighting the need for concerted social and medical services. Availability and organization of community networks of support and medical infrastructure are key in damping these social risks. Successful TB control programs need to take into consideration these larger society challenges, advocating for equity and resource distribution prioritizing high-risk groups. The interaction between environmental determinants and health services also influences TB outcomes in vulnerable populations, highlighting the importance of integrated care models. Accessibility of services, such as proximity to clinics and presence of specialist programs, mediates between chronic disease and disability, which affect older persons and other vulnerable groups. Empirical evidence establishes that better infrastructure and focused health care are able to reduce multidimensional disabilities, improve psychological status, and enhance social participation, ultimately leading to better TB control. In addition, socially inclusive community design that encourages active participation and networks of social support lead to better health and life quality (Buffel et al., 2020). Resolution of these cultural and societal determinants through integrated policy and practice frameworks is crucial for successful tuberculosis control among special populations.

10.5.1. Stigma Associated with Tuberculosis (TB) in Different Cultures

The social consequences of tuberculosis go beyond its manifestations, profoundly affecting social attitudes and beliefs. Cultural explanatory models of illness, based on temporal, religious, and social factors, frequently determine the perception of people suffering from TB in societies. In most societies, TB is linked to ideas of impurity, frailty, or the wrath of God, causing people to stigmatize those infected. This stigma breeds discrimination, leading patients to hide their diagnosis so they are not ostracized and will not suffer economically. Consequently, stigma is an obstacle to early diagnosis and treatment regimen compliance, thus extending disease transmission and making it difficult for public health interventions. It is essential to understand the cultural substrates of stigma when designing interventions that address not only the medical but also the psychosocial aspects of TB care, especially in multicultural populations whose beliefs about it vary exceedingly (Meershoek et al., 2018). Ethnic and socioeconomic inequalities add a twist to the experience of stigma among tuberculosis patients. Within minority populations, stigma is deeply embedded in larger problems of marginalization, such as restricted access to healthcare, institutional racism, and economic marginalization. These intersecting factors construct barriers to seeking and retaining TB treatment, frequently compounded by linguistic and cultural differences that impair communication with healthcare providers. Identity, both self-defined and imposed, influences individuals' response and adaptation to the diagnosis, impacting disclosure and health-seeking behavior. TB stigma in such groups requires acknowledgment of such complexities and calls for culturally appropriate strategies that include community outreach and the provision of resources to address entrenched inequities (Ahmad & Bradby, 2008). In certain cultures, stigma from tuberculosis permeates not just the individual but also his/her family or social group, influencing marriage, employment, and social status.

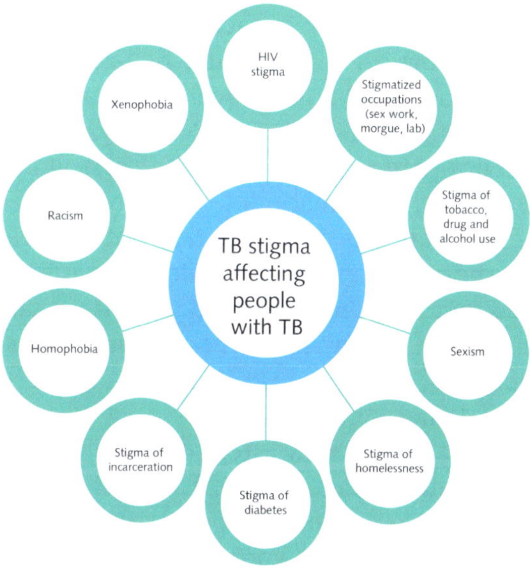

Figure 10.15. Stigmas that may impact people with TB.

Source: ResearchGate. (n.d.). *Stigmas that may impact people with TB.* https://www.researchgate.net/figure/Stigmas-that-may-impact-people-with-TB_fig2_327572824.

The threat of social exclusion promotes secrecy, which can hinder diagnosis and impede adherence to regular treatment, further worsening health outcomes. Attempts to quantify and mitigate TB stigma must thus take into account these social dynamics and the targeted cultural beliefs that drive discrimination. Stigma reduction programs must involve participation from health workers, champions, and impacted communities in building trust and familiarity. Integrating stigma measurement instruments can facilitate tracking of trends and the impacts of interventions and, in the process, create conditions under which persons are comfortable accessing care and assistance (Meershoek et al., 2018) (Figure 10.15).

10.5.2. Influence of Cultural Beliefs on Treatment Adherence

Compliance to treatment among TB patients is determined by complex factors that go beyond clinical practice, with cultural beliefs taking a central position. In most societies, local healing traditions and indigenous concepts of health influence patients' beliefs about illness and the effectiveness of treatment, often resulting in diverse reactions to biomedical intervention. These culturally embedded beliefs may promote or discourage compliance, as patients balance their faith in modern medicine against traditional concepts of disease causation. For example, the Health Belief Model illustrates how perceived benefits and barriers affect compliance, with cultural interpretations having a direct influence on these perceptions. An Indonesian study showed that patients' knowledge of TB severity and perceived self-efficacy improved heavily adherence to directly observed treatment, short-course (DOTS), while cultural misconceptions may be barriers (Pusporini et al., 2024). Awareness of the complex dynamic is crucial in the development of culturally appropriate interventions addressing local community needs and ultimately enhancing treatment outcomes in special populations. Additionally, patients' knowledge, attitudes, and behaviors regarding TB treatment are rooted deeply in their cultural context, which mostly decides upon their willingness to cooperate fully with prescribed regimens. Even where patients have high levels of biomedical knowledge, conflicting attitudes about disease and drugs in their culture can lower rates of adherence. Studies in Subulussalam City identified a paradox where good knowledge regarding TB existed in conjunction with unfavorable treatment attitudes, resulting in low overall compliance (Nursa'adah et al., 2024). This incongruence indicates that mere cognitive awareness is not enough; belief and value systems and culture need to be addressed to promote more favorable attitudes and behaviors. Customizing learning strategies to appeal to indigenous beliefs and engaging advocacy by community leaders can thereby fill this gap. The culturally adapted strategies help to improve medication compliance, and their impact on TB control programs in vulnerable groups is highly significant. Lastly, the social environment influenced by cultural activities generates unique determinants of barriers and facilitators of TB treatment compliance. TB stigma, powered by cultural contagion and moral narratives, has been known to cause patients to hide their condition or stop treatment too early. All these make the perceived barriers outlined in health behavior models worse and further emphasize the imperative of culturally competent care that takes into account patients' worldviews. Interventions that have integrated cultural sensitivity, like engaging with family members and openly confronting stigma, have shown higher rates of treatment success. As recognized in empirical literature, self-efficacy and perceived benefits correlate positively with compliance but will only be effective if reinforced under the context of patients' cultures (Pusporini et al., 2024). Therefore, TB control health programs targeting special populations should incorporate cultural aspects deeply into their programming to optimize adherence and minimize disease burden.

10.5.3. Community Engagement and Education Initiatives

Managing TB in special populations requires a multifaceted response that extends beyond the clinic to stress the critical importance of community education and participation. By instilling increased awareness and insight regarding TB transmission, symptom recognition, and medication adherence, community programs have the ability to affect significant change in health status. Especially in areas with heavy burden of MDR-TB, e.g., India, enabling community members and leaders with correct information supports fighting misinformation and stigma that frequently impede early diagnosis and compliance with treatment. Public health agency collaborations with local stakeholders allow culturally appropriate educational material to be adapted so that messages are conveyed effectively across various linguistic and social communities. Moreover, these initiatives facilitate identifying vulnerable groups who might otherwise remain outside formal healthcare systems, strengthening surveillance and early intervention efforts that are crucial to controlling disease spread and improving prognosis (Gamon, 2013). Beyond raising awareness, education initiatives serve as critical platforms for equipping individuals with the knowledge necessary to navigate healthcare services confidently. Effective programs tend to include interactive workshops, peer-support groups, and specially designed counseling sessions that target the specific obstacles experienced by special populations, such as migrants, prison inmates, and co-morbidities like HIV/AIDS. Such interventions enhance compliance with long and complicated treatment regimens, minimizing the risk of relapse or development of drug resistance. Notably, active community participation increases trust between health workers and patients, which is crucial in breaking fear and suspicion of health facilities. Active communities can further demand increased policy attention and health infrastructure investment, catalyzing systemic changes in line with international TB control strategies. Under such a setting, collaborations with non-state actors like private foundations and philanthropic bodies bring in useful resources and innovative methods, adding to national initiatives in TB management (Lundsgaarde, 2010). The control of tuberculosis among special populations depends on ongoing investment in education and empowerment of the community, underpinned by concerted multisectoral action. Local-level educational campaigns that are specific to local epidemiologic and sociocultural contexts build ownership and responsibility among healthcare communities, driving behavior change essential for effective TB prevention and treatment. In addition, the embedding of these interventions within larger public health platforms harmonizes efforts, maintains consistency, and supports synergies among other key interventions, including vaccination, nutritional supplementation, and contact tracing. The potential of technology, such as digital media and mobile health platforms, becomes more and more central to scaling up reach and engagement, particularly among youth and vulnerable populations. Finally, strengthening community networks and capacity development not only reduces TB disease but also advances general health equity and resistance to future public health threats (Gamon,Lundsgaarde, 2010; Gamon, 2013).

SUMMARY

The control of tuberculosis among special populations requires a comprehensive approach to address the specific vulnerabilities and health system issues surrounding these populations. It is clear that although the BCG vaccine has been a cornerstone of preventing tuberculosis, its inconsistent efficacy, particularly among adults and heterogeneous subpopulations, underscores the imperative for new interventions (Locht et al., 2020). The general non-specific advantages of BCG and the new vaccine contenders provide encouraging options but require careful clinical testing in varied demographic and immunologic environments. Improved vaccine regimens, complemented with increased knowledge of immunopathology in vulnerable groups, could make a marked difference. Continued fusion of cutting-edge vaccine research with public health practice is essential to combat tuberculosis's insidious burden, especially in the immunocompromised or socio-economically disadvantaged segments. Tuberculosis control among vulnerable and marginalized groups cannot be separated from the overall task of improving health systems, particularly in low- and middle-income countries (LMICs), where disease burden tends to be highest. The quality of health systems has a significant effect on diagnosis, treatment, and adherence required for successful tuberculosis control. Despite this, many challenges remain, such as diagnostic delays, poor follow-up, and poor treatment outcomes, all exacerbated by system lapses (Margaret et al., 2018). Raising the level of care involves system changes that transcend expanding access, focusing on skilled, respectful, and timely care that is adapted to meet special populations' needs. Implementing integrated strategies, including workforce training, patient-centered communication, and social determinant integration, guarantees not only better clinical outcomes but also generates trust and utilization of healthcare services, which are critical for long-term tuberculosis control. Control of tuberculosis among special groups needs to break away from traditional paradigms through the prioritization of epidemiologically appropriate vaccine strategies, inclusive system strengthening, and equity-driven care delivery. The past and continuing payoff of BCG vaccination emphasizes its central position but demonstrates the need for next-generation vaccines and additive therapeutic strategies (Locht et al., 2020). Parallel to this is the need for health systems to develop in responsiveness and quality to meet the specific vulnerabilities of these groups, reaffirming the confluence between clinical innovation and equity in health (Margaret et al., 2018). This multi-faceted approach, anchored in scientific progress and systemic reforms, presents the greatest potential for decreasing tuberculosis morbidity and mortality among special populations, eventually serving the cause of global health and the elimination of this long-lived infectious disease.

An in-depth insight into TB in vulnerable groups requires acknowledging the many-faceted issues presented by AMR. TB, particularly drug-resistant, exacerbates the challenges of handling infections in risk groups like pregnant women, the immunocompromised, and populations in resource-limited environments. The overall burden of AMR highlights how much more dangerous these issues become because resistance decreases the effectiveness of the standard drugs and raises death rates. This complexity calls for focused approaches, such as augmented diagnostic facilities and targeted therapeutic interventions, to counter the specific requirements of such populations. Further, gaps in data across different regions constrain the ability to design effective policies, reinforcing the need for better surveillance and laboratory facilities to effectively deal with resistant TB strains (Dartois & Rubin, 2022). No less critical is the strict evaluation of health system competence in treating TB in special populations. Notwithstanding improvement in healthcare outcomes across the world, disparities remain, especially in LMICs where TB burden tends to coincide with systemic vulnerabilities. Care delivery gaps in quality, including suboptimal clinical management and follow-up of patients, differentially disadvantage the vulnerable population, leading to disease advancement and spread. These gaps can be addressed by sweeping health system reforms that promote governance, workforce capability, and patient-centeredness. Strengthening these foundations guarantees that TB interventions are not only available but also effective and fair, enhancing health effects and diminishing financial costs associated with poor quality care (Margaret et al., 2018). Integrating the above points shows that addressing TB in special populations extends beyond simple clinical treatment to include systemic reforms and evidence-based policy-making. Addressing the twin menace of TB and AMR requires an integrated strategy that includes improved healthcare quality, strong infrastructure, and participatory governance. There is an urgent need to promote vulnerable populations in national health policies so that interventions are context-sensitive and culture-attuned. Sustained investment in research, surveillance, and capacity development is essential to fill knowledge gaps and reinforce health systems. Ultimately, making significant gains against TB among these groups requires concerted efforts that bring together medical, social, and policy aspects that are aligned with broader global health priorities to decrease disease burden and increase health equity (Margaret et al., 2018; Dartois & Rubin, 2022).

CLOSER LOOK

THE BURDEN OF TUBERCULOSIS (TB) IN IMMIGRANT AND REFUGEE POPULATIONS

The public health burden of TB in refugees and immigrants is a major concern worldwide because these groups tend to be at increased risk of developing the disease and of transmitting the disease relative to the general population. The overlap of migration, refugee status, and TB is multifaceted, with a number of social, environmental, and health-related factors contributing to increased risk. Refugees and immigrants frequently originate from areas with endemic TB, and their movement to nations with lower TB endemicity can lead to the dissemination of the disease in those nations.

Among the most significant drivers of increased rates of TB among these populations is exposure to TB in their home countries. Much of the refugees and immigrants migrate from regions that have high levels of TB, such as sub-Saharan Africa, Southeast Asia, and portions of Eastern Europe. In these regions, TB could be insufficiently diagnosed and treated, and TB could be endemic due to insufficient access to care. Consequently, those who move to nations with lower TB incidences could be infected with Mycobacterium tuberculosis (M. tuberculosis) already, possibly in a latent state that manifests as active TB at some point in the future. The risk of progression from latent to active TB is higher in individuals with weakened immune systems, such as those with HIV/AIDS, malnutrition, or other underlying health conditions, all of which are common in refugee populations.

In addition, social determinants of health contribute significantly to the TB burden among refugees and immigrants. Overcrowded housing, poor healthcare access, and limited socioeconomic opportunities, which enhance the spread of TB, are common among these groups. Refugees and immigrants can also have communication problems, cultural differences, and immigration-related fear of accessing healthcare, which may hinder early diagnosis and treatment. Both stigma against TB and immigration status further complicate TB control efforts because people may not want to receive medical attention in case they get deported or discriminated against.

Healthcare access is a key concern among these groups. Throughout much of the world, refugees and immigrants encounter obstacles to receiving full TB screening, diagnosis, and treatment services. Such obstacles may be lack of insurance, foreignness to healthcare systems, or discrimination on the part of healthcare providers. Moreover, poor TB surveillance in refugee camps or resource-poor settings where large numbers of displaced individuals reside raises the likelihood of TB outbreaks among these communities.

The burden of TB in immigrants and refugees necessitates specific public health interventions. Among these are universal TB screening of immigrants and refugees upon entry in a foreign country, better access to healthcare for immigrants and refugees, and education to decrease stigma and promote early treatment. A strengthened global response to TB among immigrants and refugees is needed to avoid the spread of the disease across borders and to improve the health outcomes of these patients.

REFERENCES

1. Agnes Meershoek, Alice Zwerling, Amrita Daftary, Brian Citro, Caoimhe Smyth, Dean Lewis, Deirdre Ni Cheallaigh, Elaine Byrne, Ellen M. H Mitchell, Gill Craig, Ieva Leimane, James Malar, Jens Levy, Julia van der Land, Kate Macintyre, Lisa G. Johnston, Nadine Ferris France, Nora Engel, Olive Mumba, Rajita Bhavaraju, Ronan R. Conroy, Sarah van de Berg, Stephen H-F Macdonald, Timur Abdullaev, and Tushar Nair. (2018). *TB Stigma–Measurement Guidance*. The United States Agency for International Development (USAID), !nancially supports this publication through Challenge TB under the terms of Agreement No. AID-OAA-A-14-00029. This publication was made possible by the generous support of the American people through USAID. *Core*. https://core.ac.uk/download/287580942.pdf (accessed on 10 May 2025).

2. Kumar, G. S., Pezzi, C., Wien, S., Mamo, B., Scott, K., Payton, C., Urban, K., Hughes, S., Kennedy, L., Cabanting, N., Montour, J., Titus, M., Aguirre, J., Kawasaki, B., Ford, R., & Jentes, E. S. (2020). Health of Special Immigrant Visa holders from Iraq and Afghanistan after arrival into the United States using Domestic Medical Examination data, 2014-2016: A cross-sectional analysis. *PLoS medicine*, *17*(3), e1003083. https://doi.org/10.1371/journal.pmed.1003083(accessed on 10 May 2025).

3. Ahmad, W., & Bradby, H. (2008). Ethnicity and Health: Key Themes in a Developing Field. *Current Sociology*, *56*(1), 47-56. https://doi.org/10.1177/0011392107084378 (Original work published 2008)

4. Hofman, S., Bolhuis, M. S., Koster, R. A., Akkerman, O. W., van Assen, S., Stove, C., & Alffenaar, J. W. (2015). Role of therapeutic drug monitoring in pulmonary infections: use and potential for expanded use of dried blood spot samples. *Bioanalysis*, *7*(4), 481–495. https://doi.org/10.4155/bio.14.318 (accessed on 10 May 2025).

5. Cheng, G. S., Crothers, K., Aliberti, S., Bergeron, A., Boeckh, M., Chien, J. W., Cilloniz, C., Cohen, K., Dean, N., Dela Cruz, C. S., Dickson, R. P., Greninger, A. L., Hage, C. A., Hohl, T. M., Holland, S. M., Jones, B. E., Keane, J., Metersky, M., Miller, R., Puel, A., ... Evans, S. E. (2023). Immunocompromised Host Pneumonia: Definitions and Diagnostic Criteria: An Official American Thoracic Society Workshop Report. *Annals of the American Thoracic Society*, *20*(3), 341–353. https://doi.org/10.1513/AnnalsATS.202212-1019ST

6. Ramirez, J. A., Musher, D. M., Evans, S. E., Dela Cruz, C., Crothers, K. A., Hage, C. A., Aliberti, S., Anzueto, A., Arancibia, F., Arnold, F., Azoulay, E., Blasi, F., Bordon, J., Burdette, S., Cao, B., Cavallazzi, R., Chalmers, J., Charles, P., Chastre, J., Claessens, Y. E., ... Wunderink, R. (2020). Treatment of Community-Acquired Pneumonia in Immunocompromised Adults: A Consensus Statement Regarding Initial Strategies. *Chest*, *158*(5), 1896–1911. https://doi.org/10.1016/j.chest.2020.05.598 (accessed on 10 May 2025).

7. Anand, S., Ayodele, V., Ashraf, A., Shilleh, M. A., Rahim, F., Mmbaga, B., & Rugakingira, A. (2024). Expanding healthcare access in rural sub-Saharan Africa. *Perspectives in Public Health*, *144*(6), 333–335. https://www.semanticscholar.org/paper/a9a0f0fa819dbd22ab4cea2ce618342144be64d8 (accessed on 10 May 2025).

8. Antunes, L. B., de Paula Andrade, R. L., Ribeiro, R. R., Monroe, A. A., Signor, E., Machado de Oliveira Bianchini, A. S., Veira, N. F., et al. (2024). Tuberculosis treatment during the COVID-19 pandemic: Actions offered and case profile. *Revista Gaucha de Enfermagem*, *45*, e20230127. https://www.semanticscholar.org/paper/4e9e30c60da040cd6bf3e4d688cb7ed9ecb1b654 (accessed on 10 May 2025).

9. Bogle, T., & Rakestraw, D. (2025). Access to healthcare for children and youth with special healthcare needs in Kansas. *Kansas Journal of Medicine, 18*, 1–1. https://www.semanticscholar.org/paper/12a8036c3769773cda4c6f068f33eab2f5933ff2 (accessed on 10 May 2025).

10. Buffel, T., & Phillipson, C. (2020). Age-friendly cities and communities: Policy opportunities and challenges. *Core*. https://core.ac.uk/download/326604859.pdf (accessed on 10 May 2025).

11. Cibro, N., Safrizal, Kusumawardani, E. F., Duana, M., Nursia, L. E., Umar, T., & University, T. (2024). The relationship of knowledge, attitudes and actions with medication adherence in pulmonary tuberculosis patients at the pulmonary polyclinic of Subulussalam City Hospital. *International Journal of Public Health*. https://www.semanticscholar.org/paper/000f8c67ddef0f8d692529fa7e8f076a82c17112 (accessed on 10 May 2025).

12. Devos, I., & Janssens, A. (2017). Introduction. tseg 14 (4): 5-24 doi: 10.18352/tseg.1001. (accessed on 10 May 2025).

13. Dartois, V., & Rubin, E. J. (2022). Anti-tuberculosis treatment strategies and drug development: Challenges and priorities. *Nature Reviews Microbiology, 20*, 685–701. https://doi.org/10.1038/s41579-022-00731-y.

14. Rockwood, N., du Bruyn, E., Morris, T., & Wilkinson, R. J. (2016). Assessment of treatment response in tuberculosis. *Expert review of respiratory medicine, 10*(6), 643–654. https://doi.org/10.1586/17476348.2016.1166960(accessed on 10 May 2025).

15. Ebejer, M. J. (1996). Tuberculosis in Malta in the 21st century. *Core*. https://core.ac.uk/download/46602164.pdf (accessed on 10 May 2025).

16. Gamon, Maribel, "Maribel Gamon - Multidrug-Resistant Tuberculosis in India: Solving a Problem by Reconstructing the Public Health Infrastructure" (2013). *Ronald E. McNair Scholars Program 2013*. 12. https://epublications.marquette.edu/mcnair_2013/12

17. McNerney, R., Maeurer, M., Abubakar, I., Marais, B., McHugh, T. D., Ford, N., Weyer, K., Lawn, S., Grobusch, M. P., Memish, Z., Squire, S. B., Pantaleo, G., Chakaya, J., Casenghi, M., Migliori, G. B., Mwaba, P., Zijenah, L., Hoelscher, M., Cox, H., Swaminathan, S., ... Zumla, A. (2012). Tuberculosis diagnostics and biomarkers: needs, challenges, recent advances, and opportunities. *The Journal of infectious diseases, 205 Suppl 2*, S147–S158. https://doi.org/10.1093/infdis/jir860(accessed on 10 May 2025).

18. Ismail, I., Adi, S., Basri, M., Simunati, S., & Nasrullah, N. (2025). Vitamin D receptor gene variations and tuberculosis susceptibility: Insights from Indonesian populations. *Tuberculosis and Thorax, 73*. https://www.semanticscholar.org/paper/76db079850fe5d1314f1364cfe5a1b40e440de8a (accessed on 10 May 2025).

19. Ismail, I., Nur, M., & Harliani, H. (2025). Association of ASAP1 gene polymorphisms (rs4733781 and rs10956514) with tuberculosis susceptibility in the Kaluku Bodoa Makassar population, Indonesia. *Israa University Journal for Applied Science*. https://www.semanticscholar.org/paper/968ef11b34243340c760112549149753804bc72f (accessed on 10 May 2025).

20. Kruk, M. E., Gage, A., Arsenault, C., Jordan, K., Leslie, H. H., Roder-DeWan, S., Adeyi, O., et al. (2018). High-quality health systems in the Sustainable Development Goals era: Time for a revolution. *The Lancet Global Health, 6*(12), e1196–e1252. https://doi.org/10.1016/s2214-109x(18)30386-3.

21. Livieratos, A., Gogos, C., & Akinosoglou, K. (2024). SARS-CoV-2 variants and clinical outcomes of special populations: A scoping review of the literature. *Viruses, 16*(4). https://doi.org/10.3390/v16040419.

22. Locht, C., & Lerm, M. (2020). Good old BCG–What a century-old vaccine can contribute to modern medicine. *Journal of Internal Medicine, 288*(6), 611–613. https://doi.org/10.1111/joim.13195.

23. Lundsgaarde, E. (2010). Emerging non-state actors in global development: Challenges for Europe. *Core*. https://core.ac.uk/download/75779494.pdf (accessed on 10 May 2025).

24. Manyi-Loh, C. E., Mamphweli, S., Meyer, E. L., & Okoh, A. I. (2018). Antibiotic use in agriculture and its consequential resistance in environmental sources: Potential public health implications. *Molecules, 23*(4), 795. https://doi.org/10.3390/molecules23040795.

25. Miyaji, K., Ibrahim, K., Infante, V., Megale Moreira, R., Ferreira Dos Santos, C., de Cássia Belizário, J., de Moraes Pinto, M. I., et al. (2025). Safety of two-dose schedule of COVID-19 adsorbed inactivated vaccine (CoronaVac; Sinovac/Butantan) and heterologous additional doses of mRNA BNT162b2 (Pfizer/BioNTech) in immunocompromised and immunocompetent individuals. *Revita do Instituto de Medicine Tropical de São Paulo, 67*. https://www.semanticscholar.org/paper/de3ec62e8be2f7e4abbe1604fcd3e05c5b96fb8b (accessed on 10 May 2025).

26. Murray, C. J. L., Ikuta, K. S., Sharara, F., Swetschinski, L. R., Robles Aguilar, G., Gray, A. P., Han, C., et al. (2022). Global burden of bacterial antimicrobial resistance in 2019: A systematic analysis. *The Lancet, 399*(10325), 629–655. https://doi.org/10.1016/s0140-6736(21)02724-0.

27. Niederman, M. (2003). Community-acquired pneumonia. *Annals of Internal Medicine, 151*(ITC4-1). https://www.semanticscholar.org/paper/8bbeb9dcf93b2739569f1c76f1594b9c91f5a097 (accessed on 10 May 2025).

28. Patel, A., Pundkar, A., Agarwal, A., Gadkari, C., Nagpal, A. K., & Kuttan, N. (2024). A comprehensive review of HIV-associated tuberculosis: Clinical challenges and advances in management. *Cures, 16*(5). https://doi.org/10.7759/cureus.26585.

29. Pio, I. B. (2024). Prevalence and factors associated with pulmonary tuberculosis infection among HIV/AIDS patients attending an ART clinic: A study at Fort Portal Regional Referral Hospital. *IDOSR Journal of Biochemistry, Biotechnology and Allied Fields*. https://www.semanticscholar.org/paper/adc6d177c7189236d6f737310edafd8d3ca1ebcd (accessed on 10 May 2025).

30. Potestio, L., Patruno, C., Dastoli, S., Brescia, C., & Napolitano, M. (2024). Tralokinumab for the treatment of adult atopic dermatitis in special populations. *Journal of Asthma and Allergy, 17*, 791–799. https://www.semanticscholar.org/paper/c69ee97336605aaf30749afd5ce3ab469299ee27 (accessed on 10 May 2025).

31. Pusporini, Tamtomo D, Prasetya H (2024). Adherence to Direct Observed Treatment Short-Course Treatment in Tuberculosis: Application of the Health Belief Model. J. Health Promot Behav. 09(02): 154-165. https://doi.org/10.26911/thejhpb.2024.09.02.06. (accessed on 10 May 2025).

32. Rehm, J., Gmel, G., Gmel, G., Hasan, O. S. M., Imtiaz, S., Popova, S., Probst, C., et al. (2017). The relationship between different dimensions of alcohol use and the burden of disease—An update. *Addiction, 112*(6), 968–1001. https://doi.org/10.1111/add.13757.

33. Stovner, L. J., Nichols, E., Steiner, T. J., Abd-Allah, F., Abdelalim, A., Al-Raddadi, R., Ansha, M. G.,

et al. (2018). Global, regional, and national burden of migraine and tension-type headache, 1990–2016: A systematic analysis for the Global Burden of Disease Study 2016. *The Lancet Neurology, 17*(11), 954–976. https://doi.org/10.1016/s1474-4422(18)30322-3.

34. Thromboprophylaxis Working Group on Guidelines for, COVID Management of Anticoagulation in Hospitalized Patients, Pulmonary Embolism, Society Pulmonary Vascular Diseases Group of the Chinese T, Physicians Pulmonary Vascular Disease Working Committee of China, & Prevention National Cooperation Group on Pulmonary Embolism Treatment of Pulmonary. (2023). Practice guidelines of thromboprophylaxis and management of anticoagulation in hospitalized patients with COVID-19. *Zhonghua Yi Xue Za Zhi, 103*, 1–23. https://www.semanticscholar.org/paper/c8b4d7d12ee9930831851047b062a49d13bcba35 (accessed on 10 May 2025).

35. Tiwari, J. P., B., P., & A. V., V. K. (2023). Post kidney transplant infections with special reference to cytomegalovirus. *International Journal of Research in Medical Sciences*, *11*(10), 3672–3680. https://doi.org/10.18203/2320-6012.ijrms20233017 (accessed on 10 May 2025).

36. Zhang, Y. P., Niu, Y., & Tang, P. (2023). Progress on the safety and efficacy of bedaquiline for the treatment of drug-resistant tuberculosis in special populations. *Zhonghua Jie He He Hu Xi Za Zhi = Zhonghua Jiehe He Huxi Zazhi = Chinese Journal of Tuberculosis and Respiratory Diseases, 46*(6), 619–624. https://www.semanticscholar.org/paper/ab68268a2ba0124c75fbd59dace27170913ee69c (accessed on 10 May 2025).\

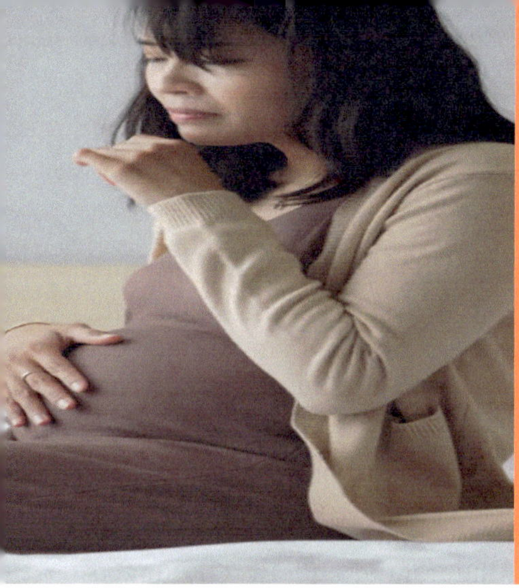

Chapter 11

TB IN PREGNANCY AND OTHER SPECIAL SITUATIONS

Contents

Introduction

The overlap of tuberculosis (TB) and pregnancy, and other rare clinical contexts, is a complex challenge in worldwide health. Pregnancy adds an element of physiological change that can potentially affect the host immune system, thus modifying susceptibility to TB infection or disease progression. Such changes make it challenging to diagnose and treat TB, requiring close attention to the mother and fetus's welfare. Furthermore, TB in pregnancy often coexists with other health complications, making treatment strategies more complex. The burden of TB remains significant in many parts of the world, particularly in regions with limited healthcare resources. Addressing TB within special populations requires an integrated approach that combines obstetric care with infectious disease expertise to optimize outcomes. It is important to set this challenge within the context of prevailing guidelines on infectious diseases and immunocompromised conditions to place the subtleties of these clinical contexts (Nast et al., 2020). The understanding of the interaction between TB and pregnancy demands a critical scrutiny of immunological modifications occurring with pregnancy. The modified immune environment of pregnant women can complicate the usual symptomatology of TB, thus withholding diagnosis and proper treatment. This delay increases the risk of unwanted outcomes like maternal morbidity, vertical transmission, and neonatal complications. Additionally, the pharmacokinetics of anti-TB drugs can differ in pregnancy, requiring appropriate dosing and monitoring to provide therapeutic effectiveness with minimal risks. Outside of pregnancy, additional special conditions like HIV co-infection, diabetes, and immunosuppression further hinder TB treatment.

These concurrent states of health demand individualized intervention guided by evidence-based practice guidelines, highlighting the need for multidisciplinary care guided by changing clinical recommendations (Lamb et al., 2019). The relevance of managing TB during pregnancy and other challenging clinical situations transcends single-patient care to higher-order public health concerns. Pregnant women with TB are part of the reservoir of infection and could influence community transmission patterns. Therefore, early detection and treatment are critical to preventing disease transmission and enhancing long-term outcomes for both mothers and children. TB screening and management must be integrated into antenatal services by health systems to ensure accessibility and continuity of care. This strategy is consistent with modern plans of personalized medicine and integrated patient care, borrowing from available systemic approaches to chronic diseases and infectious diseases (Lamb et al., 2019; Nast et al., 2020). Such convergence optimizes maternal and newborn health outcomes and promotes global TB control in high-risk populations.

Importance of Studying TB in Pregnancy

The interaction between pregnancy and tuberculosis (TB) is a clinical challenge with a need for comprehensive investigation. TB is a major infectious cause of maternal mortality and morbidity, particularly in low- and middle-income countries (LMICs), where the disease burden is further complicated by the availability of healthcare resources and infrastructure. Understanding how TB impacts pregnant patients is important because infection can impair maternal and fetal growth at the same time. Such an intersection can facilitate the creation of specific screening programs and early interventions, lowering pregnancy complications such as preterm birth, low birth weight, and mortality in the neonatal period. Additionally, the function of healthcare professionals, especially nurses, who are a core part of public health initiatives and emergency services, is critical in controlling TB in pregnancy for improved mother and child health (Denholm et al., 2012). Pregnancy specifically changes the immune system, and this affects susceptibility to infection with TB.

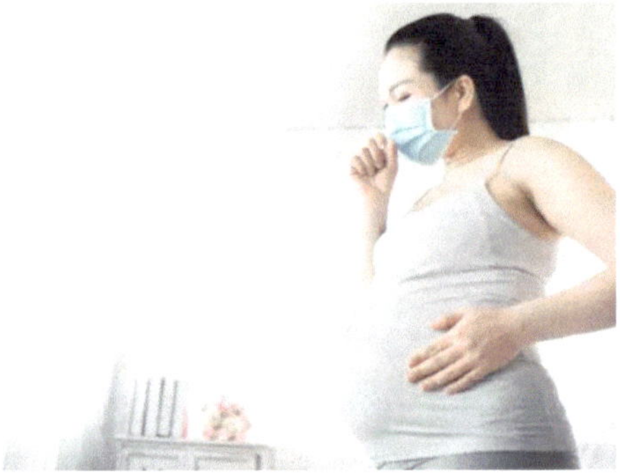

Source: The Economic Times. (n.d.). *Raising awareness about tuberculosis through community engagement.* https://etimg.etb2bimg.com/photo/90935916.cms.

During pregnancy, immune changes potentially enhance the chances of TB reactivation or re-activation in latent infection, transforming pregnant women into a high-risk population that demands special attention. Plowing research into these physiological and immunological changes has the potential to shape the optimization of diagnostic approaches, treatment schedules, and preventive interventions specific to pregnancy. Additionally, since treating TB comprises extended multidrug therapy with the possibility of teratogenicity, research into TB within the context of pregnancy allows for safer clinical practice to reconcile mother and baby well-being.

Increased understanding in this field might also inform public health policy and resource planning for preventing TB-related complications in at-risk populations as part of wider efforts addressing international disease burdens and health inequalities (Denholm et al., 2012). The significance of TB research in pregnancy goes beyond the care of individual patients to involve wider social and economic factors. Pregnant women with TB frequently suffer compounding vulnerabilities of stigma, gender inequality, and diminished access to quality care. This combination is not only a factor in poorer adherence to treatment but also in maternal mental well-being and household stability. Research in this area underpins the creation of holistic care models that bring together clinical management and social support systems so that the entire person is cared for. In addition, research on TB during pregnancy can uncover vital information regarding mother-to-child transmission dynamics that can guide preventative measures like maternal immunization or neonatal interventions early in life. Its contribution to resolving these challenges via committed research eventually enhances world health constructs and attains maternal and child health sustainable development goals (Denholm et al., 2012).

11.1. Tuberculosis (TB) in Pregnancy

Pregnancy triggers dramatic physiological changes that influence the immune system and make women immunocompromised, thereby more prone to infections like TB. The immunological adjustments intended to safeguard the fetus have the indirect effect of weakening the body's capacity to harbor latent tuberculosis infections (LTBIs), thus enhancing active disease risk during pregnancy. TB diagnosis in pregnant women is challenging because of the overlapping signs with pregnancy conditions, like fever and fatigue, that may provoke delayed treatment and recognition. Additionally, the risks involved in using diagnostic imaging for the fetus tend to postpone the application of chest radiographs, further hindering early diagnosis. These diagnostic difficulties demand a high degree of suspicion, especially in endemic areas or in women who have a history of exposure to TB, to avoid harmful maternal and neonatal outcomes. Treatment of tuberculosis during pregnancy presents clinical dilemmas where maternal health is weighed against fetal safety. First-line agents of anti-TB such as isoniazid, rifampin, and ethambutol are safe and should be used to avoid the risk of disease exacerbation. Nevertheless, the prescription of some of these second-line agents is limited because of their teratogenicity. Strict adherence to treatment is needed to avoid drug resistance, which is particularly problematic in pregnancy since multi-drug resistant tuberculosis (MDR-TB) regimens are limited and more toxic. Concurrent infection with HIV makes management even more complex, as ART needs to be optimized together with TB treatment without promoting adverse drug reactions or undermining immune recovery (Michael et al., 2018). Multidisciplinary management is essential to individualize treatments and observe maternal and fetal status throughout pregnancy. The effect on pregnancy outcome of tuberculosis highlights the need for early diagnosis and collaborative management. Untreated or poor treatment of TB during pregnancy is linked with increased miscarriage, preterm delivery, low birth weight, and perinatal death. Careful follow-up of nutritional status and comorbid conditions like other infections or chronic illnesses is crucial to maximize maternal health and fetal growth (Lamb et al., 2019). Multidisciplinary treatment regimens by obstetricians, infectious disease clinicians, and public health professionals maximize therapeutic compliance and minimize the risk of transmission. Screening initiatives among high-risk groups, within routine prenatal care, provide a strategic window of opportunity for early intervention. The resolution of the special challenge that TB represents during pregnancy ultimately calls for a greater investment in healthcare infrastructure and education to mitigate the disease burden in this at-risk group (Figure 11.1).

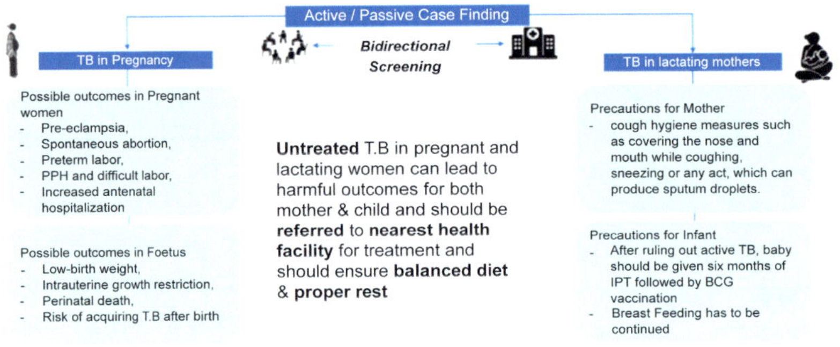

Figure 11.1. TB during pregnancy and lactation.

Source: National Tuberculosis Elimination Program (NTEP). (n.d.). *TB in pregnant and lactating women: Diagnosis and management guidelines.* https://ntep.in/node/652/CP-tb-pregnant-and-lactating-women.

11.1.1. Prevalence of Tuberculosis (TB) Among Pregnant Women

The intersection of TB and pregnancy is a special challenge to global health, especially for low- and middle-income countries (LMICs) where TB continues to be prevalent. Pregnant women, given physiological and immunological alterations, may be at increased risk of TB infection and reactivation of latent TB. The TB burden during pregnancy can be underestimated, in part because the signs and symptoms can blur with what is expected to be normal pregnancy complaints and therefore can result in underdiagnosis. Additionally, restricted access to proper healthcare fuels this situation, since diagnostic facilities are often under-equipped or unsuitable for pregnant women. Since LMICs are also the epicenter of the world's TB burden, their health systems need to reorganize to fulfill the twin needs of maternal and infectious disease treatment, to enhance detection and treatment among pregnant TB patients. Embracing the actual burden of TB among pregnant women requires credible information, which is usually lacking owing to the systemic weaknesses in health information systems within TB-high-burden countries. The absence of credible surveillance is further accentuated by social stigma and access barriers to health, hindering pregnant women from accessing timely diagnosis and treatment. As per the health care delivery analyses within LMICs, there are essential shortcomings in health outcome measurements, such as those for maternal conditions such as TB, which translate into inadequate monitoring of disease prevalence and cure. These shortcomings are indicative of more pervasive systemic failures where healthcare fails to deliver skilled care and quality user experience, both determinants of the early detection and control of TB during pregnancy (Humbert et al., 2022). Enhancing health system responsiveness and data convergence is, therefore, critical in ensuring an effective response to the burden of TB in pregnancy. The implications of the prevalence of TB among pregnant women extend beyond individual health to include maternal mortality and neonatal outcomes in a significant way. Research points out that TB complicates pregnancy by posing risk factors like preterm birth, low birth weight, and maternal morbidity. Despite the reduction of health improvements in certain settings, the recurrence of TB among pregnant populations requires that health system reforms focusing on quality and equity in care provision be championed (Humbert et al., 2022). Such reforms should incorporate the adoption of TB screening within routine antenatal care as well as ensuring that healthcare providers are trained and equipped to address TB within the context of pregnancy (Humbert et al., 2022). By integrating these strategies into larger initiatives to improve the quality of maternity and infectious disease care, it is possible to reduce the negative impacts of TB on maternal and child health outcomes (Figure 11.2).

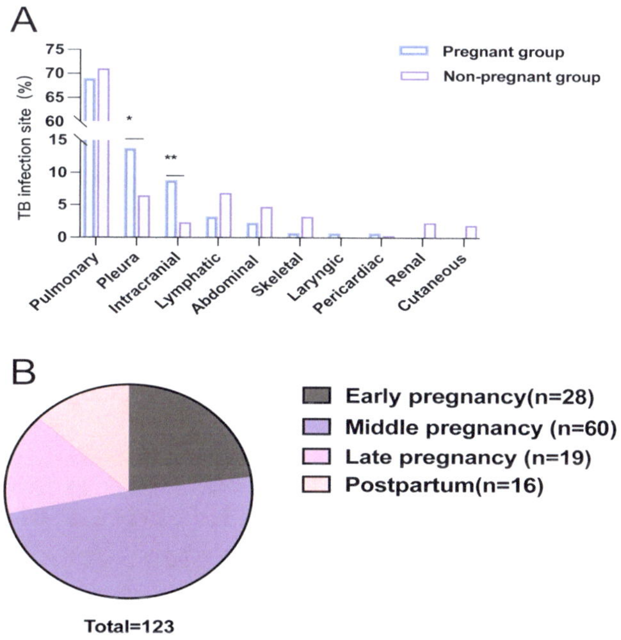

Figure 11.2. In the pregnant group, 48.8% of patients experienced TB-related clinical symptoms during the middle stage of pregnancy, as indicated by the detailed distribution provided in panel B.

Source: Taylor & Francis Online. (2024). *Tuberculosis in pregnancy: A review of current practices and challenges.* https://www.tandfonline.com/doi/full/10.1080/07853890.2024.2401108#d1e295.

11.1.2. Impact of Tuberculosis (TB) on Maternal Health

Maternal health outcomes are significantly affected by a variety of infectious diseases, and of these, TB is a major but sometimes overlooked risk. Pregnant women with TB are at increased risk of adverse outcomes of preterm labor, low birth weight, and elevated maternal mortality. This increased susceptibility stems primarily from the immunological and physiological alterations of pregnancy that impair the body's capacity to contain the infection effectively. Compounding these problems, the majority of health systems, particularly in LMICs, have insufficient quality of care, delays in diagnosis, and weak treatment support mechanisms for adherence, all of which complicate maternal health outcomes in TB-affected pregnancies negatively. If left untreated or inadequately treated, TB can worsen maternal morbidity, posing a clinical challenge that resonates beyond the pregnancy itself to impact long-term maternal and neonatal health. The overlap of TB and pregnancy also adds nuance to health delivery that demands expertise in managing dual imperatives that meet the special needs of pregnant patients. Health systems are charged not only with effective diagnosis and cure but also with coordinating care that takes into consideration the dual health imperatives of the mother and fetus. Even with improvements in healthcare facilities and treatment regimens, a lot of women remain inadequately treated for TB during pregnancy because of poor service delivery and insufficiencies in training among providers (Bhatla et al., 2018). Moreover, stigma and attendant complications during pregnancy prevent women from attending care promptly, thus exacerbating outcomes. Strengthening maternal healthcare systems to include comprehensive TB screening, counseling, and treatment adherence programs is key to minimizing maternal TB-related mortality and morbidity. Mitigating the effect of TB on maternal health requires systemic quality of care improvements and targeted interventions. At the center of this is the requirement for health systems to provide equitable access to quality TB services during pregnancy, especially among vulnerable groups who bear a disproportionate burden of disease and have restricted healthcare access (Bhatla et al., 2018). Quality maternal TB care demands integration of the most current evidence-based practices and innovations to reduce diagnostic delays and avoid poor pregnancy outcomes. Interdisciplinary collaboration between infectious disease and obstetric specialists, along with ongoing capacity development of healthcare workers, can improve quality of care and patient confidence. Ultimately, improving maternal health outcomes in TB-affected pregnancies is consistent with other global health objectives of decreasing maternal mortality and advancing equitable, high-quality care (Bhatla et al., 2018).

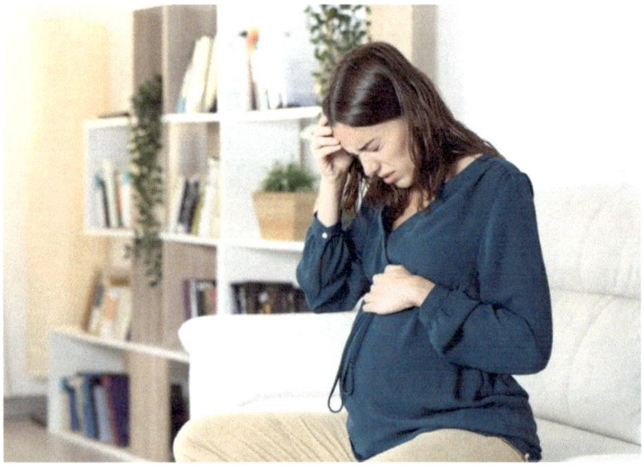

Source: News Medical. (n.d.). *Pregnant woman undergoing tuberculosis screening.* https://d2jx2rerrg6sh3.cloudfront.net/images/Article_Images/ImageForArticle_22377_16499293234115785.jpg.

11.1.3. Effects of Tuberculosis (TB) on Fetal Development

The interaction between pregnancy and infectious diseases both complicates fetal and maternal health outcomes and poses challenges in the form of TB to fetal development. Tuberculosis infection in pregnancy may disrupt normal placental function, an organ that plays a very important role in both oxygen and nutrient exchange between the fetus and mother. Disruptions in placental development and differentiation, especially in the epithelial trophoblast cells, have been associated with poor outcomes such as fetal growth restriction and preeclampsia. Placental pathologies underlying these conditions frequently originate from reduced cellular proliferation and differentiation, mechanisms controlled by pathways such as NOTCH3 signaling, critical for the preservation of trophoblast progenitor self-renewal as well as placental integrity (Dietrich et al., 2023). When TB disrupts placental function, it may result in inadequate fetal nutrition and oxygenation and eventually hinder fetal development and growth. In addition to the direct nutritional and oxygen deficiencies due to impaired placenta, TB infection has also been linked to the heightened risk of vertical transmission, whereby the pathogen penetrates the placental barrier to infect the fetus itself. Such vertical transmission has the potential to cause severe consequences, such as intrauterine fetal death or congenital infection that affects fetal organ systems. Vertical transmission mechanism of infectious disease has been highly researched in other contexts, like with the Zika virus, for which pregnancy vaccination was demonstrated to decrease placental pathology and virus transmission without negatively affecting fetal development (Kim et al., 2024). This comparison highlights the significance of immune modulation and specific therapeutic intervention in preventing infection-induced fetal complications, with the point being made that TB infection in pregnancy can likewise endanger fetal health by both direct and indirect means. In addition, the intrauterine environment modified by TB can deflect the course of fetal development by means of inflammatory and immune-mediated pathways. Chronic maternal infection causes systemic inflammation that can interfere with placental homeostasis, worsen placental insufficiency, and trigger preterm labor or low birth weight. These results lead to long-term developmental disabilities or elevated neonatal mortality. Significantly, the disruption of trophoblast stem cell renewal and differentiation in placental infections undermines the adaptive ability of the placenta to handle inflammatory insults (Dietrich et al., 2023). Therefore, making sense of TB's influence on placental biology is necessary for avoiding adverse fetal outcomes, emphasizing the necessity of comprehensive perinatal care programs that incorporate early detection, successful treatment of TB during pregnancy, and possible immunization strategies emulating successful programs from other infectious diseases (Kim et al., 2024).

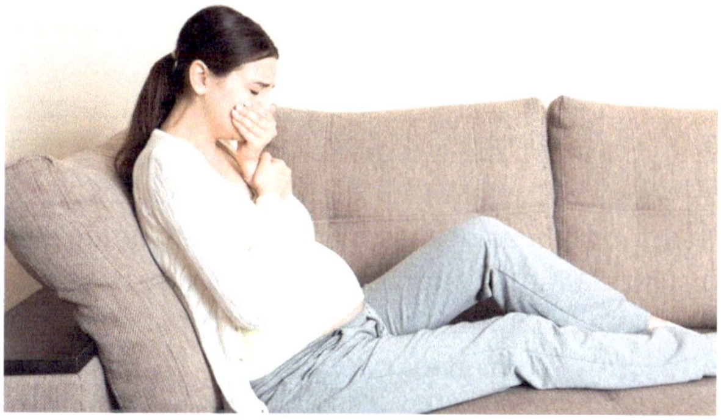

Source: OnlyMyHealth. (2024). *Pregnant woman with tuberculosis wearing a mask.* https://images.onlymyhealth.com/imported/images/2024/July/19_Jul_2024/Main_TB.jpg.

11.2. Risk Factors for Tuberculosis (TB) in Pregnant Women

The interaction between immune modulation in pregnancy and the heightened susceptibility to infectious diseases accounts for much of the risk of TB in pregnant women. Pregnancy causes a deviation toward an increased immunosuppressive state, most importantly on cell-mediated immunity, which is essential for the control of *Mycobacterium tuberculosis* (MTB) infection. Such an immunological change can predispose LTBIs to progression to active disease or worsen pre-existing TB conditions. Moreover, pregnant women with comorbid conditions like HIV or diabetes are at increased susceptibility since comorbidities compound immune vulnerability. The compound difficulty is seen in migrants from TB-endemic regions who have been found to present with untreated or undiagnosed infections. Multidisciplinary coordination for proper screening and management is necessary, but the emotional distress that comes with having a diagnosis of TB during pregnancy complicates treatment success and adherence (Zerihun et al., 2016). Hence, it is important to comprehend the physiological and socio-medical determinants of TB risk in pregnancy to plan interventions. Socioeconomic and geographical determinants are also of prime importance in raising TB risk in pregnant women. Highly populated regions with poor healthcare infrastructure, especially in Sub-Saharan Africa and Asia, show high TB prevalence among pregnant women. Poverty, undernutrition, and poor access to antenatal care aggravate vulnerability, as they restrict access to early detection and treatment. In addition, HIV co-infection significantly increases susceptibility to TB, with maternal HIV status being independently associated with TB incidence and risk of vertical transmission. The combined burden of TB and HIV establishes an unstable health situation, contributing to high maternal mortality rates and complicated pregnancies. Intervening upon these social determinants via enhanced access to healthcare, complete maternal history taking, and combined TB-HIV programs is vital to TB incidence reduction and maternal health improvement among these vulnerable populations (Adhikari et al., 2011). Direct and ongoing exposure to an infectious TB case is yet another significant risk factor for pregnant women and calls for an aggressive approach to prophylaxis and treatment. Women exposed to active pulmonary TB, particularly those with immune suppression or obstetric risk factors, are advised to receive primary Isoniazid prophylaxis to prevent disease progression. Diagnosing active TB in pregnancy is still elusive based on overlapping symptoms and limitations of diagnosis, which can lead to delays in initiating treatment and enhancing risk to both mother and fetus. Where mothers present with active TB at birth, thorough assessments of the newborn and compliance with prophylactic therapy are essential to avoid vertical transmission. The multifaceted management calls for synchronization between pulmonologists, obstetricians, and infectious disease experts to weigh effective treatment against possible adverse impact on pregnancy (Zerihun et al., 2016). Comprehensive integrated care guidelines improve TB control during pregnancy, protecting maternal and neonatal health (Figure 11.3).

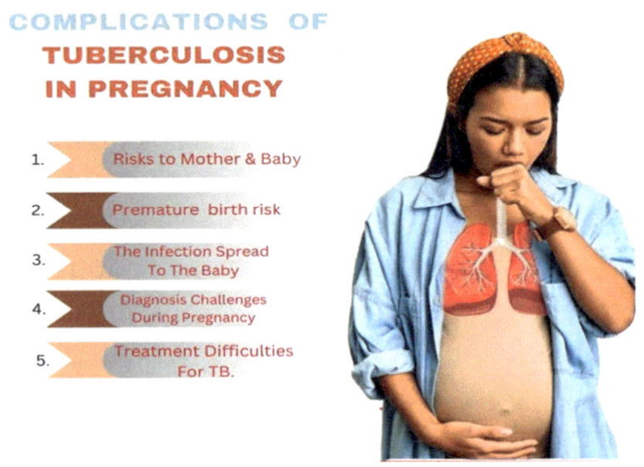

Figure 11.3. Tuberculosis (TB) in pregnancy can lead to several complications for both the mother and the fetus.

Source: Modern Hospital. (n.d.). *Tuberculosis awareness and maternal health.* https://www.instagram.com/modernhospital___/p/DFrjgOspz8K/.

11.2.1. Socioeconomic Factors

The interaction between TB and socioeconomic determinants has a significant impact on disease outcomes, especially among vulnerable groups like pregnant women. These determinants tend to determine access to healthcare services, treatment adherence, and exposure to environments that are favorable for TB transmission. In low socioeconomic environments, scarce resources often limit early diagnosis and regular treatment, aggravating the risk of pregnancy complications. In addition, poverty-related malnutrition and over-populated living also can compromise immune responses, elevating vulnerability to TB infection and disease progression. These socioeconomic limitations are further supplemented by systemic healthcare deficiencies in the form of inadequate programmatic support and ineffective patient education that together erode effective TB control. These issues underscore the importance of interventions that are specifically directed towards the clinical features as well as the determinants of social health responsible for TB's prevalence among pregnant women and other vulnerable populations (Girma et al., 2015). Pregnancy involves special physiological and immunological alterations that may affect the progression of TB disease, thus exacerbating socioeconomic inequalities even further. Women from disadvantaged socioeconomic backgrounds frequently endure extraneous stresses, such as food insecurity and restricted prenatal care, that can compromise their capacity to treat TB appropriately. The co-occurrence of MDR-TB with HIV co-infection, common in resource-poor settings, makes it even more challenging for pregnant women to treat effectively. This co-occurrence of infectious comorbidities and socioeconomic disadvantage requires holistic healthcare strategies that incorporate social support, drug adherence interventions, and increased monitoring. Resolution of these converging factors is essential to avoid negative maternal and fetal outcomes and minimize community transmission of TB, highlighting an integrated perspective of TB management that does not confine itself to pharmacological intervention (Girma et al., 2015). Loss to follow-up (LTFU), another important area of socioeconomic impact on TB treatment, predominantly affects people of marginalized communities. Research has established that LTFU among TB patients continues to persist as a strong barrier to treatment success, frequently fueled by a deficit of social support and poverty. Even though some research on LTFU in HIV-uninfected TB patients has not uniformly identified particular socioeconomic determinants, the majority of evidence suggests that factors linked to poverty, such as uncertain accommodation and transportation issues, impede ongoing interaction with healthcare services. Moreover, gender differences, with males presenting greater LTFU risk, reflect sociocultural aspects that overlap with economic issues. Measures to reduce LTFU must thus include socioeconomic factors, including patient education, social welfare interventions, and community-based support systems, to improve retention in TB care, especially among pregnant women with compounded vulnerabilities (Moyo et al., 2017) (Figure 11.4).

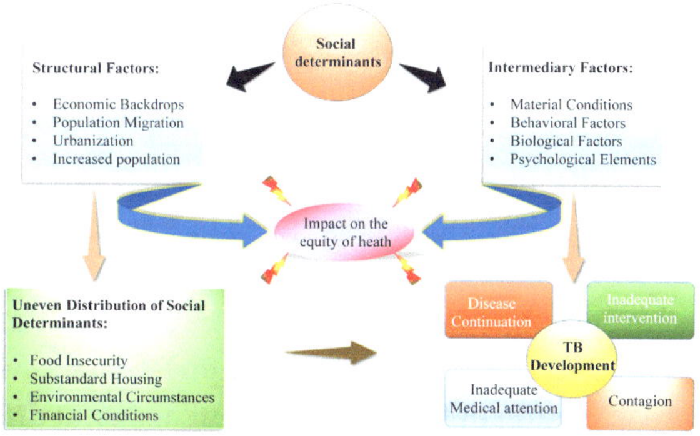

Figure 11.4. Impact of socioeconomic factors on the treatment of tuberculosis.

Source: Elsevier. (n.d.). *Management algorithm for tuberculosis in pregnancy.* https://ars.els-cdn.com/content/image/3-s2.0-B9780443240355500165-f16-01-9780443240355.jpg.

11.2.2. Pre-Existing Health Conditions

In the clinical setting, pre-existing medical conditions make treating TB in pregnancy extremely challenging, necessitating a sophisticated assessment of how such comorbidities interact with the disease process and with therapeutic interventions. The interaction between chronic conditions such as diabetes mellitus, cardiovascular diseases, and autoimmune diseases with TB is known to affect infection progression and response to treatment. Notably, immune system modification brought about by such conditions or their treatments may change TB susceptibility and outcome, particularly in pregnant women, where there are naturally occurring immunological changes. For example, the immunosuppressive action seen in some of the systemic treatments of chronic illnesses may place patients at risk for reactivation of latent TB or exacerbation of active infection and hence requires cautious risk evaluation and tailored therapeutic approaches that balance maternal and fetal safety (Nast et al., 2021). Such intricacy calls for multi-disciplinary management to maximize outcomes in this high-risk group.

In addition, some long-term pharmacologic management of pre-existing diseases could have a direct or indirect effect on TB control and pregnancy outcomes. Immunomodulatory drugs and biologics, often used for autoimmune diseases, have been found to be associated with an elevated risk of infectious complications, such as reactivation of latent TB. Although agents that act on the IL-23/Th17 inflammatory pathway have transformed the management of chronic inflammatory conditions, their safety profiles in pregnancy and concomitant TB are still being explored (Rend et al., 2019).

Methotrexate, commonly employed for autoimmune diseases, poses a further risk due to its teratogenicity and hepatotoxicity, which may be compounded by TB treatment. The physiological changes in pregnancy also alter drug pharmacokinetics, with the need for dose adjustment and close monitoring. Thus, knowing the pharmacological interaction between treatments of underlying conditions, pregnancy modifications, and TB treatment is essential for lessening side effects and maintaining therapeutic effectiveness. Finally, existing health conditions can contribute to modified diagnostic complexities and predictive outcomes of TB during pregnancy. Conditions like diabetes mellitus (DM) not only predispose to TB infection but also complicate clinical presentation, occasionally suppressing characteristic symptoms or retarding diagnosis. Similarly, renal and hepatic dysfunction prevalent in chronic diseases can restrict the application of first-line anti-TB drugs because of toxicity risks, necessitating alternative regimens with unpredictable safety profiles during pregnancy. The increased susceptibility of pregnant women with co-morbidities emphasizes the importance of comprehensive screening protocols and specially designed management strategies taking into account the combined effects of these conditions (Nast et al., 2021). Attempts to characterize these complex interactions hold the promise of decreasing maternal-fetal morbidity while refining personalized care models throughout special clinical contexts.

11.2.3. Environmental Influences

Environmental conditions contribute significantly to the vulnerability and development of TB, especially among susceptible groups like expectant women. Socioeconomic status, for example, overcrowding of the living area and poor ventilation, are factors that enhance exposure and MTB transmission. Such conditions tend to be compounded in resource-constrained environments, where the confluence of poverty and restricted access to healthcare services amplifies infection risk. Moreover, environmental contaminants and malnutrition can depress immune systems, making it more difficult for the body to suppress LTBIs. Such additive threats are particularly troublesome in pregnancy, where immune modulation to facilitate fetal development may enhance defense impairment. Thus, appreciating the broader environmental determinants is important in treating TB among pregnant women and underscores the necessity of integrative public health interventions involving both clinical and environmental determinants. Antibiotic resistance, developing as a serious environmental health problem, also adds to the difficulty of TB control during pregnancy and other special circumstances. The widespread application of antibiotics in agriculture and animal husbandry has led to the carryover of antibiotic residues in animal products, which can encourage resistant bacterial strains among human populations. These resistant pathogens can be readily spread by food chains and distributed among environmental reservoirs, increasing the risk of incurable infections. In developing nations, poor regulation and surveillance of antibiotic use accelerate this process, directly challenging successful TB treatment regimens. Pregnant women, being at elevated risk for TB complications in the first place, may experience increased morbidity from resistant infections, which emphasizes the need for antibiotic stewardship programs and greater international collaboration in the monitoring and control of antibiotic resistance (Christy et al., 2018). In addition to the complexity of managing TB in pregnancy, the management is further complicated by concomitant chronic diseases driven by environmental determinants, like inflammatory bowel disease (IBD). Rising clinical guidelines account for the need to take into consideration environmental precipitating factors and their effect on immune system dysregulation, which can coincide with TB pathogenesis. Co-morbid inflammatory disorders present require individualized therapeutic interventions that take into consideration drug metabolism changes and immune status during pregnancy. The new evidence-based frameworks put emphasis on combining environmental and clinical information to maximize outcomes among pregnant women with TB and complications. Such holistic models of care are crucial to meet the multi-level effects of environmental factors on disease presentation and treatment outcomes in special populations (Matsuoka et al., 2018).

11.3. Diagnosis of Tuberculosis (TB) in Pregnant Women

Pregnancy causes several physiological and immune alterations that make clinical diagnosis of TB more difficult. Most active TB symptoms, for example, fatigue, low-grade fever, and weight loss are very similar to common pregnancy-related aches, hence delayed suspicion and diagnosis. Secondly, radiographic imaging, a routine diagnostic procedure for pulmonary TB, tends to cause anxiety regarding fetal safety and is therefore restricted. This leads to a dependence on other diagnostic tools like sputum smear microscopy and molecular diagnostics, although these may be less sensitive in pregnancy. The issue is compounded by the common finding of smear-negative TB among pregnant women, especially those with co-infection of HIV, lowering the sensitivity of traditional diagnostic strategies and the need for more sensitive, rapid, and pregnancy-specific testing strategies. The challenge of diagnosis worsens in areas with high co-infection prevalence of HIV and TB. Sub-Saharan Africa is a case in point, where the double burden of the diseases severely impedes timely diagnosis among pregnant women. HIV infection not only makes people more susceptible to TB but also modifies the clinical presentation of the disease, concealing symptoms and resulting in higher rates of smear-negative TB. This diagnostic sophistication requires combined screening strategies that integrate symptom screening with imaging and molecular technologies to identify TB early without jeopardizing maternal or fetal well-being. The implications of delayed diagnosis go beyond maternal morbidity because untreated TB in pregnancy has been linked to poor outcomes including preterm birth, low birth weight, and excess neonatal mortality (Jo et al., 2022). Though pregnancy limits the diagnostic approaches, current developments promote safer, more efficient protocols. Imaging modalities like ultrasound and magnetic resonance imaging (MRI) have been used as adjunctive measures for detecting extrapulmonary tuberculosis (EPTB) manifestations that may not be easy to detect otherwise. Furthermore, laparoscopy, as in rare instances like suspected adnexal masses in pregnancy, presents a minimally invasive technique for direct view and biopsy where abdominal TB involvement is suspected, thereby facilitating correct diagnosis without compromising pregnancy (Jo et al., 2022). Such evolving approaches highlight the need to modify diagnostic models to suit individual pregnant women with suspected TB to enhance maternal and fetal outcomes.

11.3.1. Screening Methods

Adequate screening processes are important for the early detection and control of TB among susceptible groups like pregnant women and those in special circumstances. Pregnancy provides special challenges since immunological changes during this phase can modify the presentation and course of TB such that early diagnosis is of crucial importance.

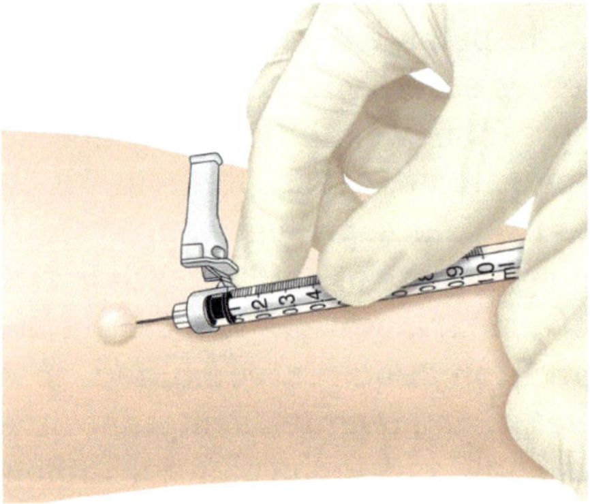

Figure 11.5. Tuberculin skin test (TST).

Source: Centers for Disease Control and Prevention (CDC). (n.d.). *Administering the Mantoux tuberculin skin test (TST).* https://www.cdc.gov/tb/media/images/Administering_the_Mantoux_TST_1200x675.jpg.

Classic screening methods such as the tuberculin skin test (TST) and interferon-gamma release assays (IGRAs) are used as first-line tools, but their sensitivity is affected by immune modulation during pregnancy. Radiographic imaging is also informative but should be used cautiously due to risks to the unborn child. The combination of clinical risk assessment with these tests improves the accuracy of the screening. Thus, a personalized strategy integrating immunologic tests, symptom assessment, and judicious radiographic use is necessary to ensure optimum results with minimal risks in these special circumstances (Nast et al., 2020) (Figure 11.5).

Outside of pregnancy, screening technologies need to be responsive to the multifaceted needs of other high-risk populations, such as migrants, immunocompromised patients, and individuals with comorbidities. Migrants tend to experience barriers to accessing healthcare, which makes it difficult for them to be screened and diagnosed for TB on time. Cultural, language, and system barriers may hinder presentation, elevating the risk of transmission and development into active disease. Therefore, screening procedures with targeted symptom screening coupled with IGRA or TST testing offer a viable strategy. Additionally, in light of differences in *Bacillus Calmette-Guérin* (BCG) vaccination status among migrants, IGRAs are useful because they have greater specificity. Providing equitable and universally accessible screening services is of utmost importance for TB control in these heterogenous groups (Lebano et al., 2020). Under special circumstances where usual screening tools may be lacking or contraindicated, novel approaches need to be applied. For instance, during pregnancy, molecular diagnostic tests like nucleic acid amplification tests (NAATs) can allow for quicker identification of MTB with improved sensitivity and specificity without exposing the fetus to radiation. Furthermore, in immunocompromised individuals, where immune-based tests can provide false-negative findings, incorporation of microbiological culture and imaging becomes crucial. Personalizing screening strategies to patient risk profiles, clinical settings, and logistical considerations boosts diagnostic yield, promotes early intervention, and ultimately leads to better maternal and fetal health outcomes. These subtle, patient-level screening strategies are the key to treating TB during pregnancy and other special populations effectively (Lebano et al., 2020; Nast et al., 2020).

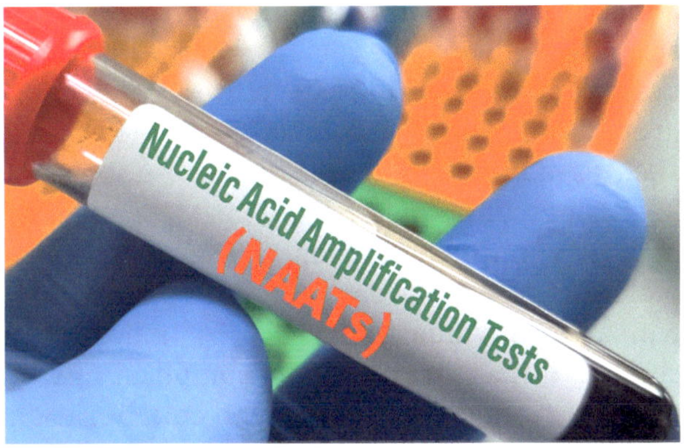

Source: Netmeds. (2023). *Nucleic acid amplification tests (NAATs) for tuberculosis diagnosis.* https://www.netmeds.com/images/cms/wysiwyg/blog/2023/10/1697541888_nucleic-acid-amplification-tests_898x450.jpg.

11.3.2. Challenges in Diagnosis

Correct diagnosis of TB in pregnancy is faced with special challenges that hinder early detection and proper control. The physiological alterations that characterize pregnancy, e.g., higher plasma volume and shifts in immune functions, are common to obscure usual manifestations of TB, rendering clinical presentations milder or uncharacteristic. In addition, overlapping signs such as tiredness, weight reduction, and low-grade fever get interpreted as manifestations of pregnancy, and thus the disease gets underestimated or misinterpreted. Therefore, clinicians will refrain from requesting thorough screening or invasive diagnostic tests to avoid causing injury to the fetus. These delays may lead to the advancement of the infection, thus elevating the risk of maternal and neonatal complications. These diagnostic issues highlight the urgent necessity for specialized training and guidelines that go against the nuances of TB among pregnant women, thus ensuring the best early detection and intervention methods (Denholm et al., 2012). Adding to the challenge of diagnosis is the compromised sensitivity and specificity of standard TB testing in pregnant patients. Routine instruments such as the TST and IGRAs can provide false-negative or indeterminate results due to pregnancy-related immune modulation. Radiologic evaluation, another pillar of TB diagnosis, is often avoided or postponed during pregnancy because of fears regarding fetal radiation exposure, limiting clinicians' ability to establish pulmonary involvement. This dependence on less specific clinical evaluation frequently inhibits timely diagnosis and the initiation of proper treatment. Besides, the presentation of EPTB among immunocompromised or pregnant women poses additional complexity as it necessitates more invasive and costly diagnostic approaches. These constraints underscore the urgent need for safer, more accurate diagnostic tools directed to the prenatal setting. Healthcare infrastructure and resource limitations further aggravate diagnostic challenges in specialized environments such as pregnancy or comorbidities. In most low-resource settings with high TB prevalence, access to sophisticated diagnostics and expert clinical assessment is not available, thereby underdiagnosing or misdiagnosing TB in pregnant women. Secondly, inter-disciplinary coordination among obstetricians, infectious disease experts, and public health experts is not often adequate, ensuing disjointed care pathways. Healthcare professionals might not have particular knowledge or practice about TB's uncommon clinical presentation in pregnancy and other special contexts, lowering the diagnostic watchfulness. Overcoming these structural barriers means not just enhancing diagnostic technology but also fortifying the workforce capability and putting in place better care models that are integrated. Through improved collaboration and education as proposed in more comprehensive public health programs, diagnostic precision can be enhanced, hence morbidity and mortality due to TB in vulnerable groups can be minimized (Suratman et al., 2014).

11.3.3. Importance of Early Detection

Early detection of TB in pregnant women is important not just for the mother's health but also for the developing child. If TB goes undetected, the disease can silently advance, resulting in severe consequences like preterm labor, low birth weight, and fetal loss. Immunological changes during pregnancy can hide initial symptoms and thus delay clinical suspicion and diagnosis. Consequently, early diagnosis enables early initiation of anti-tubercular (ATT) treatment, limiting maternal morbidity and mortality. It also prevents vertical transmission, whose neonatal effects can be debilitating. This reinforces the need for incorporating TB screening in universal antenatal care, especially among endemic areas, to improve both maternal and infant outcomes. The application of such screening programs has been found to enhance health outcomes despite infrastructural limitations regarding specialized regional autonomy as well as resource allocation (Suratman et al., 2014). Apart from the implications on individual health, early detection of TB during pregnancy also has greater public health implications. Where HIV co-infection is prevalent, for example, in parts of Sub-Saharan Africa and Asia, the interaction between TB and HIV makes both diagnosis and treatment challenging. The combination of maternal TB with HIV increases maternal mortality, exceeding that associated with conventional causes of obstetric mortality. Rapid detection of TB, together with determination of HIV status, allows for full care plans, including ART and infection control to prevent vertical transmission. Inability to diagnose TB early will result in heightened perinatal morbidity and mortality, putting additional pressure on healthcare facilities and social infrastructures. Thus, early diagnosis is a key element for attainment of global health goals for maternal and infant mortality reduction in limited-resource environments (Adhikari et al., 2011). In addition, early diagnosis of TB during pregnancy is part of solving systemic healthcare inequalities and enhancing health equity, particularly in special administrative regions. Even with raised health budgets and infrastructure construction in accordance with specific autonomy legislation, such as has been done in Papua, suboptimal health outcomes persist owing to challenges in policy implementation and access. Early diagnosis of TB prevents delay in intervention, which can reverse these gaps by limiting the chronic disease burden and complications. It also encourages intersectoral collaboration between government and non-government agencies to strengthen maternal health services and nutrition support programs that are critical during pregnancy. Therefore, early detection is a central point for coordinating the delivery of care, enhancing both epidemiological outcomes and the quality of maternal health care in multi-actor and complex socio-political contexts (Suratman et al., 2014).

11.4. Treatment Options for Tuberculosis (TB) in Pregnancy

Treating TB in pregnancy requires careful planning owing to the twin requirement of safeguarding maternal and fetal health. Treatment regimens should balance efficacy with the need to avoid the teratogenic effects of antitubercular drugs. First-line drugs such as isoniazid, rifampin, and ethambutol are generally regarded as safe and continue to be the cornerstone of treatment throughout pregnancy. Streptomycin, however, is contraindicated due to its ototoxic effects on the fetus. Initiation of therapy is important to decrease maternal morbidity and avoid vertical transmission, but also has to be watched closely for detection of adverse reactions. As pregnancy itself has an effect on drug metabolism, dosage might have to be adjusted to provide therapeutic levels. Duration of treatment usually parallels that in non-pregnancy patients, about six to nine months with close observation. This strategic equilibrium highlights the complexity of TB care during pregnancy, promoting individualized interventions to maximize mother and child outcomes (Negro et al., 2017). In addition to pharmacologic issues, TB in pregnancy should also address non-pharmacologic measures. Among them are nutrition support and adherence counseling, which are of utmost importance for coping with concomitant pregnancy and TB-related physiological and psychosocial burdens. Nutritional status has a direct effect on immunocompetence and drug metabolism, so dietary interventions are integral to overall management. Also, tight collaboration with obstetricians and infectious disease specialists enables monitoring of all aspects comprehensively, including fetal growth and maternal response to treatment. The occurrence of comorbidities like HIV infection also complicates the process of treatment decisions and makes individualized care plans more imperative. In concert with these non-pharmacologic measures, treatment adherence is promoted and complications are reduced, supporting optimal maternal and fetal health outcomes (Negro et al., 2017). Systemic access to healthcare is particularly important for the effective treatment of TB in pregnancy in vulnerable low-income groups who experience care disparities. Ensuring timely diagnosis and seamless access to care is contingent on eliminating system-level barriers like insurance coverage and access to specialized services. Advocacy and community-level support mechanisms have been found to play a critical role in helping pregnant women navigate complicated healthcare systems, with guarantees of enrollment in the right programs and retention in care. Legal and social support services also play a part in addressing non-medical determinants likely to impair treatment compliance. Thus, incorporating social support models with clinical care constitutes an integrative model of care that is crucial for this high-risk population and enhances immediate as well as long-term health outcomes in pregnant women with TB (Figure 11.6).

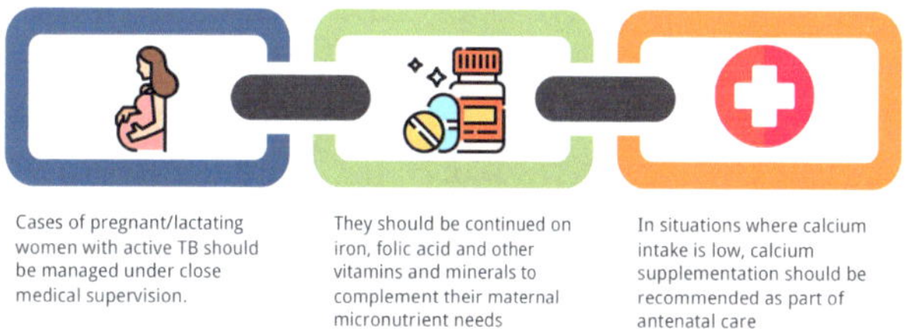

Figure 11.6. Treatment for TB in pregnant and lactating women.

Source: National Tuberculosis Elimination Program (NTEP). (n.d.). *TB in pregnant and lactating women: Diagnosis and management guidelines.* https://ntep.in/node/652/CP-tb-pregnant-and-lactating-women.

11.4.1. Recommended Medications

Treating TB in pregnancy requires a balance between optimal pathogen elimination and avoiding fetal risk, which heavily influences the choice of recommended drugs. Treatment regimens tend to favor first-line antituberculous drugs, including isoniazid, rifampicin, and ethambutol, because of their known safety in pregnancy. PZA use is more controversial, with some recommendations supporting its use to reduce the duration of treatment and others calling for caution because of scarce teratogenicity data. Drugs such as streptomycin are contraindicated secondary to ototoxic risk to the fetus. The need to manage active TB effectively in pregnancy is highlighted by the risk for vertical transmission and adverse perinatal outcome if not properly addressed. Accordingly, therapeutic guidelines are customized to limit drug-related risks without sacrificing therapeutic outcomes, depicting the complexities described in contemporary clinical guidelines that stress pragmatic approaches for diverse patient groups in TB management. In special contexts like DR-TB and concurrent infections like HIV, medication regimens have to be modified. For patients carrying MDR-TB strains, second-line medications carry greater teratogenic hazards, complicating treatment choices. In addition, ART in HIV-positive pregnant women requires harmonization with TB drugs to prevent negative pharmacokinetic interactions and cumulative toxicity. LTBI in pregnant women offers additional challenges, where the timing and selection of preventive therapy should be considered in relation to the balance between maternal protection and fetal safety. Such subtle therapeutic approaches underscore the importance of individualized management under specialist care. Such strategies resonate with expert opinion outlined in clinical guidelines that seek to negotiate the complex interface of pregnancy and TB treatment (Vassallo et al., 2007). Practical clinical experience added to drug recommendations in TB complicated by pregnancy and complicating conditions. Symptomatic presentation like chronic coughing or nasal symptoms may require the judicious application of adjunctive therapies for symptom relief without interfering with essential anti-TB drugs. The case history of the child with comorbid conditions like eczema and repeated respiratory episodes highlights the need for thorough patient evaluation to design drug regimens accordingly. Even though aimed at juvenile pediatric cases, observations from similar clinical experiences emphasize the role played by co-existent medical factors in drug selection and monitoring plans across special populations like pregnant women. This combined strategy, merging evidence-based guidelines with patient-related factors, is critical to maximize outcomes with a decrease in risks in TB treatment during pregnancy and other complicated clinical cases (Vassallo et al., 2007).

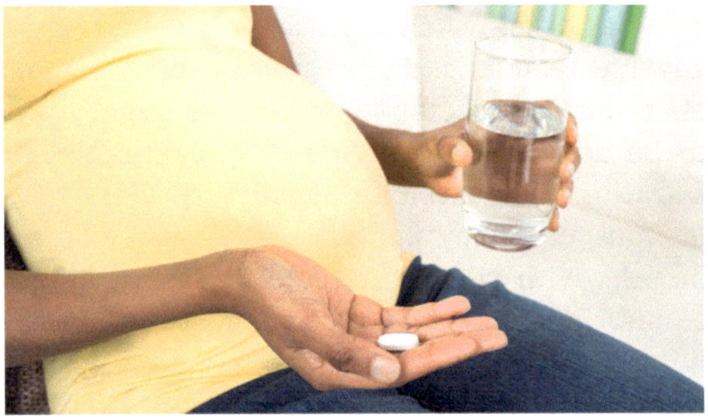

Source: Centers for Disease Control and Prevention (CDC). (2024). *TB treatment considerations during pregnancy.* https://www.cdc.gov/tb/media/images/2024/04/Pregnant_TB_Treatment_v3_1200x675.jpg.

11.4.2. Safety of Antitubercular Drugs

Successful treatment of tuberculosis in special populations requires a judicious assessment of drug safety to reduce risks while maintaining therapeutic effectiveness. Within antitubercular drugs, streptomycin use in pregnancy is particularly contraindicated because of its ototoxic action on the fetus, potentially causing permanent deafness. This precaution is also extended to second-line drugs, whose safety profiles in pregnant patients are still poorly defined, thus begging the need for cautious selection and treatment. Additionally, co-morbid conditions like diabetes, immunosuppression, or silicosis might necessitate protracted treatment with concomitant careful monitoring for the development of toxicity to maximize outcomes. The multiplicity of drug regimens, particularly in EPTB, underscores the need for specialist advice and individualized treatment to offset efficacy with safety issues (Chan et al., 1998). The interplay between tuberculosis and HIV poses extra challenges to antitubercular drug safety, mainly in co-infected subjects receiving concurrent ART. Although ART reduces mortality in HIV-associated tuberculosis patients considerably, the risk of drug-drug interactions calls for careful management. Rifampin, a mainstay of tuberculosis treatment, causes hepatic enzymes that decrease effective levels of many antiretroviral drugs, and dosing changes are required to prevent toxicity and ensure therapeutic levels.

Early ART initiation following the initiation of tuberculosis treatment has proven to have dramatic survival advantages; however, providers need to closely monitor for overlapping toxicities like hepatotoxicity and immune reconstitution inflammatory syndrome (IRIS). Therefore, the simultaneous treatment of tuberculosis and HIV demands careful balancing of drug regimens to achieve safety as well as clinical benefit (Chan et al., 1998). Given the presence of pre-existing liver or renal impairment in patients, the safety of antitubercular drugs necessitates increased caution through changes in drug metabolism and clearance. The use of hepatotoxic drugs such as isoniazid, rifampin, and PZA needs careful management with monitoring of liver function regularly and monitoring for early toxicity signs. In a similar way, streptomycin and ethambutol, which are mainly cleared renally, can build up in renal insufficiency and enhance the risk of side effects like ototoxicity and optic neuritis. Dosage adjustment and careful clinical monitoring are therefore essential to avoid drug-induced organ toxicity. These points highlight the importance of the use of individualized treatment regimens, especially in special cases when physiological changes complicate ordinary tuberculosis treatment, and stress the safety and effectiveness of antitubercular regimens (Chan et al., 1998) (Figure 11.7).

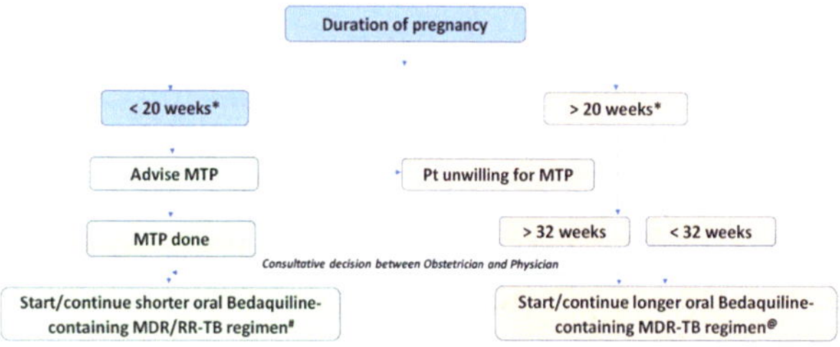

Figure 11.7. Management of M/XDR-TB patients during pregnancy based on gestation age.

Source: National Tuberculosis Elimination Program (NTEP). (n.d.). *Management of MDR/XDR-TB treatment during pregnancy.* https://ntep.in/node/1571/CP-management-mxdr-tb-treatment-during-pregnancy.

11.4.3. Monitoring and Follow-Up Care

Successful management of pregnancy with TB requires strong systems of follow-up and monitoring to guarantee both fetal and maternal safety. Pregnancy subjects a patient to physiological alterations that can modify the pharmacokinetics of anti-TB drugs, which necessitates vigilant observation to be able to easily identify adverse drug reactions (ADRs) or failure of treatment at an early stage. Additionally, the distress of diagnosis with TB during pregnancy may affect adherence, and supportive surveillance that includes psychological evaluation in addition to clinical evaluation will be required. Caregivers must proceed with caution that is inherent to pregnancy while being attentive to the potential progression or spread of TB. Such extensive monitoring supports timely adjustment of intervention and helps prevent complications like preterm labor or vertical transmission, highlighting the importance of ongoing patient interaction during pregnancy and postpartum stays (Hughes et al., 2013). Operationalizing TB treatment monitoring frameworks is particularly challenging in resource-limited settings, where constraints on the health system are likely to impede follow-up. District health management teams usually face challenges, including a lack of staff, irregular supply chains for drugs, and a lack of infrastructure to provide direct observed therapy (DOT) regularly. Moreover, systemic barriers such as delayed funding and lack of proper training further reduce the quality of antenatal TB care. Lack of consistency in political commitment at local levels directly affects resource allocation, impacting the availability of necessities like access to clean water and properly trained staff to ensure treatment protocols. These functional constraints undermine treatment compliance and integrity of follow-up, and this calls for enhanced managerial support and integrated healthcare delivery strategies to maintain treatment effectiveness (Hughes et al., 2013). Postpartum is a specially vulnerable time that demands intensive follow-up among TB-infected mothers and infants. With an increased risk of morbidity post-delivery, multidisciplinary care modules of pulmonologists, obstetricians, and specialists in infectious diseases become critical. Infants born to mothers with active TB require thorough assessments to identify latent infection or active disease and initiate appropriate prophylactic treatment to avoid tuberculosis occurrence. Repeated diagnostic testing must be included in monitoring before preventive treatment is stopped, together with prudent decisions on maternal-infant separation based on the maternal infection and response to treatment. This ongoing care model is critical in the protection of neonatal health, maternal compliance with treatment, and reducing TB transmission among households, demonstrating TB management complexity that stretches from pregnancy into early infancy (Zerihun et al., 2016).

11.5. Tuberculosis (TB) in Other Special Populations

Patients with weakened immune systems are a special group especially susceptible to TB. HIV/AIDS significantly elevates the risk for TB activation because of compromised host defense, making diagnosis and treatment more complicated. Immunosuppressive treatments for autoimmune conditions or organ transplantation also pose difficulties in treating latent or active TB disease, requiring individualized screening and prophylaxis. The shared symptomatology and potential for drug interactions in these groups necessitate an integrated strategy that satisfies immune suppression with efficacious anti-TB regimens. The risk among this population emphasizes the urgent necessity of close monitoring and specialized guidelines aimed at minimizing morbidity and mortality. Furthermore, TB management in immunocompromised patients has not just clinical but also public health aspects based on early diagnosis and prevention strategies, keeping in mind their increased susceptibility against the background of global antimicrobial resistance (AMR) issues (Dartois & Rubin, 2022). Yet another discrete group with challenges associated with TB consists of chronic IBD patients like Crohn's disease and ulcerative colitis. Such patients are usually subjected to long courses of immunosuppressive therapy, which can activate latent TB. The chronic intestinal inflammation together with immunomodulatory therapies also makes both clinical presentation and control of TB in these patients more challenging. The need to balance disease control with prevention of TB necessitates coordinated multidisciplinary care in the form of regular screening and close interaction between gastroenterologists and infectious diseases specialists. Such coordination is necessary to maximize therapeutic benefits without accelerating either disease. With the clinical guidelines adapting to meet this complexity, insight into the subtle interaction between IBD and TB further emphasizes the necessity of tailored care pathways in special groups (Lamb et al., 2019). Both pediatric and geriatric populations also represent special factors in tuberculosis treatment, mirroring physiological and immunological differences with age. Children, particularly from endemic regions, are at greater risk for disseminated and extensive forms of TB and require early detection and treatment to avoid significant morbidity. On the other hand, older adults tend to have unusual manifestations and comorbidities that make diagnosis challenging. Numerous individuals in this age category may also experience polypharmacy issues, increasing the risk of ADRs with TB treatment. These age-group-defined vulnerable groups need age-specific diagnostic standards and treatment regimens that take into account developmental or degenerative changes, maximizing efficacy and safety. Acknowledging these needs is paramount for mitigating TB burden throughout the life course and enhancing health outcomes in these special populations.

11.5.1. Tuberculosis (TB) in Immunocompromised Individuals

Immunocompromised individuals are the most vulnerable population to TB infection because they have compromised immune defenses. HIV/AIDS, cancers, organ transplants, and immunosuppressive treatment weaken the host's ability to contain MTB, usually giving rise to unusual presentations and extrapulmonary spread. This vulnerability is also complicated in pregnancy, where physiological immunosuppression can worsen the latent reactivation of TB or result in new infections with worse clinical courses. The changed immune environment can impede the timely detection of TB symptoms, thus delaying diagnosis and treatment, which increases the morbidity risk for both the mother and the fetus. Therefore, increased clinical alertness and customized screening strategies are required to enhance outcomes in this crossroads of immunocompromise and pregnancy-induced immunomodulation (Gakidi et al., 2025). Extrapulmonary TB manifestations are more common in immunocompromised hosts, often affecting unusual sites like the central nervous system (CNS). CNS tuberculomas, while uncommon, present special diagnostic problems because they can clinically and radiologically mimic neoplastic lesions. Immunosuppression allows for hematogenous spread of TB bacilli to the brain, making intracranial infections more common during such situations and necessitating multidisciplinary treatment strategies. Interestingly, the transient state of immunosuppression in pregnancy can lead to precipitous CNS TB, and therefore, TB should be kept in mind while diagnosing neurological symptoms in pregnancy. Prompt identification and management are crucial, as evidenced by reported cases in which neurosurgical resection in addition to ATT resulted in successful outcomes (Gakidi et al., 2025). This highlights the need to include immunological factors in the diagnostic and treatment protocols for TB among special groups. The convergence of TB with other infectious conditions that are common among immunocompromised individuals complicates clinical management and prognosis further. Coinfections like HIV and other tropical zoonoses, monkeypox virus, critically impair immune function and add to enhanced TB morbidity and mortality. New evidence illustrates that immunocompromised patients with no prior vaccinations or with concomitant HIV infection have increased susceptibility to severe forms and poor outcomes, which also make pregnancy management difficult. These overlapping illnesses aggravate immune dysregulation, allowing for more virulent TB disease patterns and presenting daunting challenges in resource-constrained situations. Accordingly, integrative care frameworks targeting TB in the presence of these concurrent infections—taking into account immunocompromised statuses intrinsic to pregnancy as well as other illnesses—are paramount to minimizing mortality and maximizing patient benefit (Figure 11.8).

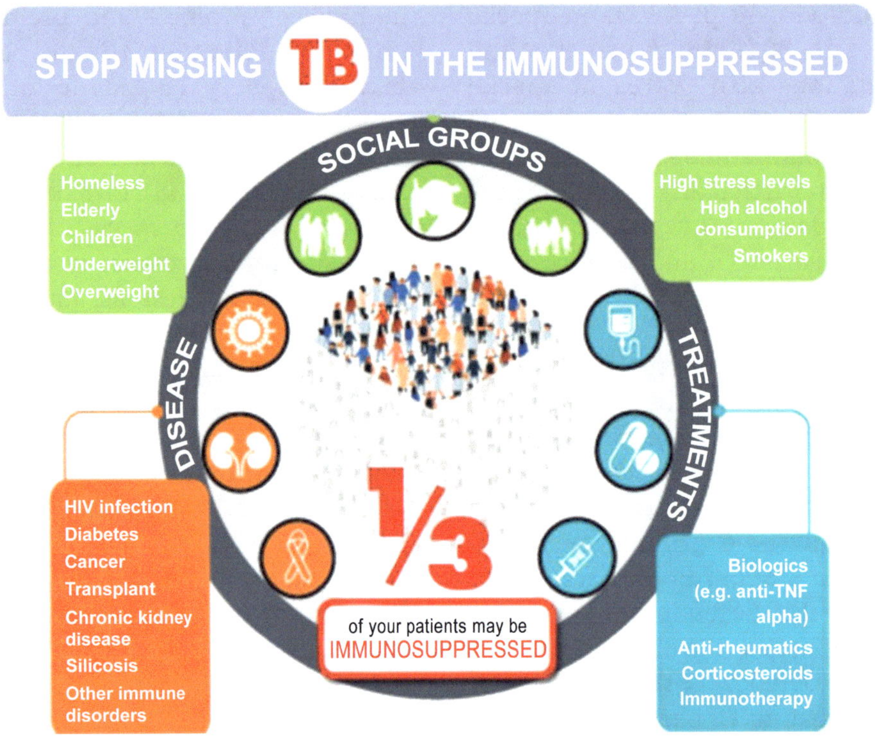

Figure 11.8. Screening for LTBI amongst the immunocompromised is crucial to the programmatic management of the disease, repercussions of LTBI misdiagnosis and test options.

Source: T-SPOT Asia. (2021). *Overview of TB diagnosis and management during pregnancy.* https://tspot.asia/wp-content/uploads/2021/07/infographic-thumbnail03.jpg.

11.5.2. Tuberculosis (TB) in Children and Adolescents

The immunology of TB infection in children and youth poses distinctive challenges relative to adults, requiring distinct clinical and public health responses. Adolescents and younger persons tend to have varying immune reactions to MTB, so diagnosing is complicated by the prevalence of paucibacillary forms of their illness. In addition, young children, particularly those less than five years of age, are more likely to have a fast course of disease following latent infection, emphasizing the need for prompt detection and treatment. Adolescents, on the other hand, increasingly form a group with high TB burden, frequently driven by social and behavioral determinants that make it difficult to comply with treatment protocols. These unique epidemiological and clinical features need to be addressed in any holistic approach dealing with TB among special groups, such as pregnancy, to maximize outcomes while lowering risks of transmission (Lebano et al., 2020). Healthcare professionals also need to address the overlap of TB among other comorbidities that are prevalent in the pediatric and adolescent age groups. Malnutrition, a prevalent condition particularly in low-resource settings, exacerbates immune suppression and worsens TB outcomes, while HIV coinfection further complicates disease management and prognosis. Additionally, the psychosocial dimensions influencing adolescents, such as peer pressure and stigma, can hinder the successful completion of lengthy TB treatment courses.

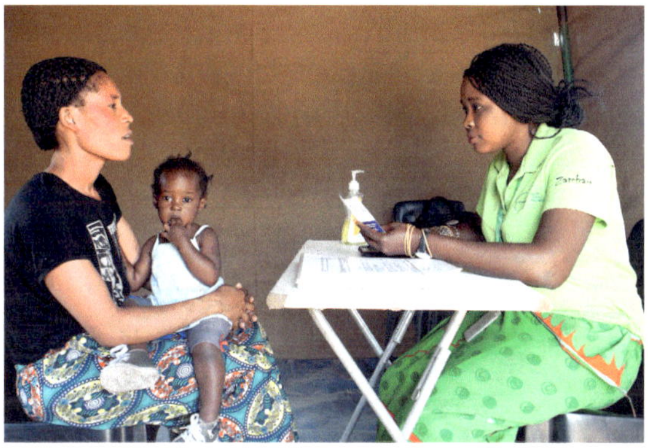

Source: The Union. (n.d.). *Healthcare worker counseling a pregnant woman about tuberculosis.* https://theunion.org/sites/default/files/inline-images/_WBP2540-Edit.jpg.

Tailored interventions that integrate nutritional support, mental health services, and patient-centered communication strategies are crucial for enhancing adherence and therapeutic efficacy. Such multicomponent care models are congruent with more general strategies proposed for other chronic conditions in which multidisciplinary treatment is an issue, with similarity seen in the management of chronic disease across vulnerable groups (Lamb et al., 2019). Prevention and control of TB in children and adolescents also necessitate strategic reforms in public health policy aimed at these age ranges. Contact tracing, preventive treatment, and vaccination policies need to be adjusted to meet the vulnerabilities specific to young people. This involves maximizing the application of the BCG vaccine and investigating new immunization strategies to provide increased protection. Health systems are also required to prioritize the balance of child-friendly diagnostic tests and formulations of anti-TB drugs to enhance access and tolerability. Maternal and child health services can integrate with TB control activities, providing potential synergies that can enhance surveillance and enable early intervention, intersectionality essential for special situations in TB management (Lebano et al., 2020).

11.5.3. Tuberculosis (TB) in the Elderly

There is a sophisticated interaction of social and physiological determinants that powerfully affects the presentation of disease in older individuals, leading to unique challenges in the diagnosis and treatment of TB among this population.

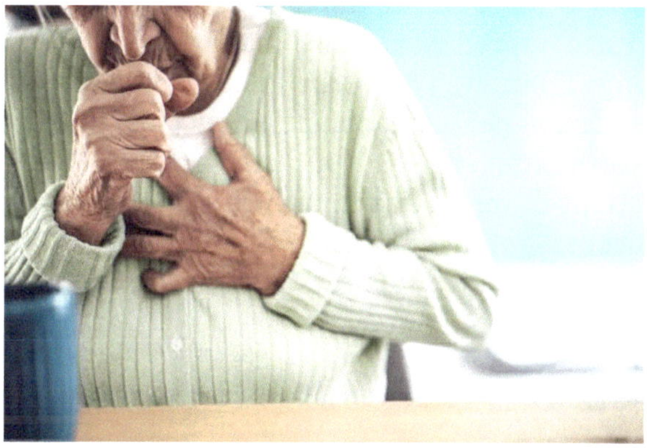

Source: RVO Health. (2023). *Symptoms of tuberculosis in adults.* https://media.post.rvohealth.io/wp-content/uploads/sites/3/2023/11/symptoms_tuberculosis_GettyImages1453186644_Header-1024x575.jpg.

Aging is associated with an alteration in immune function, referred to as immunosenescence, which distorts the classical clinical presentation of TB and encourages milder, less typical signs. Diagnosis in older patients is thus often delayed, leading to greater morbidity and mortality. Additionally, comorbidities like diabetes, chronic obstructive pulmonary disease (COPD), and malnutrition are common in the elderly and further complicate the clinical scenario and therapeutic interventions. Such complexities call for increased clinical acumen and modified diagnostic strategies to prevent underdiagnosis and initiate timely therapy, thus meeting the peculiar requirements posed by this vulnerable group.Socioeconomic determinants and housing conditions also contribute to a significant role in TB incidence and outcomes among older adults. Institutionalization within long-term care facilities or nursing home settings tends to enhance exposure risk because of the confined settings and recurrent contact with healthcare staff or other residents who might be reservoirs of latent infection. Social isolation and restricted access to health care services further add to diagnostic delays and medication compliance. In addition, age-associated cognitive impairment may interfere with comprehension and management of the long TB therapy course. These aspects are important not just for planning successful public health interventions but also for enhancing patient-centered care, thus increasing treatment success rates and decreasing transmission among older populations. TB management in the elderly is characterized by distinct clinical challenges, especially drug toxicity and polypharmacy. Elderly subjects are at greater risk of ADRs, such as hepatotoxicity and neurotoxicity, because of changes in pharmacokinetics and pharmacodynamics, along with the coadministration of other medications. This necessitates proper therapeutic monitoring and titration of doses to individual needs to balance risks against the efficacy of treatment. In addition, nutritional deficiencies prevalent among this population have the potential to compromise recovery and immune function. Providing high-quality care for older TB patients is also aligned with wider health system priorities to maximize outcomes in all groups (Margaret et al., 2018). Strategic models that involve multidisciplinary team care, patient education, and supportive care are needed to best meet these challenges and to enhance survival as well as quality of life in older groups with TB (Humbert et al., 2022).

SUMMARY

The complex interplay between tuberculosis and pregnancy necessitates a multifaceted approach to ensure both maternal and fetal safety. The physiological changes during pregnancy pose diagnostic and therapeutic challenges that can compromise the timely identification and management of TB. Moreover, coexisting health burdens and resource limitations in certain regions exacerbate these difficulties. Effective prevention of TB among pregnant women requires not just medical treatment but also the enhancement of healthcare delivery systems, most importantly antenatal care services where TB screening and treatment are integrated. This reiterates the need for workforce development and supportive policies to allow healthcare workers to respond effectively to these challenges and emphasizes the key contribution of nurses and public health programs in case coordination and education. Therefore, all-embracing strategies that address the peculiar vulnerabilities of pregnant women are essential to minimize morbidity and mortality due to TB among this special group. Outside pregnancy, extraordinary circumstances surrounding TB necessitate operational feasibility evaluations that take into account health system capabilities and contextual issues. Applying tuberculosis preventive treatment (TPT) has similarities with challenges in malaria treatment among pregnant women, whereby health management teams experience limitations in funding, personnel, and supply chain stability (Hughes et al., 2013). Such systemic challenges impact clinical compliance to treatment guidelines and access to care among patients, with the potential to lead to treatment withdrawal or poor outcomes. Political will and community participation are still crucial, as evidenced by district-level improvements in supportive infrastructure, but efforts must be scaled up equitably across diverse settings. Evaluation and understanding of these multifactorial impediments and addressing them through continued evaluation and directed allocation of resources are needed to strengthen health services for vulnerable populations faced with infectious diseases in special conditions. Effective TB management during pregnancy and similar situations requires coordinated, context-specific interventions driven by robust health systems and well-informed policies. Improving workforce capacities, guaranteeing stable supply chains, and developing multisectoral partnerships are the bases for better clinical results and public health effects (Hughes et al., 2013. Although biomedical care should be at the core, the wider determinants of quality and access to healthcare must also be considered. Subsequent studies would be aimed at streamlining implementation strategies and maximizing operational feasibility across a range of settings to reduce inequities. By solving these problems as a system, healthcare systems can maximize protection for both maternal and neonatal health and further international efforts to control TB in special populations.

The interaction of TB with pregnancy requires extensive clinical care because of the special physiological states that affect the disease course and response to treatment. Pregnancy modifies immunity, potentially making one more susceptible to infection with TB or activating latent TB, with implications for both maternal and fetal health. Early detection is essential but frequently confounded by similar symptoms of pregnancy conditions, highlighting the importance of screening protocols specific to prenatal care. The treatment regimens, too, need to be cautiously chosen to avoid teratogenic activity while successfully treating the infection, which calls for interdisciplinary solutions between obstetricians and infectious disease specialists. The assessment of these complexities emphasizes the need to incorporate TB control interventions into maternal health programs, especially in high-prevalence areas where resource limitations make diagnostic and management approaches even more difficult (Morgan et al., 1980). Complexly complicated clinical situations are presented when TB presents with other special circumstances like HIV co-infection, malnutrition, or MDR-TB, making treatment challenging and elevating the risks of mortality. In HIV-infected pregnant women, TB is still a major cause of maternal death, compounded by immunosuppression and possible drug interactions between antiretrovirals and TB drugs. Malnutrition which is common among most affected populations also weakens immune defenses, increasing recovery time and influencing fetal growth. MDR-TB poses further problems, necessitating longer and more toxic regimens that are hard to tolerate during pregnancy. These intersecting risk factors underscore the need for robust diagnostic tools and close monitoring, as well as the integration of social support services to enhance treatment adherence and outcomes among vulnerable groups (Morgan et al., 1980). Measures to tackle TB in pregnancy and other special circumstances must prioritize preventative measures, best treatment practices, and health system strengthening. Prevention through focused screening and latent TB treatment can decrease the incidence of active disease in pregnant women, eventually enhancing both maternal and neonatal prognosis. Treatment optimization requires an equilibrium between drug safety and efficacy, requiring new guidelines based on evolving evidence and pharmacovigilance. TB-endemic country health systems need to have sufficient resources and personnel with training to conduct integrated care so that maternal health programs should emphasize TB management. In addition, international health programs need to keep addressing funding and policy alignment to mitigate TB burdens among vulnerable groups. Such an integrated approach is critical for preventing TB-related morbidity and mortality during pregnancy as well as improving overall public health outcomes (Morgan et al., 1980).

CLOSER LOOK

THE ROLE OF ISONIAZID PREVENTIVE THERAPY (IPT) IN PREGNANT WOMEN

Isoniazid preventive therapy (IPT) is important in preventing the risk of tuberculosis (TB) in pregnant women, particularly in high TB burden settings. Pregnant women are highly susceptible to TB because of physiological changes during pregnancy that may influence the immune system. Furthermore, untreated latent TB can develop into active disease, which is very dangerous to the mother and the fetus. IPT, in which isoniazid is administered for a period of 6 to 9 months, is a good measure that can prevent LTBI from advancing to active TB, thus minimizing harm caused by the disease.

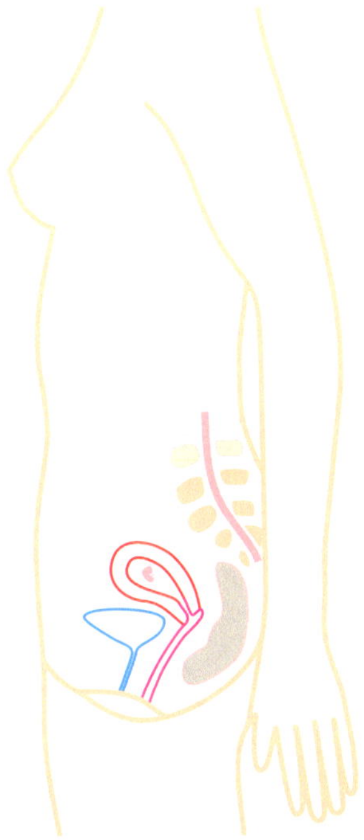

Source: By Miraceti - Freely according to images at [1] [dead link], CC BY-SA 3.0, https://commons.wikimedia.org/w/index.php?curid=904148

One of the main advantages of IPT among pregnant women is that it can prevent the risk of active TB development. Latent TB among pregnant women increases their chances of reactivating the infection, as pregnancy itself causes immune suppression. IPT kills the latent MTB bacteria within the body, preventing them from turning active and forming disease. Research has indicated that IPT reduces the occurrence of TB in people with LTBI, such as pregnant women, by a large extent, particularly when initiated early before active disease sets in.

Besides avoiding active TB, IPT is also of utmost importance for the well-being of the unborn. Pregnant women with active TB can result in adverse pregnancy outcomes such as low birth weight, prematurity, and, in limited cases, congenital TB, where the infant carries TB. Preventing active TB from developing through IPT decreases the chances of these pregnancy complications. In addition, the treatment avoids maternal TB-associated morbidity and mortality and enhances the mother's general state of health throughout pregnancy and the postpartum period.

Nonetheless, the administration of IPT during pregnancy should be handled with caution because there are reservations regarding the safety of isoniazid for both the pregnant woman and the unborn child. Although isoniazid has been studied and is indicated to be generally safe during pregnancy, risks like hepatotoxicity need to be carefully monitored. Routine liver function tests should be done during IPT so that any abnormal reaction can be recognized early. Further, the advantages of IPT should be put against the risks in women with pre-existing liver disease or other contraindications.

IPT is also a critical component of integrated HIV and TB care in pregnant women, particularly in high-burden settings where both conditions are common. In pregnant women with HIV, IPT is especially significant because HIV compromises the immune system and raises the risk of progressing from latent to active TB.

REFERENCES

1. Adhikari, M., Jeena, P., Bobat, R., Archary, M., Naidoo, K., Coutsoudis, A., Singh, R., & Nair, N. (2011). HIV-associated tuberculosis in the newborn and young infant. *International Journal of Pediatrics, 2011*, Article 354208. https://doi.org/10.1155/2011/354208.
2. Bhatla, N., Aoki, D., Sharma, D. N., & Sankaranarayanan, R. (2018). Cancer of the cervix uteri. *International Journal of Gynecology & Obstetrics, 143*, 22–36. https://doi.org/10.1002/ijgo.12611.
3. Chan, C. K., Chan, H. S., Chan, K. S., & Chan, R. C. K. (1998). Chemotherapy of tuberculosis in Hong Kong: A consensus statement. *Hong Kong Medical Journal, 4*(3), 315–320. https://core.ac.uk/download/pdf/37883904.pdf (accessed on 10 May 2025).
4. Denholm, J., Eisen, D., McBryde, E., Street, A., et al. (2012). Management of tuberculosis: A handbook for clinicians. https://core.ac.uk/download/303784777.pdf (accessed on 10 May 2025).
5. Dietrich, B., Victoria, K., Lackner, A., Meinhardt, G., Koo, B., Pollheimer, J., Haider, S., et al. (2023). NOTCH3 signalling controls human trophoblast stem cell expansion and differentiation. *bioRxiv*. https://www.semanticscholar.org/paper/87e17663bb6a3a793745e15a2b1de1b3f5dfc31c (accessed on 10 May 2025).
6. Gakidi, A., Faniadou, E., Ioannidou, D., & Boutou, A. (2025). A rare case of a solitary central nervous system tuberculoma mimicking an intracranial tumor. *Cures, 17*. https://www.semanticscholar.org/paper/65c20d10d8b6ecab533f8fa09bd61704150038b7 (accessed on 10 May 2025).
7. Girma, G. (2015). Co-infection of multidrug-resistant tuberculosis and HIV: Implication for public health (Review). Journal of Pharmacy and Alternate Medicine 4: https://iiste.org/Journals/index.php/JPAM/article/view/22978 . (accessed on 10 May 2025).
8. Hughes, A., Vallely, A., Asante, A. D., Rowe, A. K., Greenwood, B., Menendez, C., Pell, C., et al. (2013). Feasibility and coverage of implementing intermittent preventive treatment of malaria in pregnant women contacting private or public clinics in Tanzania: Experience-based viewpoints of health managers in Mkuranga and Mufindi districts. *BMC Health Services Research, 13*, Article 372. https://core.ac.uk/download/pdf/17181068.pdf (accessed on 10 May 2025).
9. Humbert, M., Kovács, G., Hoeper, M. M., Badagliacca, R., Berger, R. M. F., Brida, M., Carlsen, J., et al. (2022). 2022 ESC/ERS guidelines for the diagnosis and treatment of pulmonary hypertension. *European Respiratory Journal, 61*, 2200879. https://doi.org/10.1183/13993003.00879-2022.
10. Jo, J. Y., Cho, I., Shin, J., Lee, S., & Choi, W. (2022). Laparoscopic surgery for fallopian tube torsion due to benign tumor in the third trimester of pregnancy: A case report and literature review. *Journal of Obstetrics and Gynaecology, 42*, 2566–2572. https://www.semanticscholar.org/paper/35c06d04538f9204459ea3f1c29a69622cc34024 (accessed on 10 May 2025).
11. Keikha, M., Zandhaghighi, M., & Shahraki Zahedani, S. (2023). Death associated with human monkeypox outbreak 2022: The current perspectives–Correspondence. *International Journal of Surgery (London, England), 109*, 1806–1807. https://www.semanticscholar.org/paper/a77fc332276b4f31b9255c84cde7621f9622e95f (accessed on 10 May 2025).

12. Kim, I. J., Gonzalez, O., Tighe, M. P., Lanthier, P., Clark, M. J., Travis, K. L., Low-Beer, T. C., et al. (2024). Protective efficacy of a Zika purified inactivated virus vaccine candidate during pregnancy in marmosets. *NPJ Vaccines, 9*. https://www.semanticscholar.org/paper/e0c4e301d37db7ad1b5fa84c4e9f955f659fd740 (accessed on 10 May 2025).

13. Kruk, M. E., Gage, A., Arsenault, C., Jordan, K., Leslie, H. H., Roder-DeWan, S., Adeyi, O., et al. (2018). High-quality health systems in the Sustainable Development Goals era: Time for a revolution. *The Lancet Global Health, 6*, e1196–e1252. https://doi.org/10.1016/s2214-109x(18)30386-3.

14. Lamb, C. A., Kennedy, N. A., Raine, T., Hendy, P., Smith, P. J., Limdi, J. K., Hayee, B., et al. (2019). British Society of Gastroenterology consensus guidelines on the management of inflammatory bowel disease in adults. *Gut, 68*(Suppl 3), s1–s106. https://doi.org/10.1136/gutjnl-2019-318484.

15. Landsberg, E., Flory, J., Tawatao, M., & Sanematsu, S. (2016). Getting and keeping health coverage for low-income Californians: A guide for advocates. Western Center on Law & Poverty; https://wclp.org/wp-content/uploads/2019/07/Western_Center_2016_Health_Care_Eligibility_Guide_Full_rev.1.pdf (accessed on 10 May 2025).

16. Lebano, A., Hamed, S., Bradby, H., Gil-Salmerón, A., Durá Ferrandis, E., Garcés Ferrer, J., Azzedine, F., et al. (2020). Migrants' and refugees' health status and healthcare in Europe: A scoping literature review. *BMC Public Health, 20*, Article 1039. https://doi.org/10.1186/s12889-020-08749-8.

17. Manji, K., Sheriff, F., & Manji, M. (2011). Review of pulmonary tuberculosis and HIV co-infection among pregnant mothers in Sub-Saharan Africa. *Tanzania Medical Journal, 25*, 3–7. https://www.semanticscholar.org/paper/6b22874a910432d2b0c205d457c1805569e97d39 (accessed on 10 May 2025).

18. Manyi-Loh, C. E., Mamphweli, S., Meyer, E. L., & Okoh, A. I. (2018). Antibiotic use in agriculture and its consequential resistance in environmental sources: Potential public health implications. *Molecules, 23*(4), 795. https://doi.org/10.3390/molecules23040795.

19. Matsuoka, K., Kobayashi, T., Ueno, F., Matsui, T., Hirai, F., Inoue, N., Kato, J., et al. (2018). Evidence-based clinical practice guidelines for inflammatory bowel disease. *Journal of Gastroenterology, 53*, 305–353. https://doi.org/10.1007/s00535-018-1439-1.

20. Morgan, R. W. (1980). Basic health needs in Africa. https://open.bu.edu/bitstream/2144/40428/1/WP_29_Morgan_1980.pdf (accessed on 10 May 2025).

21. Moyo, B. (2017). Factors associated with loss to follow-up HIV-uninfected tuberculosis patients in Ekurhuleni North sub-district. A research report submitted to the Faculty of Health Sciences, University of the Witwatersrand, Johannesburg, in partial fulfilment of the requirements for the degree of MSc Epidemiology (Infectious Disease Epidemiology) . https://core.ac.uk/download/188769683.pdf (accessed on 10 May 2025).

22. Murray, C. J. L., Ikuta, K. S., Sharara, F., Swetschinski, L. R., Robles Aguilar, G., Gray, A. P., Han, C., et al. (2022). Global burden of bacterial antimicrobial resistance in 2019: A systematic analysis. *The Lancet, 399*(10325), 629–655. https://doi.org/10.1016/S0140-6736(21)02724-0.

23. Nast, A., Altenburg, A., Augustin, M., Boehncke, W. H., Härle, P., Klaus, J., Koza, J., et al. (2021). German S3-guideline on the treatment of psoriasis vulgaris, adapted from EuroGuiDerm–

Part 2: Treatment monitoring and specific clinical or comorbid situations. *JDDG: Journal der Deutschen Dermatologischen Gesellschaft, 19*(8), 1092–1115. https://doi.org/10.1111/ddg.14507.

24. Nast, A., Smith, C., Spuls, P. I., Avila Valle, G., Bata-Csörgő, Z., Boonen, H., de Jong, E. M. G. J., et al. (2020). EuroGuiDerm guideline on the systemic treatment of psoriasis vulgaris–Part 1: Treatment and monitoring recommendations. *Journal of the European Academy of Dermatology and Venereology, 34*(12), 2461–2498. https://doi.org/10.1111/jdv.16915.
25. Negro, A., Terrin, A., Raffaelli, B., Mitsikostas, D. D., Ornello, R., Khan, S., et al. (2017). Headache and pregnancy: A systematic review. *The Journal of Headache and Pain, 18*, Article 106. https://core.ac.uk/download/153369041.pdf (accessed on 10 May 2025).
26. Rendón, A., & Schäkel, K. (2019). Psoriasis pathogenesis and treatment. *International Journal of Molecular Sciences, 20*(6), 1475. https://doi.org/10.3390/ijms20061475.
27. Saag, M. S., Benson, C. A., Gandhi, R. T., Hoy, J., Landovitz, R. J., Mugavero, M. J., Sax, P. E., et al. (2018). Antiretroviral drugs for treatment and prevention of HIV infection in adults. *JAMA, 320*, 379. https://doi.org/10.1001/jama.2018.8431.
28. Suratman, A. T. (2014). Health policies under the special autonomy regime: An evaluation using health indicators. https://core.ac.uk/download/297922545.pdf (accessed on 10 May 2025).
29. Vassallo, K. (2007). Rhinitis in general practice. https://core.ac.uk/download/46602128.pdf (accessed on 10 May 2025).
30. Zerihun, A., Gudeta, A., Thomas, A., Gajjala, J., Lewis, O., Ahmed, S., & Kodadhala, V. (2016). Postpartum tuberculosis: A diagnostic and therapeutic challenge. *Case Reports in Pulmonology, 2016*, Article 3793941. https://doi.org/10.1155/2016/3793941.

Chapter 12

LATENT TUBERCULOSIS INFECTION (LTBI)

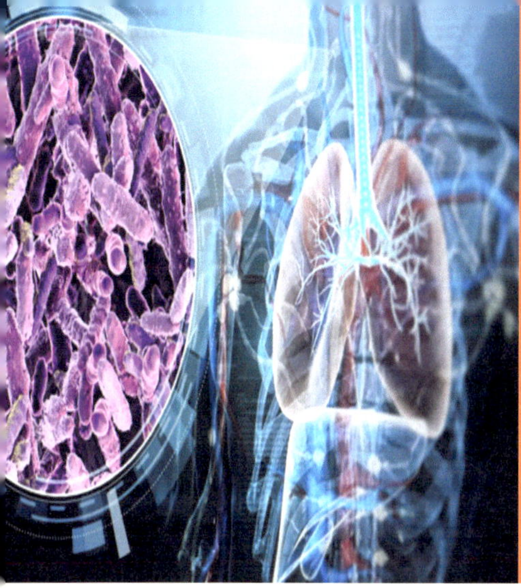

Contents

Introduction

The multifaceted nature of infectious diseases remains to affect public health worldwide, requiring a better understanding of diseases that can lie dormant but hold profound consequences. Latent tuberculosis infection (LTBI) is one such condition of particular interest because it serves as a reservoir for the reactivation of active tuberculosis (TB). Despite advances in medical diagnostics and treatment strategies, TB remains a persistent concern, particularly as it exhibits a notable prevalence in various populations worldwide. The UK, for instance, has witnessed a gradual increase in TB cases over recent decades, highlighting the urgency for improved detection and management techniques. This background highlights the relevance of LTBI management not just to prevent new active TB cases but also to mitigate the related healthcare and economic costs that can overburden health systems (Szczepura & Osipenko, unpublished). An understanding of the epidemiology of LTBI is key to designing focused interventions towards lowering the global burden of tuberculosis. A third of the world's population carries latent TB, and it is a silent but potent threat. Patients with comorbidities, including diabetes mellitus (DM), have been found to exhibit an increased risk of transitioning from latent infection to active disease. This comorbidity makes treatment results more challenging and calls for more extensive screening and control efforts. Recent research has analyzed the correlation between LTBI prevalence and glycemic control as a factor, further supporting the idea that systemic health is essential in infection dynamics. These findings are critical for public health policy aimed at reducing TB reactivation risk and improving patient outcomes among high-risk populations (Remy et al., 2016). Attempts to optimize diagnostic methods and enhance the delivery of healthcare are at the foundation of addressing LTBI successfully. Innovations in point-of-care testing offer a promising direction, with the capability to optimize detection processes and allow for early interventions. Economic analyses have shown that improving diagnostic precision and availability could substantially lower healthcare expenditures on TB care, considering the large investments needed to treat active cases. In addition, treatment of latent infections could stop transmission chains in communities, thus augmenting more general disease control goals. As such, a spend on research and development of new diagnostic technologies and the integration of multidisciplinary public health interventions are key measures for prevention of LTBI and its complications at the individual and societal levels (Szczepura & Osipenko, unpublished).

Definition of Latent Tuberculosis Infection (LTBI)

The host immune response is central to deciding the outcome after exposure to *Mycobacterium tuberculosis* (Mtb). Although most persons exposed to *Mtb* remain asymptomatic, bacteria may be present in a latent form within the host, known as LTBI. This latent phase is one where the immune system of the host has the bacteria in check without eliminating it entirely, inhibiting the occurrence of active disease. A high percentage of the world's population carries this latent infection, indicating a balance between survival of the bacteria and containment by the immune system. It is important to grasp this complex interaction, given that breaks in this equilibrium will trigger the relapse of TB, highlighting the importance of accurate definitions and enhanced diagnostic markers to detect infection risk and guide public health policy (Arisanti et al., 2024). Environmental and lifestyle determinants also shape the distribution and features of LTBI within certain groups of individuals. For example, some high-risk populations, including prisoners who reside in crowded and poorly ventilated settings, have a higher prevalence of latent infection because of increased exposure to infective droplets and lifestyle-related compromised immunity.

Research involving prisoners shows that factors such as smoking, length of stay, and drug abuse can play important roles in the risk of LTBI. These observations underscore the multifactorial etiology of LTBI, which goes beyond mere bacterial persistence to involve social and behavioral determinants that shape infection profiles among risk groups (Arisanti et al., 2024). Clinically, LTBI is characterized by the body's presence of Mtb without clinical signs and symptoms of active tuberculosis. Diagnostic tests, including the tuberculin skin test (TST) and interferon-gamma release assays (IGRAs), are used to identify immune sensitization to antigens of Mtb, confirming latent infection. Yet, these tests cannot distinguish LTBI from active disease, nor identify those who would go on to develop active TB. This test dilemma highlights the intricacy of LTBI and the need for a better grasp of its immunological and biological markers. Ongoing research is aimed at the discovery of new biomarkers and vaccine targets to enhance LTBI detection, treatment, and ultimately decrease TB incidence globally (Niu et al., 2024) (Figure 12.1).

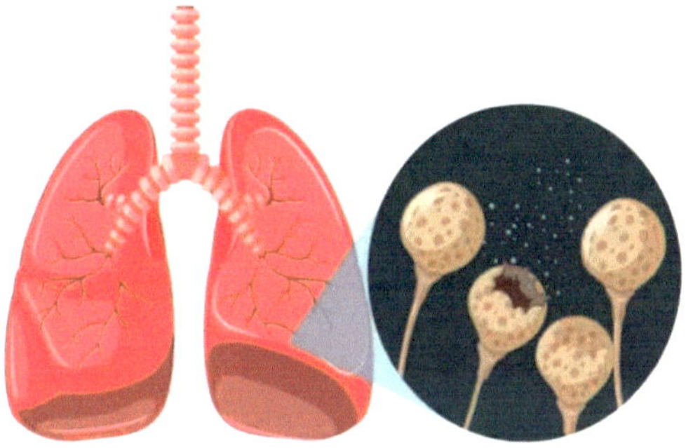

Figure 12.1. Latent tuberculosis.

Source: India.com Lifestyle Staff. (2023). *Latent Tuberculosis: Symptoms to prevention, all you need to know*. India.com. https://www.india.com/health/latent-tuberculosis-symptoms-to-prevention-all-you-need-to-know-5965008/.

Importance of Understanding Latent Tuberculosis Infection (LTBI)

The transition from LTBI to active tuberculosis disease relies on complex metabolic and immunological events that are not yet a hundred percent understood. Current proteomic investigations have shown us separate serum protein profiles that distinguish active TB patients from subjects with LTBI, especially proteins that are associated with inflammation, immune response regulation, lipid transport, and iron uptake. These findings demonstrate that LTBI is not merely a dormant phase but involves complex biological activities that could influence disease activation. By deepening our understanding of these protein signatures, medical practitioners and researchers can better predict and perhaps intervene before LTBI progresses to active TB. These findings are important for recognizing biomarkers that support early diagnosis and for the development of targeted therapies that correct the underlying alterations in metabolism during this phase of transition, thereby helping in the better control and prevention of TB (Mateos et al., 2020). Apart from the biological and molecular aspects, the sociocultural context largely influences LTBI management, especially among those high-risk groups prone to progression towards disease. Among African immigrants to the United States, for instance, reluctance to be treated for LTBI is part of wider concerns with access to healthcare, communication, and patient trust. Research points out that resistance to preventive treatment usually arises from insufficient information, perceived treatment imposition, fear of side effects, and deep-rooted fear of stigmatization and discrimination. Such factors not only inhibit the adherence to treatment but also make it difficult to prevent active TB cases resulting from latent infections. Therefore, an understanding of social determinants and patient views regarding LTBI treatment is crucial for creating culturally appropriate models of education and intervention that foster acceptance and adherence (Obatayo et al., 2024). Combining the biomedical and social understanding of LTBI highlights the need for an integrated approach to tuberculosis control. Identification of LTBI as a dynamic disease state affected by metabolic pathways and social circumstances allows for a multi-faceted public health approach. Such an approach prioritizes early detection with biomarker identification and promotes culturally sensitive patient activation to overcome treatment reluctance. By integrating science with understanding of affected populations' lived experiences, healthcare systems can strengthen preventive care, lower TB transmission, and ultimately become part of the global effort to eliminate tuberculosis. This holistic perspective not only improves clinical outcomes but also supports ethical and patient-centric care, essential in tackling one of the world's most enduring infectious diseases (Mateos et al., 2020; Obatayo et al., 2024) (Figure 12.2).

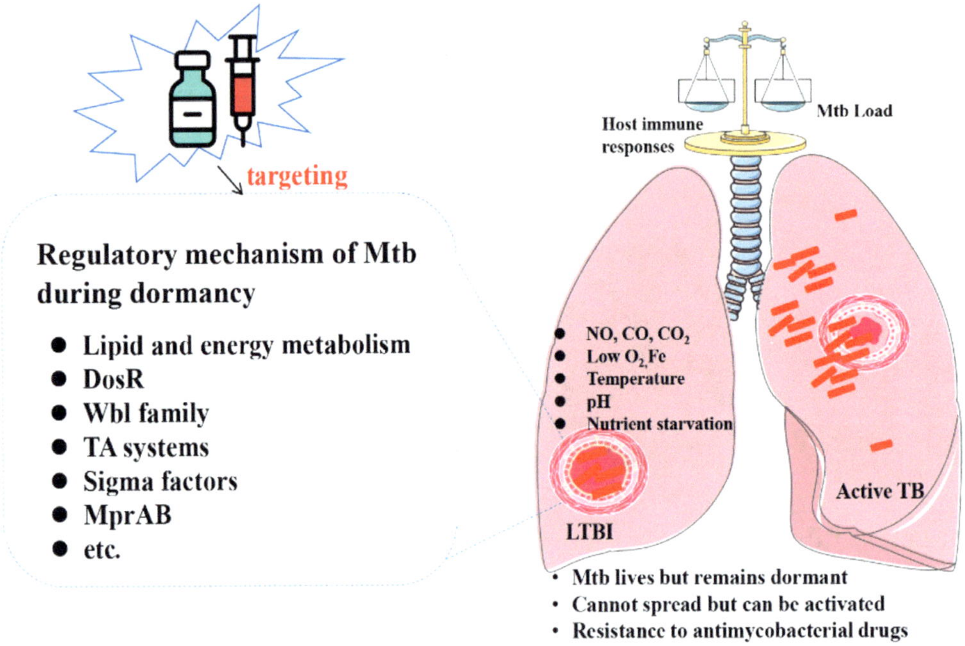

Figure 12.2. Characteristics of latent tuberculosis infection (LTBI). *M. tuberculosis* is in a dormant state, and the body does not show clinical symptoms or expel bacteria. On the one hand, the host prevents mycobacterial replication via acid stress, oxidative stress, cell surface stress, hypoxia, nutrient starvation, essential-element starvation, genotoxic stress, etc.

Source: ResearchGate. (n.d.). *Characteristics of latent tuberculosis infection: Mtb is in a dormant state and the body's immune system prevents it from developing into active disease.* https://www.researchgate.net/figure/Characteristics-of-latent-tuberculosis-infection-Mtb-is-in-a-dormant-state-and-the-body_fig1_381389387.

12.1. Epidemiology of Latent Tuberculosis Infection (LTBI)

Knowledge of the wider picture of infectious diseases sheds light on the important but little recognized contribution of LTBI to global health. Epidemiological evidence shows a complex relationship between existing conditions like diabetes mellitus (DM) and TB, especially where these two diseases are endemic. Studies projecting intervention strategies aimed at diabetic individuals show that tackling LTBI among them would potentially lower significantly the incidence and mortality from TB. The findings highlight the importance of incorporating control of LTBI into diabetes management and imply that whole-practice healthcare interventions have a significant potential to influence TB incidence in high dual disease burden nations. A whole-systems approach propels public health response by emphasizing risk factors' intersections that drive the spread of latent infections and trigger disease activation, and arguing that LTBI control cannot be achieved with TB-specific interventions alone (Sterling et al., 2020). In high-risk settings, including health facilities, the epidemiology of LTBI makes it even more challenging to effectively control tuberculosis.

Research into the prevalence of LTBI in healthcare and medical students gives important insight into occupational risk for exposure. For example, figures from a medical school at a university show that rates of LTBI are greater in postgraduate than in undergraduate students and may indicate higher exposure to clinical training. The application of diagnostic tests like the TST accompanied by more specific tests like the QuantiFERON-TB test facilitates more precise detection of cases of latent infection. The above findings emphasize the need for targeted screening and preventive measures in healthcare settings to reduce professional LTBI acquisition and prevent the development of active disease (Verso et al., 2019). Variation in LTBI epidemiology across regions underscores the difficulty of determining and managing latent infection globally. Differences in infection rates in different groups can be determined by various factors such as vaccination levels, local prevalence of TB, and success in preventive interventions. For instance, the appreciably low rate of LTBI among medical students in certain areas may imply that prompt immunization and infection prevention measures reduce exposure. However, the continued threat of LTBI as a re-emerging public health issue necessitates continued vigilance and research. Reinforcing screening programs, particularly in vulnerable and exposed populations, is critical to breaking chains of transmission and lowering latent infections that provide a reservoir for future active tuberculosis cases (Verso et al., 2019) (Figure 12.3).

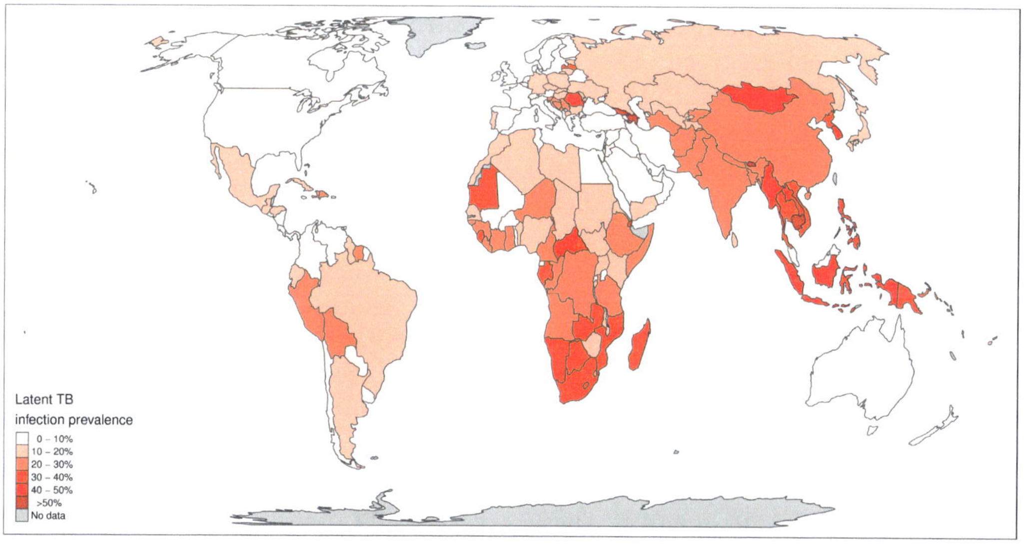

Figure 12.3. Global map of prevalence of latent tuberculosis infection (LTBI).

Source: Houben, R. M. G. J., & Dodd, P. J. (2016). *Global map of prevalence of latent TB infection: Median estimated population prevalence*. https://www.researchgate.net/publication/309454987/figure/fig3/AS:421527540768770@1477511405438/Global-map-of-prevalence-of-latent-TB-infection-Median-estimated-population-prevalence.png.

12.1.1. Global Prevalence and Incidence Rates

Despite advances in public health interventions, tuberculosis (TB) remains a considerable global health challenge, with LTBI serving as a major reservoir for future active TB cases. The global prevalence of LTBI is substantial, especially in regions with high exposure to *Mycobacterium tuberculosis* (MTB). Variability in prevalence rates corresponds closely with socioeconomic factors, population density, and HIV co-infection rates. For example, areas with low TB incidence tend to have targeted LTBI screening in high-risk groups, such as individuals with HIV (PLHIV), to prevent progression to active TB. Strategies and guidelines for LTBI screening in these groups are, however, plagued by heterogeneity, leading to uneven global control. Identifying cost-effective screening strategies is thus paramount for effective resource allocation, but existing studies indicate high variability in cost-effectiveness estimates with regard to targeted populations and protocols used (Baggaley et al., 2023). These variabilities highlight the challenge in defining a unified global strategy in addressing LTBI, despite its immense public health significance. The disparity in TB incidence and prevalence along geographic and demographic fault lines also makes control of LTBI even more challenging on the international stage. Research in varying settings, such as at Muhima District Hospital in Rwanda, demonstrates that TB prevalence may be significantly variable within and between communities and sometimes exceeds national rates reported by institutions like the World Health Organization (WHO). For instance, a 7.2% prevalence of active TB in this environment was documented, higher than the national figure of 5.2%, indicating a high localized disease burden. Moreover, the prevalence of HIV-positive carriers is relatively high, indicative of the synergistic interaction between HIV and TB infections. Notably, demographic and behavioral risk factors commonly linked to TB such as alcohol consumption and smoking were not drastically associated with TB incidence in this instance, implying that context-specific determinants also underpin LTBI and TB dynamics (Hitayezu et al., 2023). This underscores the importance of context-specific epidemiological surveillance across diverse contexts to help guide effective intervention programs. High-quality epidemiological information on LTBI prevalence and incidence is needed to inform global TB elimination programs, but significant gaps in knowledge remain, especially in lower TB incidence settings. In these countries, mass PLHIV screening has been demonstrated in a few studies to be extremely cost-effective, but others suggest more targeted interventions targeting subgroups from high-incidence settings for maximum benefit and economic value. Variations in methodological approaches to cost-effectiveness studies, ranging from differences in modeled assumptions to target populations, make studies non-comparable and restrict agreement on optimal practices (Baggaley et al., 2023). In addition, variations in data reporting and evaluation frameworks undermine standardization further, preventing the development of universally acceptable guidelines. Redressing these inequalities through collaborative research and global cooperation is essential to maximizing LTBI control interventions globally, ultimately helping to decrease the global burden of TB.

12.1.2. High-Risk Populations for Latent Tuberculosis Infection (LTBI)

Knowledge of the populations at greatest risk for LTBI is important to achieve successful public health interventions. Some groups have a disproportionately increased risk because of their socioeconomic status, geographic distribution, and inherent health status. For instance, people living in areas of high TB prevalence, like some areas of sub-Saharan Africa and Southeast Asia, are exposed to TB continuously, thereby raising their likelihood of carrying latent infection. Similarly, living conditions such as homeless shelters and correctional facilities promote transmission, setting up environments that are conducive to acquiring latent infection. Targeted testing and treatment plans based on identifying these high-risk groups can cut back on the reservoir of latent TB and limit progression to active disease, making it a necessary tool for breaking cycles of transmission and ultimately reducing tuberculosis burden overall (Churchyard & Swindells, 2019) (Figure 12.4).

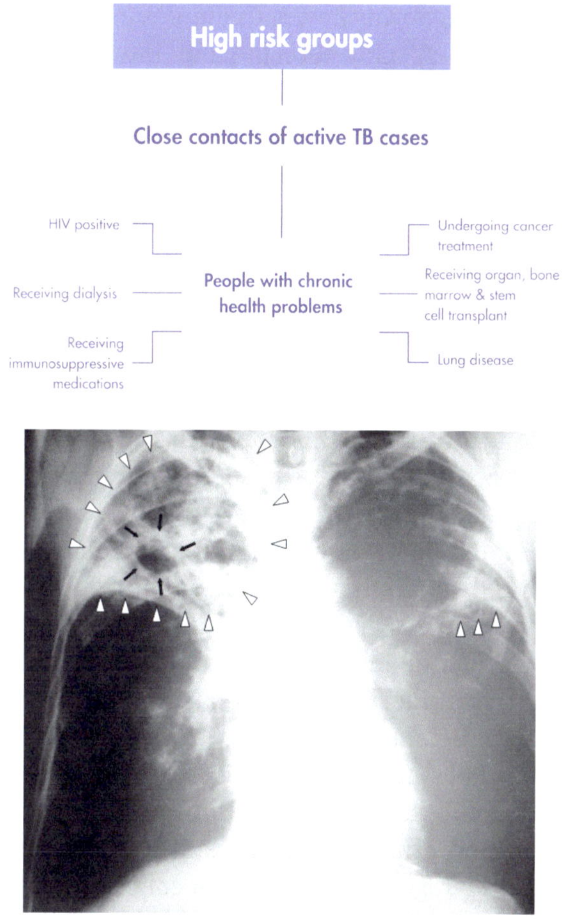

Figure 12.4. The populations most vulnerable to latent tuberculosis infection (LTBI) is crucial for effective public health interventions.

Source: By Unknown author - This media comes from the Centers for Disease Control and Prevention's Public Health Image Library (PHIL), with identification number #2543.Note: Public Domain, https://commons.wikimedia.org/w/index.php?curid=978580

Apart from geography and residence, clinical factors also define populations at higher risk for LTBI. Immunocompromised individuals, and especially those infected with HIV or on immunosuppressive treatment, are at high risk because of their compromised capacity to suppress MTB. People suffering from some chronic conditions like DM or silicosis also show heightened susceptibility to infection and reactivation. Migration to low-incidence environments from high-incidence nations also makes it more difficult to screen and manage, since latent infection also goes undetected without rigorous attempts. The Centers for Disease Control and Prevention (CDC) highlight the role of primary health care providers in detecting these risk factors to take patients in time for testing and treatment, highlighting the need for universal guidelines to meet varied patient populations (National Center for HIV/AIDS, 2025).

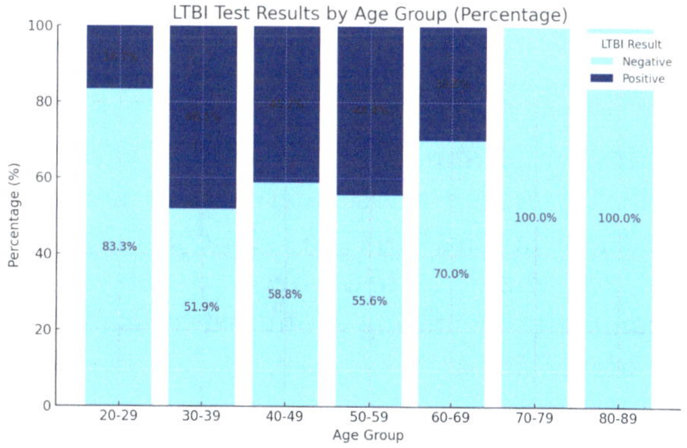

Figure 12.5. LTBI results by age group.

Source: Alene, K. A., Wangdi, K., Clements, A. C. A., Gray, D. J., & McBryde, E. S. (2023). Impact of latent tuberculosis infection on health and wellbeing: A systematic review and meta-analysis. *International Journal of Environmental Research and Public Health, 22*(3), 320.

The population with occupational exposure and social determinants also experiences a high risk for LTBI. Healthcare personnel, especially those involved in direct patient contact in high-burden environments, are repeatedly exposed to infective aerosols, which present a high chance of latent infection. Close contacts of active tuberculosis also experience heightened risk secondary to long-term exposures in close spaces. Socioeconomic determinants like poverty, overcrowding, and poor access to healthcare increase vulnerability by inhibiting early detection and treatment. Targeted testing programs in these groups are crucial, as they promote public health objectives by reducing the reservoir of latent infection. This strategic emphasis is consistent with international efforts to end tuberculosis by emphasizing prevention in those most likely to support ongoing transmission (Churchyard & Swindells, 2019; National Center for HIV/AIDS, 2025) (Figure 12.5).

12.1.3. Geographic Variations in Latent Tuberculosis Infection (LTBI) Rates

Differences in access to healthcare can have a substantial impact on geographic variation in LTBI rates. In areas where health facilities are far or in hard-to-reach locations, diagnosis and treatment of LTBI become delayed or incomplete, permitting continued transmission in communities.

For example, a study in the Philippines proved that villages with increased LTBI prevalence were significantly more distant from primary healthcare centers, both in distance and travel time (Leining, 2019). Such distance prevents prompt medical treatment, leading to increased risk for infected cases and also community transmission. These observations emphasize the critical role healthcare infrastructure plays in curbing the spread of LTBI, with geographic isolation presenting serious barriers that augment infection levels. As such, targeted outreach as a strategic intervention in remote or hard-to-reach populations is vital to LTCB control and reduction, especially among sensitive groups like children. Including geographic and demographic heterogeneity in epidemiological models enables better comprehension of LTBI patterns within various locations. Traditional models tend to simplify transmission patterns too much, ignoring how the complex interactions of location-specific determinants intersect with population attributes. New developments have demonstrated how epidemic models framed with integrated geographic, demographic, and risk-group stratifications more accurately reflect disease transmission (Worden & Porco, 2017). This can consider differences in immunity, age, and sociality, which vary geographically and impact LTBI prevalence differently in populations.

In addition, incorporating geographic organization boosts predict precision for hotspots and hotspots that are susceptible to having high latent infection rates. Such detailed modeling is precious for guiding geographically and demographically informed public health interventions, thus maximizing resource utilization and enhancing control of LTBI on regional and local levels. Environmental, social, and cultural conditions likewise underpin geographic variability in LTBI rates by affecting both susceptibility and transmission capacity. Crowded regions, lower socioeconomic status, and poor ventilation often go hand-in-hand with a higher prevalence of LTBI since they provide more exposure opportunities to MTB. Geographic isolation can likewise be accompanied by less education on health and fewer outreach programs in communities, further solidifying high infection areas (Leining, 2019).

These complex factors highlight the complexities of geographic disparities in LTBI, showing that infection rates cannot be explained by biological susceptibility alone but have to be explained within ecological and societal contexts. Fixing disparities in LTBI calls for holistic strategies incorporating enhancement of healthcare access, environmental status, and community mobilization to counteract geographic inequities that drive LTBI.

12.2. Pathophysiology of Latent Tuberculosis Infection (LTBI)

The complexity of LTBI lies in its ability to persist within the host without causing active disease, a feature that fundamentally influences its pathophysiology. *Mtb*, the pathogen responsible for TB, can infect various tissues, including lymphatic sites, where it remains contained primarily by the host's immune responses. The granulomatous structures formed during LTBI are central to its containment, acting as physical and immunological barriers that restrict bacterial proliferation.

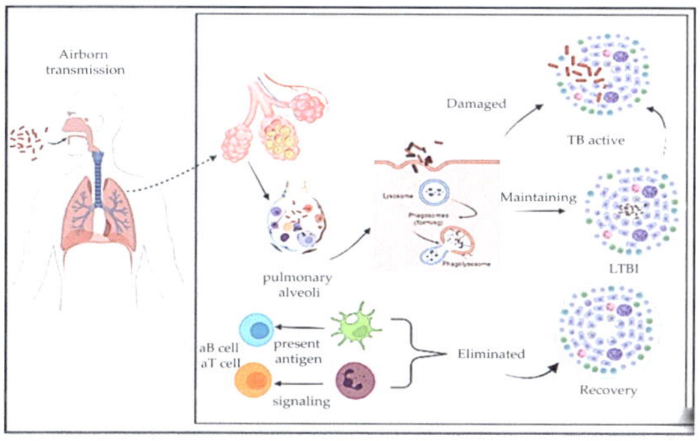

Figure 12.6. Diagram showing latent tuberculosis infection (LTBI) and its mechanism. Healthy individuals inhale *Mycobacterium tuberculosis* (*Mtb*) excreted by patients with active TB, which is recognized and phagocytized by macrophages, neutrophils, natural killer (NK) cells, and B lymphocytes.

Source: Sadeghi, J., & Saburi, A. (2016). Latent tuberculosis infection: Diagnostic approaches and treatment. *Iranian Journal of Medical Microbiology, 10*(1), 1–10.

However, such granulomas are dynamic and consist of a variety of immune cells that interact with each other in a delicate balance between bacterial persistence and host tissue integrity. Breakdown in this equilibrium, especially immune suppression, can lead to reactivation with active tuberculosis. Spatial immune cell interaction, particularly in lymph nodes (LNs), therefore, has far-reaching ramifications for unraveling the pathophysiology of LTBI and its reactivation (Miranda-Hernandez et al., 2025).

The keystone to LTBI containment is the differential function of immune cell subsets. Although $CD4^+$ T cells have long been recognized as central to *Mtb* infection control, recent evidence underscores the critical role of other immune subsets, in particular $CD8^+$ T cells, in preventing LTBI reactivation. Through immunosuppression, the redistribution and modification of immune cells within the lymphoid tissue microenvironment are implicated in the containment of latent bacteria. Interestingly, while B cells rise in infected LNs during immunosuppression, their establishment is not critical for latency maintenance. Vaccination strategies using recombinant BCG strains amplify immune-mediated LTBI control through the selective induction of $CD8^+$ T cell responses, which highlights a new paradigm of immune correlates in LTBI pathophysiology (Miranda-Hernandez et al., 2025). In addition to cellular mechanisms, inflammatory markers like the systemic inflammatory response index (SIRI) have also turned out to be critical markers in the pathophysiology as well as clinical prognosis of LTBI. Current cohort studies show an inverse association between SIRI levels and LTBI incidence, indicating that systemic inflammation may be inversely related to latent infection prevalence. Nonetheless, within infected persons with *Mtb*, elevated SIRI levels correlate with a greater risk of mortality, suggesting that systemic inflammation may mirror adverse immune activation or disease progression to active disease. Such findings not only augment the mechanistic insights into LTBI but also promise clinical utility in risk stratification and LTBI patient monitoring, possibly affecting future therapeutic approaches (Figure 12.6).

12.2.1. Mechanism of *Mycobacterium tuberculosis* (MTB) Infection

The first contact between MTB and the human host takes place in the alveolar compartments of the lung, where antigen-presenting cells (APCs) like macrophages and dendritic cells (DCs) internalize the bacilli. This is a key interaction since it determines whether there will be containment of the infection or its establishment. MTB carries a well-developed armory of genetic activity that enables it to manipulate the host's immune defenses, thereby ensuring its survival within the aggressive cellular environment of phagocytic cells. The pathogen suppresses the microbicidal activity of infected immune cells by hijacking intracellular signaling, blocking phagosome-lysosome fusion, and withstanding oxidative and nitrosative stress. These tactics guarantee the existence of the bacteria, frequently leading to the development of granulomas—organized frameworks of immune cells that seek to sequester the bacilli but also serve as niches for latent infection (Ahmad et al., 2011). After initial infection, the immune system initiates a multifaceted response that seeks to suppress MTB replication and restrict tissue damage. Yet the ability of the bacterium to modulate this response allows it to enter a state of quiescence, a characteristic of LTBI. Granulomas have a contradictory role: in containing the infection, the microenvironment within the granuloma can also sustain the survival of the bacteria in a non-replicating condition. This balance between host control and bacterial persistence is governed by host factors as well as bacterial virulence determinants, modulating the probability of disease progression to active disease or latent persistence. The complex balance presided over within granulomatous lesions underscores the dynamic nature of LTBI and the critical importance of deciphering bacterial-host interactions for designing effective interventions (Ahmad et al., 2011). The interaction between MTB infection and immunocompromising disorders, including HIV co-infection, radically modifies the natural course of latent infection. Immunopathogenesis due to HIV leads to the breakdown of controls governing the containment of the bacilli, causing more frequent reactivation of latent tuberculosis and accelerated progression after recent infection.

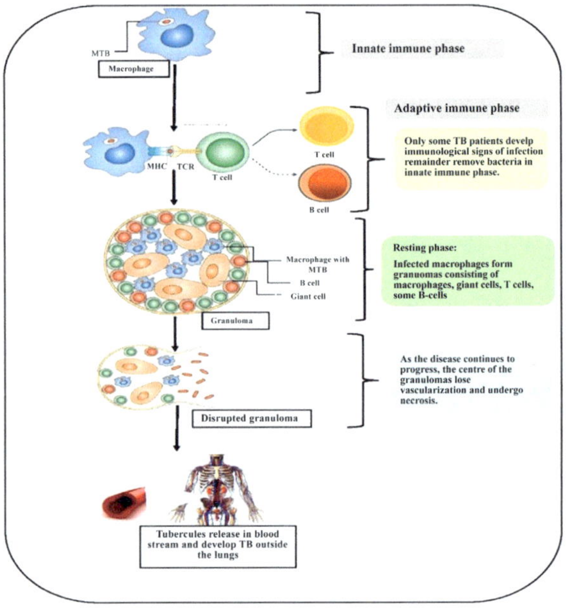

Figure 12.7. Basic mechanism of infection of *Mycobacterium tuberculosis* (MTB).

Source: ResearchGate. (n.d.). *Basic mechanism of infection of Mycobacterium tuberculosis.* https://www.researchgate.net/figure/Basic-mechanism-of-infection-of-Mycobacterium-tuberculosis_fig1_291952234.

Experiments have shown that individuals who are infected with co-pathogens have significantly enhanced risks of developing active tuberculosis, which suggests the central role of immune surveillance in latency. Disruption of the granuloma integrity and dysfunction of macrophages under HIV influence enable bacterial spread and disease progression. Understanding the molecular and immunological mechanisms underpinning these interactions remains crucial to addressing the global tuberculosis burden, especially in regions heavily impacted by the HIV pandemic (Figure 12.7).

12.2.2. Immune Response to Latent Tuberculosis Infection (LTBI)

To understand the immune response to LTBI, one must explore how the host's immune cells react to *Mtb*. Not everyone infected with *Mtb* develops active disease, with some becoming latently infected, defined by immune control of the pathogen with no symptomatic disease. This is orchestrated to a great extent by an complex web of cytokines and immune cells, led by peripheral blood mononuclear cells (PBMCs), which are instrumental in shaping the response. More recent studies utilizing live Mtb stimulation of PBMCs have emphasized unique cytokine profiles that distinguish individuals with LTBI from those exhibiting resistant phenotypes.

Certain cytokines, for example, like IL-17A and MCP-1, have been associated with categorizing immune responsiveness, proposing the idea that in addition to traditional markers like interferon-gamma (IFN-γ), a more comprehensive immune signature is important for sustaining latency as well as distinguishing it from active infection risk (Balfour et al., 2025). At the center of immune control within LTBI is T-cell subpopulation activity, most notably the Th17 subset, which plays a role in type 3 immune responses. Th17 cells are regulated by cytokines IL-6, IL-23, and IL-21; factors that induce STAT3 transcription pathways that are critical to their development and function. These cells secrete pro-inflammatory cytokines, such as IL-17, which are essential for neutrophil and other immune effector cell recruitment that harbor *Mtb* in granulomas. The equilibrium of these cytokine-driven pathways dictates the ability of the host to preserve infection latency against disease activation. This equilibrium reveals the significance of immune modulation and implies therapeutic interventions for preventing reactivation in exposed populations (Kudryavtsev et al., 2024). The heterogeneity of immune responses in individuals with LTBI uncovers a complexity that defies the binary distinction of infection status.

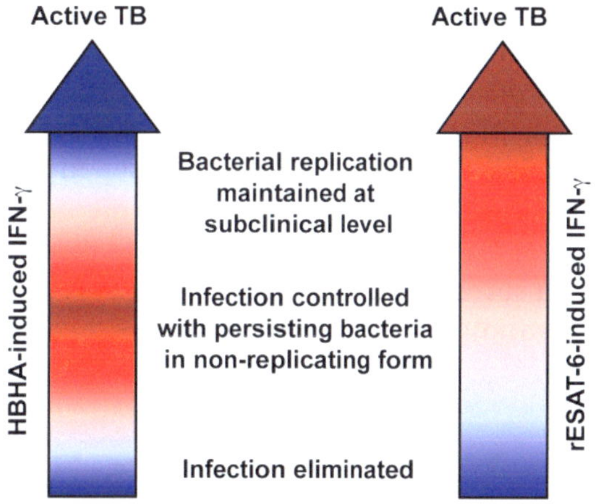

Figure 12.8. Spectrum of immune responses during LTBI. We propose to relate the spectrum of LTBI to the IFN-γ responses to two different mycobacterial antigens, HBHA represented in the left arrow, and rESAT-6 represented in the right arrow.

Source: ResearchGate. (n.d.). *Spectrum of immune responses during LTBI: We propose to relate the spectrum of LTBI to stages of TB disease as defined clinically and radiologically.* https://www.researchgate.net/figure/Spectrum-of-immune-responses-during-LTBI-We-propose-to-relate-the-spectrum-of-LTBI-to_fig13_230716469.

Recent evidence shows that even among individuals who are considered resistant or latently infected, there are separate clusters of cytokine responses, reflecting different underlying immune strategies. For instance, subsets of cytokines like TRAIL, MIP-1β, and Fractalkine have been found to clearly distinguish these immune response profiles. This immunological variability can be indicative of differential reactivation risks and underscores the limitation of existing diagnostic tools to interferon-gamma release assays (IGRAs) and TSTs. Therefore, incorporating multidimensional cytokine profiles into predictive and diagnostic models may enhance detecting real latent infection and maximize targeted interventions (Balfour et al., 2025) (Figure 12.8).

12.2.3. Transition from Latent Tuberculosis Infection (LTBI) to Active Tuberculosis

Understanding the development from LTBI to active tuberculosis disease requires consideration of both host and environmental determinants that affect immune control. Latent infection happens when MTB exists in the host without inducing signs or symptoms, held primarily by a good immune response. Still, there are conditions that alter this balance to cause reactivation of bacteria and clinical disease. In particular, chronic conditions like DM severely weaken the host's immune system, predisposing it to a greater risk of progression to active TB. Studies in sub-Saharan Africa have highlighted the interdependence of tuberculosis and diabetes, which indicate that diabetic patients have three times the susceptibility to active tuberculosis, possibly as a result of compromised immune responses and dysregulation of glucose metabolism (Faurholt-Jepsen, 2013). This association underscores the importance of addressing comorbid conditions to prevent LTBI reactivation and subsequent disease.

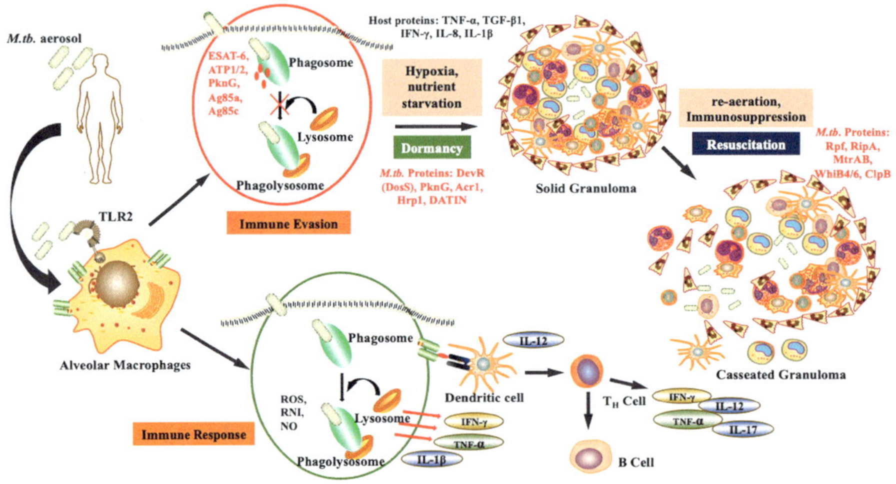

Figure 12.9. Re-activation of *M. tuberculosis* from latent stage of infection. All infected individuals are not getting into active Tuberculosis. Only 5–10% of Infected persons are getting active Tuberculosis and remaining 90–95% are remain healthy (LTBI).

Source: Verma A, Ghoshal A, Dwivedi VP and Bhaskar A (2022) Tuberculosis: The success tale of less explored dormant Mycobacterium tuberculosis. Front. Cell. Infect. Microbiol. 12:1079569. doi: 10.3389/fcimb.2022.1079569

The host immune system's ability to contain *Mtb* during latency critically depends on cytokines such as tumor necrosis factor (TNF), which orchestrate granuloma formation and maintenance. Experimental and computational studies demonstrate that TNF modulates both soluble and membrane-bound forms to regulate immune responses effectively, preventing bacterial proliferation. Therapeutic agents such as anti-TNF drugs, which are commonly applied to treat autoimmune diseases, have been associated with augmented rates of tuberculosis reactivation, highlighting the critical function of TNF in maintaining latent infection suppression (Denise et al., 2007).

These observations underscore the manner in which specific immune modulation can inadvertently disturb the fine immunological balance, leading to LTBI progression to active disease.

Clarification of such mechanisms is helpful in creating safer therapy with intact host resistance to tuberculosis. Outside host variables, outcomes of treatment and mortality risk are also influenced by conditions that promote LTBI progression. Patients co-infected with tuberculosis and diabetes gain weight slowly, have delayed hemoglobin recovery, and a much increased rate of mortality during treatment initiation phases (Faurholt-Jepsen, 2013).

Such clinical indicators imply that diabetes not only predisposes an individual to active disease but also makes therapeutic responses complicated, thus promoting an adverse disease course. The rising tide of diabetes in areas with established tuberculosis burdens presents a public health threat, risking reversal of recent improvements in tuberculosis control. As a result, integrated management models addressing both diabetes and latent tuberculosis may be critical to prevent LTBI to active infection conversion and enhance patient survival worldwide (Figure 12.9).

12.3. Diagnosis of Latent Tuberculosis Infection (LTBI)

Accurate diagnosis of LTBI is important in the control of tuberculosis dissemination, especially among populations at high risk like medical students and healthcare professionals. Screening mostly starts with the TST, a procedure that assesses the body's immune response to inhaled purified protein derivative (PPD) and serves to detect exposed persons to MTB. Although the specificity of TST can be affected by previous *Bacille Calmette-Guérin* (BCG) vaccination or past exposure to nontuberculous mycobacteria (NTM), resulting in false positives. For the sake of enhanced accuracy, positive results from TST are often confirmed by IGRAs, like the QuantiFERON-TB test (QFT). This two-step diagnostic strategy has been illustrated in research that evaluates the prevalence of LTBI in healthcare students, highlighting the need for confirmatory testing to enhance diagnosis and avoid unnecessary treatment (Verso et al., 2019). Although diagnostic strategies have improved, there are still issues in the application of LTBI testing at the population level and its cost-effectiveness, particularly in resource-limited healthcare systems. Economic analyses show that, although the up-front costs of screening programs are high, early diagnosis and treatment of LTBI have the potential to significantly lower the burden of active tuberculosis and its related healthcare costs in the long run. In the United Kingdom and other nations where tuberculosis incidence has been rising steadily, there is greater interest in the development and implementation of point-of-care diagnostic tests that are fast, low cost, and very sensitive. These innovations have the potential to increase screening effectiveness, enable timely intervention, and eventually reduce disease spread in high-risk groups (Szczepura & Osipenko, unpublished). Clinically, LTBI diagnosis occurs by combining epidemiological risk factors, clinical presentation, and test findings to ensure correct identification. Prevalence studies in healthcare trainees have reported generally low LTBI rates, yet results point to differences between undergraduate and postgraduate groups to imply differing exposure risks.

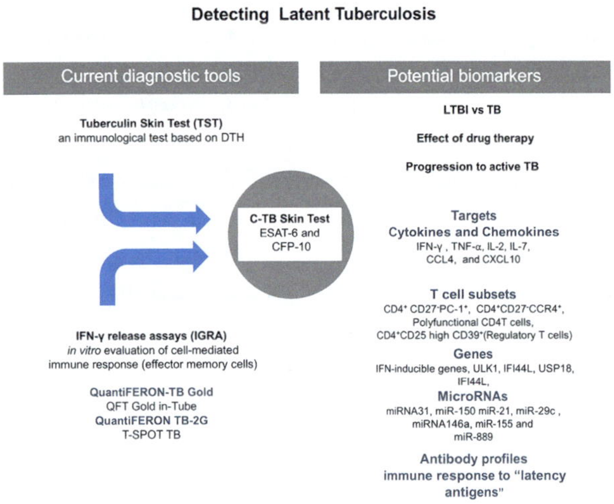

Figure 12.10. Summary of the actual and potential tools for the diagnosis of latent tuberculosis infection (LTBI). At the center of the figure, there is the C-TB skin test, which combines the sensitivity of the *in vivo* tuberculin skin test (TST) and the specificity of early secretory antigenic target (ESAT-6) and the 10-kDa culture filtrate protein (CFP-10) antigens for *M. tuberculosis* on the left side of the figure are the current diagnostic tools (TST and IGRA). On the right side of the figure are listed some of the potential biomarkers to detect LTBI.

Source: Carranza C, Pedraza-Sanchez S, de Oyarzabal-Mendez E and Torres M (2020) Diagnosis for Latent Tuberculosis Infection: New Alternatives. Front. Immunol. 11:2006. doi: 10.3389/fimmu.2020.02006

Moreover, the history of vaccination is an important determinant of test result interpretation, with an increased percentage of vaccinated cases yielding positive results among certain groups. Such subtleties highlight the importance of context-specific screening approaches that take into account local epidemiology, history of previous immunization, and occupational risk to maximize diagnosis and avert progression from latent infection to active tuberculosis (Verso et al., 2019) (Figure 12.10).

12.3.1. Tuberculin Skin Test (TST)

The proper diagnosis of LTBI is crucial to successful disease control and prevention, especially in areas with tuberculosis (TB) burden. In Iraq, where TB is still a health burden, new treatment modalities like intradermal BCG vaccine immunotherapy for viral warts have been tried. These interventions could potentially affect the validity of diagnostic tests for TB, especially the TST. The TST is also used extensively to determine BCG vaccine effectiveness and to test for LTBI, but its interpretation is problematic when prior BCG vaccination is a factor. Such interference is problematic because the resultant immune response from the vaccine can give false-positive TST results and thus potentially impair diagnostic specificity. It is thus imperative to assess the implications of using BCG-based therapies on TST interpretation prior to making general recommendations in high TB burden nations (Al-Mendalawi, 2021). Apart from the complications caused by BCG vaccination, the TST has other limitations due to patient-specific factors. Immunosuppression, for example, greatly affects test results, as evidenced by the reduced sensitivity of TST among those on corticosteroid therapy. A comparative analysis of the TST versus the QuantiFERON TB-Gold test (QFT) demonstrated a significant discordance, with TST giving a higher proportion of positive results but with fewer correlations to accepted risk factors for tuberculosis exposure. The QFT, on the other hand, was found to better correlate to true TB risk factors, illustrating its diagnostic superiority in some immunocompromised patients. These observations highlight the importance of taking into consideration patient background and immune status in interpreting

TST, as they are prone to false positives in vaccinated patients and false negatives in immunosuppressed individuals (Søborg et al., 2009). Notwithstanding its drawbacks, the TST is still a cornerstone for detecting LTBI because of its availability, low cost, and widespread clinical use. Clinicians are required to preserve a subtle insight into its issues of interpretation, especially in vaccinated populations where there is a great likelihood of cross-reactivity. Existing evidence encourages a guarded and context-dependent way of using TST, striking a balance between the advantages of early detection of LTBI with the disadvantage of misdiagnosis. Further incorporating other diagnostic means like QFT can offer supportive information, even in complicated instances of immunosuppression or previous interference vaccination. Ultimately, the best LTBI detection strategies depend on a profound evaluation of TSTs diagnostic accuracy in the overall clinical and epidemiological context (Al-Mendalawi, 2021; Søborg et al., 2009) (Figure 12.11).

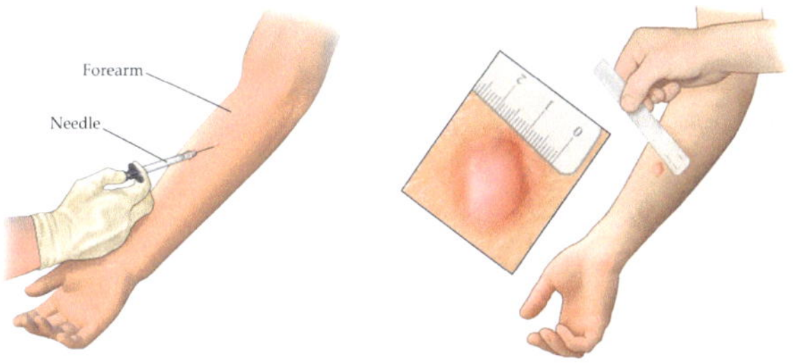

Figure 12.11. Tuberculin skin test (TST) for latent tuberculosis infection (LTBI).

Source: Healthy Lungs. (n.d.). *Mantoux test for latent tuberculosis infection.* https://www.healthylungs.in/image/blog/ltbi/mantouxtest.jpg.

12.3.2. Interferon-Gamma Release Assays (IGRAs)

Identification of LTBI continues to be an important step in tuberculosis control plans, particularly in high-risk populations that may progress to disease. The conventional method of diagnosis was mainly based on the use of the TST, which, although used extensively, has the disadvantage of cross-reactivity with the BCG vaccine and environmental NTM. The development of this limitation has generated interest in the use of IGRAs, which quantify the response to antigens of MTB. These tests, including QuantiFERON and T-SPOT.TB, provide enhanced specificity by focusing on antigens not present in BCG strains, thus reducing false-positive results prevalent with TST. Assessments of IGRA deployment among adult close contacts of active pulmonary TB cases have shown them to be cost-effective compared to TST-based approaches, especially when used as single tests, and noted their potential to maximize LTBI screening programs (Green et al., 2025). Despite the potential of IGRAs in LTBI diagnosis, their efficacy is prone to variation depending on geographical, demographic, and clinical considerations.

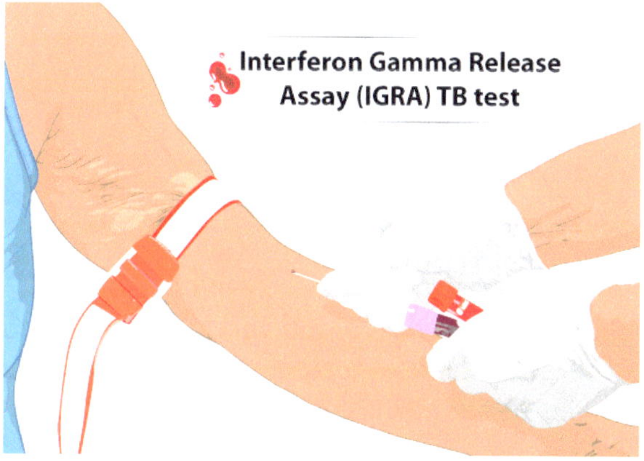

Source: MyUpchar. (n.d.). *IGRA TB test illustration.* https://image.myupchar.com/9372/original/igra-tb-test.png.

A comparative study carried out across various regions in Ghana evaluated the diagnostic performance of three IGRAs—TBF-FIA, TBF-ELISA, and QFT-Plus—in populations with different TB exposure statuses. The research showed subtle differences in sensitivity and specificity: e.g., TBF-ELISA had slightly greater sensitivity but at the cost of lower specificity than QFT-Plus, and TBF-FIA had an even diagnostic profile. These differences indicate that whereas IGRAs in general are equivalent in terms of diagnostic accuracy, selection of assays may need to be situationally dependent upon understanding population parameters and prevalence. In addition, the relative lack of in-depth data on more recent assays such as TBF-FIA means that more study is needed to confirm these results and update diagnostic algorithms (Kutame et al., 2024).

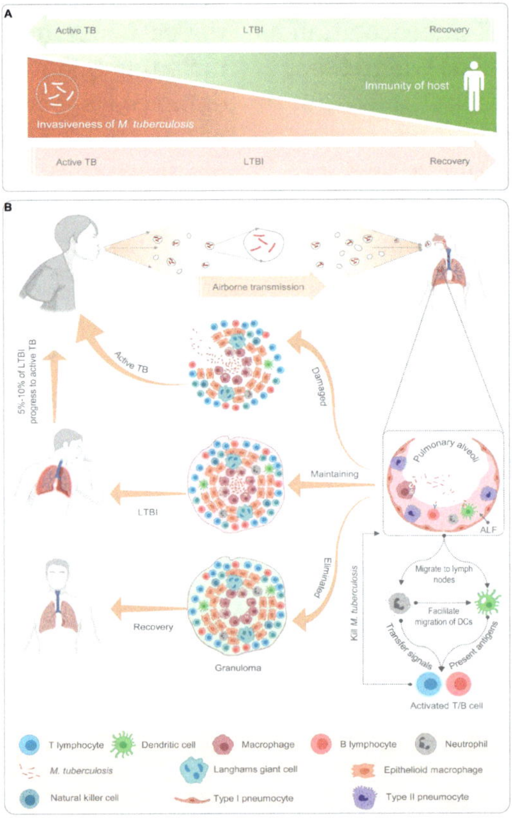

Figure 12.12. *In vivo* and *in vitro* tests for detecting *Mycobacterium tuberculosis*. (A) According to the CDC, the Mantoux test involves injecting 5 tuberculin units (TUs – 0.1 mL) intradermally into the flexor surface of the left forearm. A tuberculin syringe should be used for the injection. The test result is read after 48 hours. Individuals who have been exposed to the bacteria in the past develop an immune response to bacterial proteins on their skin. The response is a classic example of a delayed-type hypersensitivity (DTH) reaction. Inflammation is generated by T cells and myeloid cells attracted to the reaction site within 1–3 days. (B) Interferon-gamma release assay (IGRA) tests: each patient receives a positive control tube, a negative control tube, and TB antigen tubes. A heparinized human blood sample is obtained from the patient by venipuncture, and 1 mL from each sample is pipetted into three tubes: negative, positive, and TB antigen. The tubes are gently mixed by inverting and placed in a 37°C incubator overnight.

Source: Gong W and Wu X (2021) Differential Diagnosis of Latent Tuberculosis Infection and Active Tuberculosis: A Key to a Successful Tuberculosis Control Strategy. Front. Microbiol. 12:745592. doi: 10.3389/fmicb.2021.745592

The integration of IGRAs into LTBI screening programs is a major breakthrough in surmounting the drawback postulated by the TST, especially among BCG-vaccinated individuals. Economic analyses highlighted that single-step IGRA approaches, particularly the use of QuantiFERON, has positive results not only in terms of accuracy but also in terms of cost-savings when screening adult contacts of pulmonary TB patients. This result is consistent with guideline suggestions that support IGRA use in certain clinical situations to maximize the accuracy of LTBI diagnoses. However, potential limitations, e.g., requirements for specialized laboratory facilities and variability of immune responses among immunocompromised persons, need to be included in implementation plans. Ongoing improvement of IGRAs, such as assay standardization and wider validation, will be important to establishing their place in integrated tuberculosis control programs (Green et al., 2025) (Figure 12.12).

12.3.3. Challenges in Diagnosing Latent Tuberculosis Infection (LTBI)

Diagnosis of LTBI is still a sophisticated problem exacerbated by the limitations of available diagnostic tests. In contrast to active tuberculosis, LTBI is not symptomatically apparent and is non-contagious, hence the hindrance in clinical detection. The conventional tests, including the TST and IGRAs, identify immune reactions to MTB antigens but are not able to specifically differentiate between active and latent infection. This uncertainty generates diagnostic uncertainty, particularly among individuals highly exposed to non-tuberculosis mycobacteria or previously vaccinated with BCG. Furthermore, immune-compromised subjects, such as HIV co-infected patients, frequently yield false-negative or indeterminate tests, making LTBI diagnosis even more challenging. Recent discoveries investigating serum microRNA signatures propose potential non-invasive tests that may improve the accuracy and specificity of diagnoses, recognizing genetic and ethnic heterogeneity in populations (Miotto et al., 2013). A further source of complexity in the diagnosis of LTBI is its overlap with comorbidities such as DM, which changes the immune response and susceptibility of the host to tuberculosis. In the high-prevalence settings of TB and DM, the differentiation between latent infections and active disease is imperative for the maximization of treatment approaches. The occurrence of DM camouflages the subtle clinical presentation of TB progression, and this diminishes the sensitivity of immune-based diagnostic assays. Mathematical modeling research suggests that focused interventions for DM patients might substantially lower incidence and mortality from TB but will succeed only if LTBI is properly detected in this subgroup.

The diagnostic dilemma introduced by concomitant DM thus emphasizes the necessity for enhanced screening procedures that take into account metabolic effects on immune responsiveness (Sterling et al., 2020). Added to these diagnostic challenges is the heterogeneity of the presentation of LTBI among different populations, taking into consideration differences in ethnicity, geographic prevalence, and genetic susceptibility. Existing diagnostics are unable to accurately identify which person with latent infection will develop active TB, thus constraining prevention strategies. Research on serum miRNA profiles demonstrates potential ways in which LTBI can be distinguished from active pulmonary TB as well as other pulmonary infections, providing insights into population-specific biomarkers. These results underscore the value of tailoring tests to account for epidemiological and immunological variation between settings. However, implementation of such biomolecular strategies into standard clinical practice is constrained by practical considerations, such as cost, availability, and the requirement for validation in large cohorts (Miotto et al., 2013). These complex diagnostic issues must be addressed to move LTBI management forward and to bring the worldwide TB epidemic under control.

12.4. Treatment Options for Latent Tuberculosis Infection (LTBI)

Successful management of LTBI is key to avoiding disease progression, especially in groups at high risk. LTBI treatment has become more sophisticated with several WHO-authorized regimens available for individualized choice depending on patient profile and likely drug tolerance. In particular, the weekly rifapentine and isoniazid regimen (3HP) has come to the forefront because of its shortness and high completion rates. A trial of older patients with chronic obstructive pulmonary disease (COPD), a population that is at greater risk for tuberculosis, proved that 3HP was the most commonly administered regimen with an overall rate of completion of 82.0%. This is a testament to how practical and safe the regimen is, even in the elderly with comorbidities, where adverse events are still the leading cause for stopping the regimen. Involving the patient in collaborative decision-making with the provider can further improve adherence and outcomes (Huang et al., 2025). Although rifapentine and isoniazid-based regimens predominate LTBI therapy, other regimens such as daily isoniazid or rifampicin monotherapies augment the therapeutic armament. The choice of an optimal regimen usually takes into account drug interactions, current comorbid conditions, and possible side effects. For example, longer monotherapy with isoniazid can be selected when rifamycin tolerance is an issue, even though the duration of treatment is extended. Individualization of treatment is crucial for the reason that incomplete or poorly tolerated therapy jeopardizes both efficacy and resistance emergence. In addition, screening practices in different patient populations, e.g., candidates for systemic immunosuppressive therapy such as biologics in psoriasis, require careful monitoring of treatment for LTBI to prevent reactivation hazards. The inflammatory condition of patients, which can be elevated in the case of concomitant chronic diseases, adds extra points of consideration in treatment planning, pointing to the complexity of dealing with LTBI in a wide range of clinical situations (Müfide et al., 2024). Compliance with treatment protocols for LTBI is often hampered by fears of side effects, long treatment regimens, and patient comorbidities. Interventions to enhance completion rates thus need to incorporate patient education, risk-benefit counseling, and routine monitoring for toxicity.

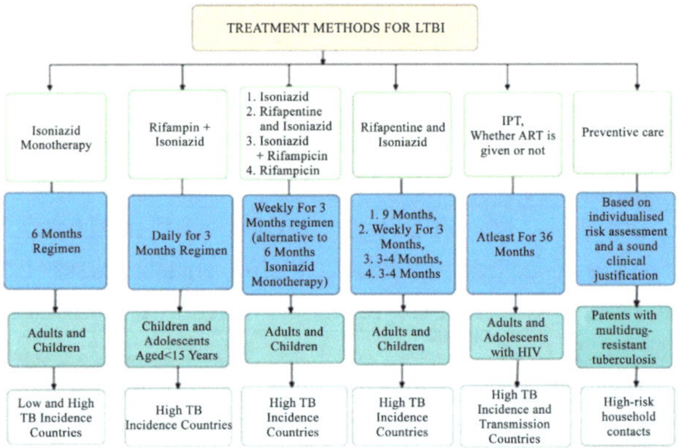

Figure 12.13. Treatment methods for LTBI. Various treatment regimens for treating LTBI.

Source: ResearchGate. (n.d.). *Treatment methods for LTBI: Various treatment regimens for treating LTBI.* https://www.researchgate.net/publication/375083384/figure/fig4/AS:11431281205456692@1700275908371/Treatment-methods-for-LTBI-Various-treatment-regimens-for-treating-LTBI.png.

The data from the elderly COPD cohort emphasize that with proper regimen selection and clinical follow-up, compliance rates of more than 80% are achievable, a threshold level of importance in lowering tuberculosis incidence. Furthermore, the promotion of research on shorter, safer regimens as well as biomarkers of treatment response may lead to further simplification of LTBI management in the years to come. Finally, effective LTBI treatment programs need not only effective pharmacologic agents but also health system capacity that can accommodate patient-specific challenges and ensure long-term follow-up. These multi-faceted interventions offer promise for successful tuberculosis control through targeted LTBI intervention (Müfide et al., 2024; Huang et al., 2025) (Figure 12.13).

12.4.1. Recommended Treatment Regimens

Successful management of LTBI depends importantly on the choice of optimal treatment regimens that maximize efficacy without increasing toxicity. Guidelines now emphasize tailoring therapy to patient risk and resource determinants, especially in intermediate and low TB-incidence settings. Several regimens have proven effective in preventing active disease progression; among them, long-term isoniazid monotherapy (6–9 months) remains a core option. However, shorter rifamycin-based regimens have also become popular due to their similar efficacy and enhanced patient compliance. In patients at increased risk, who are HIV-infected or recent contacts of new smear-positive pulmonary TB—systematic screening with immediate treatment is highly recommended. Chest radiography is warranted prior to commencing therapy to rule out active disease, making treatment of LTBI both safe and specific (Getahun et al., 2015). This strategic plan indicates a changing environment with emphasis placed on public health effects and patient individual outcomes. New developments have redirected attention to rifamycin-containing regimens because of increased tolerability and completion rates relative to classic isoniazid monotherapy. New guidelines concentrate on three optimal treatment regimens: a 12-week daily regimen of once-weekly isoniazid plus rifapentine; a 3- to 4-month daily treatment of isoniazid plus rifampin; and a 4-month daily rifampin monotherapy. These abbreviated regimens are highly recommended following high-quality clinical trials proving non-inferiority in avoiding active TB and lower hepatotoxicity risk. The precise distinction between rifampin and rifapentine is vital since they are different drugs with unique dosage needs. The shift towards rifamycin-based therapy also mirrors patient adherence and healthcare system capacity considerations, with the goal of simplifying therapy and enhancing completion in different populations (Sterling et al., 2020). Therefore, such regimens are a major step forward in LTBI management in that they both improve safety as well as efficacy. Although rifamycin-based regimens are preferred, isoniazid monotherapy is still a worthwhile option when rifamycin administration is either contraindicated or not possible. The 6- to 9-month daily regimen of isoniazid is effective but is linked with increased toxicity, especially hepatotoxicity, and reduced completion rates in comparison with shorter rifamycin regimens. Thus, it tends to be reserved for unique clinical situations, such as treating rifampin-resistant strains or in the case of drug interactions where rifamycin cannot be used. Providers should carefully balance benefits against risks, taking into account patient-specific factors like comorbidities and drug tolerability. In summary, continued studies and meta-analyses further optimize regimen choice, highlighting the importance of adaptive protocols that adapt to varying epidemiological settings and maximize treatment benefits (Sterling et al., 2020). Such detailed guidelines reflect the ever-evolving context of managing LTBI in clinical care.

12.4.2. Duration and Adherence to Treatment

Treatment adherence is also a key factor in the effective control of LTBI, where an interaction between patient behavior and duration of treatment can have a decisive impact. It has been revealed through studies that patients undergoing isoniazid therapy demonstrate inconsistent patterns of adherence based on the duration for which they have received the drug. Interestingly, individuals who have been undergoing treatment for two to four months are less likely to be non-adherent than those at the initial stages of therapy, i.e., less than two months (Simwaka et al., 2024). This is an indication that the first period of treatment is when serious challenges are likely to occur possibly attributable to side effects or drug weariness. Comprehension of these temporal compliance dynamics is necessary for healthcare workers seeking to maximize interventions and support mechanisms during the critical initial period of treatment to ensure long-term completion and ultimately enhance LTBI control. The complexities of having persistent treatment compliance are also dictated by side effects of LTBI therapy. Side effects like vomiting and peripheral neuropathy have been recognized as major hindrances, significantly raising the rate of non-adherence in patients who are taking isoniazid (Simwaka et al., 2024). Not only do these side effects weaken the physical well-being of patients, but they also discourage drug consumption, which compromises the treatment effect. Conversely, short-duration and tolerable regimens like rifamycin-based treatment have shown enhanced rates of adherence and possibly enhanced efficacy. The advent of these other treatments underscores the value of adapting therapy duration and selection to prevent side effects and enhance adherence, highlighting a patient-focused initiative in LTBI treatment regimens. Social networks come up as a key factor in LTBI treatment adherence, significantly influencing patient commitment throughout the course of therapy. Facts show that patients with strong social support are far less likely to demonstrate non-adherence than patients with weak or poor social networks (Simwaka et al., 2024). This social component not only gives emotional support but can also support practical ones like reminding medications and help with managing side effects. Therefore, enhancing patient outcomes needs to integrate approaches that enhance social support together with clinical management. By recognizing the contribution of social environments and including patient education and community resources, healthcare frameworks can assist in maintaining adherence for the whole duration of treatment, which is crucial for successful LTBI control.

12.4.3. Side Effects and Management of Treatment

Management of LTBI entails the use of preventive treatment regimens meant to eliminate latent MTB and prevent future active disease. Such regimens have been associated with side effects that can impact patient compliance. The most frequent adverse reactions reported include hepatotoxicity, gastrointestinal symptoms, and allergic reactions. While side effects are a factor for concern, research has shown that the frequency and intensity of these reactions are highly variable among individuals, and do not always correlate with worse treatment compliance. Side effect management encompasses early detection and monitoring, education of the patient as to the anticipated transient nature of mild symptoms, and prompt clinical intervention in the event of more severe adverse events. Such a strategy works towards maintaining patients active within therapy until treatment is finished, which is of particular importance due to the worldwide burden of LTBI and its tendency to become active tuberculosis if left untreated (Denholm & McBryde, 2010; Benjamin et al., 2016). In addition to targeting individual side effects, management of treatment for LTBI, in general, must take into account the complexities of patient adherence among heterogeneous populations, particularly immigrant populations in low-prevalence settings. Cultural and language barriers may impede patients' comprehension of the benefits and risks of treatments, thereby fueling fears of side effects and limiting willingness to continue therapy. Studies point out that when physicians provide culturally tailored education and unambiguous communication regarding side effect profiles, treatment aims, and the value of completion, adherence becomes much better. Also, implementing more abbreviated, well-tolerated regimens has proved to be able to reduce the severity of adverse effects, allowing for better patient compliance. Maintenance of a stable care setting with engaged providers who provide follow-up and support that is individualized is just as important in allowing management of side effects and maintenance of treatment adherence in LTBI (Benjamin et al., 2016). The continuing development of novel treatment regimens remains an evolving process as part of the challenge to balance efficacy against patient tolerance. Recent developments target the optimization of regimens to minimize duration and reduce toxicity while reducing the risk of side effects leading to early discontinuation. For instance, rifapentine-based short-course treatments with isoniazid have proven equivalent efficacy compared to conventional longer regimens while providing enhanced tolerability. Monitoring procedures involving laboratory tests of liver function and clinical assessments are critical elements of side effect management that allow for early hepatotoxicity detection. In addition, incorporating patient-level strategies, including individualized education, culturally adapted interventions, and strong adherence support systems, is an avenue towards the diminishment of the socio-economic impact of LTBI in host nations. These approaches highlight the importance of side effect management as both a clinical priority and as part of public health strategies to manage tuberculosis (Denholm & McBryde, 2010; Benjamin et al., 2016) (Figure 12.14).

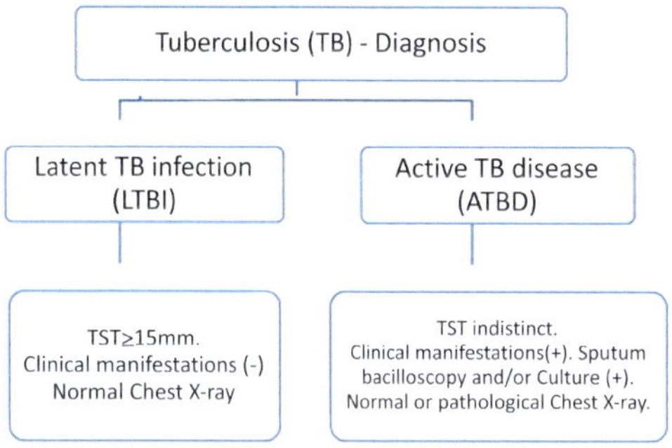

Figure 12.14. Algorithm for the management of latent tuberculosis infection (LTBI) in individuals at risk for tuberculosis (TB).

Source: Sanchez C, Jaramillo-Valverde L, Capristano S, Solis G, Soto A, Valdivia-Silva J, Poterico JA, Guio H. Antigen-Induced IL-1RA Production Discriminates Active and Latent Tuberculosis Infection. *Microorganisms*. 2023; 11(6):1385. https://doi.org/10.3390/microorganisms11061385

12.5. Socioeconomic Factors

Socioeconomic status is vital in LTBI epidemiology and control, especially in immigrant populations in low-prevalent countries. Economically disadvantaged people tend to have barriers like unstable accommodation, restricted access to healthcare, and language barriers that all compromise treatment adherence with LTBI. Research among immigrants in Western countries suggests that these social determinants can result in reduced rates of treatment completion, sustaining reservoirs of LTBI within high-need populations. In addition, cultural and linguistic barriers also complicate education and communication, which further erodes patients' assessment for preventive therapy.

Dealing with these complex socioeconomic determinants is vital in the development of proper public health interventions, as not only does treatment adherence benefit individual health status but also reduces economic and societal costs related to active tuberculosis disease (Benjamin et al., 2016). Geographic remoteness and restricted healthcare access exacerbate the socioeconomic problems that LTBI patients encounter. Studies in various settings indicate a strong association between distance to health facilities and TST positivity, suggesting that populations living in distant or resource-constrained locations are at greater risk of undiagnosed and untreated LTBI. For instance, children in geographically remote areas exhibit significantly higher rates of prevalence, partly due to poor medical outreach and delayed diagnosis. These inequalities highlight the direct impact of infrastructural and socioeconomic disparities on infection rates and effectiveness of treatment. Strengthening health care delivery using mobile clinics, community health workers, and culturally appropriate outreach programs is critical to enhance treatment uptake and completion among marginalized populations, thus pushing TB control activities forward (Leining, 2019). The interaction between socioeconomic determinants and adherence to LTBI treatment also implies that patient-specific, patient-centered strategies are required to address current barriers. Evidence indicates that conventional sociodemographic factors like age, sex, and country of origin do not play a significant role in determining treatment adherence; instead, the stability of a person's residence, the presence of well-tolerated and shorter regimens, and positive healthcare interactions are crucial. Economic instability, frequently paired with psychosocial stressors, diminishes patients' ability to interact with health care services regularly. Subsequently, measures that combine economic, social, and cultural factors, such as offering transparent, language-appropriate instruction, building trust with committed healthcare providers, and adapting treatments to limit side effects, can substantially increase adherence rates. Such strategies constitute a key investment in public health and socioeconomic equality in receiving countries among immigrants (Benjamin et al., 2016) (Figure 12.15).

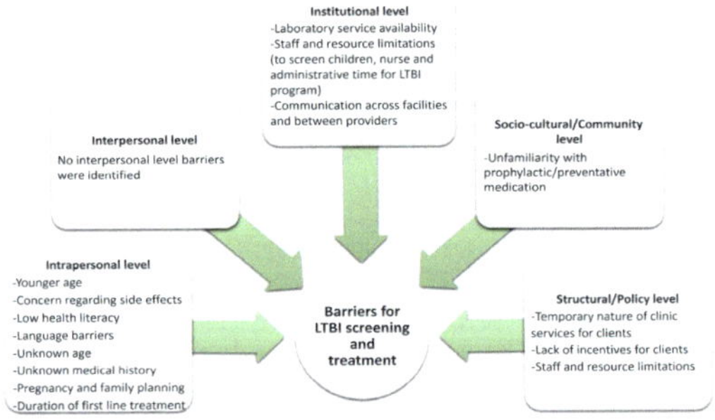

Figure 12.15. Facilitators for latent tuberculosis infection (LTBI) screening and treatment.

Source: National Collaborating Centre for Infectious Diseases (NCCID). (2017). *Latent tuberculosis infection diagram.* https://nccid.ca/wp-content/uploads/sites/2/2017/03/Fig5LTBI.png.

12.5.1. Influence of Poverty on Latent Tuberculosis Infection (LTBI) Prevalence

The complex dynamic of socioeconomic status and health results is increasingly known to be a vital component in the epidemiology of infectious diseases, such as LTBI. Poverty-stricken populations are commonly subjected to increased exposure to social determinants that enable the spread of MTB. Poor living conditions, suboptimal diet, and poor access to medical care weaken defenses and enhance susceptibility to infection. Also, the psychosocial stressors of poverty have the ability to weaken immune function, reducing the body's ability to keep latent infections at bay. Evidence suggests that negative psychosocial conditions are linked to impaired vaccine responses and changes in immune biomarkers, which have a direct effect on vulnerability to LTBI and disease progression to active tuberculosis (Hayward et al., 2019). The social and biological aspects of poverty then merge, multiplying the incidence and perpetuation of LTBI in underprivileged populations. Geographical and infrastructural limitations associated with poverty also augment the difficulties in the management of LTBI in poor-resource environments. Research has proved a robust association between indicators of community-level poverty—distance to healthcare centers, and high proportions of TST positivity among risk groups such as children. In geographically remote regions where diagnostic, preventive, and treatment services are not easily accessible, prevalence of LTBI increases exponentially, establishing the contribution of systemic barriers toward disease perpetuation (Leining, 2019). The challenge in accessing care adds to the risk of primary infection as well as the potential for untreated latent infections to develop into active tuberculosis. These geographic disparities emphasize the importance of focused health outreach and intervention efforts aimed at overcoming gaps in accessibility to help limit LTBI prevalence in low-income communities. Treatment of the effect of poverty on LTBI prevalence must be based on multiple pronged strategies that combine socioeconomic assistance with medical treatment. Apart from direct provision of healthcare services, interventions should also take into account the psychosocial context, as social disadvantage and stress erode immune competence and vaccine effectiveness, all of which are crucial to control LTBI (Hayward et al., 2019). Social protection interventions, better living conditions, and enhanced healthcare facilities in poor settings may alter the underlying determinants driving LTBI transmission. In addition, customized public health interventions that address logistical barriers and promote community engagement are necessary to end the cycle of poverty-driven vulnerability. Such holistic initiatives are critical to preventing LTBI prevalence and eventually minimizing the global tuberculosis burden.

12.5.2. Access to Healthcare and Treatment Disparities

Barriers to healthcare access tend to overlap with the complex arena of treatment acceptance, particularly in the case of LTBI. In healthcare professionals, for instance, willingness to accept LTBI therapy is strongly shaped by knowledge, attitudes, and perceived social norms. In one Malaysian teaching hospital, a study found that even with the high risk of disease reactivation, most healthcare workers had low levels of awareness and negative attitudes towards treatment of LTBI, which adversely influenced their acceptance of treatment. This suggests that knowledge gaps and social support are major causes of inequalities in the uptake of treatment even in groups that are directly exposed to infectious hazard. Closing these gaps through education and community norm interventions specifically targeted at them may increase the willingness to start therapy, which would prevent latent TB progression and transmission in healthcare facilities (Zakaria & Mansor 2024). Genetic vulnerabilities to side effects from LTBI treatment also cause healthcare disparities by impacting treatment completion rates and safety. Studies in healthcare professionals who were administered isoniazid and rifampin have identified particular HLA alleles, including HLA-A11:01 and HLA-DPB105:01, as risk factors for drug hypersensitivity and hepatotoxicity, respectively. The availability of these genetic markers complicates treatment plans, compelling clinicians to weigh efficacy against harm. Inequalities arise when patients are not properly screened for such genetic predisposition or in the event of unavailable alternative regimens due to resource limitations. Therefore, these genetic determinants highlight the value of individualized medicine in LTBI treatment, where evenhanded access to genetic testing might help minimize ADRs and enhance drug compliance (Kim et al., 2024). Socioeconomic and facility determinants also enhance inequalities in accessing LTBI treatment, especially in areas where there are no formal screening programs or policy on treatment. Healthcare environments without formal LTBI protocols tend not to offer systematic testing or follow-up treatment, leaving exposed workers at risk of untreated infection. Additionally, demographic factors like gender and clinical versus non-clinical job roles affect treatment acceptance, as evidenced by increased intention rates among female healthcare workers and those with increased exposure to clinical settings. These differences indicate that institutional policy and cultural norms collectively influence healthcare access and outcomes. To promote equity, effective LTBI management programs should integrate culturally appropriate education, inclusive screening practices, and intervention for addressing determinants of social health to ensure that treatment inequalities are reduced to a minimum within healthcare populations (Zakaria & Mansor, 2024).

12.5.3. Education and Awareness Regarding Latent Tuberculosis Infection (LTBI)

Successful interventions for communicable disease control in community settings frequently depend on the provision of correct information accompanied by focused screening programs. In the case of LTBI, educational programs carried out among adolescents from high school populations have shown encouraging potential. Thus, in San Diego County, where tuberculosis incidence remarkably exceeds the national baseline, an organized educational program among freshman students was initiated. This consisted of a single presentation on TB, and then pretest and posttest assessments to assess knowledge gain. Despite some difficulty with parental permission for additional screening, the intervention resulted in 18% higher awareness of LTBI among the students who participated. This implies that well-planned educational interventions are able to effectively engage young people and inculcate increased awareness of LTBI hazards, providing a basis for the development of stronger prevention measures in school settings (Bell, 2020). In addition to creating awareness, education needs to be coupled with practical measures like screening and treatment advice to effectively target LTBI. The San Diego program included the distribution of TB risk assessment forms and consent papers in student registration packages, along with confidential messaging inviting at-risk students' families to seek diagnostic evaluation. Despite the overall low return rate for risk assessments, a significant percentage of those returned indicated at-risk students, demonstrating a critical gap in LTBI case finding. Additionally, the program promoted the presence of shorter-duration treatment regimens like rifapentine and isoniazid (3HP), even possibly given through the school. Incentives were also used to encourage participation, highlighting the multi-step process to bring educational advancements into clinical action and ultimately minimize LTBI development within at-risk populations (Cunningham et al., 2019). However, barriers to effective education and awareness remain, particularly in achieving widespread screening compliance and parental engagement. The low return rate of TB risk assessments despite educational efforts indicates persistent obstacles in community participation and trust. Ensuring that educational programs are culturally sensitive, accessible, and coupled with clear pathways for testing and treatment may improve uptake. Also, including directly observed therapy (DOT) and on-site treatment opportunities in schools can alleviate logistical barriers experienced by families. Ongoing assessment and adjustment of these interventions are essential to maximize their effectiveness in the long term. Thus, education for LTBI should not only augment knowledge but also enable actionable public health interventions, promoting the complete management of latent tuberculosis among high-risk adolescent groups (Cunningham et al., 2019; Bell, 2020).

SUMMARY

The complexity of LTBI highlights the importance of focused intervention to decrease the future active tuberculosis burden. Improved management is initiated by identifying and treating high-risk individuals, such as immigrants and refugees, due to their disproportionate noncompletion rates of treatment. Data show that visa status individuals aged over 24 years have considerably poorer treatment adherence, and developing specific strategies for this group could significantly enhance outcomes. In addition, physical and logistical constraints, such as travel time to the point of treatment, combine with demographic characteristics to determine levels of adherence. Acknowledgment of these factors is vital in the development of targeted public health interventions that increase rates of completion and thus reduce the incidence of TB in high-risk groups. In this manner, such detailed strategies initiate social change by allocating resources according to evidence-based risk stratification as opposed to blanket procedures (Hutton, 2018). As crucial as the LTBI continuum is the place of diagnostic methods, whereby detection and, by extension, treatment have a dramatic bearing. The entry into the market of the QuantiFERON-TB gold in-tube (QFT-GIT) test has fundamentally changed the pattern of LTBI diagnosis since it offers a substitute for the classic TST. The findings indicate that implementing QFT-GIT in urban health centers such as Baltimore leads to fewer individuals being diagnosed with LTBI than with TST alone, a reversal of the tests' higher specificity and the difficulty involved in interpreting discordant results. This reversal minimizes unnecessary treatment for individuals who are not actually infected, maximizes resource distribution, and may improve compliance on the part of the patient. Yet, variable concordance between QFT-GIT and TST among foreign-born vs. U.S.-born patients suggests an urgent need for more research to tailor diagnostic algorithms for heterogeneous populations (ACET, Cellestis et al., 2012). Overall, the solution to LTBI involves an interdisciplinary approach that links enhanced screening validity with culturally and demographically attuned treatment plans. Improving treatment completion among at-risk visa holders using more accurate diagnostic tools can help significantly reduce the reservoir of latent infection driving active tuberculosis cases. Although advances such as QFT-GIT testing offer promising mechanisms for improved LTBI detection, observed gaps in completion, particularly in rural and immigrant populations, demonstrate enduring challenges. A multi-pronged approach with policy changes, community outreach, and provider training is critical to utilize diagnostic advances to achieve measurable declines in TB morbidity and mortality. The evidence indicates a focused, context-sensitive response to LTBI that strikes a balance between scientific innovation and feasible implementation (ACET, Cellestis et al., 2012; Hutton, 2018).

Knowledge of the issues of concern and informational needs of individuals with LTBI is essential for enhancing public health interventions. A study on online health sites found a broad range of questions asked by the public, reflecting general confusion about LTBI. Among the main issues are available treatments, possible side effects, infectivity, and understanding diagnostic test results. Issues of drug-related side effects like skin reactions and abnormalities of liver function were most common, emphasizing the need for open communication in terms of treatment safety. In addition, questions regarding interactions between LTBI drugs and other drugs indicate the complications patients experience in treating their disease. This patient concern insight is useful guidance for healthcare professionals to inform education and support resources, ultimately improving adherence and outcomes of LTBI treatment (Choi et al., 2024). The complexity of LTBI is further explained by a research study of biological and behavioral determinants of infection risk. Information gathered from a cohort of tuberculosis close contacts demonstrated a prevalence of LTBI of around one-third, portending a major public health issue. Factors of sociodemographic status and lifestyle like educational attainment, frequency of close contact, and eating habits (in particular consumption of animal liver and coffee), were shown to have quantifiable influences on the risk of infection. Notably, the research probed the involvement of immune signaling molecules and discovered cytokines IL-10 and TNF-α as favorable correlates of LTBI formation and CXCL5 and IFN-γ as protective. These observations emphasize the complex interconnection between host immunity and environmental interactions, pointing toward incorporating both immunologic markers and risk behaviors in extensive risk assessment to enable timely diagnosis and intervention (Razbek et al., 2024). Together, these studies highlight the need for an integrative strategy in the fight against LTBI. Education of the patient has to counteract general misconceptions and concerns gleaned through information-seeking behavior analysis so that individuals comprehend prevention through treatment despite potential side effects (Choi et al., 2024). In parallel, identifying immunological correlates and modifiable lifestyle predictors of LTBI can empower focused approaches to identifying high-risk individuals, permitting early diagnosis and individualized interventions (Razbek et al., 2024). Such an integrated system, linking patient-centered counseling with stringent biomarkers and epidemiological evidence, has the potential to lessen the global tuberculosis burden by preventing latent infection from becoming manifest disease. This integration of behavioral, clinical, and immunologic approaches constitutes the foundation of successful LTBI management (Padmapriyadarsini & Swaminathan, 2005).

CLOSER LOOK

THE ROLE OF LATENT TUBERCULOSIS INFECTION (LTBI) IN THE TUBERCULOSIS (TB) TRANSMISSION CYCLE

LTBI is central in the TB transmission cycle, even though LTBI cases do not present with active symptoms nor spread the disease. LTBI is the state where *Mycobacterium tuberculosis (M. tuberculosis)* is in the body but is not actively causing disease. The bacteria are latent in the host, generally inside of granulomas in the lungs or other organs. Even though LTBI patients do not have active TB, nor are they infectious, they have the potential to become active TB in the future and then become infectious and spread the disease.

The contribution of LTBI to the transmission of TB is mostly in terms of the reservoir of infection it provides. An overwhelming percentage of the population worldwide is estimated to carry Mtb in its latent state. The WHO estimates that about a quarter of the global population has LTBI. Although these patients do not continue to spread the bacteria, they provide a widespread reservoir. When their immune system is broken, because of causes such as malnutrition, HIV infection, or age, the latent infection may reactivate and lead to active TB. Reactivation contributes to the transmission risk to other individuals via air-borne droplets when an active TB-infected individual coughs or sneezes.

TB transmission is inextricably associated with disease progression from LTBI to active disease. This progression is a fundamental part of the disease cycle due to its role in producing the cases of infection that drive transmission within the population. Unless treated, e.g., with TB screening, preventive therapy, or vaccination, individuals with LTBI are more likely to develop active TB, especially in countries where TB is endemic or when risk factors for progression are prevalent, e.g., HIV infection. The transition from LTBI to active TB may take years or even decades from the time of initial infection and is thus a latent public health threat.

Control of transmission of TB thus involves the management of LTBI among high-risk groups, especially those close to TB-active patients. IPT and other preventions are prime measures to decrease the burden of LTBI. By treating LTBI-infected individuals before they become active cases, public health measures can lower the entire transmission cycle of TB, with fewer new cases and the eventual progress toward TB elimination.

REFERENCES

1. Getahun, H., Matteelli, A., Abubakar, I., Aziz, M. A., Baddeley, A., Barreira, D., Den Boon, S., Borroto Gutierrez, S. M., Bruchfeld, J., Burhan, E., Cavalcante, S., Cedillos, R., Chaisson, R., Chee, C. B., Chesire, L., Corbett, E., Dara, M., Denholm, J., de Vries, G., Falzon, D., ... Raviglione, M. (2015). Management of latent Mycobacterium tuberculosis infection: WHO guidelines for low tuberculosis burden countries. *The European respiratory journal*, *46*(6), 1563–1576. https://doi.org/10.1183/13993003.01245-2015 (accessed on 10 May 2025).
2. Sterling, T.R., Njie, G., Zenner, D., Cohn, D.L., Reves, R., Ahmed, A., Menzies, D., Horsburgh, C.R., Jr., Crane, C.M., Burgos, M., LoBue, P., Winston, C.A. and Belknap, R. (2020), Guidelines for the treatment of latent tuberculosis infection: Recommendations from the National Tuberculosis Controllers Association and CDC, 2020. Am J Transplant, 20: 1196-1206. https://doi.org/10.1111/ajt.15841 (accessed on 10 May 2025).
3. Awad, S. F., Critchley, J. A., & Abu-Raddad, L. J. (2019). Epidemiological impact of targeted interventions for people with diabetes mellitus on tuberculosis transmission in India: Modelling based predictions. *Epidemics*, *30*, 100381. Advance online publication. https://doi.org/10.1016/j.epidem.2019.100381 (accessed on 10 May 2025).
4. Advisory Council for the Elimination of Tuberculosis (ACET), Greenbaum, A., ATS/CDC/IDSA, ATS/CDC/IDSA, ATS/CDC/IDSA, ATS/CDC/IDSA, Cellestis, D. Kunimoto, et al. (2012). Programmatic impact of QuantiFERON-TB Gold In-Tube implementation on latent tuberculosis diagnosis and treatment in a public health clinic. https://core.ac.uk/download/pdf/8723650.pdf (accessed on 10 May 2025).
5. Ahmad, S. (2011). Pathogenesis, immunology, and diagnosis of latent *Mycobacterium tuberculosis* infection. https://core.ac.uk/download/pdf/8511457.pdf (accessed on 10 May 2025).
6. Al-Mendalawi, Mahmood D. (2021) "Re: The Bacillus Calmette-Guerin (BCG) Vaccine," Sultan Qaboos University Medical Journal: Vol. 21: e141-142. DOI: https://doi.org/10.18295/squmj.2021.21.01.023 (accessed on 10 May 2025).
7. Miotto, P., Mwangoka, G., Valente, I. C., Norbis, L., Sotgiu, G., Bosu, R., Ambrosi, A., Codecasa, L. R., Goletti, D., Matteelli, A., Ntinginya, E. N., Aloi, F., Heinrich, N., Reither, K., & Cirillo, D. M. (2013). miRNA signatures in sera of patients with active pulmonary tuberculosis. *PloS one*, *8*(11), e80149. https://doi.org/10.1371/journal.pone.0080149 (accessed on 10 May 2025).
8. Mateos, J., Estévez, O., González-Fernández, Á. *et al.* Serum proteomics of active tuberculosis patients and contacts reveals unique processes activated during *Mycobacterium tuberculosis* infection. *Sci Rep* **10**, 3844 (2020). https://doi.org/10.1038/s41598-020-60753-5 (accessed on 10 May 2025).
9. Arisanti, N. L. E., Ngurah Rai, I. B., Krisdanti, I. D. P. A., Sajinadiyasa, I., Lestari, N. N. W., Cahyani, K. M. D., Dewi, I. G. A. N. K., et al. (2024). Profile of prisoners with latent tuberculosis infection (LTBI) in correctional institution level IIA Kerobokan, Badung, Bali. *International Journal of Scientific Advances*. https://www.semanticscholar.org/paper/5a82b4ae2009c321e980c1ff4b8233fcdad1f649 (accessed on 10 May 2025).
10. Baggaley, R. F., Brown, J., Degtyareva, S., Dimala, et al. (2023). Health economic analyses of latent tuberculosis infection screening and preventive treatment among people living with HIV in lower tuberculosis incidence settings: A systematic review [version 2; peer review:

1 approved, 1 approved with reservations]. https://core.ac.uk/download/554844548.pdf (accessed on 10 May 2025).

11. Balfour, A., Masina, N., Queiroz, A. T. L., Andrade, B. B., Fukutani, E., Bekiswa, A., Lewinsohn, D. M., et al. (2025). Two distinct cytokine response clusters identified in healthcare workers with apparent resistance to infection with *Mycobacterium tuberculosis* despite sustained occupational exposure. *bioRxiv*. https://www.semanticscholar.org/paper/f0dae33a0c109f429c023bcb88a8c6030ede1a0e (accessed on 10 May 2025).
12. Bell, Andrea, "Improving Latent Tuberculosis Infection (LTBI) Screening and Treatment in a School-Based Setting" (2020). Doctor of Nursing Practice Final Manuscripts. 123. https://digital.sandiego.edu/dnp/123 (accessed on 10 May 2025).
13. Benjamin, A. (2016). Adherence to latent tuberculosis treatment among immigrants in low endemic settings: A scoping review. http://hdl.handle.net/1866/14110. https://core.ac.uk/download/151554236.pdf (accessed on 10 May 2025).
14. Hayward, S. E., Dowd, J. B., Fletcher, H., Nellums, L. B., Wurie, F., & Boccia, D. (2019). A systematic review of the impact of psychosocial factors on immunity: Implications for enhancing BCG response against tuberculosis. *SSM - population health*, *10*, 100522. https://doi.org/10.1016/j.ssmph.2019.100522 (accessed on 10 May 2025).
15. Choi, Y. S., Park, D. Y., Song, Y. K., Park, H. Y., & Kwon, J. W. (2024). On-line health counseling on latent tuberculosis infection: An analysis using text mining and machine learning. *Yakhak Hoeji*. https://www.semanticscholar.org/paper/24531afedc18a7646bafffa168af0ef511e27115 (accessed on 10 May 2025).
16. Churchyard, G. J., & Swindells, S. (2019). Controlling latent TB tuberculosis infection in high-burden countries: A neglected strategy to end TB. *PLoS medicine*, *16*(4), e1002787. https://doi.org/10.1371/journal.pmed.1002787 (accessed on 10 May 2025).
17. Verso, M. G., Serra, N., Ciccarello, A., Romanin, B., & Di Carlo, P. (2019). Latent Tuberculosis Infection among Healthcare Students and Postgraduates in a Mediterranean Italian Area: What Correlation with Work Exposure?. *International journal of environmental research and public health*, *17*(1), 137. https://doi.org/10.3390/ijerph17010137 (accessed on 10 May 2025).
18. Cunningham, I. (2019). A pilot project for school-based screening and treatment of latent TB infection among freshman high school students. https://core.ac.uk/download/214384422.pdf (accessed on 10 May 2025).
19. Denholm, J. T., & McBryde, E. S. (2010). The use of anti-tuberculosis therapy for latent TB infection. *Infection and drug resistance*, *3*, 63–72. https://doi.org/10.2147/idr.s8994 (accessed on 10 May 2025).
20. Green, N., Manalan, K., Hayama, M., O'donoghue, M., Seneviratne, S., Drey, N., Kon, O. M., et al. (2025). Latent tuberculosis infection screening of adult close contacts: A cost-utility analysis. *ERJ Open Research*. https://www.semanticscholar.org/paper/a0f112942f59eb34620d0870b495c591d64b89c0 (accessed on 10 May 2025).
21. Hitayezu, E., Kabuye, F., Ngirinshuti, V., Niyigaba, et al. (2023). Prevalence and risk factors associated with tuberculosis occurrence among patients attending Muhima District Hospital, Nyarugenge District, Rwanda. European Journal of Social Science Studies. DOI: http://dx.doi.org/10.46827/ejsss.v9i1.1519 .pdf (accessed on 10 May 2025).

22. Huang, H. L., Cheng, M. H., Lee, M. R., Chien, J. Y., Lu, P. L., Sheu, C. C., Wang, J. Y., Chong, I. W., Yang, J. M., & Huang, W. C. (2025). Prevalence and treatment outcomes of latent tuberculosis infection among older patients with chronic obstructive pulmonary disease in an area with intermediate tuberculosis burden. *Emerging microbes & infections*, *14*(1), 2497302. https://doi.org/10.1080/22221751.2025.2497302(accessed on 10 May 2025).

23. Hutton, Scott, "Latent Tuberculosis Infection Treatment Completion and Predictors of Noncompletion among Visa Holders in the Rural Setting" (2018). *Walden Dissertations and Doctoral Studies*. 5880. https://scholarworks.waldenu.edu/dissertations/5880(accessed on 10 May 2025).

24. Kim, B., Kim, J., Yoon, S. Y., Cheong, H. S., Kwon, M. J., Yeom, J. S., Kim, H. N., & Joo, E. J. (2024). *HLA-DPB1**05:01 and *HLA-A**11:01 Is Associated with Adverse Drug Reactions to Isoniazid and Rifampin for Treatment of Latent Tuberculosis Infection in South Korea. *Journal of clinical medicine*, *13*(12), 3563. https://doi.org/10.3390/jcm13123563(accessed on 10 May 2025).

25. Marino, S., Sud, D., Plessner, H., Lin, P. L., Chan, J., Flynn, J. L., & Kirschner, D. E. (2007). Differences in reactivation of tuberculosis induced from anti-TNF treatments are based on bioavailability in granulomatous tissue. *PLoS computational biology*, *3*(10), 1909–1924. https://doi.org/10.1371/journal.pcbi.0030194 (accessed on 10 May 2025).

26. Kudryavtsev I, Starshinova A, Rubinstein A, Kulpina A, Ling H, Zhuang M and Kudlay D (2024) The role of the immune response in developing tuberculosis infection: from latent infection to active tuberculosis. Front. Tuberc. 2:1438406. doi: 10.3389/ftubr.2024.1438406(accessed on 10 May 2025).

27. Kutame, R., Boateng, G., Adusi-Poku, Y., Sorvor, F., Antwi, L., Agyemang-Bioh, F., Ayensu, B., et al. (2024). Evaluation of diagnostic performance of three commercial interferon-gamma release assays for *Mycobacterium tuberculosis*. *Diagnostics, 14*. https://www.semanticscholar.org/paper/4f0860b49a0f71e50309b176819bd8359d5e7df0 (accessed on 10 May 2025).

28. Leining, Lauren M., "Geospatial Analysis Of Pediatric Tuberculosis In Bohol, Philippines: Disease Clusters And Access To Care" (2019). *Dissertations & Theses (Open Access)*. 67. https://digitalcommons.library.tmc.edu/uthsph_dissertsopen/67 (accessed on 10 May 2025).

29. Nicky J Mehtani, Sarah Puryear, Paul Pham, Kelly E Dooley, Maunank Shah, Infectious Diseases Learning Unit: Understanding Advances in the Treatment of Latent Tuberculosis Infection Among People With Human Immunodeficiency Virus, *Open Forum Infectious Diseases*, Volume 8, Issue 8, August 2021, ofab319, https://doi.org/10.1093/ofid/ofab319(accessed on 10 May 2025).

30. Miranda-Hernandez, S., Kumar, M., Henderson, A., Graham, E., Tan, X., Taylor, J., Meehan, M., et al. (2025). CD8+ T cells mediate vaccination-induced lymphatic containment of latent *Mycobacterium tuberculosis* infection following immunosuppression, while B cells are dispensable. *bioRxiv*. https://www.semanticscholar.org/paper/e669d937191503d361340c07fc0cf01888404cfd (accessed on 10 May 2025).

31. National Center for HIV/AIDS, Viral Hepatitis, STD, and TB Prevention, Division of Tuberculosis Elimination. (2025). Latent tuberculosis infection: A guide for primary health care providers. https://core.ac.uk/download/144198509.pdf (accessed on 10 May 2025).

32. Niu, L., Wang, H., Luo, G., Zhou, J., Hu, Z., & Yan, B. (2024). Advances in understanding immune homeostasis in latent tuberculosis infection. *WIREs Mechanisms of Disease*. https://www.semanticscholar.org/paper/89963c2e56db4b24b023a030e0e40436252c62b2 (accessed on 10 May 2025).

33. Obatayo, A. O. (2024). Perception of African immigrants living in the United States towards latent tuberculosis infection treatment hesitancy. https://core.ac.uk/download/616423978.pdf (accessed on 10 May 2025).

34. Szczepura, Ala and Osipenko, Leeza (2012) Point of care tests for tuberculosis (TB) : economic analysis report. Coventry: Warwick Medical School. (Unpublished) (accessed on 10 May 2025).

35. Özkarafakılı MA, Sivaz O, Altunay İ. Latent tuberculosis infection in psoriasis patients. J Health Sci Med / JHSM. January 2024;7(1):47-52. doi:10.32322/jhsm.1357532(accessed on 10 May 2025).

36. Worden, Lee, Porco, Travis C., Products of Compartmental Models in Epidemiology, *Computational and Mathematical Methods in Medicine*, 2017, 8613878, 16 pages, 2017. **https://doi.org/10.1155/2017/8613878** (accessed on 10 May 2025).

37. Razbek, J., Daken, M., Chen, Y., Ma, L., Zhang, Y., Xu, W., Wen, B., et al. (2024). Association studies of serum levels of TNF-α, IL-10, IFN-γ, and CXCL 5 with latent tuberculosis infection in close contacts. *Infection and Drug Resistance, 17*, 899–910. https://www.semanticscholar.org/paper/036b7069a5571b1197ea255020092caa761e9158 (accessed on 10 May 2025).

38. Remy, Whitney L., "The Association Between Latent Tuberculosis Infection and Diabetes Mellitus Control in the United States" (2016). Theses and Dissertations--Public Health (M.P.H. & Dr.P.H.). 122.

39. https://uknowledge.uky.edu/cph_etds/122(accessed on 10 May 2025).

40. Simwaka, M., & Chongwe, G. (2024). Adherence to tuberculosis preventive therapy in people living with HIV/AIDS. *International Journal of Scientific Research*.

41. Volume - 13 | Issue - 04 | April - 2024 | PRINT ISSN No. 2277 - 8179 | DOI : 10.36106/ (accessed on 10 May 2025).

42. Søborg, B., Ruhwald, M., Hetland, M., Jacobsen, S., Andersen, A., Milman, N., Thomsen, V., et al. (2009). Comparison of screening procedures for *Mycobacterium tuberculosis* infection among patients with inflammatory diseases. *The Journal of Rheumatology, 36*, 1876–1884. https://www.semanticscholar.org/paper/242f535aa650835bc760607172737489970aa35b (accessed on 10 May 2025).

43. Padmapriyadarsini, C., & Swaminathan, S. (2005). Preventive therapy for tuberculosis in HIV infected individuals. *The Indian journal of medical research*, *121*(4), 415–423. (accessed on 10 May 2025).

44. Wang, L., Kuang, Y., Zeng, Y., Wan, Z., Yang, S., & Li, R. (2025). Association of systemic inflammation response index with latent tuberculosis infection and all-cause mortality: A cohort study from NHANES 2011–2012. *Frontiers in Immunology, 16*. https://www.semanticscholar.org/paper/d251d1cd887b52525f4985d6a85e36015f677346 (accessed on 10 May 2025).

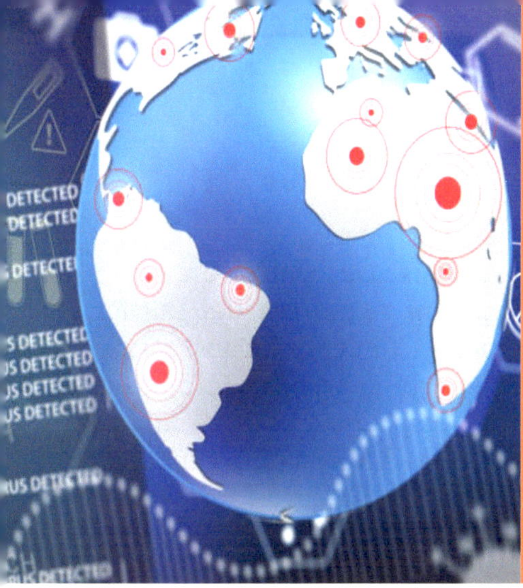

Chapter 13

TB CONTROL PROGRAMS AND GLOBAL POLICY

Contents

Introduction

The ongoing risk of tuberculosis (TB) is a deep-seated problem for health systems in the world, but most of all in low- and middle-income countries (LMICs) with the greatest burden of disease. Even with the progress of medical science, TB still kills millions of people every year, and therefore it is necessary to have a universal approach that involves successful control programs and robust global policy instruments. A recognition of the historical and present-day TB control contexts is necessary to understand the complexity of changing global health contexts. The involvement of various actors—ranging from national governments to global agencies—traces the multi-dimensional nature of TB control, which calls for concerted action to limit transmission, expand diagnosis, and promote treatment compliance. Such cooperation is conditioned within the wider global international health plans with strong levels of funds, laws, and policy directions that govern international organizations (Gostin et al.,

2010). Ensuring tuberculosis is well addressed is not only specialized public health intervention but also the positioning of such interventions within the larger global health policies that act on the fundamental social determinants of health. The political role of United States government programs and global partnerships has been indispensable in promoting TB control through technical assistance, research, and financing. The programs aim to complement national efforts by offering resources that are meant to reinforce health infrastructure, increase access to diagnostic facilities, and promote community mobilization.

In addition, international health policy frameworks call for the need to improve health systems to make control of TB sustainable given that the management of disease cannot be separated from broader socioeconomic and political determinants of health outcomes (Gostin et al., 2010). Global action to control TB illustrates an example of a paradigm encouraging collective policy-making alongside programmatic implementation, with emphasis placed on the interaction between science, governance, and funding. International organizations such as the World Health Organization (WHO) and multilateral donors have provided global guidelines and targets that will shape country TB control programs, enhancing international coherence. Global guidelines are bound to provide a template for expenditure, monitoring, and accountability systems crucial to tracking progress against the disease. An assessment for the reach and impact of such policies reveals the dynamics of providing equal access to care, preventing drug resistance, and addressing the challenge of TB among HIV/AIDS and poor populations. Control of TB thus relies on well-coordinated global policies that integrate information, resources, and expertise across borders (Gostin et al., 2010).

Importance of Tuberculosis (TB) Control Programs

The dependency of disease control on socio-economic development reinforces the call for convergent programs of TB control. Tuberculosis is among the world's major infectious diseases, one that disproportionately infects poor communities and undermines economic development. Successful TB control programs promote public health by cutting transmission rates, improving treatment compliance, and lowering drug resistance. In addition, successful initiatives achieve improved health systems that are capable of overcoming more substantial health problems than those of TB. These initiatives conform to global health governance policies aimed at sustainable, nationally driven interventions powered by international backing. As per global health finance and governance analysis, the use of the multi-dimensional strategy—cutting the allocation of funds to align with capacity building and mass involvement—guarantees TB control programs attain long-term effectiveness and equity in the provision of medical care (Gostin et al., 2010). Such a method not only ensures the resolution of immediate health issues but also supports the attainment of long-term goals for development. Tuberculosis can be fought effectively by understanding the wider impact that health has on society's stability and the productivity of citizens. Health issues like TB hinder people from participating in economic, political, and social activities to their maximum potential and thus trap them in poverty and inequality cycles. Thus, programs for TB control acquire a support role to provide welfare to society by surmounting such barriers. Strategic engagement of policy research organizations and universities is a model for the way high-quality, evidence-based methods can be translated to global health policy-making and interventions. By combining academic analysis and field application, these efforts improve conceptualization inclusive, sustainable programs with the potential to address TB in complicated health systems (Gostin et al., 2010). Such incorporation highlights the importance of cross-sectoral partnerships in developing creative solutions that target vulnerable groups and support health infrastructure globally. International policy-making, and TB control programs are key components of integrated disease prevention, and health security efforts. Programs need to be fashioned and executed considering both socio-political contexts of affected regions as well as existing epidemiological trends. Effective programs entail multisector coordination with the participation of international agencies, civil society, and the government to facilitate maximum resources and maximum benefit. Additionally, the focus on populations that are under greater vulnerability—women, children, and vulnerable groups—has the consequence of enhancing equal access to prevention and treatment. Such an emphasis on inclusiveness meets global health governance values prioritizing recipient country leadership and harmonized international support that responds to needs and circumstances at the local level (Gostin et al., 2010). Lastly, concerted efforts towards controlling TB build health system strength and inch the world closer to eliminating a disease that still imperils public health security.

Global Impact of Tuberculosis (TB)

The complexity of TB as an international health issue is compounded by its close association with socio-economic determinants and health system capacity. Poor communities typically are burdened with limitations such as unavailability of access to health care, substandard living conditions, and malnutrition, all of which make it easy to disseminate TB and prevent effective control measures. Moreover, HIV/AIDS persistence in much of the low-income world has compounded the problem because, in co-infected individuals, it leaves them immunocompromised, thereby increasing mortality. Fighting such diseases requires a well-structured and well-financed global health infrastructure, which makes governance and strategic resource allocation all the more important. In such a context, health initiatives against TB must make recipient country ownership its topmost priority and establish international partnerships responsive to the local context to achieve their maximum impact in controlling TB (Gostin et al., 2010). Alignment like this ensures that TB response is sustainable and integrated within overall health system strengthening. TB has a global impact that extends beyond health data, affecting economic productivity and social stability, particularly among heavily affected countries. Death and disease attributable to TB reduce productive working-age adult incomes in households and strain economies at the national level, entrapping individuals in poverty cycles. The stigma around TB may also stigmatize patients, making them become isolated and treatment non-adherent, with long-term public health implications at a community level. Tuberculosis policy control at an international level must therefore comprise social protection strategies and stigma-reducing and early-diagnosis-encouraging education campaigns. In addition to these interventions, a scale-up of prevention interventions focused on high-risk populations must be undertaken. Learning from the HIV pandemic reveals how increased prevention efforts, supported by governments and international donors, are key in overcoming obstacles and expanding coverage of TB control programs (Gostin et al., 2010). The battle against the global disease burden of TB must overcome the challenge of DR-TB strains that can jeopardize previous gains. The rise of multi-drug resistant tuberculosis (MDR-TB) complicates treatment regimens, increases costs, and necessitates more sophisticated healthcare infrastructure, something typically in short supply in resource-limited settings. Global policy actions must emphasize introducing advanced diagnostic technology, reliable supply chains for essential drugs, and upgrading health worker training. Further, the success of TB control interventions is highly dependent on harmonized health systems that use foreign aid reform processes to achieve maximum use of the available resources and maximize patient benefits. Strengthening these systems not only facilitates efficient TB case management but also fosters strong health infrastructures with the ability to respond to other infectious disease outbreaks (Gostin et al., 2010). Thus, interulcersive worldwide approaches addressing both medical as well as systemic concerns are essential to reduce the worldwide burden of TB.

13.1. Current State of Tuberculosis (TB) Worldwide

Despite tremendous achievements in the realm of medical science, TB continues to be an intimidating global health problem, disproportionately affecting low- and middle-income countries (LMICs). Relapse of TB is due to multifaceted determinants like socioeconomic disparities, suboptimal health infrastructure, and challenges in sustaining treatment adherence. Redoubled international efforts, such as the WHO End TB Strategy, seek to cut TB incidence and death sharply by 2035, but progress is frequently dogged by systemic bottlenecks and sociopolitical hurdles. The obstacles further worsen the disease burden, most urgently in areas plagued by HIV co-infections that weaken the immune system and complicate therapy. Additionally, the COVID-19 pandemic has also intervened in regular TB operations, delaying diagnosis and treatment and potentially exacerbating transmission. As a result, the global TB situation today is indicative of the need to accelerate effective action and maintain political will to achieve eradication targets as well as ease the disease burden worldwide. The spread of DR-TB strains through incidence and transmission has brought an added complex aspect to the existing situation of TB globally. MDR-TB and XDR-TB are dangerous threats since they have few treatment options, longer treatment duration, and increased side effects. Such resistant strains are the outcome of the misuse of antibiotics, non-adherence, and inadequate infection control practices. The problem of AMR emphasizes the complex interplay between human behavior and microbial evolution. The international rising of AMR in TB bacteria is mirrored by the wider crisis of AMR to challenge infectious disease control in the contemporary era, requiring strong surveillance and creative therapeutic advancement. DR-TB management strategies need to tap advances in diagnosis, patient-focused care, and health system improvement to avoid transmission and increase proportions of treatment success (Uddin et al., 2021; Salam et al., 2023). There is a pressing need for new strategies and international policy intervention to tackle the recalcitrant and deteriorating problem of TB control. Health systems need to be strengthened to provide universal access to high-quality diagnosis, low-cost antibiotics, and streamlined patient care. Integration of TB control into enhanced antimicrobial stewardship programs can prevent the emergence and transmission of resistance and maximize outcomes. Public health public policy must guarantee community participation, increasing awareness, reducing stigma, and treatment compliance. Research and development investment in new vaccines, improved and brief drug regimens, and rapid diagnostic tests is of utmost urgency. Global coordination and collective action between public and private sectors will fuel sustainable success needed to fight TB. In the absence of such a combined international effort, TB will continue to be the world's foremost infectious killer, threatening health gain across the world (Uddin et al., 2021; Salam et al., 2023).

13.1.1. Global Tuberculosis (TB) Statistics

TB disease burden is one of the most central global health challenges, particularly where the healthcare infrastructure is not well developed. India, like other countries, has an uneven burden of TB cases, with approximately 6,30,000 infectious cases annually, indicating systemic weaknesses in public health provision and disease control. The persistence of MDR-TB further complicates these issues, since standard regimens of treatment fail, and further complicated and expensive interventions are needed. The absence of rapid drug susceptibility testing (DST) also impedes prompt diagnosis and treatment, entrenching ongoing transmission and drug resistance. Therefore, high-prevalence countries need radical reform of their public health infrastructures, with an emphasis on early detection, efficient treatment regimens, and stronger community involvement. This strategic approach has been shown to yield better outcomes in those countries with mature programs, drawing attention to the imperative need for improved surveillance and health literacy campaigns to contain MDR-TB levels (Gamon, 2013). An examination of global TB data indicates inequalities in outcomes that frequently coincide with the strength of TB control programs and global policy settings. Quality governance and equitable funding distribution are key to determining the success of such initiatives. Global health programs highlight the need for harmonizing donor priorities with domestic ownership to facilitate sustainable advancements in TB control. In addition, harmonizing these efforts with the larger foreign aid reforms maximizes impact and eliminates duplication of effort, while a combined concentration on vulnerable groups, such as women and girls, addresses health equity gaps in access. Strengthened health infrastructures help to bring about enhanced diagnostic abilities, treatment compliance, and surveillance, all of which are pivotal to tackle TB's multifaceted epidemiology. All these inter-related factors provide an important platform for international collaborations that enable well-coordinated, responsive TB control approaches (Gostin et al., 2010). Statistical trends highlight that TB needs to be addressed through an interdisciplinary approach bringing together local, national, and global health strategies. The occurrence of resistant strains of TB emphasizes the need for culturally sensitive, population-specific programs. This includes enabling community leaders to become health literate to provide informed advocacy for early diagnosis and compliance with treatment. Enhanced laboratory capacity for rapid drug susceptibility testing will be critical to effectively individualize therapy and contain the transmission of drug resistance. Moreover, national policies must prioritize research and surveillance to track epidemiological changes and guide resource allocation appropriately. Incorporating lessons learned from successful control programs worldwide can inform adaptive strategies, particularly in high-burden countries seeking to overcome structural and social barriers to effective TB management (Gamon, 2013) (Figure 13.1).

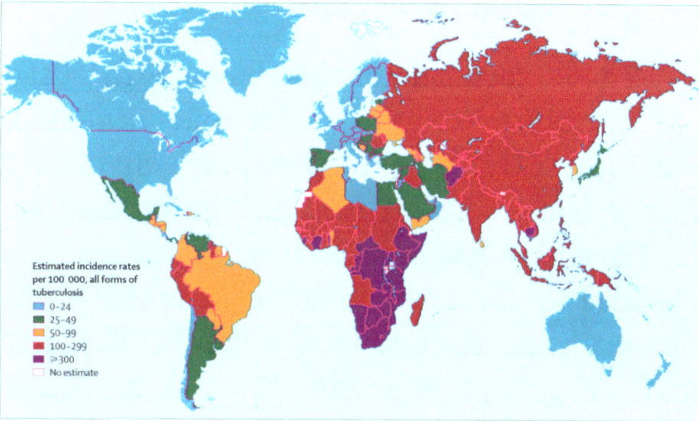

Figure 13.1. Global epidemiology of tuberculosis.

Source: The Lancet. (2006). Latent tuberculosis infection: New evidence for diagnosis and treatment. *The Lancet.* https://www.thelancet.com/journals/lancet/article/PIIS0140-6736(06)68384-0/abstract.

13.1.2. High-Burden Countries

The problems encountered by high tuberculosis (TB) burden countries are complex and deeply rooted in more extensive health system vulnerabilities. The COVID-19 pandemic has also added to these problems, derailing TB detection, treatment, and prevention programs worldwide. In most high-burden countries, health system resources were quickly diverted towards tackling COVID-19, leading to less availability of diagnostic and treatment services among TB patients. Lockdowns and other restrictions on movement also constrained patients from obtaining timely care. These disruptions resulted in a sharp decline in the number of newly diagnosed and treated TB cases in 2020, unwinding years of progress toward global TB control. The convergence of TB and COVID-19 underscores the imperative for holistic measures to effectively address similar health emergencies, including maintaining the continuity of TB services amid such pandemics (Morten et al., 2022). Socioeconomic determinants that dominate high-burden countries complicate TB control even more. Poor living conditions, malnutrition, HIV infection, and diabetes are key risk factors that enhance susceptibility to TB infection and affect disease outcomes.

These social determinants also increase susceptibility to other infectious illnesses, including COVID-19, to produce a syndemic that enhances health threats. The occurrence of TB and AMR together presents another obstacle to successful treatment, as the MDR-TB strains necessitate longer, more costly, and toxic treatment regimens. Current thorough evaluations demonstrate that AMR has a substantial contribution to mortality, particularly in resource-constrained environments with poor laboratory capability and surveillance systems. Improved laboratory infrastructure and the integration of AMR surveillance with TB programming may enhance treatment outcomes in high-burden settings (Dartois & Rubin, 2022).

As a response to these complexities, global policy efforts have increasingly focused on targeted strategies in high-burden countries to expedite TB control. Co-testing for TB and COVID-19 has also appeared to be a practical intervention in such settings by capitalizing on overlap in symptomatology to maximize diagnostic yield and make optimal use of resources. India, South Africa, and Indonesia have also tested combined screening programs, which have proved to be feasible and have the potential to detect cases that may otherwise go undetected. There are still challenges, however, like shortages of healthcare workers and protective equipment, highlighting the importance of continued investment in people and supply chains. Policy frameworks should also take into account local epidemiology, health system capacity, and social determinants to develop effective, context-appropriate TB control programs that are resilience-capable to simultaneous public health emergencies (Morten et al., 2022) (Figure 13.2).

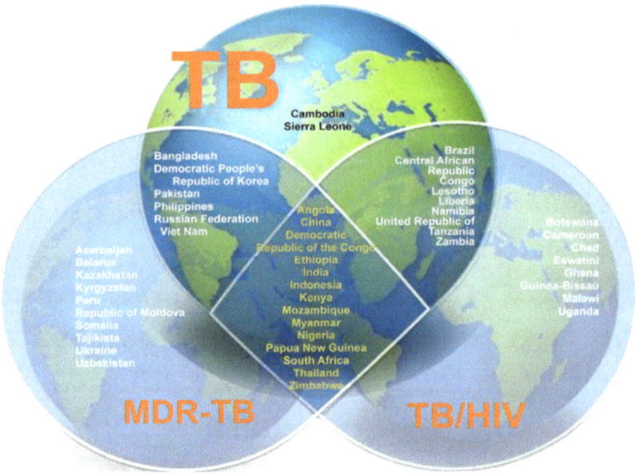

Figure 13.2. The three global HBC lists for TB, TB/HIV and MDR-TB used by WHO during the period 2016–2020, and their areas of overlap.

Source: Readkong. (n.d.). *TB, MDR/RR-TB WHO global lists of high burden countries.* https://www.readkong.com/static/90/3c/903c35f70e9c901eccc3c5d6c0850687/tb-mdr-rr-tb-who-global-lists-of-high-burden-countries-7856786-1.jpg.

13.1.3. Demographic Factors Influencing Tuberculosis (TB)

The emergence and dissemination of TB among populations are inextricably linked with demographic factors that determine individual susceptibility and exposure to healthcare services. Level of education, for instance, is important in determining exposure and prevention mechanisms against TB. A study among university students in Hainan Province, China, proves that medical students and those who have been exposed to targeted TB education have considerably superior knowledge, attitude, and practice behaviors regarding TB prevention compared to non-medical students (Xie et al., 2025). This indicates that education not only raises awareness but also promotes health-seeking behavior required for early detection and treatment adherence. Thus, education interventions designed for various demographic groups need to be incorporated within TB control programs to efficiently respond to population-level knowledge deficits and stimulate health proactive actions. As a result, demographic considerations like education level and previous education experiences are crucial determinants of TB control success. Household structure and family conditions also become critical determinants of TB spread and control success, particularly in areas with high disease burdens. Socioeconomic status, usually quantified in terms of household wealth and occupational structure, is strongly related to healthcare and preventive care access. An example can be seen in a survey of contraceptive use in Cameroon that shows household wealth, spouse occupation, and family size all play important roles in health behavior and decision-making (Amadou et al., 2025). If translated to TB control, these populations with smaller resources and bigger household sizes could be challenged in following long treatment courses or reaching diagnostic centers, worsening disease transmission. In addition, demographic factors, including the absence or presence of a spouse and the role of household heads, influence health-seeking behavior and support systems that are vital for TB control. Therefore, population considerations with regard to family and socioeconomic settings need to be incorporated into international policy platforms for the purpose of increasing the efficacy of TB control. Age and gender also complicate the situation of TB vulnerability and control, crossing over with other demographic variables to affect prevalence and treatment outcomes.

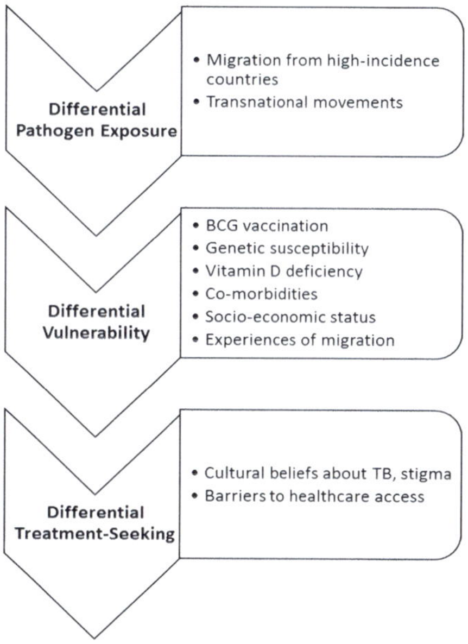

Figure 13.3. Factors contributing to the increased incidence of TB in migrant and ethnic minorities in the UK.

Source: ResearchGate. (n.d.). *Summary of factors contributing to the increased incidence of TB in migrant and ethnic minority populations.* https://www.researchgate.net/figure/Summary-of-factors-contributing-to-the-increased-incidence-of-TB-in-migrant-and-ethnic_fig1_327124213.

Women and older people who live in socioeconomically deprived or rural areas tend to face challenges when accessing healthcare services because of sociocultural expectations, caregiving duties, or restrictions on health decision-making (Amadou et al., 2025).

Such population attributes are barriers to delayed diagnosis and adherence to the drug treatment regimen and hence sustain continued transmission within communities. In addition, young, educated populations exposed to TB educational programs have shown superior preventive attitude and behavior, and early intervention is therefore paramount (Xie et al., 2025). Addressing these age- and gender-related disparities entails the deployment of differential strategies in TB control programs with respect to age- and gender-related needs, facilitating equal access and culturally relevant health communication. Strategically, such targeted interventions can reduce TB incidence dramatically and enhance world health outcomes (Figure 13.3).

13.2. Tuberculosis (TB) Control Programs: Strategies and Approaches

Efficient tuberculosis control requires a multi-faceted strategy that combines prevention, early detection, and holistic treatment. One of the greatest challenges is treating underlying health factors like malnutrition and diabetes that increase vulnerability to TB infection and complicate the recovery process. Through the introduction of specialized interventions such as tuberculosis preventive treatment (TPT) in conjunction with larger-scale health improvement programs, control programs can significantly decrease transmission rates and prevalence of the disease. Current models for TB dynamics highlight the value of such integrated strategies, illustrating that mathematically informed tactics can maximize resource utilization and intervention timing to have the maximum impact. These models also allow for cost-effectiveness analysis, important for policy planners interested in cost-effective program deployment in a resource-constrained environment. With simulation-informed insight, programs are able to balance short-term clinical management with long-term population health gain and guarantee sustainable control and eventual eradication activities (Buinwi et al., 2024). Innovation in pedagogic approaches to public health workers also strengthens TB control activity by promoting critical thinking and practical capabilities among implementers of programs. Incorporating experience-based learning, case studies, and inter-disciplinary education makes practitioners better equipped to understand TB as a multi-factorial disease with a global impact. For example, integrating findings from epidemiology, economics, and social science provides an integrated understanding of TB transmission patterns and intervention effectiveness. Online simulation and interactive learning environments further equip public health professionals to tailor approaches to various epidemiological settings. This pedagogic transformation echoes the international policy requirement for creative, evidence-based solutions in TB control. Therefore, building stronger educational foundations in health administration and policy programs directly aids in the successful design and implementation of TB control policies (Buinwi et al., 2024). International TB control programs increasingly acknowledge the value of utilizing technology and community participation to improve intervention coverage and compliance. Electronic health devices, including mobile health surveillance and telemedicine, enable ongoing patient follow-up and drug adherence, key determinants of preventing treatment failure and drug resistance, respectively. Additionally, community-oriented interventions empower affected individuals by promoting education and local healthcare engagement, achieving trust and stigma reduction regarding TB. All these approaches, when integrated with targeted screening and immediate treatment initiation, help interrupt transmission chains more efficiently. Policy frameworks integrating these strategies also have to foreground equitable access and sustainability, foregrounding both cost-effectiveness and universal health coverage objectives. These holistic approaches highlight the need for multi-sectoral collaboration and the ongoing evolution of TB control strategies according to changing epidemiological contexts (Figure 13.4) (Chhetri et al., 2024).

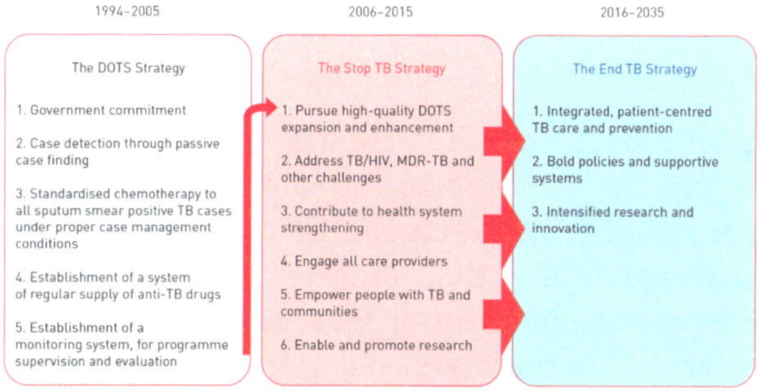

Figure 13.4. TB control programs.

Source: Insights on India. (2022). *The way to control tuberculosis.* https://www.insightsonindia.com/2022/07/06/the-way-to-control-tuberculosis/.

13.2.1. Directly Observed Treatment, Short-Course (DOTS)

International initiatives against TB have traditionally involved uniform treatment regimens to enhance patient outcomes and minimize the spread of the disease. Of these, the directly observed treatment, short-course (DOTS) strategy was a landmark method supported by the World Health Organization (WHO), which focused on supervised TB medication to raise compliance. The deployment of DOTS was instrumental in high TB burden countries by ensuring a systematic framework that included political commitment, case detection using sputum smear microscopy, standardized treatment regimens, assured drug supply, and systematic monitoring and evaluation. Most importantly, China's steep fall in smear-positive pulmonary TB from 1990 through 2010 has been mostly attributed to national coverage of DOTS, which was well implemented through its vertical TB control schemes under the aegis of the Chinese CDC. This demonstrates DOTS' potential not only to enhance the treatment success rate but also to significantly contribute to national efforts toward TB control (Long et al., 2021) (Figure 13.5).

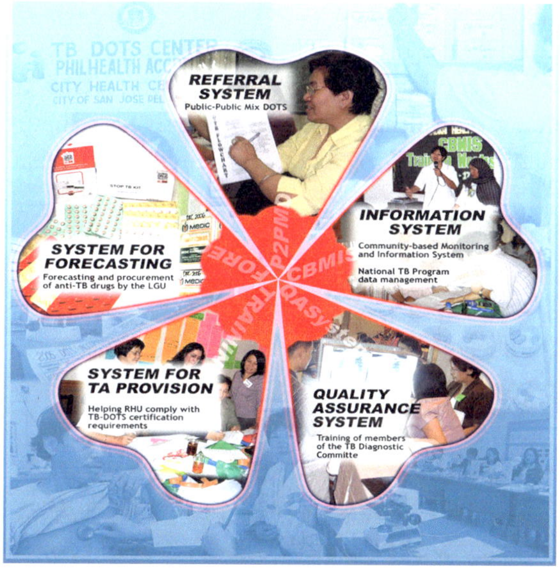

Figure 13.5. TB-DOTS: Energizing the local health system to stop TB.

Source: Pulmonary Tuberculosis (WordPress). (2012). *TB DOTS strategy illustration.* https://pulmonarytuberculosis.wordpress.com/wp-content/uploads/2012/04/tb_dots.jpg.

Notwithstanding the global spread of DOTS, debate continues in international policy circles about its relative merits compared to other forms of treatment supervision. Present evidence indicates that while DOTS targets a decline in the emergence of drug resistance and enhanced cure rates by way of direct observation of treatment, superiority over self-administered therapy has not been rigorously proved. This uncertainty calls into question assumptions regarding the universality of supervised treatment, particularly given the significant financial and social costs involved with DOTS. Patients tend to incur opportunity costs, increased stigma, and logistical difficulties that can compromise treatment uptake. Consequently, increasing demands call for pragmatic trials to rigorously test DOTS' impact under actual program situations, with a goal of maximizing TB treatment protocols by striking a balance between supervision intensity and patient-based methods (McLaren et al., 2016). New directions on TB control prioritize the need to rethink DOTS within universal health coverage and novel service delivery models.

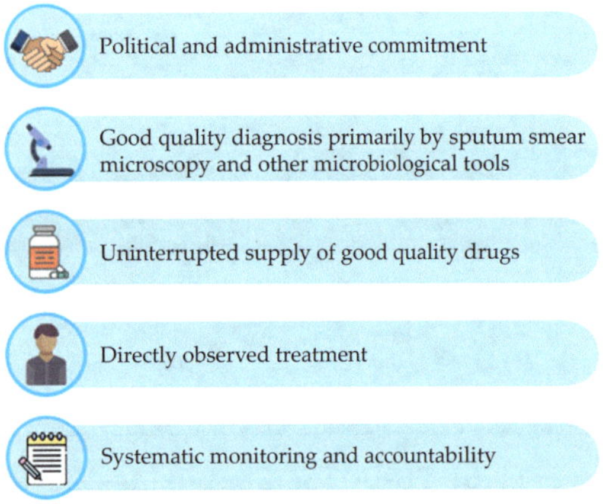

Figure 13.6. Components of the DOTS strategy.

Source: National Tuberculosis Elimination Program (NTEP). (n.d.). *CP DOTS strategy.* https://ntep.in/node/330/CP-dots-strategy.

The control programs for TB in the future might be dependent on combining new diagnostic strategies, electronic drug monitoring, and differentiated care for various patient needs instead of enforcing stringent supervision uniformly. DOTS, in this perspective, can be transformed from a strict mandate to a flexible, facilitatory system, with treatment partners and digital technologies supplementing healthcare workers for better compliance. Such reforms dovetail with international approaches that stress reducing financial misery and stigma among TB-affected groups while maintaining treatment effectiveness. Revisiting DOTS, then, both in policy and practice, may serve the twofold goals of better patient outcomes and fulfilling the lofty global target of ending the epidemic of TB (Long et al., 2021; McLaren et al., 2016) (Figure 13.6).

13.2.2. Community-Based Interventions

Successful public health interventions increasingly recognize the importance of local community involvement in disease control, acknowledging that long-term health gains frequently have their source in grassroots efforts. Community-based interventions are a prime example of this by incorporating local knowledge, resources, and social structures into overall health programs. In the case of tuberculosis (TB) control, such interventions provide support for improved case detection, treatment regimen adherence, and stigma reduction. The PATCH framework, which is a model for community organization initially developed to address chronic illness, illustrates the value of organizing collective action to empower communities to take charge in making health decisions (Heydari et al., 2025). These models can be modified to apply for TB control by engaging community health workers, local leaders, and affected groups to facilitate ownership and responsibility, thus building up the overall effectiveness of national and international TB programs. In addition to simple participation, community interventions implement more complex approaches that combine education, behavioral change, and environmental interventions to meet the multifaceted determinants of disease. Targeted education campaigns within local cultural settings raise awareness about TB transmission, symptoms, and cure, shortening delays in diagnosis and reducing transmission levels. Empirical research from chronic disease prevention programs indicates that long-term community empowerment results in better health outcomes, such as improved self-care and compliance with recommended treatments (Heydari et al., 2025). With the interconnected challenges of socioeconomic conditions, stigma, and poor healthcare infrastructure in high TB burden settings, community-based interventions constitute a comprehensive strategy. They complement international policy targets to eliminate TB by addressing not just clinical but also social determinants of health. As proven, community-based interventions against TB face various challenges that need to be resolved to maximize their long-term sustainability and impact. Problems such as logistical issues, resource limitations, and cultural resistance can hinder program implementation and assessment. Furthermore, sustainable engagement requires ongoing support from health systems and policymakers to maintain momentum and adapt to evolving community needs. Monitoring and measuring outcomes remain essential to inform policy adjustments and scalability within diverse settings. Integrating technology and telehealth platforms may enhance reach and data collection, particularly in remote areas. Hence, although community-based interventions are critical parts of integrated TB control programs, their effectiveness hinges on overcoming operational issues and integrating them into supportive global and national systems.

13.2.3. Role of Vaccination in Tuberculosis (TB) Control

TB case incidence reduction in the world depends on complex interventions, where vaccination plays an essential preventive function. With even greater improvements in health system medical care and diagnostic capabilities, the *Bacillus Calmette-Guérin* (BCG) vaccine is the only extensively utilized vaccine against TB. Its use, particularly in high-burdened countries, is an essential part of national infant and young child immunization programs. Although BCG has variable effectiveness against pulmonary TB among adults, its protective action against advanced forms of TB in children highlights vaccination's key place in disease control programs. Such a preventative measure supplements case detection and treatment work to make a triad that can help control TB transmission. Yet, issues like coverage inequalities of vaccines, cold chain management, and the capacity of the health system need to be managed to optimize vaccine benefits, particularly in rural areas with limited resources where access to healthcare is limited (Immaculata et al., 2025). In planning TB control, the effectiveness of vaccination programs tends to be limited by logistical, socio-cultural, and policy-based challenges. In several rural and underserved areas, the lack of appropriate healthcare infrastructure compromises efficient vaccine delivery, storage, and administration, which results in poor coverage rates. Socio-cultural reasons such as low awareness, deep-seated beliefs, and misinformation also play their part in causing hesitancy or refusal to accept vaccines among the population. Global and country-level policies, although sought to be incorporated with wider TB control initiatives, also often face the challenge of implementation inconsistencies due to resource constraints and competing health priorities. Breaking down such barriers calls for creative, community-led methods that integrate vaccination and health education, outreach, and mobilization with local leaders, thus engendering trust and enhancing compliance. Enhanced health systems and aligned policy measures are the keys to ensuring sustainable immunization coverage and improving TB control results (Immaculata et al., 2025). The future of TB vaccination is not just enhancing the utilization of the available BCG vaccine but also innovating the development and implementation of new vaccines with increased efficacy and additional protective benefits. Future research endeavors concentrate on novel vaccine candidates aimed at providing greater protection against adult pulmonary TB, thus extending the coverage of immunization in TB control programs. International policy guidelines prioritize the promotion of these innovations' incorporation into overall vaccination strategies that take into account the cost-effectiveness, coverage, and timeliness of the vaccine administration. Experience from vaccination campaigns for other infectious diseases teaches the crucial role of monitoring vaccine impact, dose schedules, and the provision of equitable access to all populations. With the improvement of TB vaccination initiatives through policy commitment and innovation, the international community can anticipate meaningful gains in the reduction of TB morbidity and mortality and in alignment with other health goals.

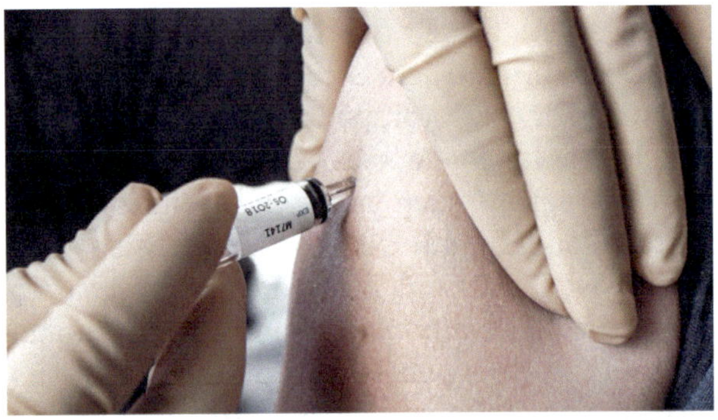

Source: Al Jazeera. (2020). *TB awareness campaign visual.* https://www.aljazeera.com/wp-content/uploads/2020/04/8af1ca3dfa1b4073a320a7673b16bd9e_18.jpeg?resize=1200%2C675.

13.3. Global Policy Frameworks

The complex task of TB control requires global policy regimes of broad sweep and adaptability that move across country borders. The success of antibiotic therapies for infectious diseases in the last decades has been eroded by the growing threat of multi-drug resistant (MDR) bacteria. This international trend calls for synchronized global policies that encourage the responsible use of antibiotics and the innovation of drug development. By incorporating synthetic biology and metagenomic advancements, policy systems can facilitate the speedy discovery of new antimicrobials specifically designed to tackle resistant forms of TB. Further, in policies, biofilms and bacterial resistance mechanisms need to be tackled since these make infection control and treatment difficult and intractable. These comprehensive frameworks must invest more in research funds, global solidarity, and fair access to improved treatments, hence strengthening the global health security platform against TB's changing threats (Uddin et al., 2021). Demographic and epidemiological changes also define the priorities under global health policies for TB control. The increase in youth populations, especially in low-income settings, increases the need for age-targeted interventions in TB programs. Young people have specific health risks related to socio-economic determinants that need to be comprehensively addressed by global policies. The crossover of infectious diseases such as TB with non-communicable diseases and risk behavior emphasizes the need for integrative policies. Screening and prevention interventions within wider adolescent health programs need to be included in health policy to limit the transmission and burden of TB. In addition, unequal health outcomes between vulnerable populations, particularly adolescent girls in multiburden nations, indicate disparities that international policies need to address to ensure equitable control of TB. Thus, integrating TB programs into broader adolescent and social health agendas guarantees a holistic response to disease prevention and long-term resilience (Helen et al., 2019). Successful global policy mechanisms need to adapt to fit complex TB control realities, calling for multisectoral coordination that extends beyond the health system. Investments in education, economic empowerment, and social protection supplement biomedical interventions by attacking underlying determinants of susceptibility to TB infection and deficient treatment adherence. Policies with integrated adolescent health services and TB screening and treatment enhance near-term outcomes while reducing long-term disease burdens. Evidence-based strategies, utilizing headline predictors of health and wellbeing, may guide country-specific, demographic, and epidemiologic context-informed interventions. Through equitable, innovative, and cross-sectoral cooperation, international policy may support evidence-based TB control that flexes in response to shifting challenges and demographic change. Political commitment and resource investment within such frameworks continue to be critical to realizing TB control as a global public health achievement (Helen et al., 2019) (Figure 13.7).

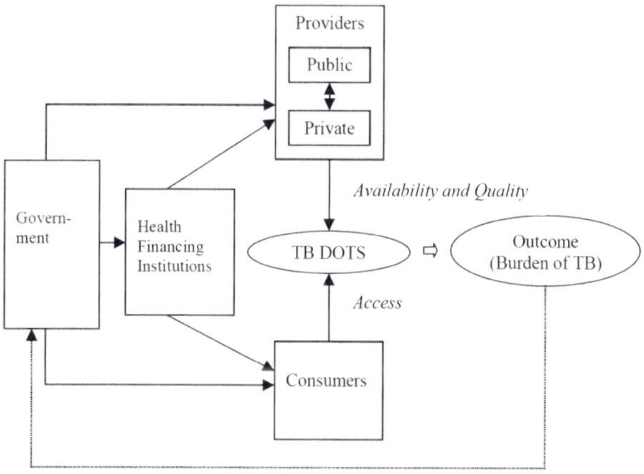

Figure 13.7. A TB policy evaluation framework.

Source: ResearchGate. (n.d.). *A TB policy evaluation framework.* https://www.researchgate.net/figure/A-TB-Policy-Evaluation-Framework_fig1_265477078.

13.3.1. World Health Organization (WHO) Guidelines

Global health programs rely significantly on standardized procedures to provide uniform and effective disease control across various settings. The WHO has set out extensive guidelines for controlling tuberculosis (TB) for long, which continue to be valuable references for national and country-level programs. These guidelines emphasize a multi-component strategy, encompassing early detection, appropriate regimens of treatment, and systematic follow-up. In establishing concrete case detection and treatment compliance parameters, WHO recommendations ensure consistency in addressing TB's public health impact. The focus of their strategy takes into account such localized issues as resource limitations and stigma, encouraging flexible interventions with engagement at the community level. Program assessment evidence shows that compliance with these standards markedly increases the coverage of case detection and treatment outcomes and diminishes the risks of transmission and drug resistance (Putri et al., 2025). Adaptability built into WHO structures allows diverse health systems globally to adjust their activity while conforming to global control missions. An important feature highlighted in the WHO guidelines is the linkage of TB control with general health services, particularly in areas hampered by high HIV prevalence. Coinfection makes diagnosis and treatment more challenging, thus requiring coordinated policies addressing both diseases simultaneously. Such integration guarantees that patients get well-rounded care, which addresses crosscutting vulnerabilities and maximizes resource allocation. It has been noted through research that there exists a positive relationship between implementing WHO-recommended combined TB and HIV control strategies and better health outcomes among affected individuals. This harmonization between TB and HIV care facilitates more effective prevention and therapeutic activities as well as enhances the enforcement of governmental policy provisions formulated to fight these dual epidemics (Musonda et al., 2024). Therefore, the WHO promotion of synergistic interventions sustains worldwide initiatives to contain TB in environments where health issues are complex and need multi-sectoral coordination. Additionally, WHO recommendations offer essential advice on monitoring and evaluation of TB control programs, which are vital to maintaining momentum and adjusting approaches with the passage of time. Proper program management, in line with WHO's input-process-output framework, allows tracking of key performance indicators like case detection rates and treatment success.

This systematic method helps health centers recognize operational constraints, including scarce human resources and inadequate diagnostic capacities, that have, in the past, hampered TB control activities in certain areas (Putri et al., 2025). The guidelines also promote community education and involvement in facing social stigma, bettering early diagnosis and treatment compliance. By encouraging evidence-based policies based on meticulous data collection and analysis, the WHO enables health systems to reconcile local programs with global TB reduction goals, so as to continuously improve and enhance program effectiveness (Figure 13.8).

To reduce *M. tuberculosis* transmission to health workers, persons attending health care facilities or other persons in settings with a high risk of transmission, the following measures are recommended:

- Administrative controls:
  - triage of people with TB signs and symptoms, or with TB disease;
  - respiratory separation or isolation of people with presumed or demonstrated infectious TB;
  - prompt initiation of effective TB treatment of people with TB disease;
  - respiratory hygiene (including cough etiquette) in people with presumed or confirmed TB.
- Environmental controls:
  - upper-room germicidal ultraviolet systems;
  - ventilation systems (including natural, mixed-mode, mechanical ventilation and recirculated air through high-efficiency particulate air filters).
- Respiratory protection:
  - particulate respirators, within the framework of a respiratory protection programme.

Figure 13.8. WHO recommendations on TB infection prevention and control.

Source: World Health Organization (WHO). (n.d.). *TB Key population strategy visual – Box 3.4.* https://tbksp.who.int/sites/default/files/inline-images/box-3-4.gif.

13.3.2. International Health Regulations (IHR)

International control of tuberculosis (TB) requires a strong legal and policy system that goes beyond national borders to effectively stem its spread and effects. The International Health Regulations (IHR) are an important element in this system, making it possible to have coordinated responses to public health emergencies, such as those caused by TB and drug-resistant TB. These regulations place a strong emphasis on the timely sharing of information, surveillance capacity, and international coordination to prevent, protect against, and control cross-border spread of disease. By enhancing national health systems' capacity to detect and respond to outbreaks of TB, countries can harmonize their policies at home with global health security goals to ensure a coherent response to control efforts. This harmonization is necessary to meet the fragmentation, often found in health governance and financing, identified by (Bultman et al., 2012) as a hindrance to implementing effective health programs. With AMR complicating TB control so significantly, the IHR acts as a framework facilitating global collaborative efforts against this urgent crisis. MDR-TB strains highlight the need for concerted international action to promote research, development, and fair distribution of new diagnostics and therapies. However, the IHR cannot alone address these issues if not supported by complementary systems that enhance innovation and stewardship. Effective good governance at all levels is needed to set priorities, monitor antibiotic use, and make them accessible, a lesson reflected in worldwide policy forums on TB. Such stewardship supports the IHR's aims by encouraging joint responsibility and bolstering health systems to decrease resistance levels and enhance cure rates (Jenner et al., 2017). The regulations therefore provide a spine that complements overarching policy actions aimed at addressing the AMR emergency under

TB control programs. Ultimately, incorporating the IHR into national and international TB control policies provides an avenue toward more harmonious, effective interventions. As nations aim to achieve universal health coverage and strengthen social protection, harmonizing health financing laws and regulatory systems with the IHR will minimize inefficiencies and enhance quality improvements in care. Creating autonomous accreditation organizations and amending laws to promote competition and cooperation among health service providers, as proposed by Bultman et al., (2012), also mirrors the IHR's focus on transparency and accountability. With this combined strategy, TB control programs are able to accomplish more robust surveillance, quick response capacity, and sustainable resource distribution. The IHR therefore not only supports global cooperation but also the policy consistency required for overcoming the sophisticated problems posed by TB globally.

13.3.3. Global Fund Initiatives

Great strides in the fight against tuberculosis have been closely linked to the development of global collaborative work, especially through funding mechanisms intended to support LMICs. Amongst these, the Global Fund programs are remarkable in that they direct considerable amounts of financial resources into TB control programs, allowing countries to expand diagnostics, treatment, and prevention efforts. These programs place great importance on recipient country ownership, which guarantees that interventions must adhere to national priorities and health systems. Also, the organizational structure of the Global Fund allows for broad partnerships among governments, civil society, and international organizations and supports a collaborative effort in TB control. This framework has driven enhanced case detection and treatment success through the targeting of both the biological and social factors of TB and, at the same time, support of strengthened health systems through system strengthening interventions (Gostin et al., 2010). Such extensive financing and management arrangements show how global policies can be transformed into productive local responses to TB. Global Fund programs' structure demonstrates a deliberate emphasis on equity, seeking to engage marginalized groups most impacted by tuberculosis. Programs intentionally include measures to respond to gender inequalities and social vulnerabilities, as they realize that women, children, and poor populations frequently experience obstacles in accessing TB care. Furthermore, these programs prioritize integration with broader health agendas, including HIV/AIDS and maternal health, ensuring more holistic and sustainable health improvements. The investment in health systems strengthening, such as improving laboratory networks, supply chains, and human resources, has been critical for sustaining long-term gains against TB. Notably, Global Fund assistance supplements interventions by national governments and other donors, aligning with foreign aid reform efforts to avoid duplication and ensure maximum efficiency (Gostin et al., 2010). This comprehensive and balanced strategy emphasizes the larger policy vision of addressing TB within a universal health perspective. Global Fund initiatives have roles beyond funding into shaping policy frameworks and global cooperation on tuberculosis control. By generating open information on disease burden and funding streams, these initiatives inform policymaking at both global and national levels. The U.S. government, as well as multilateral institutions, is an active partner with the Global Fund in streamlining financial assistance according to evolving epidemiological realities and programmatic challenges. This partnership has enabled the creation of novel strategies, including improved DR-TB treatment regimens and models of care delivered at the community level, that have been taken up in several countries. Evidence-based decision-making, facilitated through Global Fund reporting tools, allows for resource use to be both specific and responsive to changing TB patterns. Thus, the Global Fund not only finances program implementation but also facilitates dynamic policy action necessary for moving global TB control agendas forward.

13.4. Challenges in Tuberculosis (TB) Control

Successful disease control efforts are dependent on a strong healthcare infrastructure, but this is a significant challenge in most areas where TB is endemic. Inadequate human resources, insufficient health facilities, and poor management systems all compromise TB control efforts. As an example, results from the Kedaton Health Center in Indonesia demonstrate a sharp decline in case detection rates over the past few years, largely due to the lack of adequate workforce and support systems. Health workers tend to wear many hats, undermining their capacity to properly carry out case tracking, while small community cadre numbers hinder outreach and follow-up operations. These structural obstacles undermine the effectiveness of interventions aimed at the detection and treatment of TB and impede achieving national and international goals. Closing these gaps in infrastructure is essential to bolster TB control programs and enhance public health status in resource-constrained environments (Immaculata et al., 2025). In addition to structural shortcomings, socio-cultural challenges also substantially hinder TB control programs in most communities. The extensive stigma surrounding TB dissuades individuals from early diagnosis and the completion of treatment courses, further compounding disease spread and outcomes. In remote communities with poor health education, myths and misconceptions regarding TB are entrenched through traditional beliefs and misinformation. These issues lead to poor public awareness and resistance to immunization programs, making it challenging to attain comprehensive disease control. Effective interventions must therefore go beyond biomedical technology to incorporate culturally appropriate health education and community involvement. Strategies like mobilizing local leaders and community-based outreach have been promising in enhancing vaccine coverage and breaking the stigma. To create timely health-seeking actions as well as treatment compliance, holistic policies that combine the socio-cultural aspects with healthcare provision are vital (Putri et al., 2025). The added financial and logistical constraints make TB control even more difficult on an international level, especially in rural and inaccessible settings.

Poor / Delayed / Incorrect Dx (esp DRTB)	Case notification - Under-reporting/non reporting	Limited contracting capacity with private sector	Urban centricity
Variable quality - Diagnosis and treatment	Weak regulation - Enforcement	Lack of incentives / disincentives	High OOPE
Informal providers / Chemist as first point of care	Selective referral (unmanageable)	Financial flows/payment delays, costing and tariff setting	Pharmacy-diagnostics nexus
Reluctance to adhere program guidelines	Poor patient support/ adherence	Pharmacy-Diagnostics nexus	Low use of digital tech / data exchange

Figure 13.9. Challenges in engaging the private sector in TB control.

Source: National Tuberculosis Elimination Program (NTEP). (n.d.). *Challenges in engaging the private sector for TB control.* https://ntep.in/index.php/node/5394/CP-challenges-engaging-private-sector-tb-control.

Having regular vaccine supply chains, proper storage facilities, and mobile health units requires a lot of resources and coordination. The lack of transportation is a barrier to accessing diagnostic equipment and treatment facilities in most low-income countries, and as a result, early case detection and ongoing care are lowered. Moreover, intervention sustainability is a problem when programs are heavily dependent on extraneous funding or short-term solutions. Capacity building, infrastructure upgrading, and ensuring robust vaccine supply chains are essential to enhance the local health systems for long-term success. Governments, health providers, and community actors combined can develop integrated systems that can overcome logistical hurdles and provide continuous TB services, thus playing a role in global burden reduction of TB (Immaculata et al., 2025; Putri et al., 2025) (Figure 13.9).

13.4.1. Drug-Resistant Tuberculosis (DR-TB)

The international battle against tuberculosis has been amplified by the development and dissemination of drug-resistant forms, creating formidable challenges for TB control programs and international health policy efforts. In West Africa, the problem is disproportionately heightened by restricted diagnostic capabilities and limited healthcare infrastructure. These underlying conditions lead to delayed diagnosis and treatment for drug-resistant tuberculosis (DR-TB), fueling disease transmission and poor patient outcomes. Strengthening laboratory infrastructure and surveillance systems in National TB Programs (NTP) are paramount to closing these gaps. Coordination between local health authorities and global partners is more and more being directed to increase access to rapid diagnostic technology and healthcare workforce capacity building. These strategic interventions are meant to ensure early detection and optimal management of DR-TB cases, bolstering TB control efforts in resource-constrained settings (Otchere et al., 2024). Advances in molecular diagnostics have also greatly influenced present-day approaches to counter DR-TB, most notably through the understanding of the genetic mechanisms of resistance. Resistance to pyrazinamide (PZA), a central challenge in MDR-TB therapy, is largely caused by mutations in the pncA gene, but rpsA and panD gene alterations have also been involved. These molecular findings allow for more precise and timely identification of resistant strains, thus guiding more personalized and effective therapeutic regimens. The integration of genetic analysis into standard diagnostic laboratory routines can potentially maximize therapeutic outcomes and minimize treatment failure. These advancements indicate a paradigm shift toward precision medicine in TB control and enable programs worldwide to adapt interventions based on exact resistance profiles and eventually enhance the effectiveness of DR-TB treatment (Azeem et al., 2024). Despite technological and scientific advancements, the effective curtailment of DR-TB depends significantly on well-rounded policy regimes and long-term investment in healthcare systems. Subregional networks and associations, including the West African Network for TB, AIDS, and Malaria (WANETAM), are key drivers of knowledge sharing, capacity enhancement, and resource mobilization. These platforms of collaboration spur innovation in diagnostic testing, infection control measures, and drug supply, through the adoption of new agents such as bedaquiline and delamanid. Integration of these advancements into national TB control programs guarantees a synergized approach that responds to medical as well as systemic issues of drug resistance. Finally, harmonizing global policy with local realities and scientific advancements is necessary for reducing the burden of DR-TB and pursuing the larger goals of TB elimination (Otchere et al., 2024).

13.4.2. Socioeconomic Barriers

Successful disease control needs more than isolated medical measures; it needs to address the socioeconomic conditions underlying which access to care is impeded. In most TB-endemic areas, poverty levels interfere disproportionately with early diagnosis and treatment compliance. People in poor environments experience challenges of poor diets, overcrowding, and poor transportation, all of which fuel vulnerability to TB and complicate therapeutic regimens. In addition, economic limitations may limit patients' capacity to go on leave from work or travel to health facilities, causing delays in diagnosis and expanded disease transmission among communities. Awareness of these linked factors is important to inform TB control programs that not only target biomedical intervention but also include measures to mitigate poverty-driven barriers. Comparable issues have been noted within the control of other infectious diseases, highlighting the importance of socioeconomic factors in health policymaking at the global level (Bamodu et al., 2024). Education showcases itself as an important determinant in health outcomes, having an impact on both awareness and health-seeking behavior. Lower educational levels are associated with a lack of adequate information regarding TB transmission, symptoms, and significance of cure completion, and resultantly are frequently followed by delayed diagnosis and loss to follow-up (LTFU). Educational inequalities also lead to the perpetuation of stigma against TB, which can deter patients from seeking healthcare. Health communication that is adapted to break language and cultural barriers is essential among vulnerable populations to provide effective information dissemination. This strategy has been used effectively in other disease control initiatives where better awareness and community involvement have improved prevention and treatment compliance (Bamodu et al., 2024). Therefore, health policies need to include educational interventions that target these gaps as part of overall TB control measures. Gender inequality is another socioeconomic factor that hugely affects TB control worldwide. In patriarchal societies, women often have less freedom in making decisions about their health and limited economic autonomy that hinders them from accessing medical care in good time. These gender dynamics often lead to under-diagnosis and undertreatment of TB among women, hence the continued transmission and poor outcomes. To correct this imbalance, policies that support gender-sensitive delivery of healthcare, such as community outreach programs to empower women and break stigma, are necessary. Moreover, geographical disparities, especially between urban and rural areas, further exacerbate these challenges since rural areas tend to lack proper healthcare facilities and resources. Improved health systems in these poor areas are vital to the success of overcoming the complex web of socioeconomic challenges impeding proper TB control (Emmanuel, 2024).

13.4.3. Stigma and Public Perception

The complexities of tuberculosis (TB) control go beyond the realm of medical treatment, heavily entwining with the social and psychological aspects that affect the course of disease. Among such factors, the widespread stigma surrounding TB is one of major concern, which can seriously impede the process of diagnosis and treatment of those suffering from the disease. Stigma fosters an atmosphere of fear and shame, dissuading individuals from seeking timely medical assistance, thereby permitting the disease to advance uncontrollably. Such avoidance behavior not only undermines individual health outcomes but also to ongoing transmission within communities. By undermining early detection and treatment adherence protocols, stigma undermines the success of TB control initiatives, thus calling for combined approaches that work on social perceptions in addition to clinical interventions. Recognizing these societal barriers is critical to global TB policies for holistic disease management and eradication. In addition, the public perception of tuberculosis is usually influenced by myths and misinformation, which amplify stigma and fuel discrimination. The stigmatizing labels ascribed to the illness have a tendency to represent TB patients as vectors of infection, cutting them off from family and social support systems important for recovery. This stigmatization compounds health inequities as well as makes it difficult to achieve global health equity objectives. Successful TB control programs need to include stigma reduction strategies with community education and advocacy aimed at dismantling destructive narratives. Resources like the *TB Stigma – Measurement Guidance* manual allow health workers and advocates to measure levels of stigma and adapt interventions appropriately, enhancing the effect of TB programs on both clinical and social levels (N/A, 2004). These collaborative efforts help to change public attitudes towards more informed, empathetic understanding.

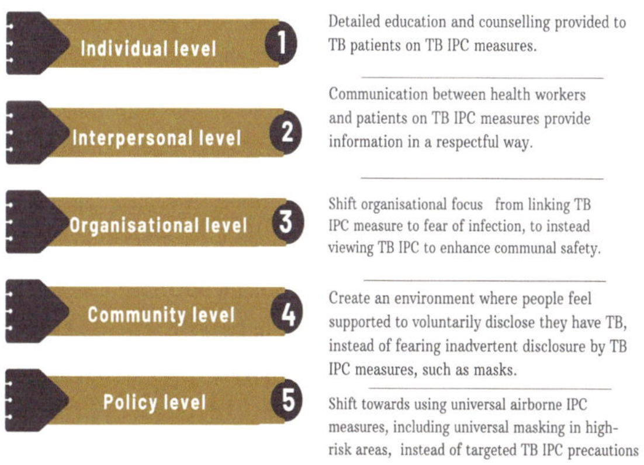

Figure 13.10. Summary of participant recommendations for multi-level, TB IPC stigma intervention targets.

Source: Gupta, A., Mishra, G. A., & Dhillon, P. K. (2024). Time to act on latent tuberculosis: Lessons from epidemiology, policy, and implementation science. *BMC Global Public Health, 2*, 97.

Along with stigma reduction at the community level, international policy guidelines need to address the interrelatedness of stigma, access to treatment, and prevention. Interventions opening up access to TB treatment in isolation cannot succeed to their full potential without contemporaneous action to decrease prejudice and discrimination, which strongly influence treatment completion and public health outcomes. Lessons learned from modeled integrated disease management, e.g., HIV/AIDS, highlight the need to integrate prevention and treatment with stigma reduction to be more effective (N/A, 2004). Inclusive policies of care atmosphere, and stigma-sensitive practice ensure stigma reduction and provide support to affected populations instead of isolating them. Accordingly, international TB control measures are increasingly turning to integrated approaches that intertwine stigma reduction with medical and social interventions with the aim of stopping transmission and enhancing patient health globally (Figure 13.10).

13.5. Role of Technology in Tuberculosis (TB) Control

The development of healthcare strategies has increasingly become entwined with technological advancements, enabling better management and control of diseases. In TB control, technological advances have greatly improved diagnostic capability and surveillance systems. Technologies like mobile health applications and electronic data systems allow for quick collection and analysis of information on patients, enabling effective interventions and real-time monitoring of drug compliance. These technologies facilitate coordination between patients and healthcare providers, minimizing operational inefficiencies in TB control programs. Additionally, applications such as machine learning algorithms and AI-based diagnostic tools aid detecting TB cases from multifaceted clinical data sources, enhancing early detection rates. Through successful incorporation of technology solutions, TB control initiatives are well-placed to tackle disease transmission and patient adherence-related challenges, attuned to global health targets to stem TB cases and deaths (Afghani,

2025). The use of artificial intelligence (AI) in public health environments is an exemplary step forward in managing infectious diseases such as tuberculosis. AI ability to analyze large datasets rapidly allows health systems to predict outbreak dynamics, streamline resource distribution, and customize treatment regimens per patient profile. In TB control, such predictive analysis not only increases situational awareness but also supports the early detection of high-risk groups to inform directed interventions. Yet, implementing AI requires a hybrid operational strategy that fuses technological efficiency and human knowledge since exclusive reliance on AI could risk ignoring contextual clinical specifics. Education of healthcare staff to critically evaluate AI-driven observations is essential in actualizing the full potential of such technology. Strategic investments and joint partnerships in AI research and application are therefore fundamental elements in underpinning the global battle against TB (Afghani, 2025). Despite the encouraging potential of technology in the control of TB, resource disparities impede equitable adoption, particularly in low-resource environments. Sustained challenges like inadequate infrastructure, exorbitant costs, and inadequate training limit the effective application of digital tools and applications of AI within TB programs. The experience with technology use in other areas of healthcare, like speech-language therapy, highlights similar challenges such as technical problems and user lack of competency that can reduce perceived performance and usability. In mitigating these barriers, proper policy frameworks must be put in place with a focus on capacity development, affordability, and equitable access. Intensive training interventions to enhance digital literacy among health workers and patients are also critical to ensure full realization of the benefits of technology. Successful technological integration in TB control programs relies on harmonized global policy measures that direct innovation toward the realities of local contexts (Figure 13.11).

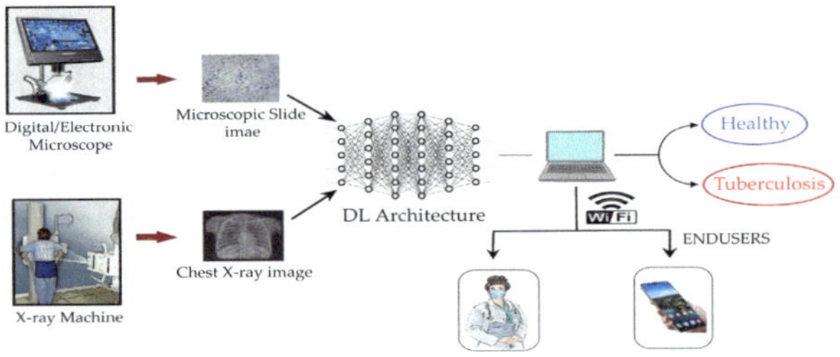

Figure 13.11. Artificial intelligent-powered detection of tuberculosis.

Source: Yadav, A., Singh, S. K., & Dewan, D. (2022). *The burden of tuberculosis infection and disease in India: A comprehensive review of current epidemiology and policy perspectives.* https://www.preprints.org/manuscript/202209.0208/v1.

13.5.1. Diagnostic Innovations

Successful control of tuberculosis is based in large measure on the ability to diagnose infections accurately and promptly, a requirement that has become increasingly important with the emergence of MDR-TB. Conventional diagnostic techniques, frequently time-consuming and resource-requiring, have posed constraints to initiating therapy promptly, particularly in settings of limited resources. New diagnostic technologies, like rapid DST, present with potential avenues the ability to close this gap through providing the possibility of faster identification of resistant strains. These technologies are essential for the adaptation of treatment regimens and inhibiting further propagation of resistant TB strains. Their adoption in public health programs has the potential to improve surveillance quality and compliance with treatment, which are key factors in controlling TB on a population level. Strengthening diagnostic tools, particularly among high-burden countries such as India, is thus a critical strategy of global TB control efforts, both clinical and public health requirements (Gamon, 2013). The complexities of putting into practice new diagnostic tools are inextricably entwined with the structural and functional realities of current public health systems. In India, for instance, attempts at integrating innovative diagnostic processes are hindered by stringent control schemes and piecemeal healthcare infrastructure. These usually act to counteract the flexibility needed to respond swiftly to new diagnostic technologies. Additionally, cultural, social, and economic constraints affect the adoption and usefulness of novel diagnostic methods. Effective integration of diagnostic innovations requires a subtle assessment of local contexts that enables localized learning and experimentation within the health system. This strategy not only enables the uptake of state-of-the-art tools but also creates an environment that is conducive to sustainable enhancement in TB detection and management (Engel et al.). Diagnostic innovation is not only a technological issue but also a policy priority that should go hand-in-hand with strategic public health capacity and education investments.

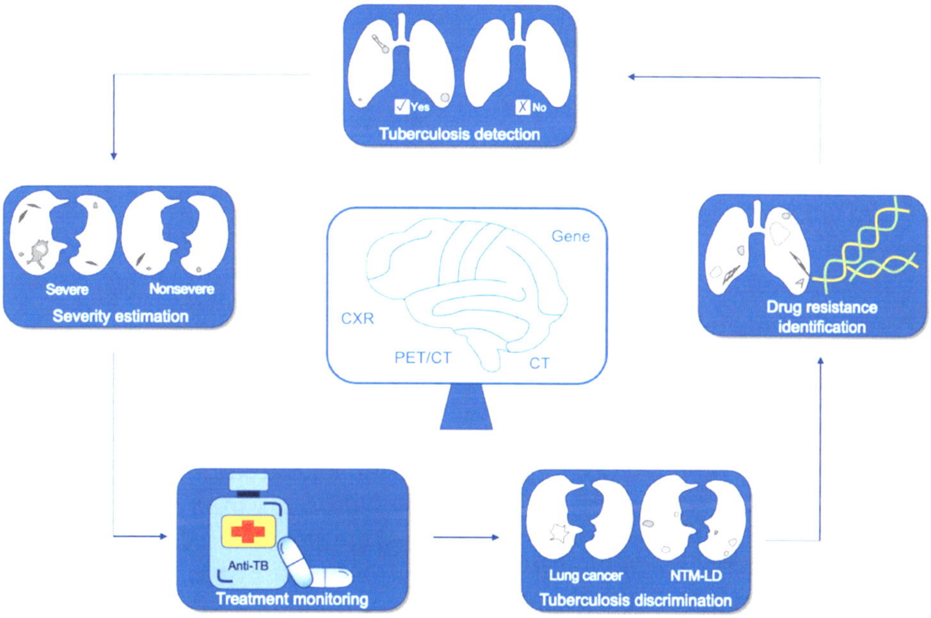

Figure 13.12. Application of artificial intelligence (AI) in tuberculosis.

Source: ResearchGate. (n.d.). *Application of artificial intelligence in tuberculosis, NTM-LD (non-tuberculous mycobacterial lung disease).* https://www.researchgate.net/figure/Application-of-artificial-intelligence-in-tuberculosis-NTM-LD-non-tuberculous_fig32_368946542. replace

Boosting diagnostic capacity requires a collaborative effort to enhance health literacy at the community and health worker levels to ensure early detection results in proper treatment compliance. Policymakers should balance diagnostic progress with successful treatment programs and strong surveillance systems to develop an integrated response to the TB epidemic. Learning from TB control model success stories in countries, with focus on quick diagnosis and access to quality drugs, can help ensure that diagnostic frameworks are culturally appropriate and operationally viable. Finally, innovation in diagnostics within a responsive and adaptive health system is critical to controlling MDR-TB and improving global TB control policies (Engel et al., 2025; Gamon, 2013) (Figure 13.12).

13.5.2. Digital Health Solutions

Integration of digital health solutions into TB control programs is a major leap in combatting the complexities of infectious disease control. Digital platforms can organize timely monitoring of patients, enhance compliance with treatment protocols, and allow for real-time data collection essential for epidemiological surveillance. With the use of mobile health technologies and electronic health records, healthcare workers can monitor the outcomes of treatment more effectively while providing targeted treatment to TB patients, thereby preventing drug resistance and transmission. Moreover, incorporating digital applications into TB programs would facilitate closing gaps in resource-constrained settings where access to the healthcare infrastructure is limited, thus increasing equity in health service delivery. These digital innovations also complement international policy objectives promoting sustainable health interventions that balance public health outcomes and environmental considerations, highlighting their potential for transformation in TB control (Gwadabe et al., 2025). Proper deployment of digital health applications in TB control involves assessing their usability and effect on patient engagement, as exemplified in other chronic disease arenas. For instance, digital interventions prescribed for patients with rheumatology have shown symptom improvement and patient satisfaction, though with differing rates of completion and improved health literacy (Albrecht et al., 2025). These findings emphasize the need to develop user-friendly digital interventions that encourage sustained use and patient activation. Using such frameworks on TB program management would make programs more resilient by promoting patient self-management, enhancing compliance to long courses of TB treatment, and eventually lowering default rates. In addition, the collection of real-world data from digital channels could inform policy and guide decision-making based on evidence of effectiveness, support the allocation of resources, and streamline treatment approaches to maximize outcomes in varying populations. Global control policies for TB increasingly see the value of incorporating innovative digital health solutions that support established methods like directly observed therapy (DOT). DOT guarantees drug adherence by supervised administration, but digital technologies present scalable options that are respectful of patient autonomy and decrease healthcare system loads.

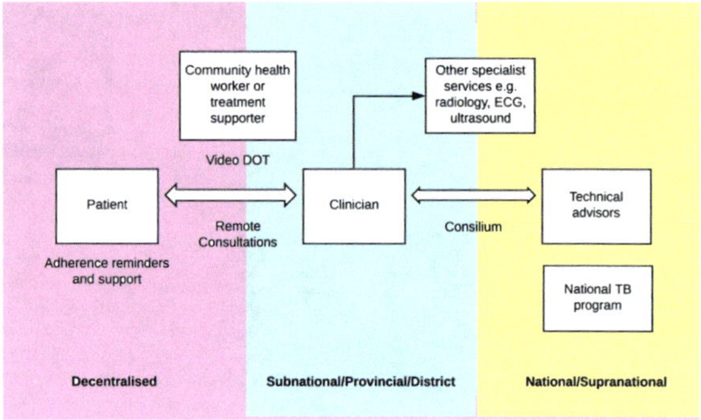

Figure 13.13. Digital health in tuberculosis program delivery.

Source: ResearchGate. (n.d.). *Digital health in tuberculosis program delivery: In many countries, TB programs are increasingly adopting digital health tools.* https://www.researchgate.net/figure/Digital-health-in-tuberculosis-program-delivery-In-many-countries-TB-programs-are_fig1_335135767.

In addition, digital tools help unconnected disease control and environmental degradation through the ability to monitor remotely and reduce travel, thus enabling sustainable healthcare provision in harmony with more extensive environmental health policy (Gwadabe et al., 2025). Policy frameworks thus need to encourage the integration of digital health tools in NTPs using financing arrangements as well as regulatory facilitation. In so doing, international TB efforts can leverage these technologies to drive equitable, effective, and sustainable disease control interventions (Figure 13.13).

13.5.3. Data Management and Surveillance

Successful TB control is dependent on the alignment of thorough data management and surveillance systems with the capability to document disease incidence and treatment outcomes precisely. The One Health philosophy's fusion of human, animal, and environmental health emphasizes the need for an interdisciplinary data model that can capture complex epidemiological patterns (Ahmed et al., 2025). Sophisticated surveillance tools allow for earlier detection of TB outbreaks, and public health interventions and allocation of resources can be made promptly. Yet data heterogeneity and completeness variability typically create major impediments, especially where healthcare infrastructure is scarce in low-resource environments. Promoting interoperability of data and real-time reporting is vital in transcending these impediments. Timely and accurate management of data not only enhances local efforts for TB control but also advances global health security by guiding international policy decisions and promoting collaborative response strategies. Upgrading laboratory and health information systems is fundamental to enhancing TB surveillance and maximizing disease management results. Laboratory management information systems (LMIS), as seen in environments like India, provide a high-tech way of streamlining diagnostic data flow—from the collection of samples to the release of results—thus improving reliability and mitigating delays in patient care (Goswami et al., 2025). Technology notwithstanding, the world outside finds practicality often bogged down by urban-rural differences in healthcare facilities, while public labs have significant challenges related to infrastructure and skilled staff. Filling these gaps through strategic investment in digital health infrastructure and workforce training is critical to securing equitable access to precise diagnostic tools. Integrate LMIS into NTPs to augment real-time surveillance capabilities so that data-based decisions can be implemented quickly to stem transmission and enhance treatment adherence. Data linkage and multisectoral partnership are critical to maximizing TB surveillance within global control programs.

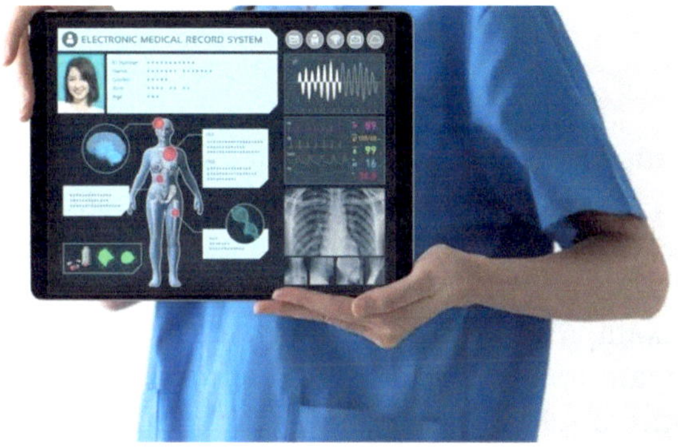

Source: Ezovion. (2023). *Portable EHR system illustration.* https://ezovion.com/wp-content/uploads/2023/08/94-portable_ehr_story.jpg__992x558_q85_crop-smart_subsampling-2_upscale-1024x568.jpg.webp.

The experiences gained from successful programs under the One Health approach, including the PREDICT project and country-level health programs, show the value in combining environmental, animal, and human health data streams to produce an enriched picture of the dynamics of disease (Ahmed et al., 2025). Such integrated surveillance improves predictability and prevention of TB outbreaks by targeting co-factors such as zoonotic disease reservoirs and AMR. In addition, international policy guidelines should focus on enhancing surveillance infrastructure through data sharing and interoperability standards, as well as ensuring sustainable funding to sustain surveillance infrastructure development. Comprehensive data management systems only contribute to improved TB control through synergistic efforts from government, health institutions, and the community.

SUMMARY

Assessment of TB control efforts worldwide discloses a complex challenge needing sustained effort and responsive strategies. Although notable strides have been achieved within nations possessing strong public health infrastructures, ongoing MDR-TB signifies glaring shortcomings in treatment compliance and diagnostic capabilities. The experiences of India, where TB remains prevalent despite ongoing interventions, underscore the necessity for reshaping health systems to prioritize rapid diagnosis, effective treatment, and continued surveillance. Strengthening these components is essential not only for improving clinical outcomes but also for preventing the emergence of drug-resistant strains that complicate global eradication efforts. Hence, global support needs to emphasize local capacity building, research, and culturally adapted programs with an aim to cater to varied community needs and enhance patient adherence (Gamon, 2013). Besides, the function of collaborative frameworks between governmental and non-governmental entities has been found to be critical in driving TB control efforts, particularly in resource-constrained environments. Examples like BRAC in Bangladesh demonstrate how stakeholder synergy, led by ideas such as value chain analysis, can maximize detection and treatment rates through full community engagement. Integrated programming guarantees not only efficient program delivery but also a durable impact by promoting local ownership and capacity development. International policies need to reflect lessons from these models, promoting flexible frameworks that appeal to country contexts and healthcare dilemmas. Encouraging these collaborative efforts at the grassroots level will increase the scale and impact of TB control efforts, eventually closing the gaps between policy development and implementation (Ravichandran, 2004). Long-term control of TB demands an interactive function of resilient health infrastructure, creative treatment approaches, and multi-sectoral collaboration. Intervening against the burden of tuberculosis, especially multi-drug resistant tuberculosis, requires that nations invest in rapid diagnostic tools, effective access to quality drugs, and strengthened surveillance systems. Additionally, global policy guidelines ought to prioritize culturally sensitive interventions and education to enhance treatment compliance and reduce transmission. Experience from successful models in different areas provides worthy lessons for the development of flexible strategies responsive to unique epidemiological and socio-economic contexts. Together, these initiatives represent the foundation of an integrated approach necessary to regulate TB and ensure long-term public health objectives on a global basis (Ravichandran, 2004; Gamon, 2013).

The struggle to master TB in the world overlaps a rich landscape of health needs and policy contexts that require a collective global effort. TB is a significant public health issue, particularly in LMICs where poverty and limited resources undermine disease control. Financing and policy strategies by both national governments and global agencies have a significant influence on TB control programs, enabling expansion in diagnostics, treatment accessibility, and monitoring. These schemes find their way into larger health programs focused on communicable diseases to maximize impact. The role of multilaterals and donor agencies has infused much-needed support, but variations in healthcare infrastructure still drive TB prevalence and treatment cure rates among regions (Gamon, 2013). These contextual considerations emphasize the imperative for localized policies that take local epidemiology, resource constraints, and health system capacity into account to maximize TB control effectiveness. The development of antibiotic resistance threatens the gains achieved in terms of global TB control efforts, making treatment more complex and more likely to fail. This is compounded by the stagnation of the discovery of new antibiotics in the past few decades, with the majority of currently available drugs being derivatives of those developed between the early 1900s and the 1980s. The gradual pace of drug innovation, coupled with the evolving ability of MTB to become resistant, especially in the scenario of MDR-TB, presents an urgent public health challenge. This serves to enforce the central necessity of new investments in research and development of new antimicrobials in conjunction with measures to maximize the use of antibiotics and avoid the dissemination of resistance. By not targeting antibiotic resistance directly, TB control programs risk negating decades of gains against this chronic infectious disease (Coukell et al., 2016). In distilling these main points, it is apparent that TB control programs are faced with the need to balance short-term clinical requirements with long-term strategic objectives within global health policy systems. Successful TB control relies on long-term funding, global cooperation, and adaptive approaches with the ability to address emerging threats like drug resistance. At the same time, the strengthening of health systems in high-burden nations is essential to increase prevention, diagnostic, and treatment services. Policymakers and global health stakeholders should focus on innovation, resource management, and equity to bridge gaps in TB care. This integrated strategy will make sure that the global efforts for TB control are strong, reactive, and compatible with broader public health goals for lowering the global disease burden (Coukell et al., 2016).

CLOSER LOOK

NATIONAL TB PROGRAMS (NTPS)

National Tuberculosis Programs (NTPs) are government-run public health activities that aim to control and ultimately eliminate tuberculosis (TB) by harmonized prevention, diagnosis, treatment, and surveillance efforts. NTPs are generally run by ministries of health in cooperation with global health bodies like the WHO, the Global Fund, and non-governmental organizations. NTPs are central to the development and coordination of national strategies in support of international TB control goals, e.g., those stated within the WHO's End TB Strategy.

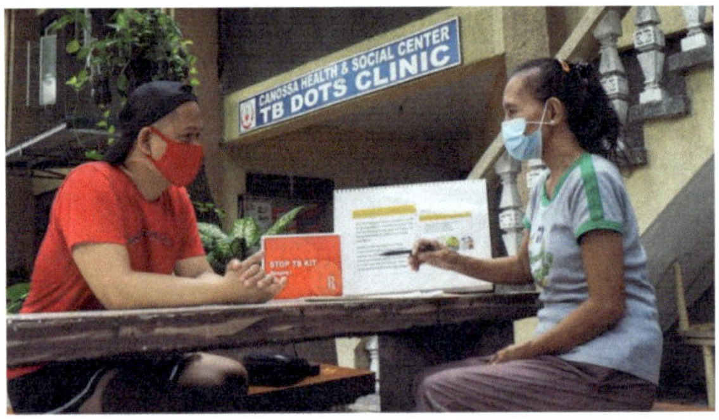

Source: DuckDuckGo. (n.d.). *TB awareness illustration.* https://external-content.duckduckgo.com/iu/?u=https%3A%2F%2Ftse4.mm.bing.net%2Fth%3Fid%3DOIP.K0O6VhbW51oE4NvaYk9OEgHaEo%26pid%3DApi&f=1&ipt=c836a15fbcbf6cafeacd235a6ef9ba2a729211aa02961c38ddbea2f02794a9c7&ipo=images.

One of the key roles of NTPs is ensuring early diagnosis and successful treatment of TB cases. This means encouraging the application of standardized diagnostic equipment, including sputum microscopy, chest X-rays, GeneXpert, and culture methods, to diagnose active TB cases, including drug-resistant TB. Following diagnosis, patients are registered into suitable treatment regimens, typically according to WHO guidelines that recommend standardized treatment lengths and drug regimens. Assuring treatment compliance with DOT is a foundation of NTPs, for the reason that poor treatment can result in relapse, treatment failure, and drug resistance.NTPs also highlight the management of MDR-TB and the integration of TB care with other health services, including HIV/AIDS programs. Since there is a strong association between TB and HIV co-infection, most NTPs provide routine HIV screening among TB patients and TB screening among HIV/AIDS patients. Preventive therapy for LTBI, particularly among the high-risk groups like PLHIV, is also included in the strategic plans of most NTPs.Another essential component of NTPs is community outreach and health education. These programs aim to decrease stigma, encourage health-seeking behavior, and make TB services available to vulnerable and underserved populations. NTPs rely heavily on using outreach workers and community health volunteers to facilitate TB care in isolated or marginalized communities.Monitoring and evaluation are also integral parts of NTPs. National programs should track, analyze, and report on TB incidence, treatment success, drug resistance, and program performance. This information informs planning, resource allocation, and measuring progress against national and international TB control objectives.

REFERENCES

1. Agnes Meershoek, Alice Zwerling, Amrita Daftary, Brian Citro, Caoimhe Smyth, Dean Lewis, Deirdre Ni Cheallaigh, Elaine Byrne, Ellen M. H Mitchell, Gill Craig, Ieva Leimane, James Malar, Jens Levy, Julia van der Land, Kate Macintyre, Lisa G. Johnston, Nadine Ferris France, Nora Engel, Olive Mumba, Rajita Bhavaraju, Ronan R. Conroy, Sarah van de Berg, Stephen H-F Macdonald, Timur Abdullaev, and Tushar Nair. (2018). *TB Stigma–Measurement Guidance*. The United States Agency for International Development (USAID), !nancially supports this publication through Challenge TB under the terms of Agreement No. AID-OAA-A-14-00029. This publication was made possible by the generous support of the American people through USAID. https://core.ac.uk/download/287580942.pdf (accessed on 10 May 2025).
2. Afghani, A. (2025). Enhancing Operational Effectiveness in Security and Defence within the UAE: The Strategic Role of Artificial Intelligence. *International Journal of Technology and Systems, 10*(1), 1–22. https://doi.org/10.47604/ijts.3194 (accessed on 10 May 2025).
3. Ahmed, M. M., Okesanya, O., Othman, Z., Ibrahim, A. M., Adigun, O. A., Ukoaka, B., Abdi, M. I., et al. (2025). Holistic approaches to zoonoses: Integrating public health, policy, and One Health in a dynamic global context. *Zoonotic Diseases*. https://www.semanticscholar.org/paper/b45c53f860c450473e6be49bbb5ae6998e16b685 (accessed on 10 May 2025).
4. Quratul Ain, & Rabia Imtiaz. (2025). The Role of Technology in Speech-Language Therapy: Perceptions, Effectiveness, and Challenges in a Resource-Limited Setting. Journal of Health and Rehabilitation Research, 5(1), 1–8. https://doi.org/10.61919/jhrr.v5i1.1754 (accessed on 10 May 2025).
5. Albrecht, A., Taubmann, J., Minopoulou, I., Hatscher, L., Kleinert, S., Mühlensiepen, F., Welcker, M., et al. (2025). Real-world evidence of digital health applications (DiGAs) in rheumatology: Insights from the DiGAReal registry. *Rheumatology and Therapy, 12*, 267–282. https://www.semanticscholar.org/paper/90b9ed14aa496faa809d9ae2205a1a2cf132af7d (accessed on 10 May 2025).
6. Alhuwayfi, S., Alwakeel, A., Alhuwayfi, A. S., & Alhuwayfi, A. (2024). Systemic review of community-based interventions for preventing chronic diseases in preventive medicine practice: Review article. *The Egyptian Journal of Hospital Medicine* (January 2024) Vol. 94, Page 291-299. https://www.semanticscholar.org/paper/90b532973f0893aeadfa5daf366759696b396f28 (accessed on 10 May 2025).
7. Al-karawi A S, Kadhim A A, Kadum M M, Recent advances in tuberculosis: A comprehensive review of emerging trends in pathogenesis, diagnostics, treatment, and prevention. Int J Clin Biochem Res 2023;10(4):262-269(accessed on 10 May 2025).
8. Amadou, S., Lee, M., Lee, J., Kim, S., & Kang, S. (2025). Family structure factors influencing modern contraceptive use in Cameroon based on analysis of 2018-2019 demographic and health survey data. *Scientific Reports, 15*(1), 14174. https://www.semanticscholar.org/paper/e4c4df2c6f51a45b7fab0c5722278ab31688be78 (accessed on 10 May 2025).
9. Atoi, A. A., Jaafar, S. J., Atil, A., Sharizman, S., Abdul, S., & Rahim, S. (2025). Factors influencing cholera vaccination effectiveness in Africa and Bangladesh: A scoping review. *Borneo Epidemiology Journal*. BEJ, VOLUME 5, ISSUE 1, DECEMBER 2024. https://www.semanticscholar.org/paper/a79e7d9890e0162783f7096ccdefe102377c64c0 (accessed on 10 May 2025).

10. Bamodu, O., & Chung, C. C. (2024). Cancer care disparities: Overcoming barriers to cancer control in low- and middle-income countries. *JCO Global Oncology, 10*, e2300439. https://www.semanticscholar.org/paper/0499bf2928b08e89c430678908d3f354535efd80 (accessed on 10 May 2025).
11. Jenner, A., Bhagwandin, N., & Kowalski, S. P. (2017). Antimicrobial resistance (AMR) and multidrug resistance (MDR): Overview of current approaches, consortia, and intellectual property issues. Global Challenges Report. https://core.ac.uk/download/215505935.pdf (accessed on 10 May 2025).
12. Buinwi, U., Okatta, C. G., Johnson, E., Buinwi, J. A., & Tuboalabo, A. (2024). Enhancing trade policy education: A review of pedagogical approaches in public administration programs. *International Journal of Applied Research in Social Sciences*. P-ISSN: 2706-9176, E-ISSN: 2706-9184 Volume 6, Issue 6, P.No. 1253-1273, June 2024 DOI: 10.51594/ijarss.v6i6.1243 Fair East Publishers Journal Homepage: www.https://doi.org/10.51594/ijarss.v6i6.1243(accessed on 10 May 2025).
13. Bultman, J., Kanywanyi, J. L., Maarifa, H., Mtei, et al. (2012). Tanzania health insurance regulatory framework review. Ministry of Health and Social WelfareandSocial Security Regulatory Authority. Final Report 30 March 2012; by Digital Library of the Tanzania Health Community
14. https://core.ac.uk/download/pdf/11307330.pdf (accessed on 10 May 2025).
15. Gostin, Lawrence O.; Cabrera, Oscar A.; and Kim, Susan C., "The O'Neill Institute for National and Global Health Law: Discovering Innovative Solutions for the Most Pressing Health Problems Facing the Nation and the World" (2010). *Georgetown Law Faculty Publications and Other Works*. 382. https://scholarship.law.georgetown.edu/facpub/382 (accessed on 10 May 2025).
16. Chhetri, S., Kiran, K., Dasu, V., Kavya, K. N., Shankar, U., Somashekar, N. E., & Chadda, V. K. (2024). Optimal intervention strategies and cost-effectiveness analysis study of tuberculosis with reference to TPT, malnutrition, and diabetes management. https://doi.org/10.48550/arXiv.2405.16500
17. (accessed on 10 May 2025).
18. Coukell, A., Shore, C., Jungman, E., Talkington, K., Kothari, P., & Urahn, S. K. (2016). A scientific roadmap for antibiotic discovery: A sustained and robust pipeline of new antibacterial drugs and therapies is critical to preserve public health. https://core.ac.uk/download/75785719.pdf (accessed on 10 May 2025).
19. Dartois, V., & Rubin, E. J. (2022). Anti-tuberculosis treatment strategies and drug development: Challenges and priorities. *Nature Reviews Microbiology, 20*, 685–701. https://doi.org/10.1038/s41579-022-00731-y.
20. Bassey Immaculata E et al (2025). Threats Analysis and Control Strategies in Immunization Programs for Rural Communities in Nigeria. Glob Acad J Med Sci; Vol-7, Iss-1 pp- 13-26(accessed on 10 May 2025).
21. Engel, N. (2025). Flexibility and innovation in response to emerging infectious diseases: Reactions to multi-drug resistant tuberculosis in India. https://core.ac.uk/download/pdf/6941410.pdf (accessed on 10 May 2025).

22. Engel, N. (2025). Innovation dynamics in tuberculosis control in India: The shift to new partnerships. https://core.ac.uk/download/pdf/6371633.pdf (accessed on 10 May 2025).

23. Gamon, Maribel, "Maribel Gamon - Multidrug-Resistant Tuberculosis in India: Solving a Problem by Reconstructing the Public Health Infrastructure" (2013). *Ronald E. McNair Scholars Program 2013.* 12. https://epublications.marquette.edu/mcnair_2013/12(accessed on 10 May 2025).

24. Goswami, M., Gopal, K. M., Kuslum, S. T., Ather, I., Nhsrc Fellow, Pha, Nhsrc MoHFW Advisor, & Pha Consultant. (2025). Laboratory management information systems in India: Challenges, opportunities, and the path forward. *International Journal for Multidisciplinary Research.* https://www.semanticscholar.org/paper/016cd1676225fbef9b6aa99fb894aaacbc16c681 (accessed on 10 May 2025).

25. Gwadabe, H. A., Elelu, S.-A., Innocent, M. O., Ibrahim, G. O., Adekunle, I. J., & Abdulsalam, M. (2025). Exploring Local-to-Global Win-Win Strategies for Infectious Disease Control: Enhancing Human Health and Sustainability. Biological Sciences, 5(1), 850–864. https://doi.org/10.55006/biolsciences.2025.5104(accessed on 10 May 2025).

26. Heydari, H., Sadeghi, R., Jamshidi, E., Rahimiforoushani, A., Nikbakht, H. A., & Mashhadsari, M. R. A. (2025). Effectiveness of community-based intervention using PATCH on disease perception, empowerment, and self-care in hypertension: A community trial protocol. *Trials, 26.* https://www.semanticscholar.org/paper/78ae71b0d965ad16861a7810a509236fae943094 (accessed on 10 May 2025).

27. Long, Q., Huang, F., Huan, ST. *et al.* Scale-up of a comprehensive model to improve tuberculosis control in China: lessons learned and the way forward. *Infect Dis Poverty* **10**, 41 (2021). https://doi.org/10.1186/s40249-021-00828-1(accessed on 10 May 2025).

28. Mahmud, A., & Parkhurst, M. (2007). The role of the health care sector in expanding economic opportunity. FSG Social Impact advisors and the Fellows of Harvad College. https://core.ac.uk/download/71341129.pdf (accessed on 10 May 2025).

29. Marme, G., Kuzma, J., Zimmerman, P. A. P., Harris, N., & Rutherford, S. (2023). Tuberculosis infection prevention and control in rural Papua New Guinea: An evaluation using the infection prevention and control assessment framework. *Antimicrobial Resistance and Infection Control, 12.* https://www.semanticscholar.org/paper/68d506a3998440c14efb97e1ac749f1bfa99d316 (accessed on 10 May 2025).

30. McLaren, Z., Milliken, A., Meyer, A., & Sharp, A. R. (2016). Does directly observed therapy improve tuberculosis treatment? More evidence is needed to guide tuberculosis policy. *BMC Infectious Diseases, 16.* https://www.semanticscholar.org/paper/27b2b4ba664b83712625c8cae84af3955904697b (accessed on 10 May 2025).

31. Mugisha Emmanuel K. (2024). The Impact of Socioeconomic Factors on HIV Prevalence and Treatment Accessibility in Nigeria: A Comprehensive Review. NEWPORT INTERNATIONAL JOURNAL OF RESEARCH IN MEDICAL SCIENCES, 5(3): 46-52. https://doi.org/10.59298/NIJRMS/2024/5.3.4652(accessed on 10 May 2025).

32. Murray, C. J. L., Ikuta, K. S., Sharara, F., Swetschinski, L. R., Robles Aguilar, G., Gray, A. P., Han, C., et al. (2022). Global burden of bacterial antimicrobial resistance in 2019: A systematic analysis. *The Lancet, 399,* 629–655. https://doi.org/10.1016/s0140-6736(21)02724-0.

33. Musonda, J. P. (2024). Effectiveness of the interventions of TB and HIV control in Zambia: A systematic review. *Texila International Journal of Academic Research.* 10.21522/TIJAR.2014.11.03.Art016(accessed on 10 May 2025).

34. Otchere, I., Asante-Poku, A., Akpadja, K., Diallo, A. B., Sanou, A., Asare, P., Osei-Wusu, S., et al. (2024). Opinion review of drug-resistant tuberculosis in West Africa: Tackling the challenges for effective control. *Frontiers in Public Health, 12.* https://www.semanticscholar.org/paper/2b395b035f05fb8c0ff8a5882e25941df7c32382 (accessed on 10 May 2025).

35. Putri, D. U. P., Hernida, H., Andani, M. T., Affrianti, N. D., Satria, M. A., & Liana, S. (2025). Assessing the effectiveness of the tuberculosis control program at Kedaton Health Center, Bandar Lampung City. *Health Dynamics.* 2 (3): 105-111. https://www.semanticscholar.org/paper/ebed83d2c87cec378ea273760258bfeef1549352 (accessed on 10 May 2025).

36. Ravichandran, N. (2004). Tuberculosis control in developing countries: A generalized community health worker-based model. Indian Institute of Management Ahmedabad May 2004. https://core.ac.uk/download/pdf/6443340.pdf (accessed on 10 May 2025).

37. Rühwald, M., Hannay, E., Sarin, S., Kao, K., Sen, R., & Chadha, S. (2022). Considerations for simultaneous testing of COVID-19 and tuberculosis in high-burden countries. *The Lancet Global Health, 10*, e465–e466. https://doi.org/10.1016/s2214-109x(22)00002-x.

38. Salam, M. A., Al-Amin, M. Y., Salam, M. T., Pawar, J. S., Akhter, N., Rabaan, A. A., & Alqumber, M. A. A. (2023). Antimicrobial resistance: A growing serious threat for global public health. *Healthcare, 11*, 1946–1946. https://doi.org/10.3390/healthcare11131946 (accessed on 10 May 2025).

39. Abdul Azeem, Tejashree A, Krishna Karthik, Nirmala A R, Geetha N, 2024. Genetic analysis of pyrazinamide resistance: mutations in the pncA gene among clinical isolates of multi-drug resistant Mycobacterium Tuberculosis. Journal of medical pharmaceutical and allied sciences, V 13 - I 2, Pages - 6479 – 6484. Doi: https://doi.org/10.55522/jmpas.V13I2.6407. (accessed on 10 May 2025).

40. Thomason, Jane, PNG Mineral Boom: Harnessing the Extractive Sector to Deliver Better Health Outcomes (January 1, 2011). Development Policy Centre Discussion Paper No. 2 , Available at SSRN: https://ssrn.com/abstract=1919304 or http://dx.doi.org/10.2139/ssrn.1919304(accessed on 10 May 2025).

41. Uddin, T. M., Chakraborty, A., Khusro, A., Zidan, B. M. R., Mitra, S., Bin Emran, T., Dhama, K., et al. (2021). Antibiotic resistance in microbes: History, mechanisms, therapeutic strategies, and future prospects. *Journal of Infection and Public Health, 14*, 1750–1766. https://doi.org/10.1016/j.jiph.2021.10.020.

42. Varambally, K. (2024). The role of social security systems in alleviating poverty among elderly populations: An evaluation of policy effectiveness and challenges. *International Journal of Commerce and Management Research Studies (IJCMRS).* https://www.semanticscholar.org/paper/855f34d2a8f27a303f47da129b105abc1333a75f (accessed on 10 May 2025).

43. Weiss, H. A., & Ferrand, R. A. (2019). Improving adolescent health: An evidence-based call to action. *The Lancet, 393*, 1073–1075. https://doi.org/10.1016/s0140-6736(18)32996-9.

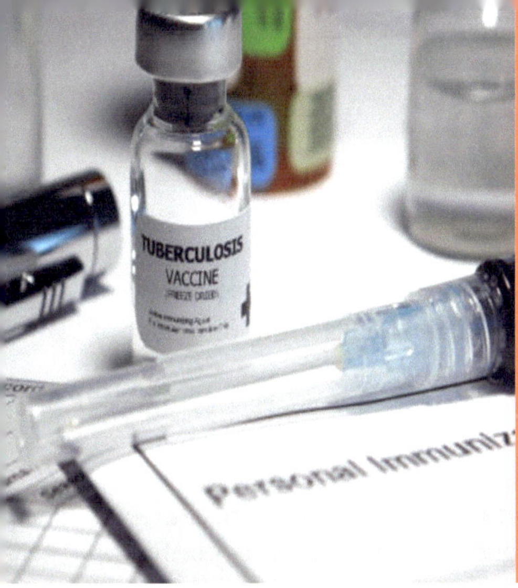

Chapter 14

VACCINATION AND PREVENTION STRATEGIES OF TUBERCULOSIS

Contents

Introduction

The global health environment has been impacted considerably by infectious diseases, which, despite advances in medical science, continue to pose great challenges. Among such diseases, TB is a persistent threat that has caused extensive morbidity and mortality across the globe. TB's persistence is also under threat from the growing problem of antimicrobial resistance (AMR), which complicates treatment and public health interventions and erodes public health programs. This silent epidemic has the potential to erode gains in infectious disease control and requires urgent, concerted action to reduce its impact. Effective control of TB requires an extensive approach that addresses new treatments and more stringent prevention to reduce spread and resistance development (Salam et al., 2023). Identification of the place of vaccination in this situation brings to the fore its central role in global health programs to regulate incidence levels and disease burden. TB control is also hampered by the ability of the bacteria to resist existing antibiotics, a situation that is a sign of an underlying crisis regarding global antimicrobial performance. The resistance not only extends disease but also increases the risk of mortality, particularly in low-resource settings where health infrastructure may be weak. The World Health Organization (WHO) and other international agencies indicate that vaccination is one of the most effective methods of disease prevention, with the potential to reduce the consumption of antibiotics and avoid resistant strain transmission. Moreover, vaccination programs are part of extensive herd immunity and control of outbreaks in risky populations. The convergence of vaccination and other public health interventions is the cornerstone of tuberculosis control, emphasizing the integration of these components into more extensive AMR action plans (Dartois & Rubin, 2022). With the complex dynamics between infectious diseases and AMR, prevention through vaccination becomes a key plank of global health policy beyond tuberculosis. Success in intervention for prevention rests not just on scientific progress but also on effective healthcare delivery, public awareness, and long-term political mobilization. As tuberculosis adapts to evade existing treatment, vaccination provides a preventive measure, capping infection levels and transmission potential. In this respect, evaluation of vaccination programs and their incorporation into broader prevention interventions holds a holistic recipe for effective control of tuberculosis. These programs need to be scientifically designed and implemented to address biological hazards as well as system determinants for the sustainable global burden of TB and AMR (Dartois & Rubin, 2022; Md. Salam et al., 2023).

Importance of Vaccination

The global health landscape is never free of infectious disease threats, which necessitate strict preventive measures to safeguard populations. Tuberculosis is caused by *Mycobacterium tuberculosis* (MTB), a leading killer even with advances in medical science. Vaccination becomes a front-line defense in this case, with a preventive shield against infection rather than relying on treatment upon onset of disease. Experience in fighting the COVID-19 pandemic over the last few years has placed the faster development and deployment of vaccines in the limelight, and this can be an example for addressing chronic threats like TB. The interplay of new vaccine platforms and faster research pipelines, witnessed during COVID-19, can quantitatively enhance the probability of developing more effective TB vaccines. These advances underscore the crucial role of vaccination not only in controlling the spread of disease but also in being in line with global health goals, such as the WHO's vision of ending TB by 2030 (Stefan, 2023). The fight against TB is also made difficult by drug resistance, which makes treatment more difficult and increases the stakes for prevention. Resistance to current antibiotics necessitates longer and more complex treatment regimens, which are also defined by high side effects and lower efficacy. Vaccination in this case becomes a major preventive intervention, with the potential to prevent the spread of drug-susceptible and DR-TB variants. The capability of vaccines to prevent infection from occurring in the first place can truncate transmission chains, reducing the reservoir from which resistance develops. In this way, vaccination complements pharmaceutical interventions in that it lessens the necessity for extended drug delivery, and consequently, also lessens the possibility of resistance development. The multiplicative benefit of vaccination extends beyond individual protection, influencing public health dynamics in terms of interrupting transmission chains and enabling global eradication (Sinha et al., 2023). Furthermore, vaccination campaigns make important contributions to global health equity by providing accessible, low-cost prevention, especially in high-burden, low-resource settings. Compared to the extensive and costly multi-drug therapy for TB disease, vaccines may be administered on a mass scale with relative ease, enabling extensive reach. Immunization strategies need to account for the complex immune response elicited by *Mtb*, necessitating vaccines that can fine-tune protective immunity without enhancing pathology. Leveraging experience from COVID-19 vaccine development, including novel platforms and efficient clinical trials, promises key solutions to overcome such challenges. Effective vaccination programs, underpinned by robust healthcare infrastructure and public health promotion, form the basis of holistic TB prevention programs that not only control existing infections but also avert new infections and resistance emergence (Sinha et al., 2023; Stefan, 2023).

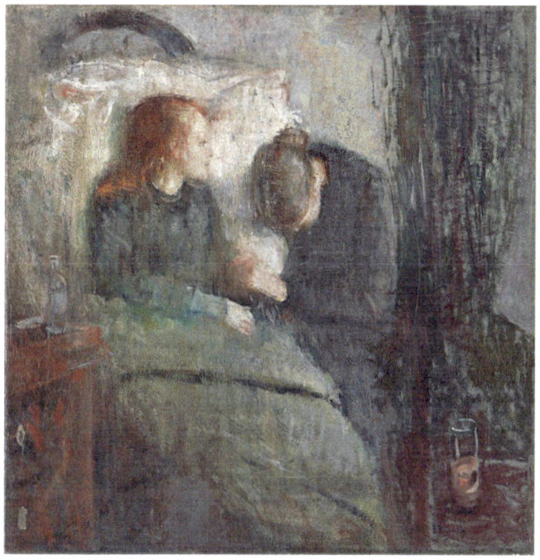

Source: By Edvard Munch - http://samling.nasjonalmuseet.no/no/object/NG.M.00839 Nasjonalmuseet / Høstland, Børre, Public Domain, https://commons.wikimedia.org/w/index.php?curid=37692571

Overview of Prevention Strategies

Effective prevention of disease is based on an assessment of both population and biological dynamics, particularly for infectious diseases such as tuberculosis. A key intervention to prevent transmission is vaccination, providing immunity in at-risk populations and breaking the infection cycle. The *Bacillus Calmette-Guérin* (BCG) vaccine is the only licensed vaccine for tuberculosis and is protective primarily against severe childhood forms of the disease but is variably effective in adults. To ensure disease control, vaccination needs to be incorporated into a total prevention strategy. This involves not only vaccinating high-risk groups but also taking into account sociocultural and economic determinants of vaccine coverage. Mathematical modeling has played an important role in illuminating such complex dynamics to enable simulating different intervention strategies and optimization of vaccination to reduce overall disease burden. Such models demonstrate the potential value of increased vaccination coverage in at-risk populations to control tuberculosis transmission efficiently, underlining the relevance of targeted prevention policies. Combined with vaccination, complete prevention of tuberculosis involves early detection and treatment of latent infection, with a priority on the reduction of the reservoir of infective individuals. Public health interventions frequently involve screening programs, particularly in high-risk individuals, to identify latent tuberculosis infections (LTBIs) before they become active disease. This is a preventive intervention that reduces transmission potential and complements vaccination. Infection control in healthcare and congregate settings reduces airborne transmission, an important aspect of tuberculosis prevention. Such multi-component interventions reduce disease incidence, however, but there are issues with healthcare infrastructure and resource allocation. A balance between vaccine-induced immunity and other prevention interventions underlines the relevance of an integrated strategy. Mathematical modeling indicates that combined vaccination and early treatment, along with public health interventions, is better than single-intervention strategies, proposing holistic models of tuberculosis control. These developments in vaccination science recently offer a vision to improve respect for the effectiveness of preventive immunization, particularly through new vaccine designs and targeted delivery strategies. Although current vaccines are far from ideal, new clinical trials aim to increase immunogenicity and duration of protection. Success with maternal immunization against other respiratory pathogens, respiratory syncytial virus, has lessons to inform maternal or neonatal tuberculosis vaccine development to induce early-life immunity (Papazisis et al., 2024). The strategy is founded on passive antibody transfer methods, increasing protection at high-risk infancy ages when the immune system continues to mature. Evaluation of these new strategies must pass through rigorous safety and efficacy testing, necessary to gain public acceptance and policy adoption. Therefore, continued research and surveillance are needed to propel tuberculosis prevention strategies to keep pace with shifting epidemiological trends and vaccine technology to inch towards disease eradication goals (Papazisis et al., 2024).

14.1. Bacillus Calmette-Guérin (BCG) Vaccine: Efficacy and Limitations

The worldwide struggle against tuberculosis has, for decades, been dependent on vaccination as the bedrock of prevention efforts, with the BCG vaccine at its core. Though it is the sole licensed tuberculosis vaccine, the efficacy of the BCG vaccine is not consistent in various populations and age categories. The observed differences in efficacy are both reflective of the biological and epidemiological nuances surrounding tuberculosis infection and immunity (Van Goethem et al., 2019). Although BCG vaccination provides significant protection against severe manifestations of TB in children, its protective efficacy against pulmonary tuberculosis (PTB) in adults, the most prevalent and transmissible form, is significantly lower. This limitation has led to policy changes regarding vaccination globally, particularly in countries with a decreasing trend in TB cases, where cost-effectiveness is now a critical factor in vaccination policy (Machlaurin et al., 2019). As such, the dynamics highlight the need to establish better vaccine formulations or booster vaccines to boost the overall protective effect of tuberculosis. Different BCG strains of vaccine from various nations vary in their protective efficacy, making standardization of the vaccine programs all over the world a complex endeavor. A comparative assessment conducted in Kazakhstan using Japanese, Serbian, and Russian strains showed wide variations in protection against clinical and culture-confirmed cases of TB. Preferably, the Japanese BCG strain showed maximum efficacy at 69% against clinical tuberculosis and 92% against culture-confirmed tuberculosis. In comparison, the Russian preparation showed comparatively low protection. Nevertheless, all vaccines provided high protection against TB meningitis. The results underscore the value of careful choice of vaccine strain in national immunization programs to maximize the outcomes of prevention (Favorov et al., 2012). In addition, methodological limitations, including retrospective analysis and possible confounding risk factors, were identified by the study as requiring careful interpretation but not reducing the value of strain-specific effectiveness data in policy-making. Although BCG vaccine protection is established, its inherent weaknesses limit the attainment of global tuberculosis control. The vaccine's unreliability in adults and regional differences in immune responses based on environmental and genetic factors hinder its universal usage. In addition, the lack of sustained immunity requires revaccination planning, yet cost-effectiveness proof and enhanced protection through booster approaches remain inconclusive (Machlaurin et al., 2019). This uncertain terrain highlights the need for continued investigation of new tuberculosis vaccines that would potentially replace or complement BCG, especially in adult groups at greater risk of transmission. Improved vaccine candidates provide great potential for bolstering global prevention regimens but also need careful clinical testing to confirm enhanced efficacy and long-lasting immunity, ultimately aiming to curb the disease burden of tuberculosis globally.

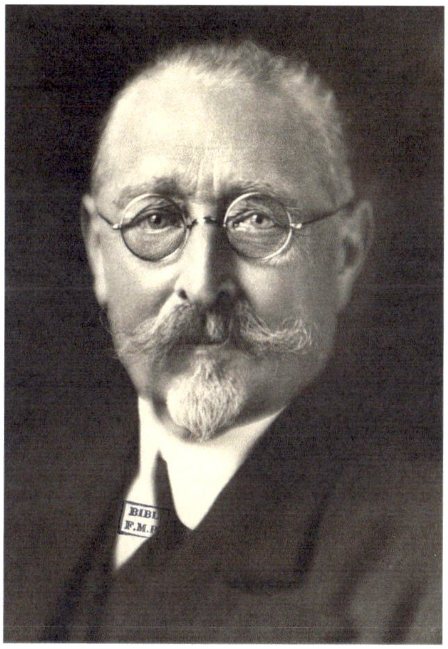

Source: By This document belongs to the collections of the Bibliothèque interuniversitaire de santé. It was uploaded to Commons through a partnership with Wikimedia France., Licence Ouverte, https://commons.wikimedia.org/w/index.php?curid=165680079

14.1.1. Overview of Bacillus Calmette-Guérin (BCG) Vaccine

The construction of efficacious vaccination methods for tuberculosis (TB) has been a cornerstone of public health interventions for decreasing disease burden for decades worldwide. Amongst these, the BCG vaccine is the only vaccine in use that has a broad distribution against TB and has been used for nearly a century. Despite protection heterogeneity between populations and geographic locations, data from recent meta-analyses highlight BCG's significant contribution in preventing severe tuberculosis forms, such as miliary and meningeal TB, among young children. These results advocate for infant BCG vaccination as essential in the early years of life, noting that immunization provides approximately 37% protection against all TB types in children under five and 42% protection against pulmonary TB in children under three (Hatherill et al., 2022). Although adult protection is still minimal, the vaccine's effectiveness on early childhood morbidity and mortality secures its cornerstone position in TB prevention measures. However, the persistence of BCG protection presents major threats to long-term control of TB. Protection is seen to be lost after childhood, with little to no effect in adolescents and adults after infant BCG immunization based on recent cohort studies (Hatherill et al., 2022) (Figure 14.1).

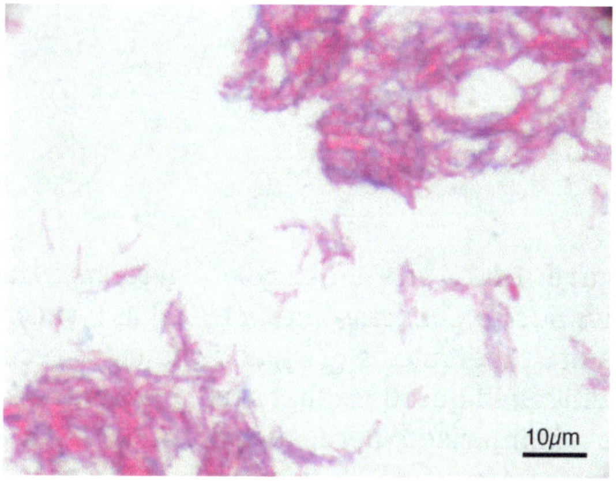

Figure 14.1. BCG vaccine.

Source: By Y tambe - Y tambe's file, CC BY-SA 3.0, https://commons.wikimedia.org/w/index.php?curid=1827666

A number of hypotheses explain this phenomenon, such as the possible attenuation of contemporary BCG strains compared to the older ones and the effects of host and environmental variables that may reduce the efficacy of the vaccine over time. Furthermore, the challenge in distinguishing MTB infection from BCG-induced immunity makes it challenging to comprehend the role played by the vaccine in protecting against infection versus active disease progression. These complexities imply that although the BCG vaccine is crucial, in isolation it might not be enough to prevent TB transmission or incidence across all age ranges, making boosted or different vaccination strategies necessary to maintain immunity in adolescents and adults. Interestingly, the BCG vaccine could provide advantages on top of direct tuberculosis protection.

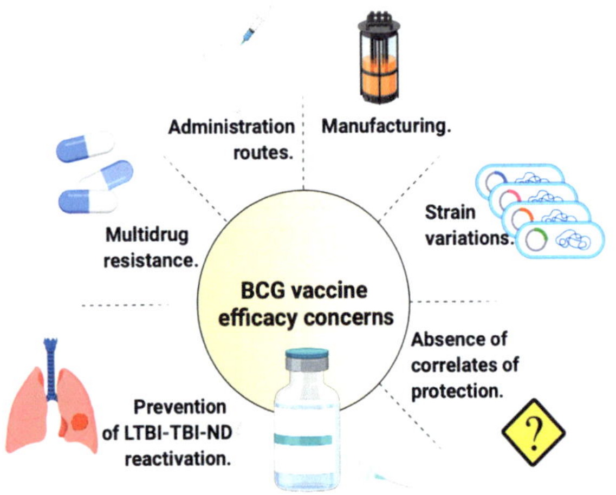

Figure 14.2. The efficacy of *Mycobacterium bovis Bacille Calmette-Guérin* (BCG) as a vaccine against tuberculosis (TB), and the most recent findings and questions that need to be addressed are summarized here, as potential areas of research for novel TB vaccine candidates.

Source: Flores-Valdez MA. After 100 Years of BCG Immunization against Tuberculosis, What Is New and Still Outstanding for This Vaccine? *Vaccines*. 2022; 10(1):57. https://doi.org/10.3390/vaccines10010057

Observational evidence points to a substantial decrease in all-cause mortality in vaccinated children for as long as 14 years, an effect above and beyond expectations in terms of TB prevention (Hatherill et al., 2022). One such explanation is through the concept of trained immunity, whereby BCG vaccination triggers nonspecific immunological improvements elicited by broad immunological changes that offer protection against other infections, including even viral infections. This immunomodulatory function mirrors lessons from other global vaccination campaigns, like the rapid advancement of COVID-19 vaccines, which have highlighted the need to understand innate and adaptive immune pathways to maximize vaccine performance and longevity. These findings about BCG's wider-ranging immunological role may stimulate integrated vaccination approaches, combining disease-specific and nonspecific protective mechanisms to better suppress childhood mortality and infectious disease burden globally (Figure 14.2).

14.1.2. Efficacy in Different Populations

Understanding the variable effectiveness of tuberculosis (TB) vaccines across populations is relevant in evaluating their net impact on world health. The widely administered BCG vaccine holds strong protective efficacy against infant disseminated TB but shows varied immune response across geographical and demographic populations. Gambian infant studies present the entire spectrum of interferon-gamma (IFN-γ) responses to BCG vaccination, pointing towards inter-individual variability that may be based on genetic, environmental, or nutritional factors. The heterogeneity implies that although BCG still forms the foundation in neonatal immunization schedules, its protective function might vary widely, making it challenging to employ universal vaccination tactics. Furthermore, immune markers like IL-5 and IL-13 cytokines present with heterogeneic patterns, confirming the challenge of interpreting immunogenicity among the population (Lalvani et al., 2008). Physiological and anatomic differences that occur naturally in target groups also play a role in the effectiveness of vaccines. The respiratory tract, where MTB infection commonly occurs, has minor variations between ages and environmental exposures and impacts immune responses accordingly. For instance, the infant and aging body's lung architecture and mucosal immunity might change vaccine protection levels. Nonhuman primate models, highly comparable to human pulmonary anatomy and immune system function, suggest that environmental determinants and concurrent respiratory disease can alter immune response to TB vaccines. These results show that host physiology and environmental exposures underlie observed heterogeneity in vaccine performance beyond the vaccine agent itself, particularly in high respiratory disease burden populations (Miller et al., 2017).

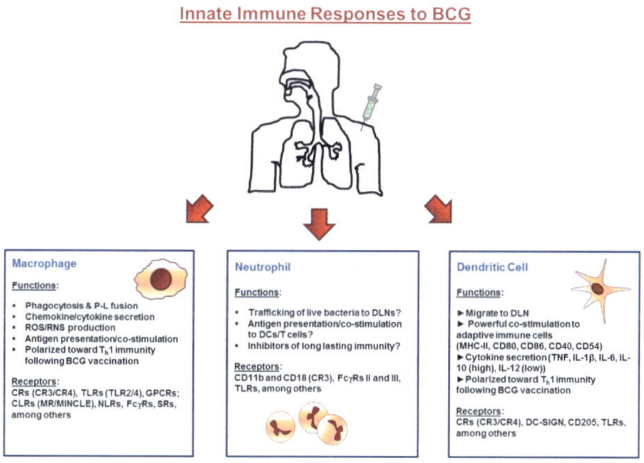

Figure 14.3. Innate immune cell responses to *Bacillus Calmette-Guérin* (BCG) vaccination.

Source: Moliva JI, Turner J and Torrelles JB (2017) Immune Responses to Bacillus Calmette–Guérin Vaccination: Why Do They Fail to Protect against Mycobacterium tuberculosis? Front. Immunol. 8:407. doi: 10.3389/fimmu.2017.00407

TB vaccine effectiveness must also account for interaction between local epidemiology and host immunity. Environmental organism-induced immune priming blunts or enhances vaccine-induced immunity in high TB prevalence or high environmental mycobacteria exposure settings. The complex host-pathogen interactions can diminish the efficacy of BCG or recombinant vaccines, necessitating regional studies to identify immune correlates of vaccine protection. These arguments favor region-specific prevention regimens that take into account immunological, environmental, and socio-economic factors to optimize vaccine efficacy in diverse populations. Thus, while BCG remains the cornerstone of TB prevention, ongoing investigation of population-dependent immunogenicity is essential to next-generation vaccine and immunization strategy design (Lalvani et al., 2008) (Figure 14.3).

14.1.3. Limitations and Challenges

Despite major progress with tuberculosis vaccination and prevention methodologies, a number of shortcomings prevent their widespread application. One major impediment is the geographical and logistical constraints that limit access to healthcare, most notably among isolated populations. Research undertaken in regions like the Philippines illustrates a clear relationship between greater distance from healthcare centers and increased rates of tuberculosis infection among children and highlights how isolation magnifies late diagnosis and treatment. These geographic inequalities compromise the potential for timely vaccination and ongoing preventive treatment, facilitating continued transmission in hard-to-reach groups. Thus, improving healthcare outreach and facilities is essential to overcoming disparities in access and better controlling pediatric and adult tuberculosis (Leining, 2019). This spatial factor highlights the ongoing challenge of putting uniform prevention measures into action globally. Further, tuberculosis program work is made complex by the changing nature of epidemiological approaches and the incorporation of new science. Changes from old models of chronic disease work to infectious disease epidemiology have brought new challenges in collecting data, analyzing data, and applying data. New technologies related to molecular and digital surveillance, the latest developments, promise much but require immense adjustment in public health programs. Complex data set assimilation into predictive models demands interdisciplinary skill and sound infrastructure that is frequently wanting in resource-constrained environments of maximal tuberculosis burden. Beyond this, synthesizing varied causal inference paradigms to infectious disease assessment, e.g., understanding microbial etiology amidst complex clinical syndromes, is still an intimidating methodological challenge. These novel needs point to the need for ongoing training and investment aimed at sharpening epidemiological tools that are relevant to vaccine efficacy and prevention mechanisms for tuberculosis (Lewnard et al., 2019).

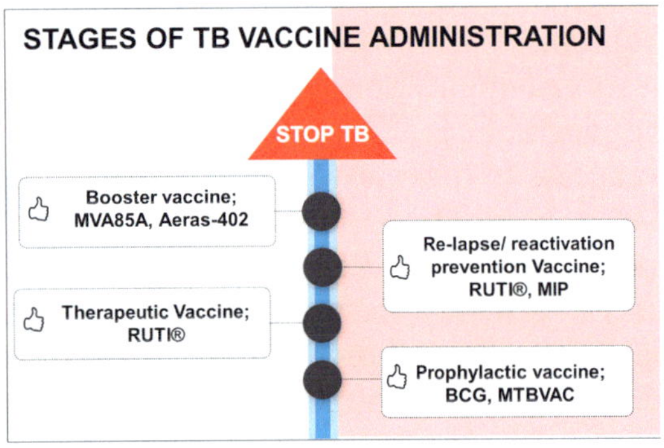

Figure 14.4. Stages of TB vaccine administration: TB exhibits variability in disease manifestations; thus, vaccine candidates should be developed to target specific forms of the disease rather than relying solely on a general vaccine (e.g., BCG).

Source: Mangla, M., Singla, R., & Kumar, A. (2023). BCG vaccine: Tuberculosis prevention versus therapeutic potential and limitations. *Vaccines, 11*(5), 1013.

Another key limitation regarding tuberculous prevention is based on the biological and immunological limitations of current vaccines, especially the BCG vaccine. Although BCG protects against severe forms of pediatric TB, its protection is highly variable in different populations and does not consistently prevent adult pulmonary TB, the source of most transmission. This incomplete and variable immunity makes control of disease transmission more difficult, requiring additional preventive interventions like screening and chemoprophylaxis, which have their own challenges with logistics and adherence. In addition, socio-economic conditions, such as poverty, malnourishment, and high population density, aggravate the challenge in tuberculosis control, while reducing the effectiveness of vaccination by itself. Therefore, strategies with multiple dimensions involving the development of vaccines, health accessibility, epidemiological innovation, and social intervention must be employed to address the complicated nature of tuberculosis prevention holistically (Figure 14.4).

14.2. Alternative Vaccine Research

TB control progress ever more recognizes the shortfalls of the BCG vaccine, calling forth substantial research into novel vaccination strategies. The most important challenge is to differentiate vaccinated from infected subjects, particularly in livestock populations, where cattle tuberculosis poses a dual threat to agriculture economies and public health. Immunological methods like intracellular IFN-γ expression in $CD4^+$ T cells provide encouraging diagnostic refinement for studying this. By correctly distinguishing infected cattle from BCG vaccinates, the strategy not only improves disease surveillance but also enables the viability of introducing vaccination into existing control systems that incorporate testing and culling (Sopp et al., 2006). The strategies are indicative of the use of complementary diagnostic systems and alternative vaccines to ensure accurate disease management and avoid the accidental spread of disease. The mucosal route of vaccine administration presents itself as a new frontier with promise for TB prevention in consideration of the respiratory mode of MTB transmission. In contrast to conventional systemic vaccines, mucosal immunization addresses the site of pathogen entry primarily and may elicit optimal localized immunity. Recent reviews summarize evidence favoring aerosolized or mucosal vaccine candidates that engage native mucosal immune mechanisms, which could promote more effective prevention of primary infection and progression to disease (Kaufmann, 2023)). Yet, notwithstanding its theoretic appeal, mucosal vaccine development will face technical hurdles regarding delivery systems as well as a fuller understanding of mucosal immune responses to TB.

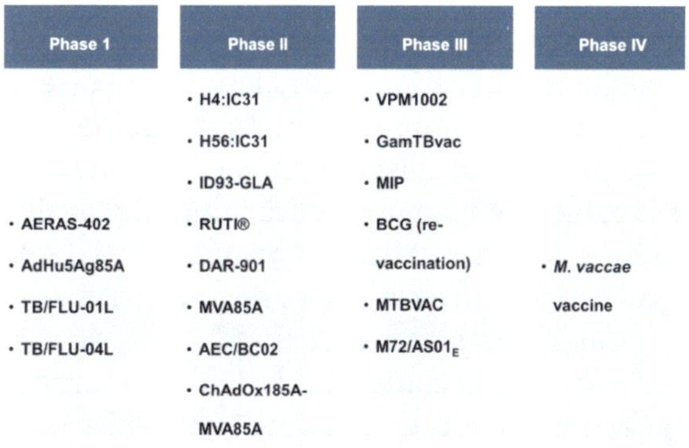

Figure 14.5. Clinical trial status of vaccine candidates against tuberculosis.

Source: Srivastava S, Dey S, Mukhopadhyay S. Vaccines against Tuberculosis: Where Are We Now? *Vaccines*. 2023; 11(5):1013. https://doi.org/10.3390/vaccines11051013

These considerations highlight a pressing need for continued research to improve both the immunogenicity and practical administration of such vaccines. Emerging research underscores a multifaceted approach to alternative vaccine development, where immunological precision, delivery innovation, and operational feasibility converge. Combining new diagnostic assays with mucosal vaccine candidates may transform TB prevention strategies by facilitating early and correct infection detection as well as more protection at the site of infection. Beyond BCG means overcoming biological efficacy, safety, and implementation issues in a variety of epidemiological contexts. As preclinical and clinical advancement of alternative vaccines continues, collaborations between scientists, policymakers, and public health professionals will be essential to bring these innovations to fruition in the form of successful, scalable TB control interventions. They represent collectively a decisive step toward TB eradication through more sensitive, targeted, and responsive vaccination techniques (Sopp et al., 2006; WR et al., 2019) (Figure 14.5).

14.2.1. Current Research Initiatives

Breakthroughs in TB research have picked up pace over the past few years, with major emphasis laid on strengthening detection, treatment, and prevention measures to counter this longstanding global health menace. New diagnostic tests based on molecular and genomic methods have transformed the diagnosis of TB and drug-resistant TB. These advances make diagnosis quicker and more precise, allowing early therapeutic interventions that are invaluable in controlling TB spread. Furthermore, recent studies highlight the synergy of artificial intelligence (AI) and whole-genome sequencing (WGS) to enhance knowledge on pathogen evolution and better customize treatment regimens. These advances in technology not only support clinical performance but also enhance public health interventions, reflecting a unification of biotechnological advances and epidemiologic monitoring. Such holistic strategies underlie current efforts to stem TB incidence and deaths, highlighting the imperative of integrating sophisticated diagnostics with effective prevention and vaccination measures. Concurrent with diagnostic innovation, significant research focuses on the creation of more potent TB vaccines and preventive tools.

Limitations of the BCG vaccine, primarily its inconsistent efficacy in adults, have driven the search for new vaccine candidates with greater and longer-term immunity. Recent efforts investigate new antigen forms and delivery routes with the goal of inducing strong immunity in a wide range of populations. In addition, research is evaluating the potential role of booster vaccination and combination vaccine regimens for maximizing protection, especially in vulnerable populations. Prevention also includes behavioral and socioeconomic determinants of TB transmission and vaccination program take-up. Through the tackling of both biological as well as contextual determinants of infection, these research activities aim to create holistic prevention systems that can be tailored to fit regional epidemiology and public health demands (Chanpitakkul, 2024).

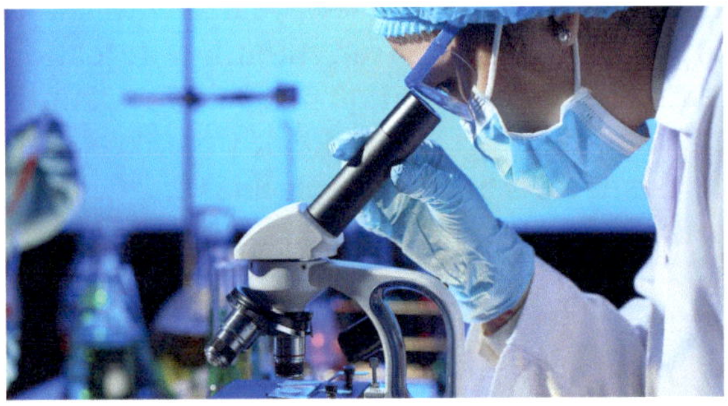

Source: TheHealthSite. (2023). *Tuberculosis awareness visual.* https://sc0.blr1.cdn.digitaloceanspaces.com/article/190961-nglcfwaywz-1686054556.jpg.

Apart from biomedical research, concerted public health efforts have been instrumental in pushing TB control forward on the international scene. Multinational study and programmatic implementation through collaborative platforms ensure the exchange of knowledge and harmonized approaches to TB elimination. The government-driven campaigns like the Pradhan Mantri TB Mukt Bharat Abhiyaan illustrate how political will coupled with scientific advancements can transform research advances into policy-effective community interventions. In addition, these efforts emphasize the necessity of a one health strategy taking into account zoonotic spread and environmental influences on TB dynamics. The interaction between leading scientific research, policy formulation, and integrated prevention strategies upholds global initiative measures in subduing TB's impact toward ultimately achieving the objective of eradication (Chanpitakkul, 2024).

14.2.2. Promising Candidates in Development

Progress in the development of a tuberculosis vaccine has picked up pace as a result of the continued worldwide burden of the disease and shortcomings of the BCG vaccine, which despite its common utilization, has failed to stop disease transmission or impede resistant strains. New strategies aim at developing vaccines that will be capable of giving protective immunity against all clinical manifestations of tuberculosis, such as pulmonary disease due to drug-sensitive and drug-resistant strains. A number of vaccine candidates are in clinical trials, with encouraging suggestions that they can boost immunity more than what BCG can do. The new vaccines not only aim to prevent infection but also to inhibit reactivation and transmission of disease, thus filling key gaps in existing prevention measures. Construction of such vaccines is critical in the face of growing antimicrobial resistance (AMR) because they may be capable of breaking the resistance emergence and disease transmission cycle (Martin et al., 2020). The public health burden of tuberculosis is multiplied by the emergence of multi-drug resistant (MDR) strains and by the synergistic effect of co-infection like HIV, which increase susceptibility and complicate the outcome of treatment. To address such obstacles, vaccine development focuses on candidates with the potential to induce strong and long-lasting immune responses that can overcome the immunosuppressive mechanisms linked to coinfections. Innovative vaccine platforms involve subunit vaccines, viral vectored vaccines, and enhanced live attenuated strains aimed at enhancing or substituting BCG. These approaches demonstrate greater insight into tuberculosis immunopathology and utilize new antigen targets and delivery systems. Resolution of such biological complexities is pivotal to furthering vaccine effectiveness and achieving greater protection in multicultural populations impacted by tuberculosis (Thaiss et al., 2012).

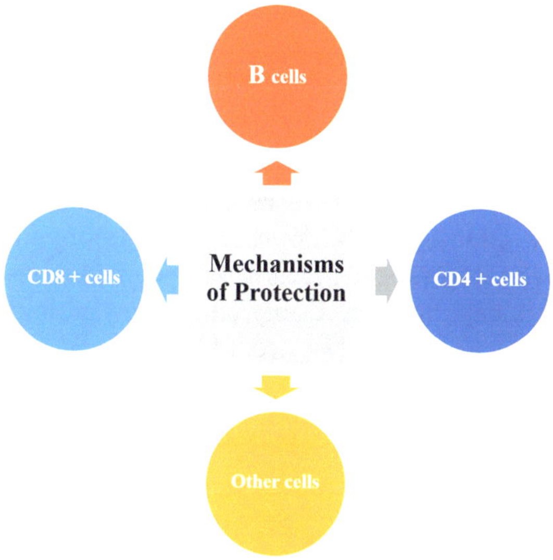

Figure 14.6. Putative mechanisms of vaccine-induced protective immunity against TB. An ideal TB vaccine will possibly require to engage multiple mechanisms and should aim to elicit a balanced immune response involving $CD4^+$ T cells, $CD8^+$ T cells, B cells and other immune cells such as NK cells and unconventional T cells.

Source: Zhou F and Zhang D (2023) Recent advance in the development of tuberculosis vaccines in clinical trials and virus-like particle-based vaccine candidates. Front. Immunol. 14:1238649. doi: 10.3389/fimmu.2023.1238649

Public-private partnerships have fueled advances in the development of vaccine candidates with potential to revolutionize tuberculosis control strategies across the world. Such candidates focus not only on preventing primary infection but also on the potential to confer immunotherapeutic benefits in already infected individuals to slow down disease progression. CANDIDATES of promise in the pipeline are vaccines with early-phase clinical trial efficacy, which could lower infection rates and disease severity significantly if implemented successfully. Introduction of these vaccines into integrated tuberculosis prevention programs, with enhanced diagnostics and treatment regimens, offers hope for seeing substantial decreases in global morbidity and death. Sustained investment in vaccine research continues to be crucial to dealing with the enduring challenges of tuberculosis and its multidrug-resistant forms (Thaiss et al., 2012; Martin et al., 2020) (Figure 14.6).

14.2.3. Future Directions in Vaccine Research

The constant development of infectious diseases calls for ongoing development of vaccine research to further improve prevention measures, especially with TB. Present challenges such as drug-resistant organisms and inconsistent vaccine efficacy unveil the weakness of current immunization procedures. Future strategies must prioritize the introduction of new vaccine candidates using innovative techniques like mRNA platforms, which have been proven effective in recent viral epidemics. These novel strategies hold the promise of increased flexibility, making it possible to make quick decisions based on the evolving TB variants. Further, making the immune response more specific and long-lasting is essential, requiring thorough insights into the host-pathogen interactions at both molecular and cellular levels. Coupled with strong epidemiological insights, this would propel targeted vaccination strategies for high-risk groups. With changing global health priorities, integrating vaccine development with overall public health paradigms is the need of the hour to combat TBs impact more effectively (Alize et al., 2024). Concurrently, the future of TB vaccine research relies on harnessing big data and advanced modeling methods to frame design and deployment strategies. The Global Burden of Diseases dataset illustrates complex patterns of disease that need to be addressed when creating and deploying vaccines, particularly in heterogeneously demographic and geographic contexts (Alize et al., 2024). Through including dense datasets that reflect age, sex, and socioeconomic status, researchers can identify vaccine candidates best suited to treat the hardest-hit regions and subpopulations. Predictive modeling also allows vaccine distribution logistics to be maximized for equitable access and coverage. This data-intensive strategy is critical to bridging disparities that continue in TB morbidity and mortality levels, especially in low-resource environments. As such, interdisciplinary collaborations that integrate immunology, epidemiology, and computational sciences are central to defining next-generation vaccines and intervention strategies. Ultimately, vaccine science for tuberculosis in the future must also address socio-political and economic factors driving vaccine acceptance and utilization. Despite advances in science, obstacles like misinformation, logistical limitations, and shortages of healthcare infrastructure hamper effective vaccination drives. The research approach thus has to combine behavioral and social sciences to comprehend and counteract vaccine resistance, particularly among high-burden groups. Moreover, long-term investment in public health infrastructure and community interactions is critical to turn scientific breakthroughs into effective health gains. Having adaptive regulatory frameworks in place for the evolving vaccine technologies will also enable timely approval and deployment. Incorporating a systematic approach that balances technological innovation with considerations of society and policies, future TB vaccine development is capable of not only enhancing biological efficacy but also optimizing global health impact (Alize et al., 2024) (Figure 14.7).

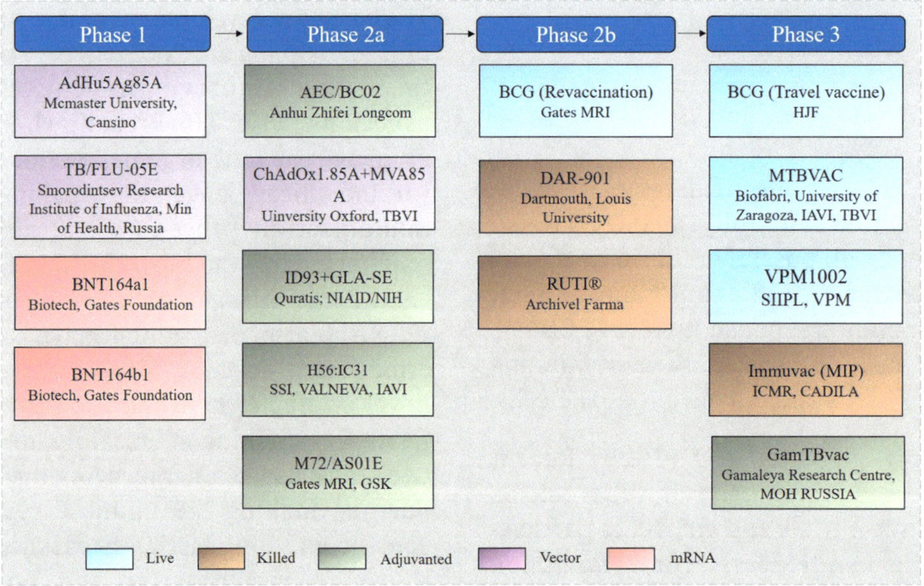

Figure 14.7. TB vaccine candidates in the clinical pipeline.

Source: Zhou F and Zhang D (2023) Recent advance in the development of tuberculosis vaccines in clinical trials and virus-like particle-based vaccine candidates. Front. Immunol. 14:1238649. doi: 10.3389/fimmu.2023.1238649

14.3. Public Health Strategies for Tuberculosis (TB) Prevention

Successful public health measures for preventing tuberculosis depend significantly on strong immunization programs backed by full-scale public health infrastructure. As far as tuberculosis is concerned, vaccination with the BCG vaccine continues to be a mainstay preventive measure, especially in high-risk groups.

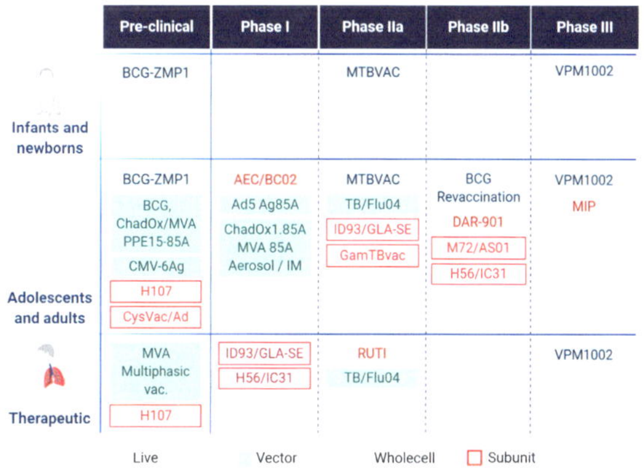

Figure 14.8. Embedding TB IPC within broader health system initiatives that link with components of a high-quality health system.

Source: Bellini C, Horváti K. Recent Advances in the Development of Protein- and Peptide-Based Subunit Vaccines against Tuberculosis. *Cells.* 2020; 9(12):2673. https://doi.org/10.3390/cells9122673

Prevention, however, goes beyond vaccination and entails education, advocacy, and collaboration between healthcare professionals and communities to provide extensive vaccine coverage. Public health agencies are crucial to this system in raising awareness and making vaccination services accessible. The Bureau of Immunization and Tuberculosis's Immunization Program is such an example, providing a model that harmonizes the delivery of vaccination with disease surveillance, reporting, and outbreak control. This systemic process is crucial to achieving long-term tuberculosis incidence reduction and enhanced overall community health outcomes (Alize et al., 2024) (Figure 14.8).

Sustained tuberculosis prevention also hinges on the filling of gaps in vaccination coverage and timely detection of cases, particularly among under-served and vulnerable populations. Intervening in under-vaccinated populations through targeted outreach programs strengthens vaccination equity and arrests tuberculosis transmission. Moreover, the timely reporting and proper investigation of suspected cases of tuberculosis allow for rapid intervention to avert outbreaks. The Iowa Department of Public Health Division of Acute Disease Prevention and Emergency Response is a prime example of the combination of education, technical assistance, and coordination of emergency response to aid local health agencies. Via collaborative partnerships and systems like the Immunization Registry Information System, the division enhances public health capacity in real-time, guaranteeing prompt response measures to be taken effectively (Alize et al., 2024). Another critical ingredient in preventing tuberculosis is ongoing public health preparedness combined with evidence-based decision making. Leverage use of information technology platforms to monitor vaccination status, observe disease trends, and assess program effectiveness enables health authorities to locate risk hotspots and modify strategies accordingly. Additionally, community mobilization and advocacy are key determinants in maintaining high vaccination levels by overcoming vaccine hesitancy and generating confidence in populations. Education and healthcare provider training programs ensure that correct information filters down to the population, promoting informed consent and adherence. The synergy of these strategic interventions, supported by institutional backing from public health bureaus, provides a solid basis for minimizing tuberculosis burden through effective prevention strategies (Alize et al., 2024) (Figure 14.9).

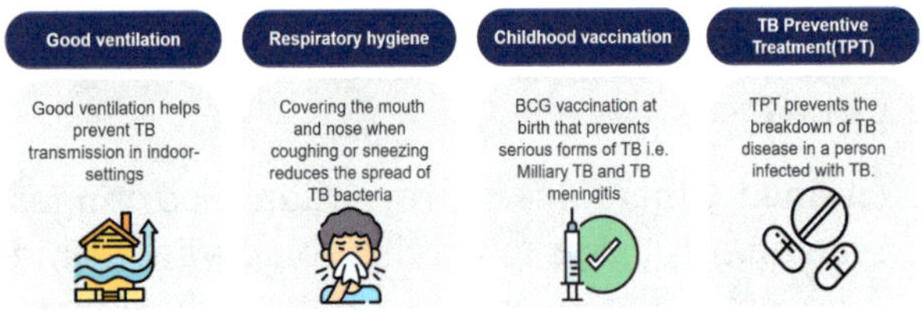

Figure 14.9. Measures for control and prevention of tuberculosis.

Source: National Tuberculosis Elimination Program (NTEP). (n.d.). *Prevention of TB.* https://ntep.in/node/552/CP-prevention-tb.

14.3.1. Screening and Early Detection

Successful disease control not only depends on prevention via vaccination but also on early detection of infection to curb transmission and enhance patient outcomes. For TB, screening and early detection are essential approaches to reinforce vaccination efforts. Early diagnosis enables early treatment initiation, slows disease advancement, and reduces contagiousness, thus disrupting chains of infection in communities. Especially among immune-compromised individuals, such as children and patients on immunosuppressive therapy, the task of effective screening is aggravated with atypical immune reactions. New diagnostic tests like interferon-gamma release assays (IGRAs) have become available that are more specific than conventional tuberculin skin tests (TSTs) by identifying immune sensitization to MTB antigens that the BCG vaccines and environmental mycobacteria lack. These advancements optimize the accuracy of latent tuberculosis infection (LTBI) detection, which is crucial for early intervention in high-risk populations (Figure 14.10).

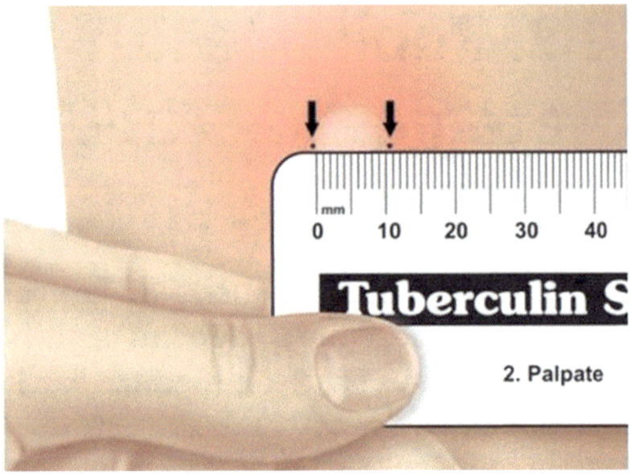

Figure 14.10. A trained healthcare provider reads a TB skin test between 48 and 72 hours after placement.

Source: Centers for Disease Control and Prevention (CDC). (n.d.). *Reading the TB skin test.* https://www.cdc.gov/tb/media/images/Reading_the_TB_skin_test_1200x675.jpg.

Despite technical advances, the efficacy and utility of different screening assays are still in question. Research has shown mixed sensitivity and specificity between tests; for example, TS-TB test based on ELISPOT is more sensitive compared to ELISA-based QuantiFERON TB Gold assays and TST but also produces a significant percentage of indeterminate results. The interpretation of this result is confounded by the lack of a perfect gold standard test for latent TB and potential cross-reactivity with nontuberculous mycobacteria (NTM) that are endemic to some regions. Moreover, immune suppression, such as that experienced by patients on tumor necrosis factor-alpha (TNF-α) blockers or patients with rheumatologic diseases, may decrease the accuracy of these tests. As such, clinical decisions typically necessitate a careful comparison of test outcomes with patient history and epidemiological background, highlighting an important gap in standardized screening procedures (Mata-Espinosa et al., 2023). Incorporation of screening and early detection into overall TB control interventions necessitates a system-level response aware of demographic and environmental determinants of disease patterns. Epidemiological data reveal that early detection efforts must adapt to local population dynamics, such as age distributions and prevalent risk factors like immunosuppression or malnutrition. Furthermore, as with other infectious diseases whose burden escalates in resource-limited settings, cancer screening exemplifies how structured surveillance programs can uncover rising incidence trends and direct preventive measures effectively (Mata-Espinosa et al., 2023). Analogously, TB prevention programs benefit from coordinated screening campaigns, especially in vulnerable groups. Improved laboratory facilities, combined with health education and follow-up treatment, is essential to make early detection ring true in terms of decreased morbidity and mortality. Therefore, an interplay between vaccination, screening, and prompt treatment is the pillar of comprehensive TB control.

14.3.2. Treatment of Latent Tuberculosis Infection (LTBI)

Efficient control of TB depends not only on the cure of active disease but also on treating LTBI, where individuals carry MTB without showing signs of symptoms. LTBI is a large pool of latent future active cases and is therefore an important target for management in TB prevention. Current management of LTBI usually consists of long-term antibiotic treatment to avoid reactivation, although problems of patient adherence and drug toxicity remain. Recent developments investigate adjunct treatments, with gene therapy using recombinant adenoviruses expressing immune-modulating cytokines such as IFN-γ and IL-12 being under investigation. These methods can help increase host immunity and decrease the risk of reactivation by more actively targeting occult mycobacterial populations. These innovations provide encouraging directions not only for treating LTBI but also for enabling general TB control programs by controlling transmission from latent infection to active disease (Mata-Espinosa et al., 2023). The COVID-19 pandemic has made it even harder to manage LTBI, as disrupted healthcare services resulted in reduced screening and initiation of treatment. Research shows latent TB detection and treatment to be substantially reduced during the pandemic, further increasing risks of subsequent TB outbreaks. Approaches to counteract these effects focus on sustaining critical health services and conducting catch-up screening operations for LTBI to cover gaps as a result of service disruptions. In addition, utilizing integrated diagnostic platforms testing for TB and COVID-19 concurrently has been suggested for enhancing case-finding efficiency. Digital health technologies also provide potential avenues for monitoring adherence to treatment and supporting contact tracing, thus enabling sustained prevention efforts in the face of adversity brought about by the pandemic (Jeong & Min, 2023). Such adaptive interventions are instrumental in maintaining achievements toward controlling latent TB. New vaccine strategies are increasingly seen as critical additions to LTBI treatment in prevention. Beyond the standard BCG vaccine, newer vaccines presenting mycobacterial antigens from viral vectors or nanoparticles are being tested for their ability to produce enhanced and more long-lived immunity. These vaccines would have multiple functions, preventing new infection as well as reducing the reactivation of latent infection. In addition, adjunctive immunotherapies that support the immune system's capacity to downregulate latent bacilli hold tremendous promise. Gene therapy models involving cytokine-coding adenoviruses are representative of this innovative strategy, holding very promising adjunctive therapies for boosting protective host immunity. Incorporating these novel therapeutics into traditional antibiotic regimens could end up transforming LTBI treatment and making a significant contribution to worldwide TB eradication (Mata-Espinosa et al., 2023).

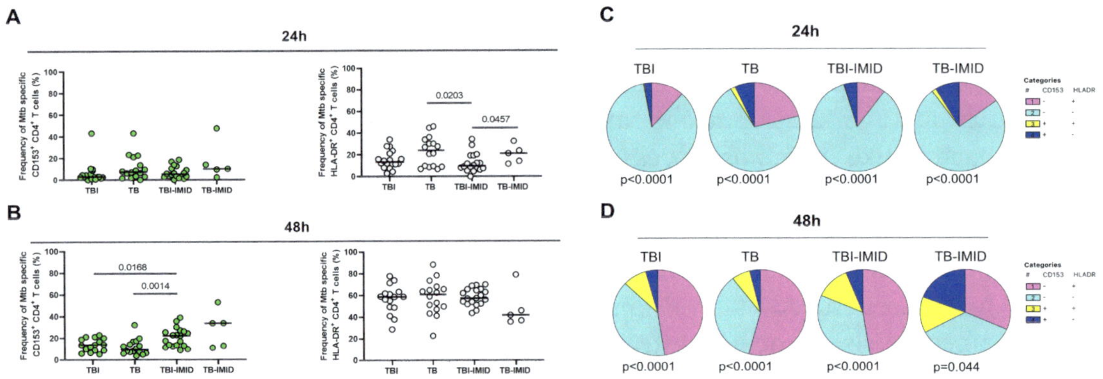

Source: Farroni C, Altera AMG, Salmi A, Vanini V, Cuzzi G, Lindestam Arlehamn CS, Sette A, Delogu G, Palucci I, Sbarra S, Aiello A, Picchianti-Diamanti A, Gualano G, Palmieri F, Goletti D and Petruccioli E (2025) Specific immune response to M. tuberculosis and ability to in vitro control mycobacterial replication are not impaired in subjects with immune-mediated inflammatory disease and tuberculosis infection. Front. Immunol. 15:1484143. doi: 10.3389/fimmu.2024.1484143

14.3.3. Community Education and Awareness

Effective vaccination and prevention work goes beyond clinical care and is highly dependent on community education and sensitization initiatives. Public education on the hazards of tuberculosis, the advantages of vaccines, and the need to complete a treatment course promotes evidence-based decision-making. Community education interventions can remove misconceptions and vaccine refusal, both critical impediments to achieving high levels of immunization coverage. Adaptation of educational content to the cultural and linguistic environments of diverse groups heightens understanding and acceptance. In addition, community outreach programs facilitate a partnership process, enabling participants to become champions for tuberculosis prevention in their social networks. This participatory process is essential, as evidenced in other infectious disease initiatives, where health fairs and targeted efforts were effective in raising awareness and improving vaccine uptake (Hulstine et al., 2017). Educational efforts are therefore a core component that supports medical measures to provide long-term community-level protection against tuberculosis. Implementation of community-oriented education campaigns has to traverse multifaceted socio-political contexts and diverse health infrastructures. Implications from policy advocacy campaigns for infectious disease control highlight the imperative for continuous and integrative modes of communication to guide public conduct and legislative backing. For instance, focused interventions have involved the creation of detailed educational packages for caregivers and community outreach to local events, both revealing higher public participation and acceptability (Hulstine et al., 2017). These strategies underscore how policy advocacy and grassroots awareness combined are essential to facilitating vaccination acceptance. Further, incorporating educational interventions within surveillance and infection control policies helps to develop an all-encompassing prevention model. Evidence indicates that policy interventions need to be responsive to local socioeconomic conditions to achieve optimal reach and impact, and the complex balance between national guidelines and local needs. The One Health strategy emphasizes the need to integrate community education into a more holistic framework that is responsive to the interconnectedness of human, animal, and environmental health in addressing tuberculosis. This view supports sector-sensitive policies and awareness initiatives that foster concerted action while avoiding sector-specific challenges. Public awareness of tuberculosis must therefore go beyond health at the individual level to include environmental determinants and good practices limiting disease spread between populations. By promoting community awareness of these connections, education programs can empower people to engage constructively in prevention measures such as vaccination and hygiene habits. Finally, consistent community consciousness campaigns in parallel with integrated policy systems are necessary to attain successful tuberculosis control and prevention globally.

14.4. Role of Governments in Tuberculosis (TB) Control

Successful TB control relies not just on advances in medicine but also on the critical role of government institutions, which must coordinate large-scale vaccination and prevention efforts across the country. Governments must create strong public health infrastructures that make widespread access to BCG vaccine and repeated screening programs readily available to especially high-risk populations. These programs involve elaborate planning and mobilization of resources such as finance, training of health personnel, and vaccine stockpiling. Governments also establish surveillance systems required to track tuberculosis cases and drug resistance outbreaks to enable intervention promptly. Through collaboration among different actors such as international bodies and local communities, governments ensure that tuberculosis control interventions are context-dependent and sustainable (Nell & van Vugt, 2011). Thus, political commitment is a critical factor in converting scientific evidence into effective, population-level prevention interventions that eventually curtail tuberculosis prevalence. Besides coordinating vaccination efforts, governments have an important contribution to make to public education and awareness, which are essential components of tuberculosis prevention measures. The stigma usually linked with the disease can hinder early detection and treatment compliance. To do this, policymakers can adopt countrywide health education initiatives that educate the public on tuberculosis transmission, signs of the disease, and the need for early medical treatment. Such programs enable earlier detection of cases and lower transmission rates by inspiring individuals to access care early. Government programs also enhance intersectoral collaboration in health sectors, combining tuberculosis control with more comprehensive healthcare services addressing social determinants of vulnerability to the disease. Health equity ensured by outreach to marginalized groups highlights the active responsibility governments have to control tuberculosis successfully (Adjei et al., 2006). Governments use prevention measures other than vaccination by creating an educated, compliant population, significantly helping to control tuberculosis. Governments affect tuberculosis control also through policy-making and global coordination, developing an overarching framework for continued prevention. Regulatory and legal actions can streamline protocols for treatment compliance, vaccination, and infection control within healthcare settings and communities. Policies allow for integration of emerging diagnostic technologies and therapeutic interventions as scientific breakthroughs occur. Governments are also crucial for mobilizing funding and technical support from international programs aimed at the elimination of tuberculosis. Cross-border cooperation in tackling tuberculosis transmission occurs in areas impacted by migration and socio-economic inequalities. By placing tuberculosis at the top of national health agendas, governments show political will that encourages ongoing investment in research, training, and health system strengthening.

In this concerted action, the critical role of governments is emphasized not only for the delivery of vaccination campaigns but also for the maintenance of integrated prevention strategies to fight tuberculosis (Adjei et al., 2006; Nell and van Vugt, 2025) (Figure 14.11).

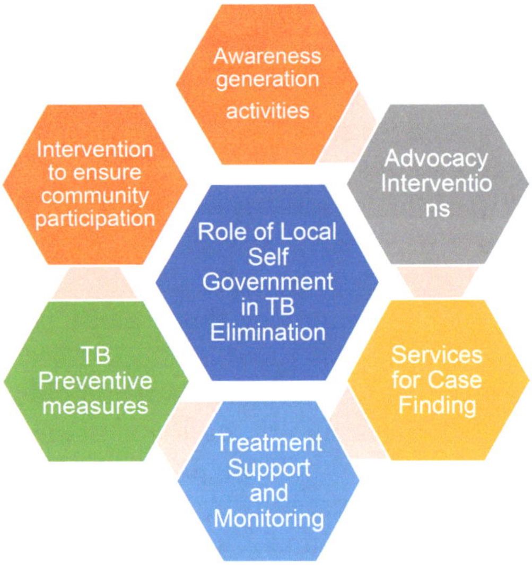

Figure 14.11. Role of local self-government in TB elimination.

Source: National Tuberculosis Elimination Program (NTEP). (n.d.). *Role of Local Self-Governments (LSG) in TB elimination.* https://www.ntep.in/gu/node/1594/CP-role-lsg-tb-elimination.

14.4.1. Policy Development and Implementation

Successful public health interventions depend on building strong policies that tackle both medical and socio-economic determinants of illness. In such areas as Eastern Sudan, where tuberculosis is still endemic because of issues like limited access to healthcare, population displacement, and poor infrastructure, policy frameworks are critical. These frameworks need to incorporate disease surveillance, diagnostic strength, and treatment approaches appropriate to the local environment. An overall policy in this direction not only streamlines TB control efforts but also optimizes the mobilization of resources to specifically address multi-drug resistant strains. In being aligned with international health agendas, such policies have synergistic benefits in enhancing case-finding and patient retention, both of which are very important in curbing transmission of TB. The success that has been witnessed in Sudan highlights the significance of policy formulation at the grassroots level that considers epidemiological information, public participation, and building capacity (Elshayeb et al., 2020). It is essential to apply this method in reshaping health landscapes where traditional measures have not shown notable effects. Apart from policy development, the process of implementation brings complex challenges that require multidisciplinary cooperation and ongoing assessment. Effective roll-outs of vaccination and prevention interventions are contingent upon coordinating healthcare infrastructure, education programs, and socio-cultural approval. The control of zoonotic diseases, for instance, provides useful lessons on how to tackle such complexities. Disease prevalence and public health responses are influenced by variability in ecological, economic, and social determinants worldwide. Policies need to be responsive with consideration of vector ecology data, community behavior patterns, and availability of resources. Preventive interventions for illnesses such as tuberculosis are enhanced by this integrative perspective through pre-empting obstacles in the form of vaccine resistance, geographical remoteness, and logistical limitations. Furthermore, including monitoring frameworks assures that policy guidelines remain evidence-informed and adaptive to emergent threats or service gaps (Torrence, 2007). This adaptive process of implementation promotes the sustainability of tuberculosis prevention programs, particularly in low-resource environments. The interaction between policy creation and deployment is central to the elimination of tuberculosis, requiring cyclical feedback systems refining both strategy and practice. Success is contingent upon reconciling national health priorities with international frameworks and driving innovation in diagnosis and treatment delivery. Effective policy also requires systematic assessment to quantify short- and long-term impact, such as enhanced case detection rates and diminished disease burden. Sudan's experience, underpinned by implementation research agendas, underscores the way high-level political commitment in conjunction with community-level participation brings about significant change (Elshayeb et al., 2020). These policies have to be framed with flexibility in mind to respond to varied epidemiological settings as well as challenges posed by concomitant zoonotic diseases and socio-economic inequalities (Torrence, 2007). Finally, sustained political will, proper funding, and intersectoral collaboration are required to guarantee that vaccination and prevention strategies transcend theoretical models into actual public health triumphs (Figure 14.12).

Vaccine type	Vaccine Candidates	Mycobacterial strains	Modification	Clinical stages
Live	VPM1002	*Mycobacterium bovis BCG-Prague*	addition of a listeriolysin gene, deletion of a urease gene	Phase 3
	MTBVAC	*M. tuberculosis*	Deletions of virulence genes phoP and fadD26	Phase 3
	BCG (Travel vaccine)	*BCG (Tokyo 172)*	-	Phase 3
	BCG (Revaccination)	*AJVaccines' BCG (Danish 1331)*	-	Phase 2b
Inactivated	M.*vaccae*	*Mycobacterium vaccae*	Heat-killed	Phase 3 (completed, data not published)
	RUTI	*Mycobacterium indicus pranii*	Heat-killed	Phase 2b
	MIP	*Mycobacterium obuense*	Heat-killed	Phase 3
	DAR-901	*Mycobacterium kyogaense* sp. *nov.*	Heat-killed	Phase 2b

Figure 14.12. Strategic actions for accelerating progress to achieve the End TB goals.

Source: Zhou F and Zhang D (2023) Recent advance in the development of tuberculosis vaccines in clinical trials and virus-like particle-based vaccine candidates. Front. Immunol. 14:1238649. doi: 10.3389/fimmu.2023.1238649

14.4.2. Funding and Resource Allocation

Financial resource allocation in international health interventions has been found to significantly determine the success of immunization programs, particularly for conditions such as TB. Despite the advancement achieved, funding disparity still threatens the consistent application of TB prevention measures. Investment is not only required to fund vaccine development but also to enhance healthcare infrastructure to enable mass immunization coverage. The inequity in mortality rates, as reflected through differential performance across the regions, highlights the importance of targeted resource allocation that is responsive to local epidemiological and socio-economic conditions. In the absence of strategic investment into both vaccine availability and integrated healthcare services, TB control efforts are likely to plateau. Assessing worldwide disease burden statistics emphasizes the role of resource allocation in life expectancy and mortality decrease, promoting an equally balanced strategy of prioritizing both innovation and scale in vaccination (Naghavi et al., 2024). This tiered funding can fill gaps in TB prevention and improve overall population health outcomes.

Allocation of policy-influenced resources is essential in projecting upcoming health issues and bolstering vaccination systems against tuberculosis. Epidemiological trend projections indicate that sustainable financing addressed to changing epidemiological settings increases disease resurgence resilience. The application of economic growth predictors and investments specifically in health is expected to predict impending gains in the decline of mortality due to TB, highlighting the importance of ongoing financial support. Interestingly, projections indicate that increasing intervention coverage and lessening socio-economic risk factors can significantly reduce the influence of tuberculosis during the next few decades. In contrast, poor resource allocation may undermine gains, especially in low-income communities where the burden of disease is still disproportionately high. Strategic budget prioritization towards full-coverage vaccination approaches, health education, and infrastructure investments will be critical to leverage predictable health gains, preventing TB from eroding improvements in life expectancy (Kyle et al., 2018). This strategy guarantees that prevention interventions are efficient and responsive to fluid health terrain. In addition, the intricacy of tuberculosis prevention requires that funding systems are flexible enough to tackle biomedical as well as social determinants of health. The appropriation of all resources for vaccine delivery ignores the larger environment in which TB persists, such as housing, nutrition, and accessibility to healthcare (Dar et al., 2016). Increased financial assistance must therefore include community-based interventions and public health efforts that promote preventive practices in conjunction with immunization strategies. Evidence of concentrated mortality in certain areas calls for targeted investment to redress localized vulnerabilities and, therefore, maximize the effectiveness of resource allocation. In this perspective, diversified funding sources that are synergistic among government, international, and private sector sources can maximize TB vaccination efficacy. Finally, efficient and fair distribution of resources is critical for maintaining progress in TB prevention so that the effects of vaccination can be translated into long-term reductions in incidence and mortality from the disease (Kyle et al., 2018; Naghavi et al., 2024).

14.4.3. International Collaboration Efforts

The complexities of tuberculosis control cut across international boundaries, calling for extensive global coordination to optimize vaccination and prevention mechanisms. In a more connected global environment, infectious diseases like tuberculosis become a major threat not only in one's local environment but worldwide, underscored by the need for collaborative health endeavors. Interventions such as the One Health approach highlight the convergence of human, animal, and environmental health viewpoints to address disease issues holistically. This strategy supports inter-disciplinary collaborations between veterinarians, epidemiologists, and public health professionals to exchange information and expertise and, ultimately, increase tuberculosis prevention effectiveness in various populations (Conrad et al., 2009). Such integrated systems can be embraced by international efforts to more effectively address both direct and indirect transmission routes, and enhance overall capacity for global tuberculosis burden reduction through unified vaccination campaigns and innovative public health initiatives. In addition to theoretical principles, cross-country and institutional practical collaboration is key to tuberculosis research and control progress. For instance, collaborations across various stakeholders ranging from ministries of health to universities enable cross-fertilization of skills, staff, and training that is critical to building country-level capacity. Through such collaborations, comparative analyses on disease patterns and vaccine efficacy in varying epidemiological settings become possible, with cross-border knowledge transfer. In addition, regional networks offer forums for harmonizing surveillance systems and aligning prevention efforts, which is essential in eliminating disparities in tuberculosis control. Efficient communication among cooperating players guarantees that research and intervention initiatives supplement but do not replicate efforts, maximizing the use of available resources and the overall effect of vaccination efforts globally (Bourhy et al., 2012). Continuous global cooperation also aims to fill particular knowledge gaps through coordinated projects specific to diverse regional requirements. It is only through harmonized multidisciplinary research activities across nations, for example, that the contribution of wildlife reservoirs and the eco-social determinants of tuberculosis transmission can be comprehensively understood. It places equal emphasis on capacity building as well as scientific investigation, which allows the formulation of evidence-based policies that include ecological and social determinants of tuberculosis risk. In addition, training modules and exchange programs enable the development of qualified personnel who can transfer sophisticated vaccination and prevention techniques to their home countries. Through investments in these international collaborations, the global community unleashes synergistic gains that hasten tuberculosis eradication efforts, highlighting the invaluable contribution of global coordination in public health (Conrad et al., 2009; Bourhy et al., 2012).

SUMMARY

The recurring problem of TB control highlights the intricacy of infectious disease control across different sociopolitical settings. Areas of conflict, where healthcare infrastructures are degraded and population mobility is high, significantly increase the risk of TB transmission. Not only do such conditions interfere with customary vaccination regimens, but they also inhibit disease surveillance and access to early cure, fostering the continuity and outbreaks of tuberculosis. Successful prevention efforts must then be multi-pronged, not just accelerating vaccination campaigns but also building the resilience of healthcare systems in these risk-prone areas. With efforts to overcome the structural barriers that conflict and instability pose, public health efforts can reduce TB spread and enhance overall disease control, underlining the critical role of adaptive policy and international coordination in protecting vulnerable groups (Marou et al., 2024). In a review of the effectiveness of particular TB control programs, the establishment of the DOTS approach demonstrates considerable advancements in diminishing infectious disease burden. Mathematical modeling of the transmission of TB in China demonstrates that although complete DOTS coverage has resulted in a considerable decrease in basic reproduction number, meaning decreased transmission, it is still greater than the threshold for eliminating disease. This indicates that vaccination has to be combined with improved diagnostic and treatment regimens to promote complete control. Optimal control theory also promotes targeted interventions for exposed and infected individuals, reaffirming that vaccination, when supplemented with careful treatment schemes, lies at the foundation of sustainable TB control and long-term public health gain (Liu et al., 2020). Finally, the conclusion based on empirical data and theoretical models confirms that vaccination itself is not enough to eliminate tuberculosis. A comprehensive strategy combining vaccination campaigns, strong treatment programs, and cutting-edge public health interventions is essential. Political will, intersectoral coordination, and continuing investment in health infrastructure are just as essential to establish an environment for successful TB control. The integration of these interventions not only boosts immunity but also targets social determinants and disease transmission barriers. As the international community persists in tackling tuberculosis, particularly in challenging environments such as conflict-affected areas, adherence to evidence-based adaptive prevention methods must be unwavering if meaningful reductions in TB prevalence and deaths are to be registered (Liu et al., 2020; Marou et al., 2024).

Dynamic modeling of tuberculosis transmission gives important information about how vaccination and other control interventions affect disease outcomes. The initial analyses usually address the determination of the equilibrium states, such as disease-free and endemic equilibria, which represent stable states of the system under certain conditions. Stability calculations of such equilibria show that the healthy state is locally and globally stable when the basic reproduction number, $\Re0$, is less than one, which means that there are chances of successful eradication of the disease with effective interventions. This is the basis on which vaccination programs are based, as lowering $\Re0$ emphasizes the need for sustaining high immunization coverage and the use of complementary control measures. Mathematical models also confirm that unless $\Re0$ is adequately decreased, tuberculosis infection remains endemically, reinforcing the importance of an integrated strategy including vaccination, treatment, and environmental controls as key to effective disease control (Al-Hdaibat et al., 2025). Additional investigation into the contribution of vaccination in particular reinforces the central role it plays in tuberculosis prevalence and transmission patterns. The addition of a vaccinated compartment in epidemiological models verifies that an increase in the portion of susceptible persons entering vaccination diminishes the burden of total infections by having a negative impact on $\mathfrak{R}0$. This is an effect that highlights the role of vaccination policy and practice in preventing the spread of tuberculosis effectively. Numerical computations validate this by showing improvements in population health with increased vaccine coverage, which confirms that vaccination serves as a keystone in prevention efforts. Sensitivity analyses indicate that vaccine parameters, including coverage rate and vaccine efficacy, have significant impacts on the epidemic trajectory, hence offering policymakers quantitative evidence for maximizing public health benefit and optimizing resource allocation (Ma et al., 2024). Finally, the combination of mathematical modeling and empirical evidence supports a comprehensive approach to tuberculosis prevention. Optimal control research posits that the combined use of vaccination, public education, active screening, and environmental pathogen removal yields the highest rates of exposed and infected population decreases. The synergy between preventive interventions is recognized in this combined approach, as it recognizes that individual interventions are not enough when applied alone. The entire examination of tuberculosis control points towards the fact that vaccination by itself, although important, has to be supplemented by other interventions for the effective containment of disease impact. These findings emphasize the value of multidisciplinary approaches to public health measures involved in tuberculosis elimination, calling for persistent investment and adaptable control measures in endemic environments (Al-Hdaibat et al., 2025).

CLOSER LOOK

GLOBAL BACILLUS CALMETTE-GUÉRIN (BCG) VACCINATION POLICIES

Policies of BCG vaccination all over the world differ greatly from nation to nation based on variations in TB burden, healthcare system, and public health strategies. BCG vaccine, which is a product of the attenuated *Mycobacterium bovis* strain, has been used since the 1920s and is currently the only licensed vaccine against TB. Its main function is to guard against advanced forms of TB in young children, including miliary TB and TB meningitis, and not pulmonary TB in adults. Due to its inconsistent protection against adult TB and disease epidemiology shifts, worldwide BCG vaccination policy has developed and branched out considerably.

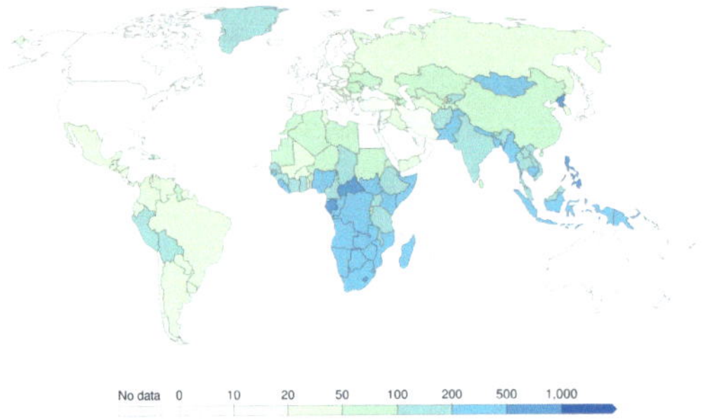

Source: By Our World In Data - https://ourworldindata.org/grapher/incidence-of-tuberculosis-sdgs, CC BY 3.0, https://commons.wikimedia.org/w/index.php?curid=86956073

In countries with high TB burden, like India, Indonesia, Nigeria, and most of the countries in sub-Saharan Africa and Southeast Asia, BCG is administered universally at birth or shortly thereafter. This is endorsed by the World Health Organization (WHO), which advises that high TB incidence countries incorporate BCG into their national immunization programs. Universal infant BCG vaccination in these settings is aimed at reducing childhood mortality and morbidity from TB and is often administered in hospitals or during routine immunization visits.Alternatively, in countries with low TB burdens like the United States, the Netherlands, and certain areas of Northern and Western Europe, routine BCG vaccines have been abandoned. These countries generally adopt focused vaccination in high-risk groups like immigrants from TB-endemic areas, healthcare workers, or those exposed to DR-TB. The reasoning for this strategy is that the overall risk of transmitting TB is low, and the advantages of widespread BCG vaccination do not outweigh the cost and possible complications.A few nations have implemented modified or phased-out policies due to evolving TB epidemiology. Such as, universal BCG vaccination of school-going children was halted in the United Kingdom in 2005 and was replaced with a selective program for infants in high-risk settings. Some nations, such as Canada, have policy variations at the regional level according to the regional TB burden, especially in indigenous or isolated communities.The worldwide BCG policy landscape persists in adapting to TB control interventions and the construction of new TB vaccines. Investigations persist in creating more potent vaccines that might confer more expansive protection, notably for pulmonary TB in adults (Dar et al., 2016).

REFERENCES

1. Dar, O. A., Hasan, R., Schlundt, J., Harbarth, S., Caleo, G., Dar, F. K., Littmann, J., Rweyemamu, M., Buckley, E. J., Shahid, M., Kock, R., Li, H. L., Giha, H., Khan, M., So, A. D., Bindayna, K. M., Kessel, A., Pedersen, H. B., Permanand, G., Zumla, A., ... Heymann, D. L. (2016). Exploring the evidence base for national and regional policy interventions to combat resistance. *Lancet (London, England)*, *387*(10015), 285–295. https://doi.org/10.1016/S0140-6736(15)00520-6 (accessed on 10 May 2025).
2. Adjei, O. K., Amofah, G. K., Andries, K., Aujoulat, I., Bentoucha, M., Darie, M., et al. (2006). *Mycobacterium ulcerans* infection: Control, diagnosis, and treatment. https://core.ac.uk/download/pdf/9416615.pdf (accessed on 10 May 2025).
3. Martin C, Aguilo N, Marinova D, Gonzalo-Asensio J. Update on TB Vaccine Pipeline. *Applied Sciences*. 2020; 10(7):2632. https://doi.org/10.3390/app10072632 (accessed on 10 May 2025).
4. Al-Hdaibat, B., DarAssi, M.H., Ahmad, I., Altaf Khan, M. and Algethamie, R. (2025), Investigating Tuberculosis Dynamics Under Various Control Strategies: A Comprehensive Analysis Using Real Statistical Data. Math. Meth. Appl. Sci. https://doi.org/10.1002/mma.10779(accessed on 10 May 2025).
5. Stylianou, E., Paul, M. J., Reljic, R., & McShane, H. (2019). Mucosal delivery of tuberculosis vaccines: a review of current approaches and challenges. *Expert review of vaccines*, *18*(12), 1271–1284. https://doi.org/10.1080/14760584.2019.1692657 Van Goethem, N., Descamps, T., Devleesschauwer, B., Roosens, N. H. C., Boon, N. A. M., Van Oyen, H., & Robert, A. (2019). Status and potential of bacterial genomics for public health practice: a scoping review. *Implementation science : IS*, *14*(1), 79. https://doi.org/10.1186/s13012-019-0930-2 (accessed on 10 May 2025).
6. Bourhy, H., Gaidet, N., & Molia, S. (2012). Mission to Indonesia to participate in the 1st Indonesia-France Seminar in Medicine & Public Health and investigate potential collaborations on animal health: 2nd–9th of November 2012. http://agritrop.cirad.fr/567354/1/document_567354.pdf (accessed on 10 May 2025).
7. Bruzzese, E., Bocchino, M., Assante, L., Alessio, M., Bellofiore, B., Bruzzese, D., Iorio, R., et al. (2009). Gamma interferon release assays for diagnosis of tuberculosis infection in immune-compromised children in a country in which the prevalence of tuberculosis is low. *Journal of Clinical Microbiology, 47*, 2355–2357. https://www.semanticscholar.org/paper/8a63324c7e02bcf69f3c0f2b7b091c463df57b02 (accessed on 10 May 2025).
8. Chanpitakkul, J. (2024). MPOX (Monkeypox): Current epidemiology, clinical manifestations, and advances in treatment and prevention strategies. *International Journal of Current Science Research and Review*. https://doi.org/10.9734/ijcsrr/2024/v7i3/70188.
9. Conrad, P. A., Mazet, J. A., Clifford, D., Scott, C., & Wilkes, M. (2009). Evolution of a transdisciplinary "One Medicine-One Health" approach to global health education at the University of California, Davis. *Preventive veterinary medicine*, *92*(4), 268–274. https://doi.org/10.1016/j.prevetmed.2009.09.002 (accessed on 10 May 2025).
10. Huchko, M. J., Maloba, M., Nakalembe, M., & Cohen, C. R. (2015). The time has come to make cervical cancer prevention an essential part of comprehensive sexual and reproductive health

services for HIV-positive women in low-income countries. *Journal of the International AIDS Society, 18*(Suppl 5), 20282. https://doi.org/10.7448/IAS.18.6.20282(accessed on 10 May 2025).

11. Elshayeb, A., Ahmed, N., Salih, K. M., Nugoud, O. A. Z., Yagoub, A. A. E., & Ali, A. K. S. (2020). Innovative strategies for developing tuberculosis implementation research in Sudan. Preprint. DOI: https://doi.org/10.21203/rs.3.rs-97758/v1(accessed on 10 May 2025).

12. Ferrari, A. J., Santomauro, D., Aali, A., Abate, Y. H., Abbafati, C., Abbastabar, H., Abd ElHafeez, S., et al. (2024). Global incidence, prevalence, years lived with disability (YLDs), disability-adjusted life-years (DALYs), and healthy life expectancy (HALE) for 371 diseases and injuries in 204 countries and territories and 811 subnational locations, 1990–2021: A systematic analysis for the Global Burden of Disease Study 2021. *The Lancet, 403*, 2133–2161. https://doi.org/10.1016/s0140-6736(24)00757-8.

13. Foreman, K. J., Marquez, N., Dolgert, A. J., Fukutaki, K., Fullman, N., McGaughey, M., Pletcher, M. A., et al. (2018). Forecasting life expectancy, years of life lost, and all-cause and cause-specific mortality for 250 causes of death: Reference and alternative scenarios for 2016–40 for 195 countries and territories. *The Lancet, 392*(10159), 2052–2090. https://doi.org/10.1016/s0140-6736(18)31694-5.

14. Gopalan, Narendran and Ariarathinam, Newtonraj and Elizabeth Hanna, Luke and Shanmugam, Siva Kumar and Ranganathan, Uma Devi and Malaisamy, Muniyandi and Ramraj, Balaji and Devaleenal, Bella and Venkataraman, Aishwarya and Nagarajan, Karikalan and Bethunaickan, Ramalingam and Sathya Narayanan, Mukesh Kumar and Deka, Mrigen and Selvaraju, Sriram and Santhanakrishnan, Ramesh Kumar and Krishnan, Rajendran and Chinnaiyan, Ponnuraja and Palaniyandi, Kannan and Vetrivel, Umashankar and Shanmugam Murugaiha, Jeyakumar and Natarajan, Saravanan and Mathur, Alok (2024) *Current challenges and future development of India's healthcare system' towards tuberculosis free India – research evidence and programmatic initiatives.* Current challenges and future development of India's healthcare system' towards tuberculosis free India – research evidence and programmatic initiatives, 1(1) (1). pp. 35-38.(accessed on 10 May 2025).

15. Hatherill, M., & Cobelens, F. (2022). Infant BCG vaccination is beneficial, but not sufficient. *The Lancet Global Health, 10*, e1220–e1221. https://doi.org/10.1016/s2214-109x(22)00325-4.

16. Sopp P, Howard CJ, Hope JC 2006. Flow Cytometric Detection of Gamma Interferon Can Effectively Discriminate *Mycobacterium bovis* BCG-Vaccinated Cattle from *M. bovis*-Infected Cattle. Clin Vaccine Immunol 13:.

17. Hulstine, A. (2017). Vaccine implementation: Alaska 2017. A Project Submitted in Partial Fulfillment of the Requirements for the Degree of MASTER OF SCIENCE in Nursing Science University of Alaska Anchorage May 2017. https://core.ac.uk/download/286607590.pdf (accessed on 10 May 2025).

18. Jeong, Y., & Min, J. (2023). Impact of COVID-19 Pandemic on Tuberculosis Preventive Services and Their Post-Pandemic Recovery Strategies: A Rapid Review of Literature. *Journal of Korean medical science, 38*(5), e43. https://doi.org/10.3346/jkms.2023.38.e43 (accessed on 10 May 2025).

19. Jeyanathan, M., Afkhami, S., Smaill, F., Miller, M. S., Lichty, B. D., & Xing, Z. (2020). Immunological considerations for COVID-19 vaccine strategies. *Nature Reviews Immunology, 20*, 615–632. https://doi.org/10.1038/s41577-020-00434-6.

20. Kaufmann S. H. E. (2023). Vaccine development against tuberculosis before and after Covid-19. *Frontiers in immunology, 14*, 1273938. https://doi.org/10.3389/fimmu.2023.1273938 (accessed on 10 May 2025).

21. Lalvani, A., Marchant, A., Cooper, A. M., Soares, A. P., Marchant, A., Pym, A. S., Hill, A. V., et al. (2008). Natural variation in immune responses to neonatal *Mycobacterium bovis Bacillus Calmette-Guérin* (BCG) vaccination in a cohort of Gambian infants. https://core.ac.uk/download/2709729.pdf (accessed on 10 May 2025).

22. Leining, Lauren M., "Geospatial Analysis Of Pediatric Tuberculosis In Bohol, Philippines: Disease Clusters And Access To Care" (2019). *Dissertations & Theses (Open Access)*. 67. https://digitalcommons.library.tmc.edu/uthsph_dissertsopen/67 (accessed on 10 May 2025).

23. Lewnard, J. A., & Reingold, A. L. (2019). Emerging Challenges and Opportunities in Infectious Disease Epidemiology. *American journal of epidemiology, 188*(5), 873–882. https://doi.org/10.1093/aje/kwy264 (accessed on 10 May 2025).

24. Liu, S., Bi, Y., & Liu, Y. (2020). Modeling and dynamic analysis of tuberculosis in mainland China from 1998 to 2017: The effect of DOTS strategy and further control. *Theoretical Biology and Medical Modelling, 17*. https://doi.org/10.1186/s12976-020-00124-9.

25. Ma, R., Sugiarto, S., & Nurwijaya, S. (2024). Dynamical system for tuberculosis outbreak with vaccination treatment and different interventions on the burden of drug resistance. *Jambura Journal of Biomathematics (JJBM)*. https://www.semanticscholar.org/paper/6452ed6fa537c4d85a3ed2b0a1b0b48d7bd8feb4 (accessed on 10 May 2025).

26. Machlaurin, A., Pol, S. V., Setiawan, D., van der Werf, T. S., & Postma, M. J. (2019). Health economic evaluation of current vaccination strategies and new vaccines against tuberculosis: a systematic review. *Expert review of vaccines, 18*(9), 897–911. https://doi.org/10.1080/14760584.2019.1651650 (accessed on 10 May 2025).

27. Marou, V., Vardavas, C., Aslanoglou, K., Nikitara, K., Plyta, Z., Leonardi-Bee, J., Atkins, K., et al. (2024). The impact of conflict on infectious disease: A systematic literature review. *Conflict and Health, 18*. https://doi.org/10.1186/s13031-023-00568-z.

28. Mata-Espinosa, D., Lara-Espinosa, J. V., Barrios-Payán, J., & Hernández-Pando, R. (2023). The Use of Viral Vectors for Gene Therapy and Vaccination in Tuberculosis. *Pharmaceuticals (Basel, Switzerland), 16*(10), 1475. https://doi.org/10.3390/ph16101475 (accessed on 10 May 2025).

29. Miller, L. A., Royer, C. M., Pinkerton, K. E., & Schelegle, E. S. (2017). Nonhuman Primate Models of Respiratory Disease: Past, Present, and Future. *ILAR journal, 58*(2), 269–280. https://doi.org/10.1093/ilar/ilx030 (accessed on 10 May 2025).

30. Murray, C. J. L., Ikuta, K. S., Sharara, F., Swetschinski, L. R., Robles Aguilar, G., Gray, A. P., Han, C., et al. (2022). Global burden of bacterial antimicrobial resistance in 2019: A systematic analysis. *The Lancet, 399*, 629–655. https://doi.org/10.1016/s0140-6736(21)02724-0.

31. Naghavi, M., Ong, K. L., Aali, A., Ababneh, H., Abate, Y. H., Abbafati, C., Abbasgholizadeh, R., et al. (2024). Global burden of 288 causes of death and life expectancy decomposition in 204 countries and territories and 811 subnational locations, 1990–2021: A systematic analysis for the Global Burden of Disease Study 2021. *The Lancet, 403*, 2100–2132. https://doi.org/10.1016/s0140-6736(24)00367-2.

32. Nell, A. J., & van Vugt, F. (2011). *BOCI-Egypt : Brucellosis and Tuberculosis control 21- 25 March 2011*. (Mission Report). Centre for Development Innovation. https://edepot.wur.nl/173913 (accessed on 10 May 2025).

33. Papazisis, G., & Topalidou, X. (2024). Maternal vaccination for the prevention of infantile RSV disease: An overview of the authorized, in-progress, and rejected vaccine candidates. *Vaccines, 12*. https://doi.org/10.3390/vaccines12030456.

34. Salam, M. A., Al-Amin, M. Y., Salam, M. T., Pawar, J. S., Akhter, N., Rabaan, A. A., & Alqumber, M. A. A. (2023). Antimicrobial resistance: A growing serious threat for global public health. *Healthcare, 11*(13), 1946. https://doi.org/10.3390/healthcare11131946.

35. Sinha, A., Kethar, J. ., & Appavu,Ph.d, D. (2023). Prevention of Drug-resistant Tuberculosis. *Journal of Student Research, 12*(3). https://doi.org/10.47611/jsrhs.v12i3.5100(accessed on 10 May 2025).

36. Thaiss, W. M., Thaiss, C. C., & Thaiss, C. A. (2012). Recent developments in the epidemiology and management of tuberculosis - new solutions to old problems?. *Infection and drug resistance, 5*, 1–8. https://doi.org/10.2147/IDR.S27604 (accessed on 10 May 2025).

37. Torrence, M. (2007). Zoonoses. *Zoonoses and Public Health, 54*. https://doi.org/10.1111/j.1863-2378.2007.01020.x.

38. Favorov, M., Ali, M., Tursunbayeva, A., Aitmagambetova, I., Kilgore, P., Ismailov, S., & Chorba, T. (2012). Comparative tuberculosis (TB) prevention effectiveness in children of Bacillus Calmette-Guérin (BCG) vaccines from different sources, Kazakhstan. *PloS one, 7*(3), e32567. https://doi.org/10.1371/journal.pone.0032567 (accessed on 10 May 2025).

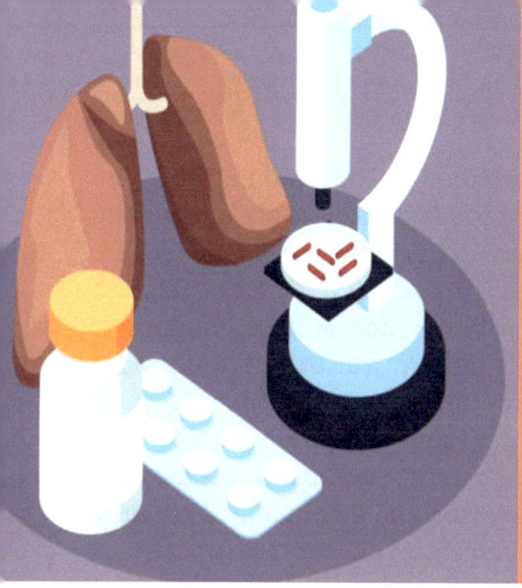

Chapter 15

ADVANCES IN TB DIAGNOSTICS AND TREATMENT

Contents

Introduction

The persistent challenge posed by tuberculosis (TB) underscores a critical public health imperative demanding continual innovation in both diagnostics and treatment. The disease, despite being preventable and curable, remains endemic in various regions, necessitating updated clinical guidelines that reflect recent advancements and localized contexts. In Singapore, for example, the clinical management of TB has evolved significantly since the initial practice guidelines published in 2016, encompassing improvements from diagnostic modalities to therapeutic regimens. These updates have been informed by multidisciplinary panels employing systematic review methods and consensus-building techniques to address drug-susceptible tuberculosis (DS-TB) effectively. Incorporating novel technologies such as artificial intelligence (AI)-assisted radiological screening and next-generation sequencing (NGS) reinforces the commitment to enhancing early detection and tailored treatment strategies vital for limiting transmission and improving patient outcomes (Ang et al., 2024). The global burden of TB is further complicated by the rise of drug-resistant strains, notably multi-drug resistant (MDR) and extensively drug-resistant (XDR) variants of *Mycobacterium tuberculosis* (MTB). This evolving resistance threatens to undermine progress made in TB control and necessitates a deeper understanding of the genetic mechanisms underpinning drug resistance. Modern diagnostic tools, including WGS and CRISPR-based assays, have emerged as pivotal innovations that allow for rapid, precise identification of resistant strains, thereby informing treatment decisions that are more individualized and potentially more effective. The complex interplay between pathogen genetics and treatment efficacy highlights the importance of integrating advanced molecular diagnostics into standard TB control protocols to combat resistance and improve therapeutic outcomes globally (Deshpande et al., 2024). Advances in TB diagnostics and treatment also emphasize the importance of collaborative, multidisciplinary approaches that bridge clinical practice, laboratory research, and public health policy. Recognizing that equitable access to cutting-edge diagnostic and treatment tools remains uneven across different regions, there is a pressing need for strategies that address these global disparities. The integration of shorter treatment regimens, digital health technologies such as video observed therapy, and AI for screening represents promising developments that could transform TB care worldwide. Future efforts must focus on enhancing these innovations while ensuring that resource-limited settings receive adequate support to implement them effectively, thus advancing toward the ultimate goal of TB eradication with a more personalized, precise medical approach (Ang et al., 2024; Deshpande et al., 2024).

Importance of Advances in Diagnostics and Treatment

Striving for effective tuberculosis control depends on the resolution of major diagnostic challenges that have long prevented timely and accurate diagnosis. Conventional laboratory-based techniques, although trustworthy, usually involve lengthy waiting times and multiple testing levels that prolong diagnosis and treatment initiation. This delay not only sustains transmission cycles but also complicates patient outcome. Improvements in molecular methods and automated liquid culture platforms enhanced the rapid detection of drug-resistant strains, allowing clinicians to better individualize treatments. These new developments meet the key demand for diagnostic devices that balance precision with speed and flexibility in diverse healthcare environments. Widespread access to these advanced diagnostic tools in resource-constrained settings is crucial, considering the worldwide spread of TB and its drug-resistant forms. The innovation and spread of these technologies constitute an imperative first step in limiting morbidity and mortality from tuberculosis (O'Grady et al., 2011). Another critical aspect is the combination of sophisticated diagnostic functions with effective treatment regimens to stem the emerging danger of drug-resistant tuberculosis (DR-TB). First-line and second-line drug resistance complicates clinical care and requires accurate susceptibility testing to direct therapy. Existing WHO-recommended methods for drug susceptibility testing (DST), such as automated liquid cultures and molecular testing, set a higher standard for resistance pattern detection. Nevertheless, there are still limitations, particularly in the case of less-studied second-line medicines, where test reliability is inconsistent. This highlights the need for ongoing improvement in diagnostic precision and treatment regimens to avoid the intensification of resistance. Finally, diagnostic gains need to be accompanied by affordable, evidence-driven treatment options to bring about significant improvement in TB containment and public health protection (O'Grady et al., 2011). Beyond technological advances, the larger value of progress in TB diagnostics and treatment is their ability to alter world health outcomes by facilitating earlier diagnosis and more successful interventions. Rapid and accurate diagnoses allow for early initiation of suitable therapies, lowering the spread of disease and enhancing the patient prognosis. Additionally, point-of-care testing development, while still problematic, is an essential TB control frontier, with the potential to provide decentralized testing and instant results. This has the potential to significantly increase case detection in resource-poor, high-burden environments where laboratory facilities are weak. Parallel to such technical progress, continued political dedication and investment are necessary to ensure that diagnostic and treatment innovation is converted into scalable, sustainable healthcare solutions. These multifaceted challenges need to be addressed for controlling tuberculosis in the midst of chronic epidemics, especially where HIV co-infection and drug resistance complicate the situation.

15.1. Current Diagnostic Methods

Despite the compelling necessity for high-speed and precise diagnosis of tuberculosis (TB), existing diagnostic tests have not been able to keep up with the rising complexity of drug-resistant strains. The use of conventional techniques like sputum smear microscopy is prevalent in most resource-poor environments because of their cost-effectiveness and ease of application. However, these are not sensitive tests, particularly in HIV co-infected children and adults, and hence they result in false negatives and ongoing transmission. Culture-based assays are more sensitive and deliver drug susceptibility results but are time-consuming, requiring weeks before they can deliver results. Molecular tests like nucleic acid amplification tests (NAATs) have enhanced detection speed and drug resistance profiling but their application remains unequal between regions, especially in high-burden developing nations. Strengthening diagnostic infrastructure is critical to counter the increasing incidence of multi-drug resistant tuberculosis (MDR-TB), which compromises TB control programs globally (Migliori et al., 2010). Implementation of new diagnostics with available health services needs to be a priority to improve early detection and treatment initiation. The problems facing TB diagnostics are most acute in nations with fractured public health systems. Countries such as India have a dual burden of infectious and chronic diseases in addition to constrained access to effective diagnostic tests and treatment programs. Rapid DST is pivotal to the control of MDR-TB, avoiding the spread of resistance, and implementing individualized treatment regimens. However, poor surveillance frameworks and uneven laboratory capacities prevent early diagnosis. Evidence indicates that populations with well-organized health programs and prompt diagnosis have notably higher treatment outcomes and adherence rates, highlighting the significance of speedy and accessible diagnostics (Gamon, 2013). Enhancing community-level health literacy and culturally appropriate interventions can promote diagnostic uptake and treatment compliance, key determinants in reducing MDR-TB cases in high-burden contexts. New technologies have the potential to revolutionize TB diagnosis by enabling faster, more accurate detection at the point of care. Progress in molecular platforms like GeneXpert MTB/RIF has already transformed screening by diagnosing both TB and rifampicin resistance simultaneously in hours, significantly reducing diagnostic delays. Even so, with its success, it is hampered by a high price tag and technical complexity that restricts broader availability to low-income areas. More recent assays for other resistance markers and host biomarkers are being tested to offer complete drug susceptibility profiles and to distinguish latent from active TB. These advances, combined with improving health infrastructure and political will to finance, are crucial to address the increasingly growing menace of MDR-TB and extensively drug-resistant tuberculosis (XDR-TB) (Migliori et al., 2010). A multifaceted approach incorporating cutting-edge diagnostics, strengthened reporting, and community engagement will be instrumental in advancing global TB control efforts (Figure 15.1).

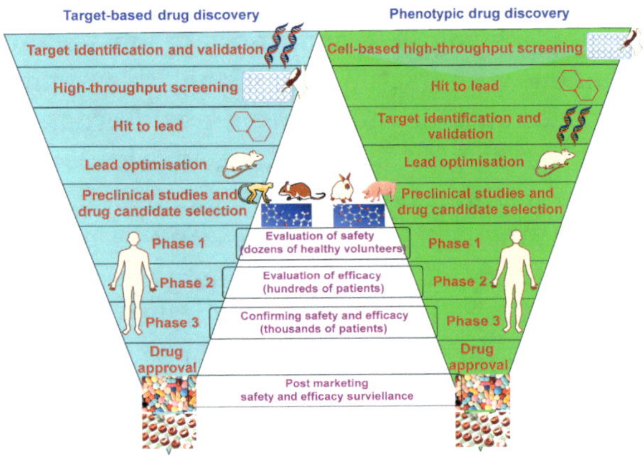

Figure 15.1. Pathology-based diagnosis of tuberculosis.

Source: Alsayed SSR, Gunosewoyo H. Tuberculosis: Pathogenesis, Current Treatment Regimens and New Drug Targets. *International Journal of Molecular Sciences.* 2023; 24(6):5202. https://doi.org/10.3390/ijms24065202

15.1.1. Sputum Smear Microscopy

Identification of infectious cases of tuberculosis relies most importantly on diagnostic technologies that are able to provide timely and precise output. Throughout much of the globe, sputum smear microscopy has been the standard for detecting active pulmonary tuberculosis (PTB) based on its comparative simplicity and affordability. While it allows for the visualization of acid-fast bacilli (AFB) from patient specimens directly, the technique has significant shortcomings, such as reduced sensitivity to culture or molecular testing, particularly in samples with a low bacterial load. The built-in time and technical delay of diagnosing tuberculosis by conventional laboratory techniques add to transmission, highlighting the immediate need for better diagnostic methods. Improving sputum smear microscopy's effectiveness or coupling it with new modalities might fill in the gap between current approaches and the ultimate rapid point-of-care tests that are critical for global tuberculosis control strategies (McNerney et al., 2012). Owing to the introduction of modern molecular diagnostics and rapid tests for detecting antigens, sputum smear microscopy remains extensively used, particularly in resource-poor environments where access is limited to complex laboratory facilities. Its simplicity of operation renders it flexible, but its diagnostic yield is greatly compromised in HIV-co-infected or pediatric patients with low bacillary load. Attempts at optimizing microscopy are fluorescence staining methods and automated digital microscopy that improve sensitivity and decrease subjective variation in examining slides. Challenged by these issues, concerted efforts by public health professionals, scientists, and policymakers have prioritized the continued need to enhance sputum smear microscopy procedures in more comprehensive tuberculosis control programs (Nahid et al., 2012). These enhancements need to be weighed against cost, access, and simplicity of application to gain the largest public health benefit in various healthcare environments. When looking at the pattern of tuberculosis diagnostic development, sputum smear microscopy continues as a key, though not flawless, diagnostic tool in the arsenal. Its quick turn-around time promotes early detection of cases and treatment, which are crucial to breaking transmission chains. Yet using this method in isolation is not adequate, especially with rising awareness of MDR-TB strains that necessitate the more complex detection techniques. Combining smear microscopy with other diagnostic technologies, including NAATs and biomarkers, has the potential for thorough patient assessment. Clinical and programmatic studies continue to investigate how sputum smear microscopy may be maximized so that advances in tuberculosis diagnostics are translated into real treatment benefits and public health impact (McNerney et al., 2012; Nahid et al., 2012) (Figure 15.2).

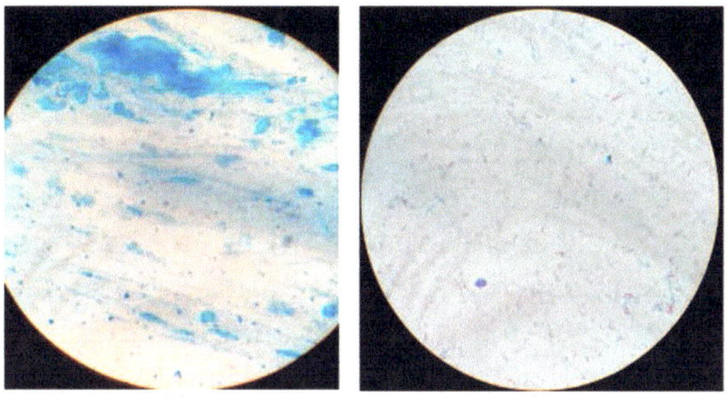

(a) (b)

Figure 15.2. Negative smear microscopy for sputum sample 4475. (a) Directed SSM: 297 AFB, 2+ (b) The bleach SSM: 401 AFB, 3+. Magnification: 100× in immersion.

Source: Liu, Y., Bi, X., Chen, S., & Mao, Y. (2023). Analysis of the status quo and influencing factors of tuberculosis knowledge among elderly people in Shenzhen, China. *International Journal of Environmental Research and Public Health, 20*(1), 135.

15.1.2. Culture Techniques

Diagnosis of tuberculosis has traditionally depended on several laboratory tests, with culture methods being a stronghold even after the advent of molecular tests. Cultivation of *Mycobacterium tuberculosis* (MTB) from clinical material not only proves infection but also permits DST, which plays a key role in treating resistant organisms. Solid medium cultures can be classically prized for their specificity and sensitivity, and they yield clearly defined colony morphology that is helpful for identification. Nonetheless, these procedures are time-consuming, taking several weeks before diagnosis because the bacterium is slow-growing. Techniques involving liquid media are more sensitive and have lower turnaround times, which allow quicker detection and consequently earlier initiation of treatment. Despite this, there has been an ever-growing realization of the importance of a holistic approach involving both culture types, in addition to rapid molecular diagnostics, to maximize sensitivity and accuracy in TB diagnosis (Zaporojan et al., 2024). Although culture methods are beneficial, they are practically challenged in their use, especially in resource-constrained environments where TB prevalence is greatest. It is challenging to maintain specialized machinery, implement biosafety measures, and the long incubation periods that are required for the growth of cultures in widespread applications. Recent technologies like automated liquid culture systems have improved diagnostic effectiveness by giving constant monitoring and faster detection of bacterial growth. Such systems not only enhance laboratory throughput but also allow for early detection of drug-resistant strains, aiding in customized therapeutic measures. Implementation of such advances in National TB Programs (NTPs) is key to overcoming logistical challenges, and achieving cost-effectiveness while improving the accuracy of diagnosis in a variety of clinical settings. Culture procedures, thus, continue to be essential even as molecular instruments gain increased importance (Solanki et al., 2024). Looking ahead, culture methods continue to evolve in the face of advancements in TB diagnosis and treatment models. The combination of culture data with molecular and genomic testing provides an impressive platform for directing personalized therapy. WGS of cultured isolates gives them profound insights into drug resistance mutations, transmission dynamics, and bacterial evolution. In addition, new technologies such as the molybdenum blue assay (MBLA) are being tested in clinical trials to assess response to treatment, illustrating that culture techniques still retain meaningful clinical utility beyond mere diagnosis. Although molecular tests provide speed, culture techniques provide the requisite biological material for extensive investigations and verification of novel diagnostics. Finally, it is critical to maintain and enhance culture-based diagnostics in parallel with new technologies to effectively decrease TB morbidity and mortality (Solanki et al., 2024; Zaporojan et al., 2024).

15.1.3. Molecular Diagnostics

Tuberculosis diagnosis has been driven heavily by improvements in molecular technologies, which provide unprecedented speed and specificity in detecting MTB as well as drug resistance patterns. Conventional diagnostic methods tend to be based on culture techniques that take weeks to produce results, hindering timely clinical intervention. Molecular testing, on the other hand, leverages nucleic acid amplification technologies and genotyping methods to identify tuberculosis bacilli and separate multi-drug resistant (MDR) and extensively drug-resistant (XDR) strains within hours to days. Such advances have revolutionized clinical management by facilitating prompt case detection and proper treatment regimen choice, vital in preventing transmission and minimizing death. The recent scientific literature emphasizes that using molecular tests enables not just a more precise diagnosis but also a nuanced epidemiological interpretation of tuberculosis transmission and resistance patterns (O'Grady et al., 2011).

AFB smear microscopy result	Indigen MTB/DR-TB	MTB culture positive	MTB culture negative	Sensitivity, % (95% CI)	Specificity, % (95% CI)	PPV (95% CI)	NPV (95% CI)	Accuracy (95% CI)	κ-value ± SE
Overall (N = 610)	MTB positive	288	5	94.1 (90.9–96.5)	98.4 (96.2–99.5)	98.3 (96.0–99.3)	94.4 (91.4–96.3)	96.2 (94.4–97.6)	0.9 ± 0.02 0.9–1
	MTB negative	18	299						
Positive (N = 224)	MTB positive	222	0	100 (98.4–100)	100 (15.8–100)	100 (98.4–100)	100 (15.8–100)	100 (98.4–100)	1 ± 0 1–1
	MTB negative	0	2						
Negative (N = 386)	MTB positive	66	5	78.6 (68.3–86.8)	98.3 (96.2–99.5)	93 (84.6–97)	94.3 (91.6–96.1)	94 (91.2–96.2)	0.8 ± 0.04 0.7 ± 0.9
	MTB negative	18	297						

PPV, positive predictive value; NPV, negative predictive value.

Figure 15.3. The model for optimizing molecular diagnostic capacity to fight tuberculosis. Aligning national and international partnerships, research and development and community empowerment will lead to better financing of health systems and research, production of effective diagnostics and strong communities that can seek and afford medical attention, and adhere to prescribed medical interventions.

Source: Parwati I, Chaidir L, Yunus M, Montain MM, Budhiarko D, Selasih SF, Ristandi RB, Rachman RW, Nurhayati RD, Pambudi I and Budiyati AD (2024) Evaluation of a real-time PCR assay performance to detect Mycobacterium tuberculosis, rifampicin, and isoniazid resistance in sputum specimens: a multicenter study in two major cities of Indonesia. Front. Microbiol. 15:1372647. doi: 10.3389/fmicb.2024.1372647

These innovations represent a major step toward breaking the diagnostic bottlenecks that have typically weakened tuberculosis control. Despite these encouraging advances, routine use of molecular diagnostics in tuberculosis care is confronted with a number of practical and technical issues. The definitive diagnostic test for tuberculosis does not yet exist, especially for point-of-care use in resource-constrained environments where the disease burden is greatest. Current gold-standard tests are accurate in controlled laboratory environments but tend to have sophisticated protocols and infrastructure demands that make them inaccessible and time-consuming to use in areas of high endemicity. In addition, identifying new biomarkers for diagnosis of tuberculosis and drug resistance remains a significant challenge, hindering efforts toward fast, affordable molecular tests deployable at scale. The intersection of test performance, price, and operational viability highlights the importance of ongoing innovation and political will to deploy these technologies equitably. Without overcoming these systemic barriers, the full potential of molecular diagnostics to speed up tuberculosis detection and outcome improvement is unfulfilled (McNerney et al., 2012). In addition, molecular diagnostics have provided new opportunities to distinguish tuberculosis from nontuberculous mycobacteria (NTM) infections, which frequently need different treatments. Traditional diagnostic methods have been challenged by specificity and have resulted in misdiagnosis and inappropriate treatment. Molecular methods like polymerase chain reaction (PCR) tests and genotyping have facilitated accelerated identification of mycobacterial species to the strain level, which benefits clinical decision-making. Notably, this specificity is essential in the management of complicated presentations or co-infection patients, enabling individualized interventions and more accurate prognosis. Clinical trials focusing on molecular diagnostics also help refine recommendations and treatment guidelines, especially for challenging-to-diagnose diseases like tuberculous pericarditis. Together, these developments indicate an increased integration of molecular techniques into the diagnostic process and research paradigms, marking a revolutionary change in tuberculosis treatment and management (O'Grady et al., 2011) (Figure 15.3).

15.2. Novel Diagnostic Technologies

The problem of timely and correct tuberculosis diagnosis is closely interconnected with the shortcomings of traditional lab-based tests, which usually postpone treatment beginning and facilitate ongoing disease transmission. Existing gold standards demand repeated invasions during long timeframes, demonstrating a pressing need for fast point-of-care diagnostics. New technologies have provided innovative assays sensitive enough to identify active tuberculosis and latent infections. These new technologies hold the promise of enhanced speed and accuracy in diagnosis, albeit still held back by the complexities of MTB biology and the heterogeneity of immune responses. Furthermore, such innovation must be translated into reality through tremendous political will and investment to implement these in healthcare systems, especially in countries affected by both tuberculosis and HIV epidemics (McNerney et al., 2012). MDR-TB and XDR-TB have made global control of tuberculosis more complex, urging the urgent requirement for sophisticated diagnostics that quickly detect patterns of resistance. Misuse of the principal therapeutic agents has driven the emergence of resistant strains that are becoming widespread in various geographic locations such as Asia and sub-Saharan Africa. New molecular diagnostic technologies are now allowing quick detection of mutations of resistance, promoting early targeted regimens of treatment and minimizing transmission of resistant strains. If applied with strong screening in HIV co-infected populations, these instruments are promising for enhancing clinical outcomes. The absence of extended diagnostic capability in settings of poverty, however, hinders these advances to adequately respond to the complicated epidemiology of DR-TB (Migliori et al., 2010). Despite the potential of new diagnostic technologies, significant roadblocks persist in their deployment for use and integration into public health systems. The search for point-of-care testing with sensitivity, specificity, and cost-effectiveness persists, as numerous current assays demand advanced laboratory settings and trained labor. Additionally, biomarker discovery, critical for the creation of next-generation diagnostics, is hindered by inherent limitations due to the heterogeneous nature of tuberculosis infection and disease presentation. Tackling these challenges requires interdisciplinary studies combined with continuous funding and policy endorsement to increase test availability, affordability, and scalability. In the end, driving diagnostic innovations must not only be technical in nature but include attention to implementation strategies prioritizing high-burden, resource-limited environments to realize meaningful global tuberculosis control (McNerney et al., 2012).

15.2.1. GeneXpert MTB/RIF Technology

Classic TB diagnosis approaches commonly suffer from major constraints, including long turnaround times and inability to distinguish between MTB and NTM. Delays in proper treatment may be caused by such limitations, especially in the case of acid-fast smear-positive TB where differentiation of the causative organism is important. The advent of GeneXpert MTB/RIF technology, a real-time fluorescence NAAT, has significantly improved diagnostic accuracy. Not only does this technology identify MTB with great sensitivity but it also identifies rifampicin resistance at the same time, allowing for prompt implementation of individualized therapy. On bronchoalveolar lavage fluid (BALF) specimens from acid-fast smear-positive patients, GeneXpert showed almost perfect sensitivity and specificity and was able to distinguish pulmonary TB from NTM infections successfully. This ability closes a significant diagnostic gap, enhancing clinical decision-making in patients with mycobacterial lung diseases and reducing inappropriate treatments (Wu et al., 2025) (Figure 15.4).

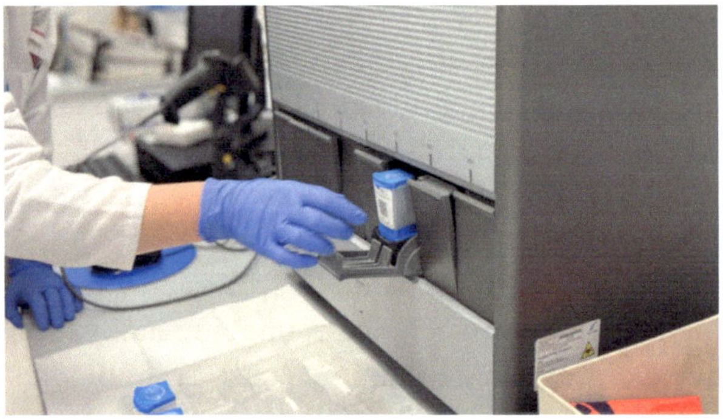

Figure 15.4. Xpert MTB/RIF assay.

Source: Centers for Disease Control and Prevention (CDC). (2024). *Nucleic acid amplification (NAA) test for TB.* https://www.cdc.gov/tb/media/images/2024/04/NAA_Test_1200x675.jpg.

Comparative analyses of GeneXpert MTB/RIF with alternate diagnostic methods point to its better performance in regard to sensitivity and speed. In smear-negative presumptive pulmonary TB, GeneXpert outperformed modified culture techniques and gene chip technologies consistently by yielding the highest positive detection rates and minimizing turnaround time appreciably. It is crucial in deciding on timely treatment for such patients who would otherwise risk delay due to inconclusive results from smear examination. While it had lower specificity than gene chip technology, GeneXpert's aggregate diagnostic sensitivity and predictive value best matched clinical diagnosis. Additionally, its ability to detect drug resistance concurrently increases clinical utility through early detection of rifampicin-resistant cases and adequate guide of treatment regimens (Xie et al., 2022). In addition to detection, GeneXpert MTB/RIF technology significantly enhances drug susceptibility testing (DST), a cornerstone of current TB management in the context of increasing antimicrobial resistance (AMR). Head-to-head comparisons of GeneXpert with conventional culture-based approaches and with molecular methods reveal that it compares favourably in detecting resistance to rifampicin and isoniazid. This enables clinicians to reformulate regimens quickly, forestalling the danger of treatment failure and continued transmission. However, combining GeneXpert with other complementary molecular diagnostics is recommended to further improve diagnostic precision and overcome the limitations of single-method testing. Therefore, GeneXpert is a crucial development, not just by accelerating MTB detection but also by yielding essential drug resistance information needed for personalized treatment strategies (Xie et al., 2022).

15.2.2. Liquid Culture Systems

The difficulty of diagnosing TB, especially drug-resistant TB, requires highly sensitive and accurate laboratory methods that are able to yield timely results. Standard solid agar culture techniques, although valuable, meet some limitations when it comes to speed and sensitivity and tend to time diagnosis and treatment starting. To counteract these limitations, automated liquid culture technology has become a breakthrough in TB diagnostic technology. These systems enable the quick growth and detection of MTB by offering a favorable liquid environment that accelerates bacterial multiplication. The increased sensitivity and lower turnaround time of liquid culture systems greatly enhance detection of both drug-susceptible and DR-TB strains. Based on recent guidelines, automated liquid culture systems represent the gold standard for initial DST today, emphasizing their pivotal role in contemporary TB control strategies (Affolabi et al., 2011). By reducing diagnostic delays, these systems are responsible for quicker clinical decision-making and enhanced patient outcomes. Irrespective of the progress made with molecular diagnostics, phenotypic tools like liquid culture systems are still unreplaceable for thorough drug resistance profiling in TB. Although molecular tests are able to quickly identify prevalent resistance mutations, they might not capture the entire range of second-line drug resistance. Automated liquid culture systems, in contrast, offer a direct measure of bacterial growth with the presence of a variety of antimicrobial drugs, allowing accurate susceptibility determination. Significantly, liquid culture DST has revealed high reproducibility and reliability for major second-line drugs such as aminoglycosides, polypeptides, and fluoroquinolones that are paramount to treating extensively DR-TB. Testing for other second-line drugs is, however, less standardized because of varying performance and complexity (Affolabi et al., 2011). This emphasizes the need to sustain liquid culture systems as key tools within TB diagnosis algorithms while further optimizing their uses for more therapeutics. The dissemination of liquid culture systems is hindered by cost, requirements for infrastructure, and technical expertise, particularly in resource-constrained settings with the greatest TB burden. Although these systems enormously shorten diagnostic delay over conventional solid media, operational and cost constraints limit availability to much of the high-incidence world. Therefore, realization of an ultra-rapid point-of-care test that leverages liquid culture's sensitivity with ease of molecular detection remains an ideal in TB diagnosis. However, liquid culture platforms offer a necessary link in modern diagnostic strategies, providing strong phenotypic drug resistance confirmation necessary for successful treatment regimens. Therefore, in conjunction with emerging technologies, liquid culture systems remain a cornerstone for further tuberculosis control efforts by providing proper diagnosis and individualized therapy (Figure 15.5).

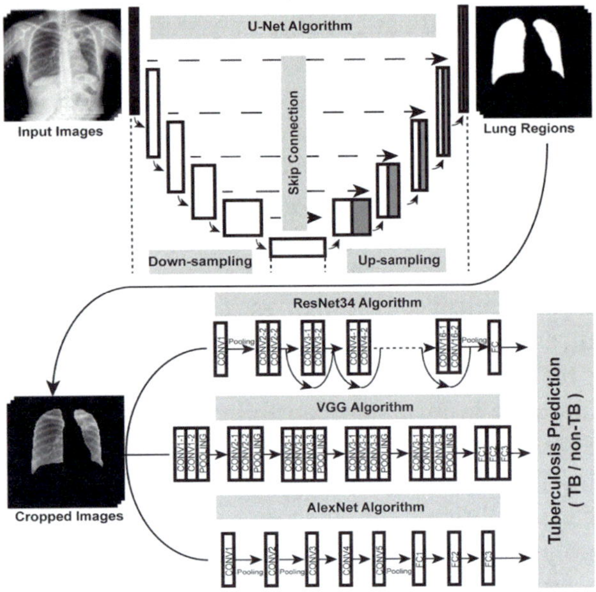

Figure 15.5. Overall structure of the DCNN-based AI diagnosis system. The workflow of the system could be divided into two parts: image segmentation network (U-Net), image classification network (ResNet or VGG or AlexNet). Regions of the lung in the original chest X-ray photographs were recognized by the U-Net. Then, the cropped and resized lung region images served as an input for image classification algorithms, which generated diagnoses.*Source:* Nijiati M, Ma J, Hu C, Tuersun A, Abulizi A, Kelimu A, Zhang D, Li G and Zou X (2022) Artificial Intelligence Assisting the Early Detection of Active Pulmonary Tuberculosis From Chest X-Rays: A Population-Based Study. Front. Mol. Biosci. 9:874475. doi: 10.3389/fmolb.2022.874475

15.2.3. Serological Tests

The history of tuberculosis diagnosis has emphasized the importance of rapid, sensitive, and accessible methods, especially in resource-poor environments. Serological tests have gained attention among these for their ability to identify host antibody responses to MTB antigens. Being less invasive or time-consuming than other methods, serological tests have the benefit of simplicity and expediency and in most cases use easily accessed blood samples. These tests may supplement classical tools for diagnosis by detecting exposed or infected persons who may not yet present symptoms of active disease. Yet, obstacles like fluctuating patient antibody levels and cross-reactivity with NTM have created impediments to their reproducibility and accuracy. Despite these challenges, recent advances in microfluidic technologies and point-of-care platforms are already starting to overcome these challenges, with potentially more reliable and transportable serological diagnostics on the horizon (Mejía-Salazar et al., 2020). The integration of serological testing into the larger context of TB diagnostics complements molecular and culture-based approaches by offering a host immune response view. Current serological platforms more and more utilize biosensing components combined with microengineering to provide rapid and accurate detection of tuberculosis-specific antibodies. This bridge between immunology and microfluidics allows for the production of lab-on-a-chip devices with low sample volume requirements and real-time feedback. This is consistent with progress in other infectious disease tests, where portability, affordability, and connectivity via wireless data make it more clinically useful. Notably, the convergence of big data analytics and artificial intelligence (AI) can help sharpen test interpretation, enhancing specificity and sensitivity through the ability to identify trends in serological markers. Such technological convergence highlights the enhanced potential of serological tests for use in future TB diagnosis and monitoring protocols (Mejía-Salazar et al., 2020). Although promising in terms of technology, clinical use of serological tests for tuberculosis is uncertain owing to diagnostic performance variability in endemic areas and patient groups. Heterogeneity in the antibody response, determined by HIV co-infection and immunosuppression, makes test reliability challenging, and region-specific assessments and adjusted cutoffs are required. Lessons from other infectious diseases like visceral leishmaniasis show that serological and molecular diagnostics need to be tailored to epidemiologic situations and patient immune status to achieve optimum treatment outcomes. Therefore, future efforts should be directed towards the standardization of serological assays, their validation in various clinical settings, and their integration into established diagnostic algorithms. The integration of new diagnostic technologies with knowledge of host immune variability will be crucial to strengthening the contribution of serological tests to integrated TB control programs.

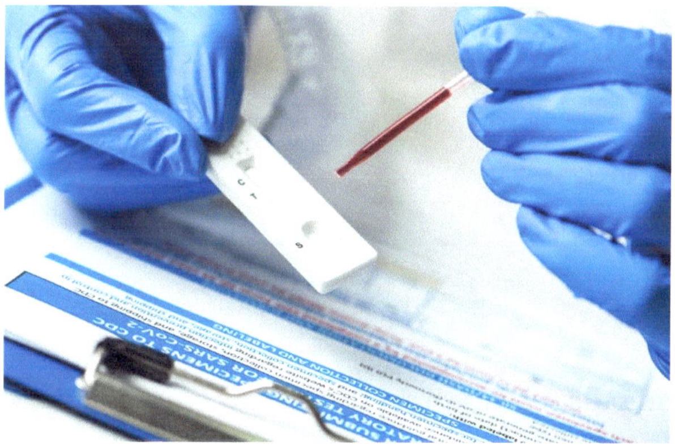

Source: News Medical. (n.d.). *TB diagnostic laboratory setup.* https://d2jx2rerrg6sh3.cloudfront.net/images/news/ImageForNews_705943_16462272081747550.jpg.

15.3. Advances in Tuberculosis (TB) Treatment

The treatment landscape of TB has been largely transformed with the advent of new therapeutic strategies and better drug regimens that aim to improve efficacy and shorten the course of treatment. Latest developments target molecular diagnostics to allow quick detection of drug-resistant strains to enable the timely initiation of specific therapies. Precision medicine strategies are key to overcoming difficulties posed by multi-drug resistant and extensively DR-TB cases. Moreover, shorter-course therapy and new drug combinations have shown similar efficacy in reducing adverse effects, and solving the issues of patient adherence and abandonment of treatment. These therapeutic advances are integrated into clinical practice, however, only unevenly, because of the lack of healthcare infrastructure and socioeconomic obstacles in high-burden areas. Strengthening healthcare delivery systems and increasing access to these innovations are essential to convert scientific advances into better patient outcomes and decreased transmission rates (Wulandari et al., 2025). Immunocompromised groups, especially HIV-infected individuals, pose complex challenges in treating TB due to possible drug interactions and complications from comorbid conditions. Treating TB in such patients requires cautious planning of antiretroviral therapy (ART) regimens in addition to anti-TB medications to prevent toxicity and optimize treatment outcomes. New evidence describes elevated rates of kidney dysfunction in these individuals, which are partly due to TB infection itself and the drug-induced nephrotoxicity of agents such as tenofovir disoproxil fumarate. To address these challenges involves integrated strategies that include augmented diagnostic tools for opportunistic infections, intensified monitoring for adverse effects of treatment, and multidisciplinary models of care that unite TB and HIV management. This effort re-emphasizes the role of individualized approaches to medicine and the discovery of new drugs that target minimal harm and maximal efficacy (Wearne & Davidson, 2024). Despite encouraging progress in therapeutic approaches and drug research, delayed diagnosis and restricted access to healthcare persist as barriers to the best TB treatment outcomes in the world. The intersection of biological complexities and socioeconomic factors necessitates a comprehensive approach that harmonizes medical innovation with health systems strengthening. There is promise in emerging treatments, such as host-directed therapies and vaccines in clinical trials, to transform TB care by enhancing immune responses and averting the recurrence of infection. In addition, health policies that emphasize early detection of cases, equitable distribution of medicines, and patient-focused support structures must be put in place to curb care barriers. An integrated approach to meet structural disparities along with scientific advancements will be crucial in moving towards the international target of TB control and ultimate elimination (Wulandari et al., 2025) (Figure 15.6).

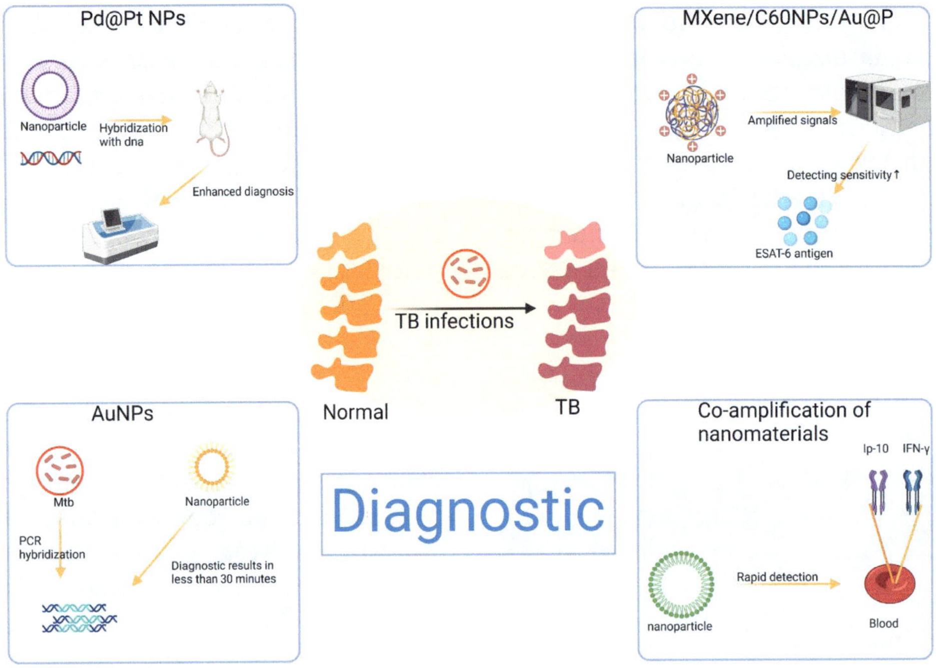

Figure 15.6. Advances in conventional and nanomedicines for the treatment of pulmonary tuberculosis (PTB).

Source: Ding Y, Li B, Yi Y, Liu C, Wen J, Jian X and Li Y (2025) Progress in the role of nanoparticles in the diagnosis and treatment of bone and joint tuberculosis. Front. Med. 12:1536547. doi: 10.3389/fmed.2025.1536547

15.3.1. Standard Treatment Regimens

Successful management of tuberculosis relies on the use of uniform treatment regimens, extended multidrug therapy for six months being a common practice. The regimen has been formulated to limit drug resistance and ensure sterilizing cure, balancing efficacy and patient compliance. Problems continue, particularly in high-burden countries, as socioeconomic conditions and healthcare infrastructure preclude continuity of care. Modern progress highlights individualizing these regimens according to patient profiles and patterns of drug susceptibility, taking advantage of advanced diagnostic methods to direct therapy in a more targeted fashion. The traditional six-month treatment regimen for drug-susceptible tuberculosis (DS-TB) continues to be the backbone of therapy, but new developments target streamlining drug combinations and doses to improve efficacy while minimizing side effects. These advances mirror the larger movement toward personalized medicine to counteract treatment failure and drug resistance as it occurs while keeping in mind the public health program feasibility (Hsu et al., 2025) (Figure 15.7).

TB Treatment Regimens				
Intensive phase treatment		Continuation phase		Comments
Medicines	Dosing Frequency	Medicines	Dosing Frequency	
Two months of isoniazid, rifampicin, pyrazinamide, and ethambutol	Daily[a]	Four months of isoniazid and rifampicin	Daily[a]	a = Optimal
	Daily[b]	Four months of isoniazid and rifampicin	3 times a week[b]	b = Acceptable alternative for any new TB patient
	3 times a week[c]		3 times a week[c]	c = Acceptable alternative EXCEPT for patients who— Are living with HIV OR Live in HIV prevalent settings

Figure 15.7. Standard regimens for new TB patients.

Source: ResearchGate. (n.d.). *Standard regimens for new TB patients.* https://www.researchgate.net/profile/Hernan-Reyes-3/publication/281115087/figure/tbl4/AS:651116060631040@1532249574167/standard-regimens-for-new-Tb-Patients.png.

More recent treatment approaches increasingly feature shorter, more specific regimens based on resistance patterns detected by sophisticated diagnostic tests. With the increasing frequency of drug-resistant tuberculosis (DR-TB) strains, reference regimens are being reassessed to include new agents and shorter treatment durations without sacrificing successful outcomes. Pharmacokinetics and pharmacodynamics have guided changes in dosage and frequency with the aim of optimizing bacterial killing while limiting toxicity. Furthermore, incorporating flexible clinical trial designs expedites the assessment of innovative combinations, enabling a faster shift from research to practice. This development harmonizes with modern paradigms in antimicrobial stewardship, which promote evidence-informed prescribing practice based on considerations of pathogen resistance patterns, patient compliance, and total treatment outcomes. Such a paradigm honors principles seen in other infectious disease treatments, highlighting the merits of evidence-based alterations of traditional regimens (Hsu et al., 2025; Warner et al., 2023). Despite these advances, the efficacy of traditional treatment regimens continues to be dependent upon timely and accurate diagnosis, highlighting the indistinguishability of diagnostics and therapeutics in tuberculosis treatment. Advancements in molecular diagnostics, such as resistance detection and WGS, allow clinicians to start appropriate regimens early and modify them according to real-time information. This accuracy lowers the risk of inappropriate treatment that leads to resistance and failure of treatment. Additionally, investigating shorter treatment lengths and the addition of new drugs promises relief from lengthy therapy burdens, enhancing patient compliance and clinical outcomes. Combined with stewardship practices that maximize diagnosis, drug choice, dosing, and treatment duration, these developments create an integrated approach to controlling TB. Ultimately, the improvement of standard treatment regimens through diagnostic innovation and stewardship principles is a necessary frontier to fight tuberculosis worldwide (Warner et al., 2023; Hsu et al., 2025).

15.3.2. Shorter Treatment Courses

Emerging developments in treating TB have been more concerned with refining treatment regimens to maximize patient compliance and minimize adverse reactions. Conventional TB treatment involves long periods of use of multiple drugs lasting six months or longer, which poses problems of drug toxicity, poor compliance, and heightened risk of drug resistance. Therefore, studies have investigated whether shorter regimens have the ability to achieve comparable efficacy in reducing these challenges. More effective utilization of healthcare resources could be achieved through shorter regimens as well, particularly in high-burden, low-resource settings where extended treatment oversight presents considerable logistical challenges. These initiatives are in line with wider objectives of improving TB diagnostics and treatment through increased availability and accessibility of care for various patient populations with the aim of achieving better treatment outcomes and reduced transmission rates. Reducing TB treatment duration has support from advancing pharmacological technology and clinical evidence supporting the effectiveness of new drug combinations and dosing regimens. For example, recent antimycobacterial agents with strong bactericidal activity have the potential to shorten the time taken for mycobacterial clearance. Such novel drugs can be incorporated into regimens that sustain or enhance cure rates but with shorter therapy durations. Molecular diagnostic methods have also enhanced treatment tailoring with drug susceptibility profiles so that clinicians can prescribe short courses with confidence for drug-sensitive TB. Rapid and accurate diagnosis is also a key element in safely reducing therapy duration without sacrificing efficacy, pointing to the synergistic relationship between diagnostic and therapeutic progress in contemporary TB treatment. Implementing shorter treatment regimens could thus revolutionize the quality of care, bringing therapeutic duration into congruence with personalized patient requirements. Notwithstanding the advantages, however, the application of shorter TB treatment regimens must be cautiously weighed against a number of variables to guarantee safety and efficacy. Treating mycobacterial infection, especially difficult infections like cutaneous tuberculosis, frequently involves long-term multidrug therapy, and any deviations from recommended procedures need to be well-documented and closely monitored (Gardini et al., 2022). Additionally, the perceived burden of treatment can affect patient adherence, and therefore shorter durations may enhance compliance but must be supported with firm clinical support. Surgical procedures continue to have a place in some manifestations of TB, noting that short-course drug regimens are not automatically transferable (Gardini et al., 2022). Additionally, health systems have to respond to incorporate new protocols and diagnostics effectively, being mindful of possible differences in patient groups and co-morbidities like liver illness. These arguments further serve to emphasize the necessity for continued multidisciplinary measures to maximize the benefits of shorter treatment regimens in TB treatment.

15.3.3. New Drug Developments

Major advances in the creation of new medications have appeared as a major part of fighting the global issue of TB, particularly drug-resistant TB. Conventional treatment regimens, more often than not long and onerous, have destroyed patient compliance and helped to fuel the growth of resistant MTB strains. New technologies are oriented toward the use of new pharmacological tools, like bedaquiline and linezolid, which are especially effective against MDR-TB and XDR-TB. These emerging drugs not only expand therapeutic choices but also facilitate briefer, more tolerable treatment regimens that enhance patient outcomes and lower transmission rates. Such advancements are key to overcoming the constraints put in place by older treatments and addressing the challenges of drug-resistant TB infections that continue to thrive worldwide (Abubakar et al., 2016; Tiberi et al., 2022). The combination of newly created anti-TB drugs with better diagnostic tools has revolutionized the disease control map. Technologies such as WGS allow for quick identification of resistance profiles, enabling clinicians to best match drug regimens. This precision medicine strategy maximizes the application of new agents, enabling the highest efficacy treatments to be given to the patient while limiting the generation of additional resistance. Notwithstanding these breakthroughs, there are still challenges, such as guaranteeing the accessibility and affordability of these medicines in high-burden, resource-constrained environments. Increased research and investment are needed to bring access further and to develop more therapeutics targeting both drug-sensitive and DR-TB strains, encouraging global collaboration toward TB elimination (Abubakar et al., 2016; Tiberi et al., 2022).

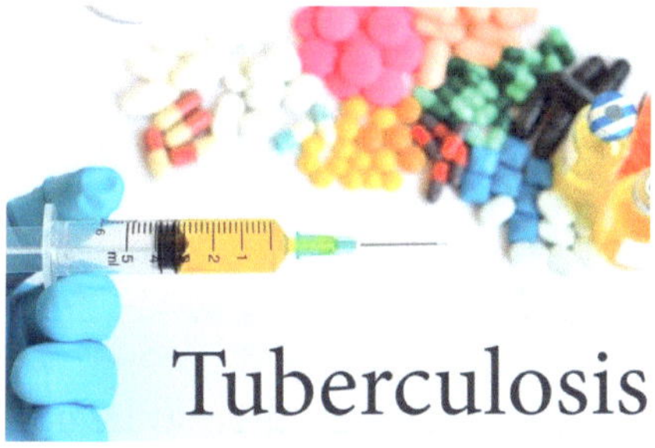

Source: Paras Hospitals. (2019). *Tuberculosis injection illustration.* https://api.parashospitals.com/uploads/2019/03/tuberculosis_needle.jpg.

Attempts to decrease TB treatment length rely on the effective application of these new drug treatments, which are essential to minimize the long waits currently necessary to establish patient cure. The absence of good biomarkers for cure has traditionally held up assessing treatment effectiveness in clinical trials, but the introduction of highly effective new drugs opens the door to shorter, more potent treatment regimens. These abbreviated regimens are expected to improve compliance, decrease side effects, and minimize treatment costs, all of which are critical to TB epidemic control on the global level. Finally, new drug development continues to be a cornerstone of integrated TB control programs, combating drug resistance while simplifying care delivery to better enhance public health outcomes globally (Abubakar et al., 2016; Tiberi et al., 2022).

15.4. Role of Vaccines in Tuberculosis (TB) Control

The world drive to control TB has increasingly noted the vital importance of vaccines in controlling the disease spread. While diagnostics and therapies have significantly improved, vaccination continues to be a cornerstone in avoiding infection, particularly in high-burden areas. The *Bacillus Calmette-Guérin* (BCG) vaccine, which was constructed almost a century ago, offers partial protection against TB severe forms in children but demonstrates poor efficacy in adults, evidencing the compelling need for better vaccine candidates. The evolution of immunology and molecular biology has led to the innovation of novel vaccine approaches to boost immune responses and minimize latent infections. These new vaccines promise not just preventing TB but also better outcomes when given with current diagnostic and therapeutic tools, filling gaps in existing TB control programs. The combination of these tools is necessary to fight transmission and stem the spread of resistant forms. Along with traditional vaccination activities, the combination of new vaccine platforms with enhanced diagnostic approaches is critical to attaining a complete control of TB. Vaccines aimed at preventing various phases of MTB infection are being investigated to supplement diagnostics that can detect active and latent infection with increased specificity. Vaccines, through prevention of infection development and spread, can reduce disease incidence and take care of the burden on health systems, particularly in poor settings. Additionally, vaccine strategies need to be integrated with international AMR control since misuse of antibiotics in TB is leading to MDR-TB problems. Building and releasing effective vaccines has the potential to minimize antibiotic dependency, thus being a crucial step in controlling AMR and promoting sustainable treatment outcomes (Jenner et al., 2017). Collaborative action on vaccine development and stewardship is the key to long-term success in TB control.

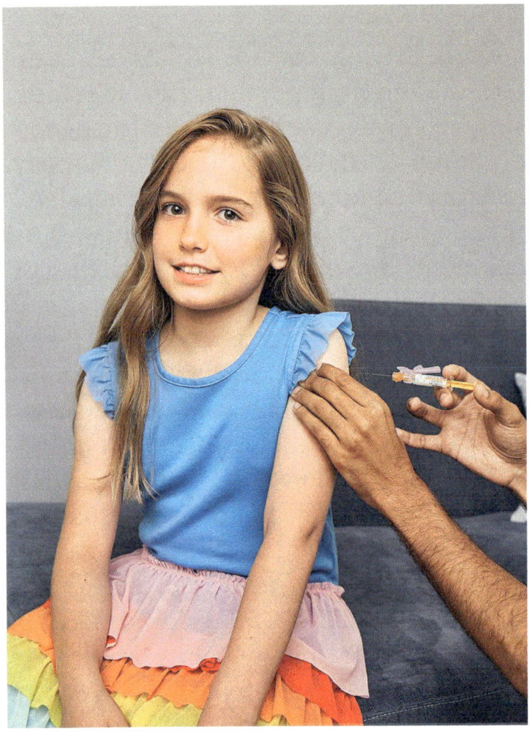

Figure 15.8. Vaccine development is currently one of the biggest challenges of research into tuberculosis.

Source: By SELF Magazine - Young girl about to receive a vaccine in her upper arm, CC BY 2.0, https://commons.wikimedia.org/w/index.php?curid=81631650

The upscaling of vaccine research and delivery calls for significant economic investment and strong systems of governance to guarantee inclusive access to diverse populations. Institutions participating in TB treatment and research, including academic institutions as represented by annual overviews, offer valuable information on advancements and efficient allocation of resources (London School of Hygiene and Tropical Medicine, 2013). Strategic funding goes towards clinical trials in candidates for advanced vaccines, while policy structures facilitate integration with diagnostics and treatment regimens. Furthermore, intellectual property and public-private partnership can enhance the motivations for the pharmaceutical sector to bring TB vaccine development to the forefront, overcoming market failures due to low commercial returns. An efficient, multi-level strategy, not only speeding up technological progress but also equitably distributing it around the world, is crucial for vaccines to realize their promise in TB control in a more general diagnostics and treatment framework (Figure 15.8).

15.4.1. Current Vaccination Strategies

The development of vaccination strategies against TB is an essential part of global measures towards controlling this chronic infectious disease. The conventional cornerstone of TB prevention has been the BCG vaccine, yet its unpredictable effectiveness, particularly among adults, makes the development of new immunization strategies essential. Today's approaches more and more center on the development of vaccines that act on multiple phases of MTB infection to not just prevent disease, but to also decrease the reactivation of latent infection. These involve recombinant protein-based vaccines, viral vector platforms, and live attenuated strains that induce strong and long-lasting immunity. Further, the combination of vaccination with current diagnostics and timely therapeutic modalities constitutes an integrated approach to preventing TB transmission and disease burden globally, emphasizing the need for changing immunization paradigms in TB control programs (Figure 15.9).

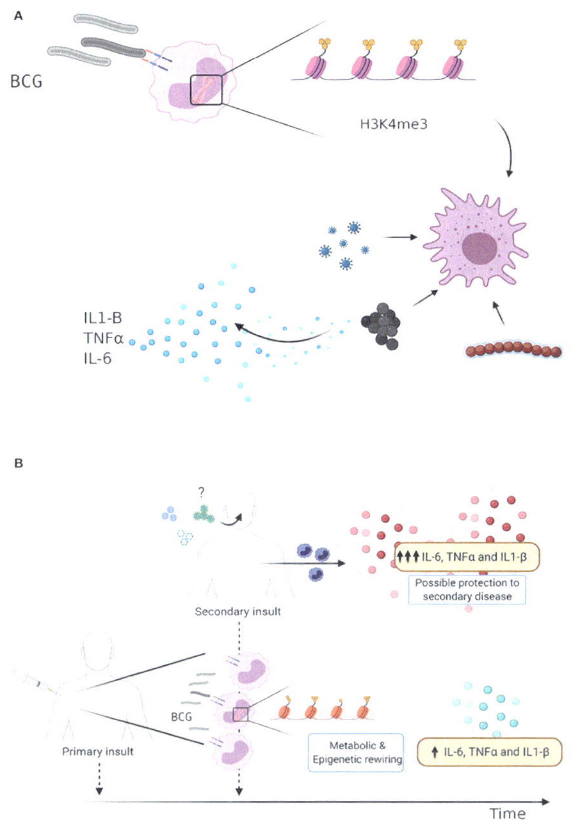

Figure 15.9. *Bacillus Calmette-Guérin* (BCG) vaccine.

Source: Gonzalez-Perez M, Sanchez-Tarjuelo R, Shor B, Nistal-Villan E and Ochando J (2021) The BCG Vaccine for COVID-19: First Verdict and Future Directions. Front. Immunol. 12:632478. doi: 10.3389/fimmu.2021.632478

Recent advances focus on multistage vaccine candidates that can induce immune responses in both early infection and the latent phase, a new direction away from the conventional BCG model. These vaccines attempt to overcome efficacy limitations by targeting particular mycobacterial antigens present at various stages of infection, possibly providing greater protection in highly prevalent disease populations. Prime-boost vaccination regimens using BCG with new formulations are also being clinically assessed to increase immune memory and prolong protection duration. Advancements in immunological and molecular research also facilitate the discovery of correlates of protection, essential in informing target product profile-based tailoring of vaccine-induced immunity to varied demographic and epidemiologic contexts. Incorporating vaccination approaches within large-scale public health frameworks places the importance on multidisciplinary partnership and ongoing adjustment according to unfolding science and actual effectiveness findings (Lamb et al., 2019). In the face of the danger of AMR that complicates treating TB, vaccination is revealed as a tactical measure to modulate disease incidence and restrain the over-reliance on long-course antibiotic therapy. By averting infection and reactivation alike, useful vaccines can decrease the selective pressure for resistant MTB strains to emerge, complementing drug-related advances. This strategy is in concordance with global health strategies that approach AMR as a multicausal problem for which both pharmaceutical development and preventive options like immunization are necessary. The convergence of vaccine research with enhanced diagnostic specificity and drug regimens constitutes an integrated strategy that is essential for sustainable control of TB. Therefore, today's vaccination campaigns are not only taking forward immunoprophylaxis but are part of preventing larger public health complications arising from resistant tuberculosis strains (O'Grady et al., 2011).

15.4.2. Research on New Vaccines

The quest for novel vaccines is central to strengthening global health security, especially when responding to emerging infectious disease threats like TB. Conventional TB vaccines have shown inadequate immunity, particularly among adults, creating a need to pursue novel research approaches in vaccine development. Emerging advancements in molecular and immunological biology have enabled the discovery of new antigens and delivery vehicles, which are likely to yield better protective immune responses. In addition, merging genomic and proteomic information has speeded up candidate vaccine development, with specially designed immune targets that would obviate previous setbacks. These advances in science are matched by institutional determination and investment, as shown in the broad-ranging range of research activities captured yearly that represent the School's dedication to public health innovation and capacity development (London School of Hygiene and Tropical Medicine, 2013). This changing landscape emphasizes the need for continued investment in vaccine development to fight TB effectively, as well as other issues of AMR. The threat posed by AMR has highlighted the imperative of new vaccines that can decrease dependency on current antimicrobials and therefore prevent the emergence of drug-resistant strains of TB. Shortages in supplies of effective diagnostics and therapeutics compound the issue, highlighting the catalytic role of vaccines in disrupting transmission chains. Global and local governance frameworks play critical roles in setting research priorities, with developments tailored to varied epidemiological settings and made available globally. Coordinated public-private efforts, complemented by stewardship policies, can foster an environment for innovation where intellectual property rights are strategically used to encourage research while ensuring equitable access. The multiple-pronged strategy resonates with the outcomes from recent global challenge reports that promote an integrated approach to stimulate and sustain the development of vaccines as part of a critical component to fight MDR-TB (Jenner et al., 2017). In addition, the incentive design for vaccine innovation must be grounded in a subtle assessment of market forces and risk factors inherent to TB vaccine development. Unlike more marketable drugs, vaccines usually encounter financial and regulatory challenges that discourage investment even when the public health value is certain. To overcome these obstacles, new mechanisms like prize funds, advance market commitments, and public-private partnerships have been recommended to de-risk research and speed up vaccine availability. These mechanisms can supplement conventional intellectual property regimes so that promising candidates for vaccines make it through clinical trials and regulatory approval smoothly. Such approaches are critical, in fact, to addressing the pressing demand for new-generation TB vaccines, which have the potential to significantly decrease the global burden of the disease and be entirely in line with the School's current mission to translate research advances into useful solutions for infectious disease control (London School of Hygiene and Tropical Medicine, 2013; Jenner et al., 2017).

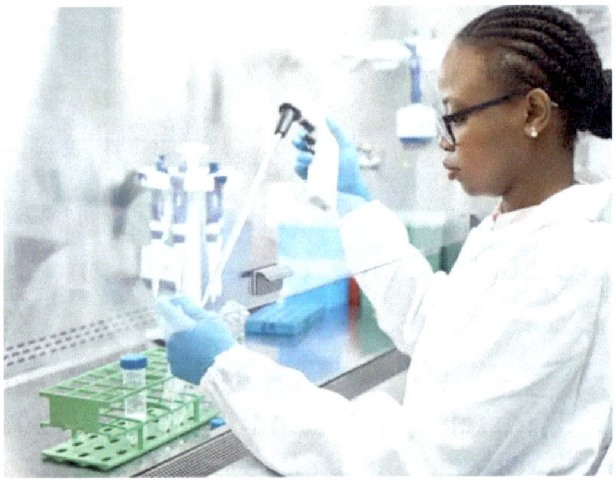

Source: ETHealthworld. (2024). *Tuberculosis treatment awareness visual.* https://etimg.etb2bimg.com/photo/108748690.cms.

15.4.3. Challenges in Vaccine Development

The complexity of MTB contributes significantly to the challenges faced in developing an effective vaccine. Unlike many infectious agents, MTB has developed sophisticated mechanisms to evade the host immune system, making it difficult to identify vaccine targets that consistently elicit protective immunity. The difficulty is compounded by the bacterium's ability to persist in a latent state, which current vaccines struggle to address. Furthermore, the genetic heterogeneity of tuberculosis strains among geographic regions necessitates a vaccine that will be effective across a broad geographic area, adding to the difficulty of design and testing. Such biological challenges are coupled with operations challenges, including the absence of rapid, sensitive diagnostic tests that detect distinct infection stages, making it difficult to evaluate vaccine efficacy quickly in clinical trials (McNerney et al., 2012). Unless these inherent scientific obstacles are overcome, gains in treatment and diagnostics could fail to achieve control of TB on a population basis. Economic and infrastructure barriers also prevent the development of vaccines, reflecting the complexity of the public health issue. Restrictions caused by limited funds on long-term research studies, especially on new vaccine candidates that may involve very expensive and long clinical trials, also impede efforts. This disparity is worsened by the unequal availability of healthcare resources, particularly in areas where the burden of tuberculosis is greatest but where infrastructures to deliver vaccines are weakest. Political will is important in marshaling financial investments and prioritizing vaccine research in global health agendas. As identified in recent institutional reports, continued financing and concerted global cooperation are the necessary key elements for surmounting these barriers (London School of Hygiene and Tropical Medicine, 2013). Absence of strong financial backing and infrastructure spells uncertainty to the deployment of an effective TB vaccine despite advances in laboratory science for diagnostics and treatment regimens. Additionally, the regulatory landscape adds another layer of complexity to vaccine development against tuberculosis. Vaccine candidates will have to go through intense stages of clinical trials to prove safety, efficacy, and scalability, processes that are of a fundamentally time- and cost-intensive nature. It is made more difficult by the absence of valid biomarkers for early markers of vaccine efficacy, an issue directly related to diagnostic problems. Without accurate tools for the measurement of immune responses or distinguishing between latent infection and active disease, trials can produce ambiguous results or take longer to determine outcomes. As a result, the interconnected problems of inadequate biomarkers, long regulatory processes, and constrained diagnostic capacity retard the rate of innovation. Overcoming these system barriers through improved research into immune correlates and streamlined regulatory structures is needed to speed up the introduction of successful TB vaccines (McNerney et al., 2012).

15.5. Future Directions in Tuberculosis (TB) Research

Next-generation technological developments promise brighter prospects for the diagnosis of TB with faster and more accurate detection of the disease. Conventional techniques, though age-old, are plagued by drawbacks like long turnaround times and decreased sensitivity in specific patient groups. The future of research lies in harnessing the power of advanced molecular methods, such as next-generation sequencing (NGS), to mitigate these shortcomings. Clinical metagenomic next-generation sequencing (mNGS) is one such method that fully examines microbial genetic material directly from patient samples, potentially allowing for a diagnostic breakthrough. The method not only allows for faster detection but also gives insightful information on pathogen resistance profiles as well as host-pathogen interactions, which are critical for designing effective treatments. The deployment of mNGS into standard clinical care is challenging but quickly advancing, heralding a revolutionary prospect for TB diagnosis with potential to expedite turnaround times and enhance therapy outcomes (London School of Hygiene and Tropical Medicine, 2013). Of equal importance to the future of TB research are the establishment of new therapeutic approaches countering the emerging threat of drug resistance. With rising MDR-TB and XDR-TB cases across the world, there is a growing need for novel drug regimens and tailored treatment regimens. With breakthroughs in genomic science, it becomes possible to gain a better insight into resistance mechanisms and design targeted therapy that can bypass past treatment failures. The integration of host immune response modulation with traditional antimicrobial therapy is increasingly seen as the way forward, with the intention of increasing efficacy and diminishing toxicity. To maintain momentum in therapeutic development, interdisciplinary research is critical, which includes findings from immunology, pharmacology, and systems biology. Such collaborative research will close existing knowledge gaps and translate findings from the laboratory into successful clinical interventions (Chiu & Miller, 2019). For the future, the future of TB research is in a multidisciplinary approach that will synergize state-of-the-art diagnostics, personalized therapy, and worldwide epidemiological surveillance. Integration of data from high-throughput sequencing, advanced imaging, and real-time surveillance systems will facilitate more accurate detection of TB transmission patterns and prediction of outbreaks. Also, the application of AI and machine learning in the analysis of complex datasets promises to speed discovery and optimize patient-specific treatment regimens. Together with integration of these technological advances with improved knowledge of the pathogen's biology and host determinants, these advances will accelerate TB control efforts. Yet continued research infrastructure and capacity investments in high-burden areas continue to be essential. These strategic imperatives highlight an integrated vision for TB research that will not only enhance the care of individual patients but also improve global public health outcomes (London School of Hygiene and Tropical Medicine, 2013; Chiu & Miller, 2019) (Figure 15.10).

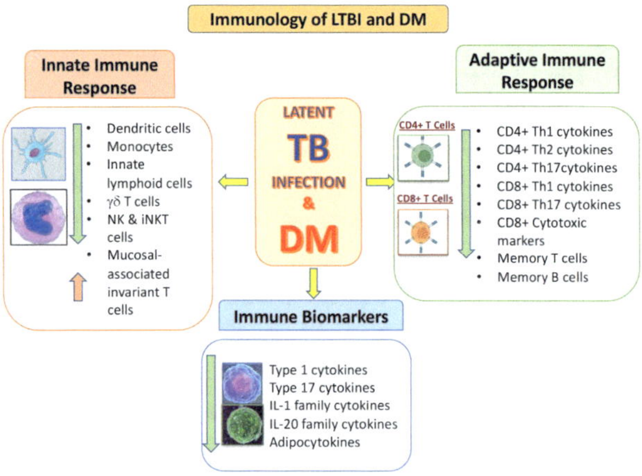

Figure 15.10. Challenges and future directions for DM-TB control. First, further research is needed to understand the mechanisms linking DM and LTBI reactivation, potentially providing immunological targets for preventing TB in DM patients. Early screening and intervention for LTBI in DM patients is proposed, utilizing TST and IGRA for screening and implementing TPT treatment as early intervention.

Source: Kumar NP and Babu S (2023) Impact of diabetes mellitus on immunity to latent tuberculosis infection. Front. Clin. Diabetes Healthc. 4:1095467. doi: 10.3389/fcdhc.2023.1095467

15.5.1. Innovations in Diagnostic Technologies

Prompt and precise diagnosis is a mainstay of successful TB control, but conventional diagnostic techniques have long been slow and labor-consuming, restricting intervention promptly. Diagnosis has in the past depended on sputum smear microscopy and culture methods, which take weeks to produce results and need well-equipped laboratories. The limitations restrict early detection and enable continued transmission among infected communities. Recent developments have aimed to revolutionize this paradigm by creating diagnostic technologies that not only are faster but also can be used at the point of care in resource-constrained environments. These are molecular tests that target MTB DNA, and they decrease diagnostic times markedly while increasing sensitivity over traditional procedures. Even so, while encouraging progress has been made, challenges remain in the development of genuinely affordable, precise, and field-friendly diagnostic devices that can be scaled internationally to effectively address the TB epidemic (McNerney et al., 2012). The technical complexity of TB diagnostics is also increased by the necessity of detecting not just active infection but also latent tuberculosis infection (LTBI), which is a large reservoir for future disease. New diagnostic platforms combine host immune response profiling with biomarker detection to distinguish latent infection from active disease, with potential enhanced patient management. New developments have also targeted identifying drug-resistant strains by incorporating rapid molecular DST, hence informing timely and appropriate therapeutic interventions. Despite such advances, the full incorporation of new technologies into standard clinical practice continues to be limited by expense, infrastructure needs, and the requirement for trained human resources. Supporting these innovations to lead to minimized transmission rates and better patient outcomes requires holistic approaches involving political will and durable funding mechanisms (McNerney et al., 2012). In the future, the emphasis of current research is on the discovery of point-of-care diagnostic tests that are simultaneously accurate, cheap, and easy to use, so that they can be deployed even in the most peripheral environments. New biomarker discovery remains a key thrust, with activities to find host or pathogen signatures that are identified by non-invasive sampling. Such tests have the potential to transform TB control by providing real-time diagnosis and initiation of treatment, interrupting infectious periods and disease progression. In addition, the integration of digital health technologies and AI into diagnostic pathways promises increased diagnostic accuracy and data handling. However, it is still crucial to overcome technical and operational challenges in test validation, manufacturability, and field implementation. Intersectoral coordinated action between scientific, public health, and funding areas is required to support these innovative advances to meet their full potential effect in controlling the world's tuberculosis burden (McNerney et al., 2012) (Figure 15.11).

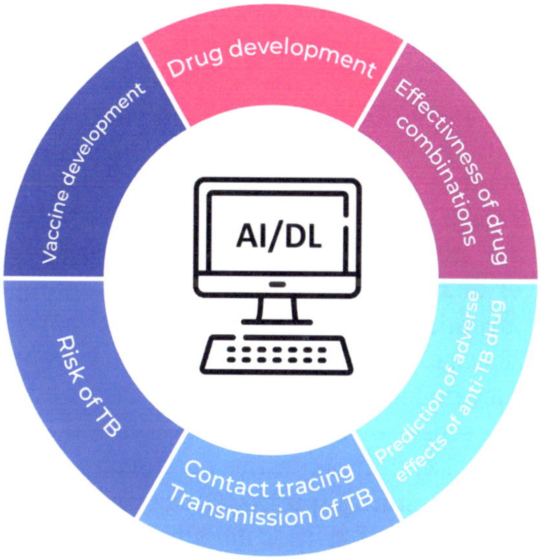

Figure 15.11. Seven transitions that can transform how TB is diagnosed and close the diagnostic gap.

Source: Dohál M, Porvazník I, Solovič I and Mokrý J (2023) Advancing tuberculosis management: the role of predictive, preventive, and personalized medicine. Front. Microbiol. 14:1225438. doi: 10.3389/fmicb.2023.1225438

15.5.2. Emerging Treatment Modalities

Current advances in treating TB represent a vital counteraction to the ongoing threat of multi-drug resistant forms of MTB. Emerging treatment strategies involve augmenting the number of effective antibiotics and maximizing therapeutic approaches to provide better patient outcomes. New agents have exhibited encouraging clinical activity, targeting resistant organisms more specifically than traditional agents. Nonetheless, the initiation of new pharmacological alternatives has to be supported by thorough mortality risk assessment and patient safety profiles. Notably, molecular diagnostic advances, in the form of PCR-based TB tests, are enabling detection at earlier stages and timely treatment initiation, potentially curbing disease progression and transmission. Although these diagnostic devices are presently undergoing further validation for particular types of TB, including intestinal infections, their development represents a substantial step toward combining diagnostics with targeted treatment interventions (Bourke et al., 2015). Such collaboration between novel drugs and rapid diagnostics highlights the promise to overcome traditional barriers in TB care. Beside pharmacological advances, adjunct imaging modalities have also become useful tools to augment decision-making in treating TB, differentiating TB infections from the confounding pathologies like Crohn's disease. Such modalities augment the accuracy of detecting sites of active disease so that clinicians can better individualize therapeutic interventions. In addition, the tailoring of treatment regimens to comorbidities and immune status is becoming increasingly important, given that patients with secondary or primary immunodeficiencies can benefit from specialist approaches. The combination of prolonged antibiotic courses and sophisticated therapeutic monitoring plays a key role in treating complicated cases such as disseminated TB. Overall, these measures constitute a move from mass treatments to more tailored and dynamic regimens. The build-up of such methodologies attests to the multidisciplinary collaboration required to tackle the biological heterogeneity of TB manifestations and the rise of resistant strains (Bourke et al., 2015). These notwithstanding, there are still challenges to maintaining a vigorous pipeline of new therapeutics and to bringing advances in science into broad clinical practice. The 2013 Pittsburgh Lung Conference underscored concerns at the glacial pace of antibiotic discovery in the face of the global burden of pulmonary infections such as TB. It underlined the call for novel drug development platforms, enhanced vaccines, and combination regimens to effectively counteract drug resistance. Multidisciplinary research efforts by academic investigators, clinicians, industry partners, and policymakers are key to hastening these advances. Additionally, it is believed that insights into how TB pathogens interact with the host lung microbiome can hold the key to novel treatment strategies, potentially even the next modalities moving beyond traditional antibiotics being the only option. Such trends demonstrate the complex reality of TB treatment innovation, as translational research and clinical practice intersect to combat emerging health challenges (Kontsevaya et al., 2024).

15.5.3. Global Health Initiatives and Collaborations

The complexities of TB, especially in terms of increasing multidrug resistance, call for synergistic global action that is national-boundary-cutting. Health programs that combine research, financing, and knowledge sharing are the crux of addressing the interrelated TB challenges. International partnerships allow for the sharing of resources and expertise to facilitate the development and dissemination of new diagnostics and treatments. Such efforts also promote the development of harmonized standards of surveillance, diagnosis, and treatment regimens that are needed to monitor and contain the transmission of resistant TB strains. Public-private sector efforts globally mirror the value of collaborative partnerships that bridge innovation with practice, where advances reach high-burden areas early and equitably. The development of resistance highlights the interdependence of countries in health security, where poor responses anywhere can undermine everywhere, emphasizing the necessity of shared governance and stewardship (Jenner et al., 2017). In high TB-burden nations, the success of global health efforts is frequently dependent upon local adaptation of strategies to circumstances and needs. In nations like India, where fragmented public health infrastructure complicates disease management, international partnerships can provide not only technological advancements but also models for strengthening health systems. This includes capacity building for rapid DST and fostering community engagement to improve treatment adherence. Learning from nations with effective public health programs provides a model for incorporating culturally appropriate interventions addressing social determinants of health to stem the transmission of MDR-TB. Reporting and surveillance systems built through partnerships facilitate timely data sharing to inform policy and resource allocation effectively. Alignment of global and local action is hence essential to ensure that innovation in TB diagnosis and treatment is converted into quantifiable health impact among vulnerable populations (Gamon, 2013). The issue of governance and intellectual property regimes in international collaborations again highlights the complexity of stimulating innovation and ensuring access. The creation of new TB treatments and diagnostics entails long-term investment, and systems that reward research while preserving fair access are essential. Joint efforts highlight the need for harmonizing intellectual property rights with public health needs, suggesting innovative reward models that encourage research without precluding availability. In addition, stewardship initiatives in these networks focus on limiting AMR by encouraging rational use and reducing antibiotic overexposure. Coordination of policies at the global, regional, and national levels promotes accountability and guarantees that TB treatment progress is sustainable. Thus, international efforts for health not only accelerate scientific advances but also incorporate ethical and regulatory aspects necessary in the fight against TB on a global level (Jenner et al., 2017).

SUMMARY

The continuous struggle against tuberculosis has also brought to light the indispensable role of incorporating novel diagnostic techniques and treatment strategies in coping with both clinical and socio-economic aspects of disease control. Recent developments, especially the use of machine learning models like the Extreme Gradient Boosting Classifier, have brought outstanding precision in predicting drug resistance rates in MTB strains. This accuracy in diagnostics allows for earlier and more individualized treatment protocols, with the potential to slow the development of DR-TB and enhance patient outcomes. The use of detailed genomic information to drive these models represents a large step over the older phenotypic methods, pointing toward a future in which TB diagnostics are rapid as well as very specific. Such advancements reflect not only technological advancement but also hold the promise of remaking clinical practice by offering healthcare providers solutions to predict treatment issues prior to them occurring (Paredes-Gutierrez et al., 2025). The promise of sophisticated diagnostics and treatment, however, is moderated by ongoing difficulties with patient retention and compliance in the care continuum. Qualitative research points out that despite leading-edge medical therapies, conditions including stigma, poverty, side effects of drugs, and mental distress significantly affect patients' capacity to remain on treatment. These social determinants tend to pose barriers that counter the impact of biomedical progress, curtailing the full capacity of enhanced therapies. A sole clinical emphasis is therefore not enough; healthcare systems need to embrace holistic approaches that recognize the socioeconomic conditions of patients with DR-TB. By building improved patient-healthcare worker relationships, augmented support networks, and socioeconomic support tailored to the needs of the individual, treatment programs can enhance retention, which is still paramount in meeting global control targets for TB (Mphothulo et al., 2025). The intersection of next-generation diagnostic tools with a sophisticated assessment for patient-centered care is the foundation upon which future breakthroughs in the management of tuberculosis will be achieved. As machine learning provides unparalleled precision in the prediction of drug resistance, however, achieving positive treatment outcomes hinges on confronting the larger environment in which patients exist and must manage their care. Multidisciplinary strategies that align technological innovation with integrated systems of support hold the most promise for decreasing the TB burden globally. Future initiatives should focus on the combination of genomic data-driven interventions with efforts to overcome psychosocial and economic obstacles, thus increasing both the effectiveness and availability of TB treatment services. Through such well-rounded strategies, the global community can continue to advance toward ending the longstanding menace of tuberculosis (Mphothulo et al., 2025; Paredes-Gutierrez et al., 2025).

Recent advances in tuberculosis diagnosis indicate substantial progress towards faster and more precise detection, essentially transforming clinical practice and public health policy. Advances in molecular tests, for example, NAATs like the widely used Xpert MTB/RIF, have had a substantial impact in decreasing diagnostic lags so that intervention and commencement of treatment are earlier (Kontsevaya et al., 2024). The technologies allow for simultaneous detection of TB and drug resistance, essential for individualized prescription of effective therapeutic regimens. Beyond laboratory improvements, modeling studies have underscored the importance of optimizing diagnostic pathways to enhance system efficiency and reduce the infectious period before treatment initiation. However, despite these technological gains, models indicate considerable variability in cost-effectiveness depending on the epidemiological context, underscoring the need for locale-specific approaches that integrate healthcare infrastructure dynamics and patient pathways (Omidian

& Mfoafo, 2023). Such understanding guides policy and resource allocation decisions aimed at optimizing the public health value of diagnostic innovation. At the same time, improvements in therapy have been driven by greater knowledge of mechanisms of drug delivery and treatment optimization, with nanotechnology increasingly playing a key role in this area. Through nanoscale manipulation of drug carriers, enhanced bioavailability and targeted delivery have been attained, leading to increased efficacy and decreased systemic toxicity; a key factor in pediatric populations as well as DR-TB. Several nanoparticle-based platforms have been investigated to penetrate biological barriers including the blood-brain barrier, enabling treatment of extrapulmonary presentations such as medulloblastoma-associated TB infection. Although promising, nanotechnology use must carefully assess possible risks of nanoparticle exposure, warranting a balance between innovative drug delivery systems and safety in patients. The thorough assessment of these new therapeutic systems represents a critical step toward the development of personalized TB treatment and reduction of treatment-related side effects (Omidian & Mfoafo, 2023). Broadening tuberculosis control, mathematical modeling has increasingly had a key function in assessing the potential epidemiological benefit and cost-effectiveness of new diagnostics and treatment interventions. Using advanced frameworks, these models estimate disease transmission patterns and interactions between the healthcare system, projecting essential evidence for policymakers. Of particular note, they identify gaps such as multi-parameter sensitivity analysis needs and including pre-diagnostic infectious periods that affect transmission risk. Additionally, models uncover that effective application of new diagnostics requires local context taking into account resources, patient involvement, and so on to provide real-world applicability. As the models become more sophisticated, their merging with empirical information will improve predictive value as well as inform effective resource allocation of interventions, thereby speeding toward TB elimination targets as well as enhancing health outcomes (Zwerling et al., 2014).

CLOSER LOOK

LINE PROBE ASSAYS (LPAS)

LPAs are DNA hybridization-based molecular diagnostic tests employed for quick detection of MTB and co-existent drug resistance, especially to first- and second-line anti-tuberculosis medications. The LPAs enable simultaneous detection of the causative bacteria of TB and the drug resistance-conferring genetic mutations through simultaneous detection. The WHO recommends the use of LPAs in TB control programs, particularly in countries with high TB burden, owing to their high speed and accuracy in MDR-TB detection.

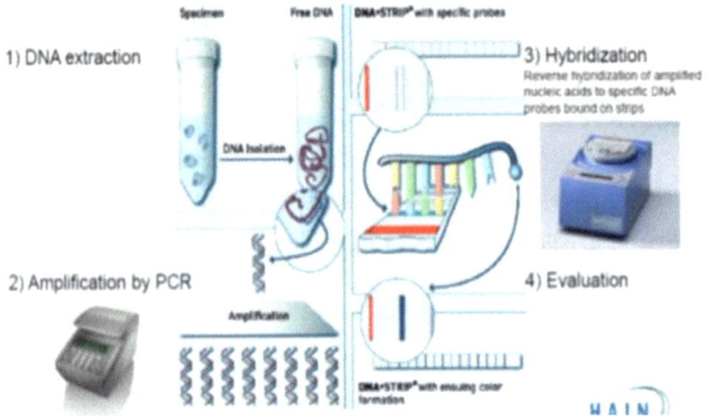

Source: Bokop C, Faye LM, Apalata T. Analysis of Discordance between Genotypic and Phenotypic Assays for Rifampicin-Resistant *Mycobacterium tuberculosis* Isolated from Healthcare Facilities in Mthatha. *Pathogens*. 2023; 12(7):909. https://doi.org/10.3390/pathogens12070909

The mechanism underlying LPAs entailthe isolation of DNA from a TB sample (most commonly sputum or cultured isolates), followed by PCR amplification of gene segments with known associations with drug resistance. The amplified fragments are then hybridized with particular oligonucleotide probes captured on a nitrocellulose strip. Such probes are used to detect wild-type sequences and established mutations in genes like rpoB (for resistance to rifampicin), katG, and in the inhA promoter region (for isoniazid resistance). The presence or absence of hybridization signals on the strip can be used to interpret the results.One of the key benefits of LPAs is their quick turnaround time, with results usually available within 1–2 days, whereas traditional culture-based DST can take weeks. Such prompt detection allows for earlier initiation of the correct treatment regimens, curbing the risk of transmission and enhancing outcomes in patients. LPAs are especially useful in the diagnosis of rifampicin-resistant tuberculosis (RR-TB), as a surrogate marker of MDR-TB, allowing for timely management of resistant cases.In addition, LPAs are very sensitive and specific when applied to smear-positive specimens or culture isolates. That said, their performance is not as optimal in smear-negative specimens because of the lower bacterial load, and this can restrict their use in specific patient groups, e.g., children or those co-infected with HIV.Despite their advantages, implementing LPAs requires laboratory infrastructure and trained personnel, making them less feasible in resource-limited settings without external support. Additionally, LPAs only detect known mutations, so resistance due to rare or novel genetic changes may be missed.

REFERENCES

1. Migliori, G. B., Dheda, K., Centis, R., Mwaba, P., Bates, M., O'Grady, J., Hoelscher, M., & Zumla, A. (2010). Review of multidrug-resistant and extensively drug-resistant TB: global perspectives with a focus on sub-Saharan Africa. *Tropical medicine & international health : TM & IH, 15*(9), 1052–1066. https://doi.org/10.1111/j.1365-3156.2010.02581.x (accessed on 10 May 2025).

2. Abubakar, I., Lipman, M., McHugh, T. D., & Fletcher, H. (2016). Uniting to end the TB epidemic: advances in disease control from prevention to better diagnosis and treatment. *BMC medicine, 14*, 47. https://doi.org/10.1186/s12916-016-0599-1(accessed on 10 May 2025).

3. O'Grady, Justin[a,b]; Maeurer, Markus[c]; Mwaba, Peter[b,d]; Kapata, Nathan[b,d]; Bates, Matthew[a,b]; Hoelscher, Michael[e]; Zumla, Alimuddin[a,b]. New and improved diagnostics for detection of drug-resistant pulmonary tuberculosis. Current Opinion in Pulmonary Medicine 17(3):p 134-141, May 2011. | DOI: 10.1097/MCP.0b013e3283452346 (accessed on 10 May 2025).

4. Nahid, P., Kim, P. S., Evans, C. A., Alland, D., Barer, M., Diefenbach, J., Ellner, J., Hafner, R., Hamilton, C. D., Iademarco, M. F., Ireton, G., Kimerling, M. E., Lienhardt, C., MacKenzie, W. R., Murray, M., Perkins, M. D., Posey, J. E., Roberts, T., Sizemore, C., Stevens, W. S., ... Swindells, S. (2012). Clinical research and development of tuberculosis diagnostics: moving from silos to synergy. *The Journal of infectious diseases, 205 Suppl 2*(Suppl 2), S159–S168. https://doi.org/10.1093/infdis/jis194 (accessed on 10 May 2025).

5. Ang, M., Chan, S. M., Cheng, L. T., Cheong, H. Y., Chew, K. L., Chlebicki, P., Hsu, L. Y., et al. (2024). Singapore tuberculosis (TB) clinical management guidelines 2024: A modified Delphi adaptation of international guidelines for drug-susceptible TB infection and pulmonary disease. *Annals of the Academy of Medicine, Singapore, 53*(3), 170–186. https://www.semanticscholar.org/paper/4b00e154fb4f0e6890eed0119bee8d0453c5ba9a (accessed on 10 May 2025).

6. Jenner, A., Bhagwandin, N., & Kowalski, S. P. (2017). Antimicrobial resistance (AMR) and multidrug resistance (MDR): Overview of current approaches, consortia, and intellectual property issues. Global Challenges Report. https://www.wipo.int/publications/en/details.jsp?id=4210 (accessed on 10 May 2025).

7. Biggins, S. W., Angeli, P., García-Tsao, G., Ginés, P., Ling, S. C., Nadim, M. K., Wong, F., et al. (2021). Diagnosis, evaluation, and management of ascites, spontaneous bacterial peritonitis and hepatorenal syndrome: 2021 practice guidance by the American Association for the Study of Liver Diseases. *Hepatology, 74*, 1014–1048. https://doi.org/10.1002/hep.31884.

8. Bourke, B., & Hussey, S. (2015). Chronic infections of the small intestine. *Current Opinion in Gastroenterology, 31*, 104–110. https://www.semanticscholar.org/paper/61ef7042dbbbccb3168eac00d4c2a6674ca8eda1 (accessed on 10 May 2025).

9. Kontsevaya, I., Cabibbe, A. M., Cirillo, D. M., DiNardo, A. R., Frahm, N., Gillespie, S. H., Holtzman, D., Meiwes, L., Petruccioli, E., Reimann, M., Ruhwald, M., Sabiiti, W., Saluzzo, F., Tagliani, E., & Goletti, D. (2024). Update on the diagnosis of tuberculosis. *Clinical microbiology and infection : the official publication of the European Society of Clinical Microbiology and Infectious Diseases, 30*(9), 1115–1122. https://doi.org/10.1016/j.cmi.2023.07.014 (accessed on 10 May 2025).

10. Tiberi, S., Utjesanovic, N., Galvin, J., Centis, R., D'Ambrosio, L., van den Boom, M., Zumla, A., & Migliori, G. B. (2022). Drug resistant TB - latest developments in epidemiology, diagnostics

and management. *International journal of infectious diseases : IJID : official publication of the International Society for Infectious Diseases, 124 Suppl 1*, S20–S25. https://doi.org/10.1016/j.ijid.2022.03.026 (accessed on 10 May 2025).

11. Chiu, C.Y., Miller, S.A. Clinical metagenomics. *Nat Rev Genet* **20**, 341–355 (2019). https://doi.org/10.1038/s41576-019-0113-7 (accessed on 10 May 2025).
12. Zwerling, A., White, R. G., Vassall, A., Cohen, T., Dowdy, D. W., & Houben, R. M. (2014). Modeling of novel diagnostic strategies for active tuberculosis - a systematic review: current practices and recommendations. *PloS one*, *9*(10), e110558. https://doi.org/10.1371/journal.pone.0110558 (accessed on 10 May 2025).
13. Deshpande, A., Likhar, R., Khan, T., & Omri, A. (2024). Decoding drug resistance in *Mycobacterium tuberculosis* complex: Genetic insights and future challenges. *Expert Review of Anti-Infective Therapy*. https://www.semanticscholar.org/paper/a010f5007989178ffc7d53e0b337a7dca05f1189 (accessed on 10 May 2025).
14. Gamon, Maribel, "Maribel Gamon - Multidrug-Resistant Tuberculosis in India: Solving a Problem by Reconstructing the Public Health Infrastructure" (2013). *Ronald E. McNair Scholars Program 2013*. 12. https://epublications.marquette.edu/mcnair_2013/12(accessed on 10 May 2025).
15. Gardini, G., Gregori, N., Matteelli, A., & Castelli, F. (2022). Mycobacterial skin infection. *Current Opinion in Infectious Diseases, 35*, 79–87. https://doi.org/10.1097/qco.0000000000000820.
16. McNerney, R., Maeurer, M., Abubakar, I., Marais, B., McHugh, T. D., Ford, N., Weyer, K., Lawn, S., Grobusch, M. P., Memish, Z., Squire, S. B., Pantaleo, G., Chakaya, J., Casenghi, M., Migliori, G. B., Mwaba, P., Zijenah, L., Hoelscher, M., Cox, H., Swaminathan, S., ... Zumla, A. (2012). Tuberculosis diagnostics and biomarkers: needs, challenges, recent advances, and opportunities. *The Journal of infectious diseases, 205 Suppl 2*, S147–S158. https://doi.org/10.1093/infdis/jir860 (accessed on 10 May 2025).
17. Hsu, J. Y., Wu, U. I., Wang, J. T., Sheng, W. H., Chen, Y. C., & Chang, S. C. (2025). Managing *Helicobacter pylori* as an infectious disease: Implementation of antimicrobial stewardship. *Helicobacter, 30*(1), e70013. https://www.semanticscholar.org/paper/a6a8475303d838cdda86b1793dd997e2d16257a6 (accessed on 10 May 2025).
18. Lamb, C. A., Kennedy, N. A., Raine, T., Hendy, P., Smith, P. J., Limdi, J. K., Hayee, B., et al. (2019). British Society of Gastroenterology consensus guidelines on the management of inflammatory bowel disease in adults. *Gut, 68*, s1–s106. https://doi.org/10.1136/gutjnl-2019-318484.
19. London School of Hygiene & Tropical Medicine. (2013). Annual report 2013. https://core.ac.uk/download/19452766.pdf (accessed on 10 May 2025).
20. Mejía-Salazar, J. R., Rodrigues Cruz, K., Materón Vásques, E. M., & Oliveira, O. N. (2020). Microfluidic point-of-care devices: New trends and future prospects for eHealth diagnostics. *Sensors, 20*, 1951. https://doi.org/10.3390/s20071951.
21. Omidian, H., & Mfoafo, K. (2023). Exploring the Potential of Nanotechnology in Pediatric Healthcare: Advances, Challenges, and Future Directions. *Pharmaceutics, 15*(6), 1583. https://doi.org/10.3390/pharmaceutics15061583 (accessed on 10 May 2025).
22. Morris, A., Norris, K., & Gladwin, M. (2014). Acute and chronic lung infections. Novel pathogens, diagnostics, and therapeutics. *Annals of the American Thoracic Society, 11*(Suppl 4), S187–

S188. https://www.semanticscholar.org/paper/4e1dc1e4f0744a36f2404fa4262120005715a98b (accessed on 10 May 2025).

23. Mphothulo, N., Hlangu, S., Furin, J., Moshabela, M., & Loveday, M. (2025). Navigating DR-TB Treatment care: a qualitative exploration of barriers and facilitators to retention in care among people with history of early disengagement from drug-resistant tuberculosis treatment in Johannesburg, South Africa. *BMC health services research*, *25*(1), 122. https://doi.org/10.1186/s12913-025-12265-z(accessed on 10 May 2025).
24. Paredes-Gutierrez, G., Perea-Jacobo, R., Acosta-Mesa, H. G., Mezura-Montes, E., Morales Morales Reyes, J. L., Zenteno-Cuevas, R., Guerrero-Chevannier, M., et al. (2025). Predicting drug resistance in *Mycobacterium tuberculosis*: A machine learning approach to genomic mutation analysis. *Diagnostics, 15*. https://www.semanticscholar.org/paper/ae2593e5e0f0d88ef84fc2fadc181d3459aca751 (accessed on 10 May 2025).
25. Solanki, P., Elton, L., Honeyborne, I., Park, M., Satta, G., & McHugh, T. D. (2024). Improving the diagnosis of tuberculosis: old and new laboratory tools. *Expert review of molecular diagnostics*, *24*(6), 487–496. https://doi.org/10.1080/14737159.2024.2362165 (accessed on 10 May 2025).
26. van Griensven, J., & Diro, E. (2019). Visceral leishmaniasis. *Infectious Disease Clinics of North America, 33*, 79–99. https://doi.org/10.1016/j.idc.2018.10.005.
27. Warner, D., & Wood, R. (2023). New tricks for an old dog: Opportunities for better tuberculosis control. *Journal of the International AIDS Society, 26*. https://www.semanticscholar.org/paper/47b82af3d380a9e9bac805c5583e1a9f7fd66db4 (accessed on 10 May 2025).
28. Wearne, N., & Davidson, B. (2024). HIV-associated kidney disease: the changing spectrum and treatment priorities. *Current opinion in nephrology and hypertension*, *33*(6), 603–612. https://doi.org/10.1097/MNH.0000000000001018 (accessed on 10 May 2025).
29. Wu, Z. X., Shi, J., Qiu, C. C., Zhou, Y., Pan, N., Wu, L., & Jiang, X. (2025). Diagnostic value of GeneXpert MTB/RIF in bronchoalveolar lavage fluid for pulmonary non-tuberculosis mycobacterial in acid-fast stain smear-positive and GeneXpert MTB/RIF-negative cases. *Journal of Thoracic Disease, 17*, 1444–1451. https://www.semanticscholar.org/paper/7dc175c1a69d93b59a936bae454c50abcde2c145 (accessed on 10 May 2025).
30. Wulandari, R., & Mega, M. C. (2025). Diagnosis, management and complications of tuberculosis: A comprehensive systematic review. *The Indonesian Journal of General Medicine*. 11(1):11-30
31. DOI:10.70070/r7ve2h33(accessed on 10 May 2025).
32. Xie, C., Hu, X., Liu, Y., & Shu, C. (2022). Performance Comparison of GeneXpert MTB/RIF, Gene Chip Technology, and Modified Roche Culture Method in Detecting *Mycobacterium tuberculosis* and Drug Susceptibility in Sputum. *Contrast media & molecular imaging*, *2022*, 2995464. https://doi.org/10.1155/2022/2995464 (accessed on 10 May 2025).
33. Zaporojan, N., Negrean, R. A., Hodișan, R., Zaporojan, C., Csep, A., & Zaha, D. C. (2024). Evolution of Laboratory Diagnosis of Tuberculosis. *Clinics and practice*, *14*(2), 388–416. https://doi.org/10.3390/clinpract14020030 (accessed on 10 May 2025).

INDEX

D

E

I

L

M